Middle Ear Diseases

Salah Mansour • Jacques Magnan
Karen Nicolas • Hassan Haidar

Middle Ear Diseases

Advances in Diagnosis and Management

Springer

Salah Mansour
Lebanese University
Department of Otolaryngology
HNS Amoudi Center Boulevard Mazraa
Beirut
Lebanon

Karen Nicolas
Department of Radiology
Middle East Institute of Health
Bsalim
Lebanon

Lebanese University
Beirut
Lebanon

Jacques Magnan
Aix-Marseille University
Marseille
France

Hassan Haidar
Department of Otolaryngology
Hamad Medical Corporation
Weill Cornell Medical College
Doha
Qatar

ISBN 978-3-030-10292-0 ISBN 978-3-319-72962-6 (eBook)
https://doi.org/10.1007/978-3-319-72962-6

Softcover re-print of the Hardcover 1st edition 2018

This Springer imprint is published by Springer Nature, under the registered company Springer International Publishing AG
The registered company address is: Gewerbestrasse 11, 6330 Cham, Switzerland

To Ruth, my partner in life, for her love and constant support.
To my three sons, Jana, Ryhan and Fady, for filling me with pride.

Salah Mansour

Preface

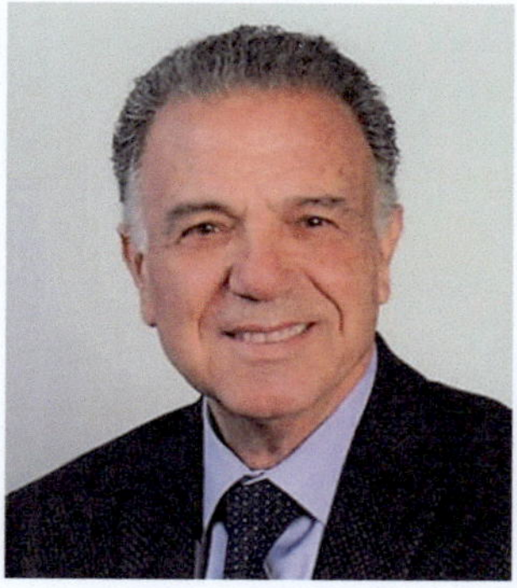

In recent years, most studies on ear-related illnesses and their treatment have focused on the latest advances in implants, especially cochlear implants, with their particular technical and rehabilitation requirements. While positive in one sense, this situation has unfortunately negatively impacted the current body of available resources and innovative studies on middle ear pathologies; specifically for the purposes of teaching medical candidates and other academic and clinical users in Otology.

This book has been produced to shed light on the latest advances that have been achieved in relevant complementary disciplines addressing the middle ear, such as innovations in the understanding of its functional anatomy and breakthroughs in physiopathology which candidates are rarely exposed to. In addition, new audiological investigative methods and advanced technical approaches in imaging which have had formidable impacts in the diagnosis and therapeutic processes of these pathologies have also now been made available. In preparing this book, we have drawn on many sources that seemed to have advanced applicable merit and we reported these sources accurately in the references.

As a result, a rich and diverse evidentiary base has allowed us to build a new multidimensional methodology in the diagnosis of middle ear ailments and their treatment.

As such, this book is equally timely for candidates, academics, and specialists as it represents a valuable up-to-date learning resource, based on demonstrated clinico-radiological correlations. It also gathers, under one single cover, most illnesses that relate to the middle ear and their treatments. The reader will find this book to be a valuable tool when faced with a difficult diagnosis and when needing to determine next steps before a complex pathology of the middle ear, especially if contemplating proceeding with surgery.

In closing I want to thank warmly my colleagues, the co-authors, for their devotion and dedication in working closely together to end up with such achievement. My special thanks go to my friend Prof Jacques Magnan who, with his unique expertise, his wide experience and huge knowledge, gave to this work an invaluable contribution.

Beirut, Lebanon Salah Mansour

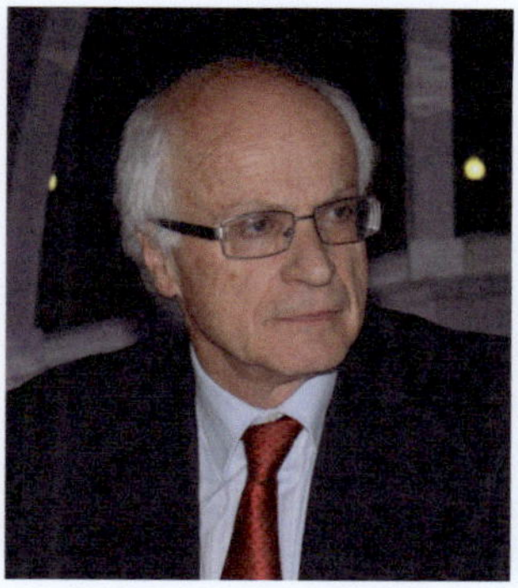

Over the past two decades, progress in otology largely derived from technological improvements, rather than the accomplishments of clinicians and pathologists. Among such improvements imaging technology has dominated the field, sometimes to the detriment of clinical observations, with some practitioners forgetting that radiological exams are intended to complement clinical work. Indeed, radiologists were trained to look to the clinician's inputs in order to guide their radiological analyses and draw diagnostic conclusions.

This evolution highlights the increasing value of correlations drawn from combined clinical and radiological efforts, as strategic vectors that guide therapeutic attitudes and otological management.

It is in light of this new reality that Professor Salah Mansour called us back to work in order to assemble and harmonize (conveniently into a single book) the achievements of basic sciences, together with the clinical, pathological and radiological data that lead to enlightened diagnostics and surgical decisions. Our ambition is to provide an update on recent developments regarding the diseases of the middle ear, and outline the space within which the rules of surgical otology will continue to evolve. We hope that talented individuals will benefit from such outline and contribute to the progress of our practice.

Colombiers, France Jacques Magnan

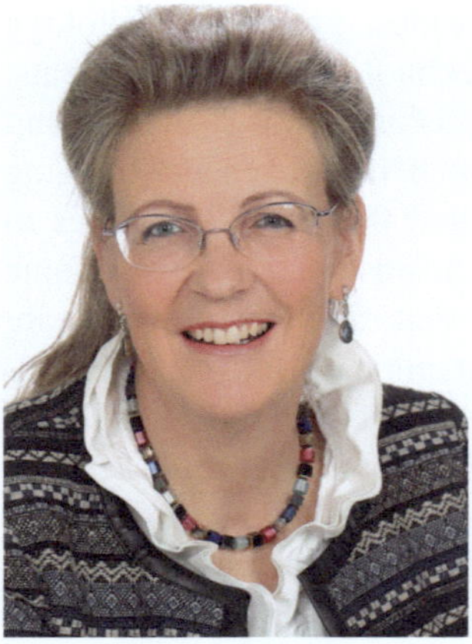

Nowadays the close correlation between clinical evaluation and radiological observation is the key to successful diagnostic and follow up inquiries regarding most middle ear diseases.

By combining advanced anatomical knowledge with clinical and scannographic findings, radiologists were able to develop useful algorithms that placed modern imaging techniques into the stream of disease management. My commitment to oto-radiology during the past 15 years has allowed me to tackle the challenge of illustrating most pathologic entities, and I strongly believe that excellent and comprehensive imaging has an important impact in otology practice.

Working on this book was a unique opportunity for me to learn from the great experience of my respectful co-authors, and I am proud to have contributed to this great work.

Beirut, Lebanon Karen Nicolas

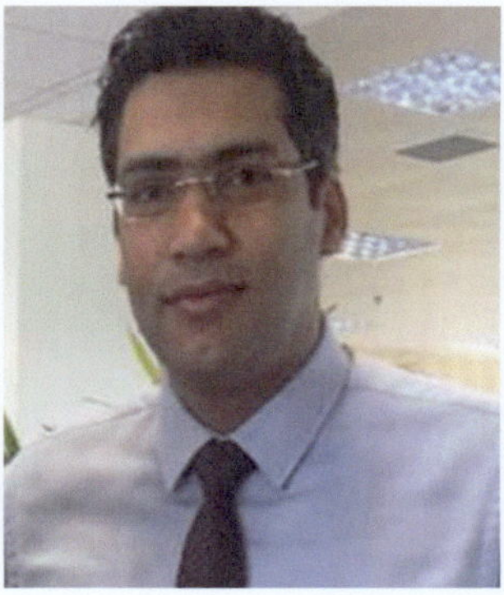

I was honored to participate in the production of this state of the art otology book with Prof. Salah Mansour and Prof. Jacques Magnan, who are two leading pioneers in the field of otology. I have learned a great deal from them, and owe my professional success to their teaching and mentorship. This book would not exist as it is without the great contribution of Dr. Karen Nicolas, a brilliant otoradiologist who is expert in the field of temporal bone imaging.

This book is the happy culmination of our keen and long-drawn focus on middle ear diseases. It addresses complex facts and controversial issues in the field. Lucid presentation was of particular importance when approaching each subject, as we intended to facilitate the easy recall and reproduction of concepts by students and practitioners.

We intended this book for our departments, residents and fellows, our colleagues, and the patients who will ultimately benefit from advances in our field. We hope our readers can build upon the achievements described in this book.

I owe my own achievements to my wife Fatima, my daughter Hawraa, my family, and friends. I cannot thank them enough.

Doha, Qatar Hassan Haidar

Contents

Otosclerosis

1

Contents

S. Mansour et al., *Middle Ear Diseases*,
https://doi.org/10.1007/978-3-319-72962-6_1

1.1 Introduction

Otosclerosis is a progressive temporal bone dysplasia that affects selectively the human otic capsule and is characterized by excessive bone remodeling in the otic capsule (bone resorption and reactive bone deposition). It was first identified and reported by Adam Politzer [1, 2]. The hallmark of the disease is stapes fixation with resultant conductive hearing loss. Otosclerosis is the most common cause of conductive hearing loss in adults with normal appearing tympanic membrane. The age of onset of hearing loss is commonly in the third decade of life.

Advanced molecular biology studies and genetic works helped otologists to understand some etiological factors behind the disease, even though these intensive researches failed yet to fully explain the etiopathogenesis of otosclerosis.

Nowadays, the diagnostic tests for otosclerosis have greatly improved, especially the imaging techniques, making the preoperative diagnosis almost 100% accurate. In addition, surgical techniques refinement permitted easier and safer surgeries with better outcome and much lower complications rate. Moreover, cochlear implants offered a great progress in the hearing rehabilitation for the far advanced disease.

In this chapter the latest updates will be discussed, encompassing all the aspects of otosclerosis from its histopathology, molecular biology, genetics, the different clinical courses, its diagnostic and preoperative workup, to the advanced inputs of clinico-radiological correlations along with their surgical impact. Also surgical treatments of otosclerosis and their relative concerns are discussed in depth.

Fig. 1.1 Epidemiology of otosclerosis

Epidemiology of Otosclerosis

- 10 % overall prevalence of histological otosclerosis
- 1 % overall prevalence of clinical otosclerosis
- Clinical otosclerosis–2:1 (F:M)
- Possible progression during pregnancy
- Most common age of presentation 25-45 years

1.2 Epidemiology

Otosclerosis was classified by Schuknecht and Barber as clinical and histological [3]. 'Histologic otosclerosis' refers to a disease process without clinical symptoms or manifestations that can only be discovered by routine sectioning of the temporal bone at autopsy. 'Clinical otosclerosis' concerns the presence of otosclerosis at a site where it causes conductive hearing loss by interfering with the motion of the stapes or of the round window membrane [4, 5]. The incidence of histological otosclerosis in the general population ranges from 5 to 15% as reported by several autopsy studies [6–12].

Histological otosclerosis occurs in 10% of Caucasians but only 1% of them develop clinical manifestations of otosclerosis (Fig. 1.1). Histologic otosclerosis is as common in the Japanese population (2.5%) as in European populations (2.5%), the otosclerotic foci are less frequent around the oval window, which can explain the lower incidence of clinical otosclerosis in Japenese population (very rare) compared to European population (0.4%) [13, 14].

The incidence of clinical otosclerosis varies worldwide with the highest rate reported in Southern India and the lowest rate in Africa [15]. It is common in white races and in Indians, but very rare in Africans, Japenese, and Chinese. Approximately 0.2–1% of light skin populations have clinical otosclerosis [4, 7, 16–25].

Family history of otosclerosis is reported in almost half of affected patients. Women are more frequently affected than men (female/male = 2/1) [18, 26].

The incidence of clinical otosclerosis has declined significantly in the recent years. This decline is mainly attributed to the massive measles vaccination; however, paradoxically, there is even a drop in the incidence of otosclerosis in undeveloped countries where measles continue to be widespread [19, 27].

In addition, the severity of otosclerosis is changing; the incidence of advanced disease has also diminished as measured by the percentage of cases requiring a drill out of the oval window for obliterative otosclerosis. The incidence of obliterative otosclerosis dropped from 20 to 5% [28, 29]. This decline in incidence and severity affects the surgical practice of this disease and its training availability.

1.3 Etiopathogenesis

It is hypothesized that in response to various gene defects, the physiological inhibition of bone turnover in the otic capsule is overruled due to a greater susceptibility to environmental factors, resulting in a localized bone dysplasia

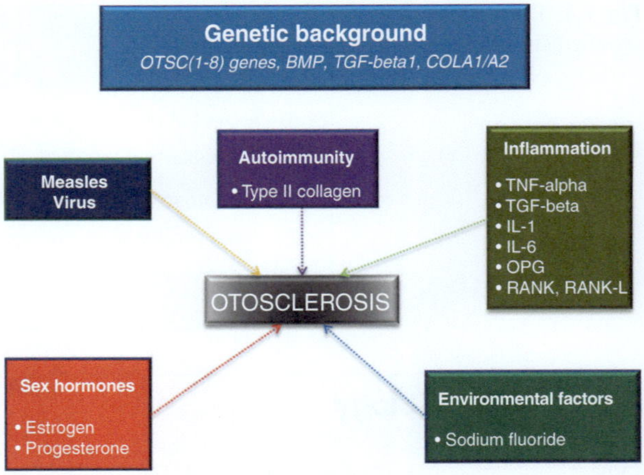

Fig. 1.2 Factors involved in the etiopathogenesis of otosclerosis

known as otosclerosis [30]. Several factors are involved in the etiopathogenesis of otosclerosis (Fig. 1.2)

1.3.1 Biology of the Otic Capsule

The bone of the otic capsule is unique: it exhibits two main features not found in other bones of the human skeleton:

1. Very low bone remodeling rate because of its special OPG/RANK/RANK-L system.
2. It contains small regions of immature cartilaginous tissue called the *Globuli Interossei.*

These two unique features may explain the fact that otosclerosis is exclusive to the otic capsule (**organotropism**):

1.3.1.1 OPG/RANK/RANK-L System

Bone metabolism of the otic capsule differs fundamentally from the rest of the skeleton. Bone remodeling (or bone metabolism) is a lifelong process where mature bone tissue is removed from the skeleton (bone resorption) and new bone tissue is formed (bone formation). These processes control the reshaping or replacement of bone following injuries like fractures but also micro-damage, which occurs during normal activity. Remodeling responds also to functional demands of the mechanical loading. In adults, remodeling proceeds at about 10% per year. In contrary, bone remodeling is normally highly restricted in the otic capsule to less than 0.15% per year. A local inner ear mechanism is responsible for the inhibition of capsular remodeling activity. The mechanism responsible for this *inhibition of bone remodeling* is the inner ear OPG/RANK/RANKL signaling system [31–33].

Osteoprotegerin (OPG), also known as osteoclastogenesis inhibitory factor (OCIF), is an anti-resorptive cytokine named from its ability to "protect" bone against resorption. By binding RANKL, OPG prevents RANK-mediated nuclear

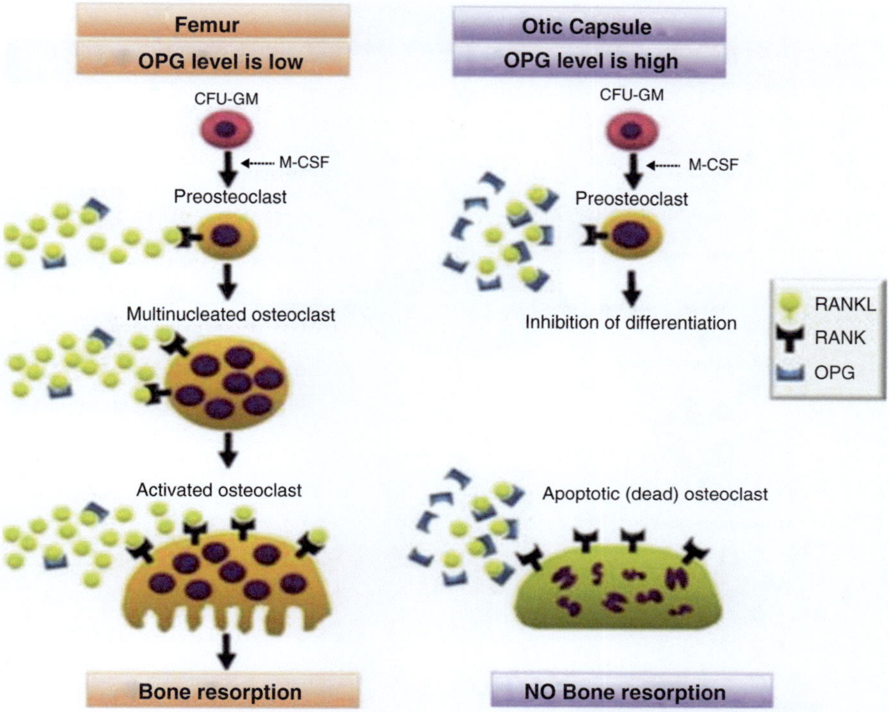

Fig. 1.3 High level of OPG in the otic capsule binds to RANK-L; inhibiting RANK/RANK-L interaction thus prevents osteoclast differentiation and reduces bone resorption

factor kappa B (NF-κB) activation which is central for osteoclast activation and bone resorption. OPG is expressed in high levels (>1000× normal bone levels) by the inner ear structures to inhibit otic capsule bone remodeling [31–33] (Fig. 1.3). What could be the mechanism behind the development of otosclerosis? The bone turnover is highly suppressed in normal otic capsules, probably due to a local inner ear mechanism for which OPG seems to be an important factor. It is most likely that otosclerosis develops due to a relief of this specific inhibition of bone remodeling, rather than a more general activation of bone turnover.

OPG/RANK/RANK-L System Dysregulation

The importance of the inner ear OPG dysregulation was shown in a study on mice: after knocking out of OPG, they developed an excessive and disorganized capsular bone remodeling, stapes fixation, and progressive hearing loss [31–33].

Measles virus infection, in a genetically predisposed patient, may trigger the process of otosclerosis via activation of T-lymphocytes and resultant increased secretion of RANKL. [34–36] (Fig. 1.4).

Pregnancy and lactation induce a status of hyperprolactinemia which is known to downregulate OPG [37]. This may explain the increased risk and acceleration of otosclerosis during pregnancy.

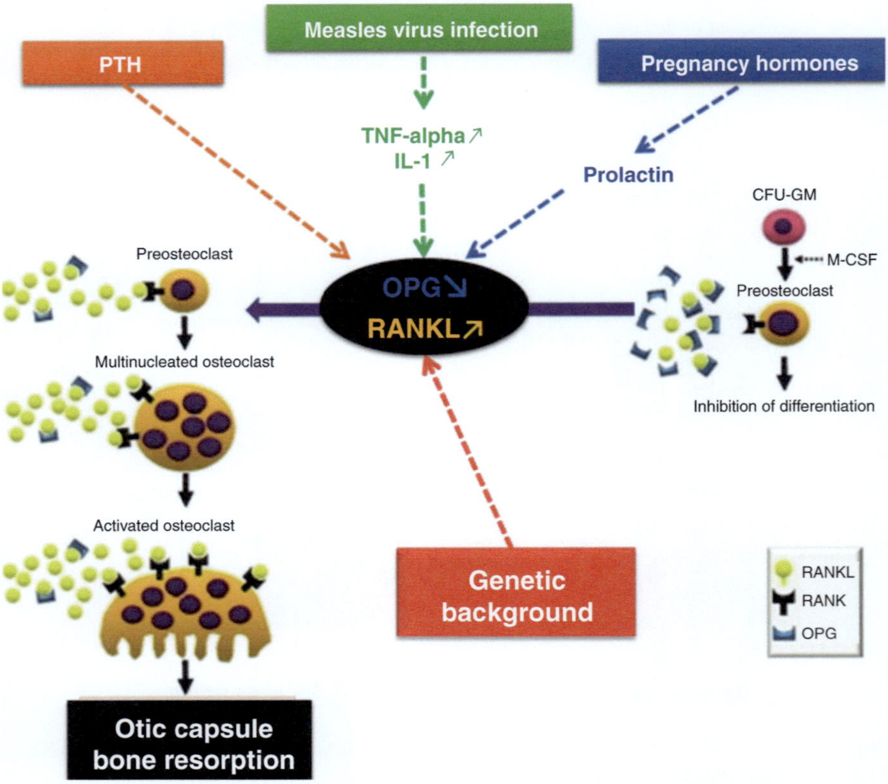

Fig. 1.4 OPG/RANK/RANK-L System could be dysregulated in genetically predisposed individuals by measles virus infection through increased secretions of TNF-alpha and IL-1, or by pregnancy hormones, mainly Prolactin. Dysregulation of OPG/RANK/RANK-L System stimulates bone resorption in the otic capsule with the resultant capsular remodeling and possible stapes fixation

Genetic and racial factors affect the levels of OPG and the settings of the OPG/RANKL/RANK signaling system and consequently the vulnerability of the bony otic capsule to otosclerosis.

1.3.1.2 Globuli Interossei

Another unique feature of otic capsule is its unique bony development. It consists of an inner endosteal layer, an intermediate endochondral layer, and an outer periosteal layer. The otic capsule arises during the fetal development through endochondral ossification, a bone formation process in which first a cartilage model is made, which is then replaced by bone. During this process, cartilaginous remnants are often not removed when the lacunae of degenerating cartilage cells are being replaced by primary bone. These remnants are called globuli interossei and are located in the intermediate endochondral layer. (Fig. 1.5). "Globuli Interossei" form a layer which demonstrates embryonic immature cartilage remnants. The otic

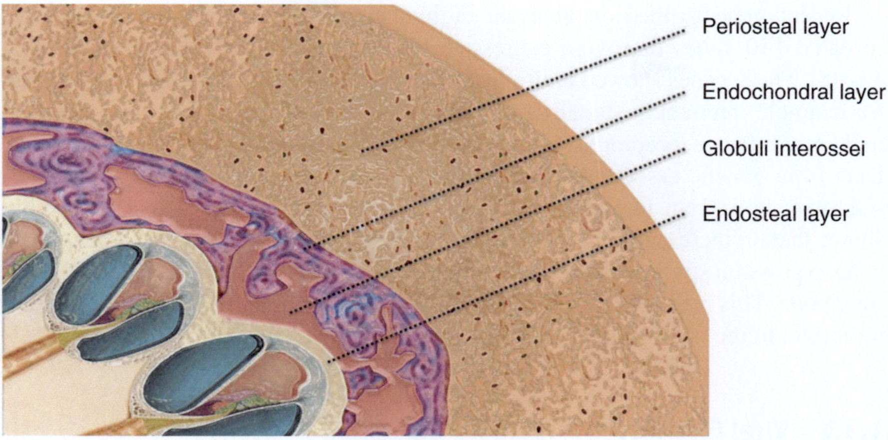

Fig. 1.5 A unique feature of the otic capsule is the presence of *globuli interossei* between the endosteal layer and the external periosteal layer of the otic capsule. "Globuli Interossei" form a layer which demonstrates immature embryonic cartilage remnants and could be the site of the earliest otosclerotic foci

capsule is the only organ of the human skeleton that contains such a layer. It is assumed that these "*interosseous globules*" could be the site of the earliest otosclerotic foci after being infected by measles virus and explain why otosclerosis would be limited only to the otic capsule [38, 39].

1.3.2 Genetic Inheritance

From a genetic viewpoint, otosclerosis can be seen as a complex disease where both genetic and environmental factors confer disease susceptibility, with rare autosomal dominant forms in which one gene causes otosclerosis. About 60% of patients with clinical otosclerosis report a family history of the disease [40]. It can be considered as an autosomal dominant disease with incomplete penetrance. Reduced penetrance of the otosclerosis gene means that the abnormal gene does not always dominate over the normal gene. The probability for a person, who has one parent affected by the disease, to develop otosclerosis is about 25%. If both parents have the disease, the probability for the child to develop otosclerosis raises to 50%.

Many family linkage studies and candidate gene association studies have been performed; however disease-causing mutations remain elusive [41]. One gene associated with otosclerosis is *COLA1*; an error in this gene leads to osteogenesis imperfecta (type I). Histological similarities exist between these two entities, and some authors have suggested that otosclerosis is a local manifestation of osteogenesis imperfecta (type I) [42].

Recent gene expression analysis of human otosclerotic stapedial footplates revealed 110 genes that were expressed differently compared with controls [41, 43–45]. These genes showed multiple pathways that could lead to bone remodeling, for example interleukin signaling, inflammation, p53 signaling, apoptosis, epidermal growth factor receptor signaling (EGFR) and an oxidative stress response [46]. Data from genetic association studies and from gene expression analysis for otosclerosis showed an important role for TGF-β1 pathway. The association study shows that an increased TGF-β1 activity protects against otosclerosis, whereas the gene expression study showed evidence for decreased TGF-β1 signaling in otosclerotic bone. This means that TGF-β1 and genes involved in the TGF-β1 signaling are important in the pathogenesis of otosclerosis [47].

1.3.3 Viral Etiology

Some authors have suggested an inflammatory etiology for otosclerosis due to a persistent measles virus infection of the otic capsule [34, 48]. In a study of 116 patients with stapedectomy, Karosi et al. observed measles virus RNA in all footplates with a histological otosclerotic focus [49]. Similarly, the expression of a virus binding receptor (CD46) was increased substantially in footplates with a histological focus [49]. Epidemiological reports of a decreased incidence of otosclerosis after a measles vaccination program also support its viral aetiology [50, 51]. Elevated anti-measles antibodies have been detected in perilymph samples collected during stapedectomy [52]. On the other hand, lower levels of circulating anti-measles antibodies have been found in patients with otosclerosis [53]. This finding is thought to demonstrate specific immune reactions stemming from the endolymphatic sac, which are evoked by measles antigens near the perilymphatic space [52].

1.3.4 Endocrinological Factors

1.3.4.1 Pregnancy

Pregnancy is an evident predisposing factor to cause the onset or the progression of otosclerosis [54, 55]. Shambaugh found that 50% of 475 female patients suffering from otosclerosis, showed onset of hearing loss during pregnancy. Symptoms seem to accelerate in some women after their second or third pregnancy.

1.3.4.2 Parathyroid Hormone

Studies showed that the expression and the function of PTH receptors in otosclerotic stapes footplates are lower than in the bone collected from the external ear canal. PTH is probably not the triggering factor in the pathogenesis, but a consequence of abnormal regulation of the bone matrix protein metabolism caused by another factor [56].

1.3.5 Immunological Factors

Otosclerosis was hypothesized to be an autoimmune disease because elevated levels of collagen II autoantibody were detected in otosclerotic patients compared to a control group [57]. As otosclerosis may be considered as an autoimmune bone remodeling disorder, immunosuppressive, anti-inflammatory therapy including NSAIDs, corticosteroids or anti-TNF have been used in order to control the disease, but without positive results. In addition, anti-osteoporotic agents including vitamin D, bisphosphonates, calcitonin and fluorides failed to control the pathological bone process.

1.4 Histopathology

Otosclerosis is a disease affecting the endochondral bone of the otic capsule, characterized by dysregulated resorption and deposition of bone. Otosclerosis is also called 'otospongiosis' since the normal ivory-like endochondral bone is being replaced by spongy vascular bone. The progression of otosclerosis can be divided into 4 stages. In the first stage, the resorptive or active inflammatory phase, the endochondral bone of the otic capsule is resorbed by osteoclasts. This is initiated by an unknown pathologic stimulus and affects certain anatomic sites such as the fissula ante fenestram and the globuli interossei near the oval window. The bone is then replaced with a highly vascular cellular and fibrous tissue. Subsequently, new bone is formed. This second phase is characterized by the production of a dysplastic, immature basophilic bone and the filling of the vascular spaces with connective tissue and the synthesis of collagen fibrils. The third phase is the remodeling phase in which the basophilic bone is remodeled and becomes a less vascular and more mature acidophilic bone with a laminated matrix. In the fourth and last phase, the mature or otosclerotic phase, mineralization of the dysplastic bone results in a new dense compact bone with a characteristic woven pattern.

Classically, two histologic phases are described in otosclerosis:

1. ***active phase***: characterized by bone resorption (spongiosis),
2. ***stabilized phase***: characterized by bone deposition (sclerosis)

During the active phase, the hypervascularized lesion shows usually dark blue staining on hematoxylin–eosin staining (Fig. 1.6). An important feature of active otosclerotic foci is the woven pattern of collagenous fibrils, which run in an entirely irregular crisscross fashion through the otosclerotic focus. A distinct boundary between the normal and dystrophic bone is described [58].

In the remission phase of otosclerosis, osteoclasts disappear, while osteoblasts or osteocytes are still present within the affected area (Fig. 1.6). The vascular spaces become narrow or obliterated by apposition of lamellar bone and appear as pink or red on hematoxylin–eosin staining [59].

Histologically, the sites of predilection of otosclerosis are the window regions OW (80–95%), RW (40%), and pericochlear areas (35%) [12].

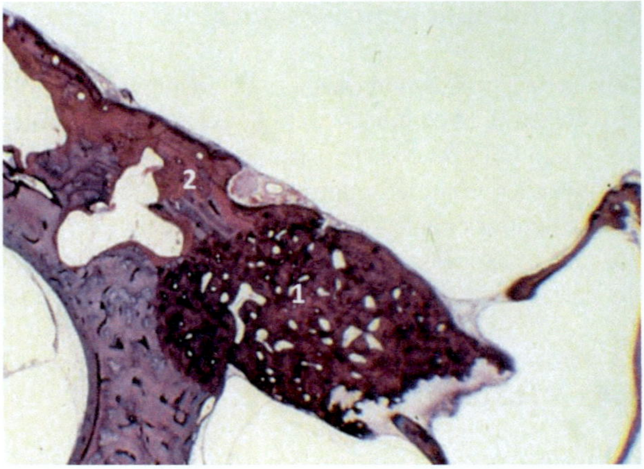

Fig. 1.6 Axial cut of left temporal bone at the level of fissula ante-fenestram showing the two phases of otosclerosis at the same time, active phase (1) and stabilized phase (2). The active focus shows spongiotic bone in contact with the footplate with disappearance of the annular ligament. The stabilized focus shows dense bone

1.5 Sites of Localization of Otosclerosis

In otosclerosis, foci of abnormal bone deposition are particularly frequent around the oval and round window and in the otic capsule close to the cochlea, three places of the otic capsule which are rich in globuli interossei and where the inhibition of bone remodeling is most prominent. Two types of otosclerosis are described based on the localization of the disease: ***fenestral*** and ***retrofenestral*** otosclerosis. As the name suggests (fenestra is the Latin word for window), fenestral otosclerosis affects the lateral labyrinthine wall, including both the oval and round window niche. Retrofenestral otosclerosis involves the pericochlear otic capsule and is commonly associated with the fenestral otosclerosis (Fig. 1.7).

1.5.1 Fenestral Otosclerosis

1.5.1.1 The Oval Window

Fenestral Otosclerosis is the most frequent type of otosclerosis that involves the stapes and the oval window causing a fixity and secondary conductive hearing loss. The site of predilection is the *fissula ante-fenestram* in front of the vestibule in 80–90% of cases (Fig. 1.7).

Stapes fixation starts with the calcification and narrowing of the annular ligament. In this process, the otosclerotic lesion of the oval window fuses with the stapedial footplate. The stapes subsequently becomes fixed by this lesion. The process extends across the ligament onto the footplate until there is no remnant of the original annular ligament (Fig. 1.8). Relative to the histological maturation phase of the disease process, the degree of conductive hearing loss varies from 20 to 50 dB. Complete obliteration of the oval window may occur in 5% of cases (obliterative otosclerosis). In the obliterative type of otosclerosis, the stapes footplate is greatly thickened and diffusely replaced by a massive otosclerotic deposit that fills the oval window niche.

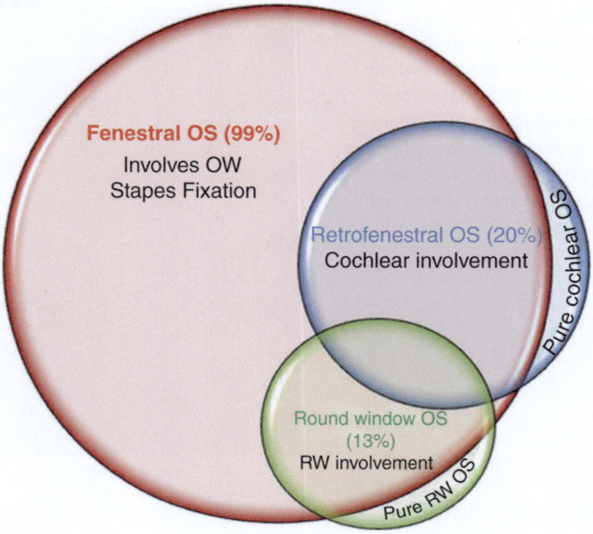

Fig. 1.7 Types of otosclerosis

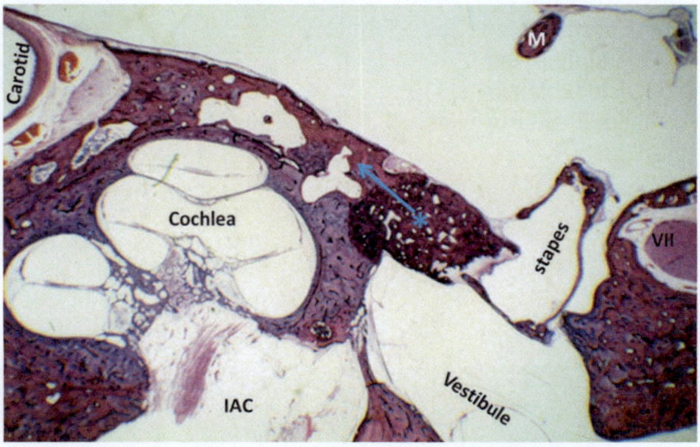

Fig. 1.8 Histological transverse cut of left ear showing otosclerotic focus involving the fissula ante fenestram (*) extending to the footplate and to the pericochlear region (arrow). *VII* facial nerve, *M* malleus handle, *IAC* internal auditory canal

1.5.1.2 The Round Window

Round window involvement is found histologically in 40% of patients with otosclerosis [12] (Fig. 1.9). In a clinico-radiological study, RW otosclerosis was observed in 13% of patients with conductive hearing loss and stapedial otosclerosis; cases of isolated RW otosclerosis without any other focus found in the otic capsule have been reported [60] (Fig. 1.7).

1.5.2 Retrofenestral (Pericochlear) Otosclerosis

Histologically, foci of demineralised spongy vascular bone could be seen in the cochlear capsule, and may extend around the vestibule, the semicircular canals and the internal auditory canal (Figs. 1.10 and 1.11). Pure **cochlear otosclerosis** is a

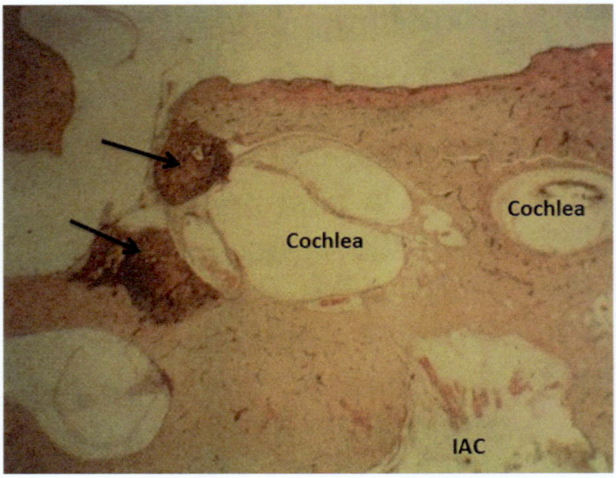

Fig. 1.9 Histologic transverse cut of the otic capsule at the level of the round window showing otosclerotic involvement of the round window edges (arrows). *IAC:* Internal auditory canal (Document P. Roulleau, C. Martin)

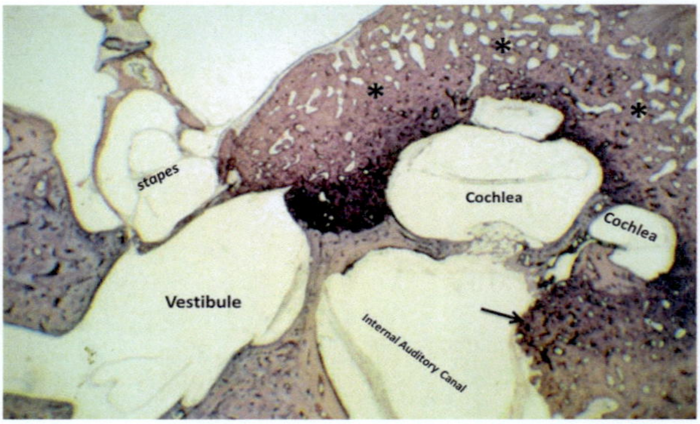

Fig. 1.10 Transverse histological cut of right ear showing stapedial otosclerosis and pericochlear involvement (*) extending to the endocochlear lumen and to the internal auditory canal (black arrow)

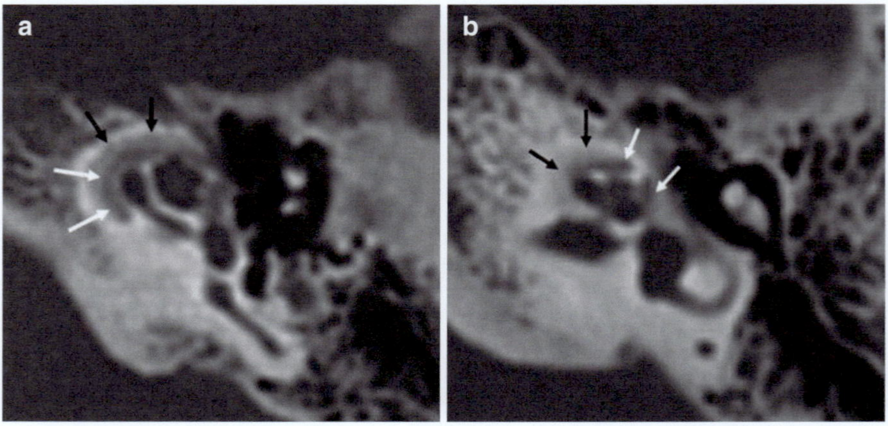

Fig. 1.11 Axial CT-views of left ears of different patients with longstanding otosclerosis: a very hypodense rim of otosclerosis (white arrows) is in intimate contact with the cochlear endosteum, the more peripheral ring (black arrows) is only mildly hypodense corresponding to the maturation process of otospongiosis into otosclerosis

term used in cases when the otosclerotic lesion spares the footplate and invades the cochlear endosteum and manifests usually as a pure sensorineural hearing loss without any conductive component [8]. Direct injury to the cochlea and to the spiral ligament, due to direct invasion by an otosclerotic focus itself or by the proteolytic enzymes and cytokines released from a nearby focus, are incriminated as the most probable cause for the SNHL. The earlier the cochlear disease starts, the more severe it will become later.

1.6 Clinical Manifestations

1.6.1 Hearing Loss

Progressive conductive hearing loss in an adult without history of recurrent ear infections or head trauma and with normal otoscopic examination is typical of otosclerosis. In approximately 70–80% of cases, both ears are affected over time. Hearing loss is usually noticed when it reaches 15–25 dB.

Patients may report that they hear better in the presence of a background noise, the so called phenomenon of paracusis of Willis. This phenomenon occurs because the conductive hearing loss attenuates the background noise and renders the dynamic range of the ear at the level of the speaker's voice, thus effectively increasing the signal to noise ratio.

In 10% of the patients, a sensorineural component arises with the conductive component with a resultant mixed hearing loss. It is due to stapes fixation and cochlear involvement. Patients with long-term otosclerosis accompanied by severe mixed hearing loss can eventually develop far-advanced otosclerosis [61]. Very rarely, otosclerosis may manifest as a pure sensorineural hearing loss because of cochlear damage without stapes fixation (pure cochlear otosclerosis). A sensorineural hearing loss that cannot be correlated with the patient's age warrants investigation for otosclerosis.

1.6.2 Tinnitus

The incidence of subjective tinnitus in otosclerosis patients is reported to be between 65–92% [62, 63]. It may be of a roaring or hissing character in the majority of cases. Pulsatile tinnitus is less common and is due to the hypervascularisation status in the early stages of the disease. It usually disappears when the lesion matures and the spongy vascular bone is replaced by the hard sclerotic bone.

Tinnitus may be unilateral or bilateral. In patients with unilateral tinnitus, the likelihood that tinnitus will be localized to the poorer hearing ear is correlated with the magnitude of interaural asymmetry. When the interaural difference is greater than 15 dB, tinnitus will be localized in the poorer ear in more than 75% of patients [64].

Several theories have been proposed to explain the existence of tinnitus in otosclerosis: [63, 65]:

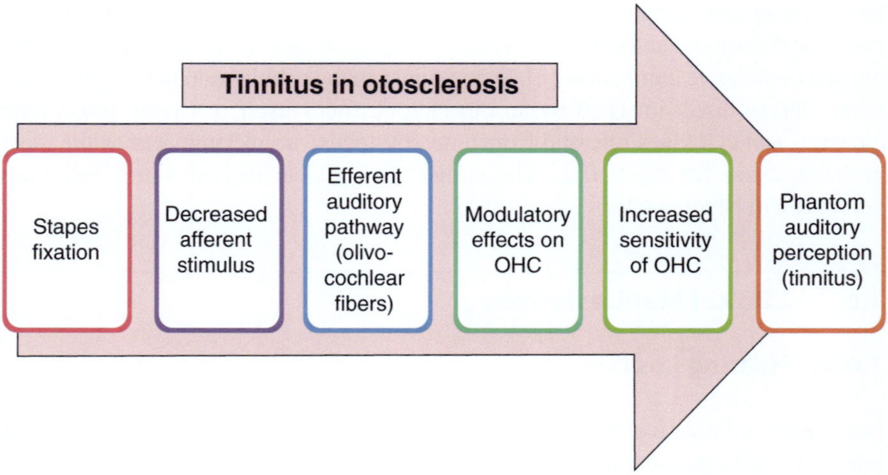

Fig. 1.12 Modulatory theory of tinnitus in otosclerosis; OHC: outer hair cells

1.6.2.1 Toxicity Theory

In active stages of otosclerosis, a high amount of cytotoxic enzymes (elastase, collagenase, cathepsin-D/B, etc.), inflammatory cytokine mediators, and complement fragments are suspected to be released from the otosclerotic foci. These substances could flow into the perilymph and change the electromotility of the outer hair cells.

1.6.2.2 Modulatory Theory

The efferent auditory pathway (olivocochlear fibers) could have a modulatory effect on the outer hair cells; the efferent pathway could buffer or amplify the message in response to the suffering outer hair cells (Fig. 1.12) [65].

1.6.3 Dizziness

Dizziness is reported in almost 25–30% of patients with otosclerosis before surgery [21, 66]. In most cases, dizziness is due to otolithic dysfunction induced by otosclerosis itself. Occasionally, dizziness may be the expression of an associated pathology like Meniere's disease. In such scenario, the indication for the surgical treatment of otosclerosis is challenging.

Dizziness due to an otolithic dysfunction is a major cause of balance problems in patients with otosclerosis. Changes in utricular and saccular end organs were seen in autopsy studies from patients with otosclerosis, such as absent otoconia located near an otosclerotic focus [67]. Otolith damage in otosclerosis appears more in the saccule than in the utricle as shown by different VEMP studies: cVEMP is usually affected when oVEMP is preserved. Anatomically, the saccule lies more closer to the footplate than the utricle, so the released toxins from the otosclerotic focus might affect the saccule easier and earlier before reaching the utricle [68] (Fig. 1.13).

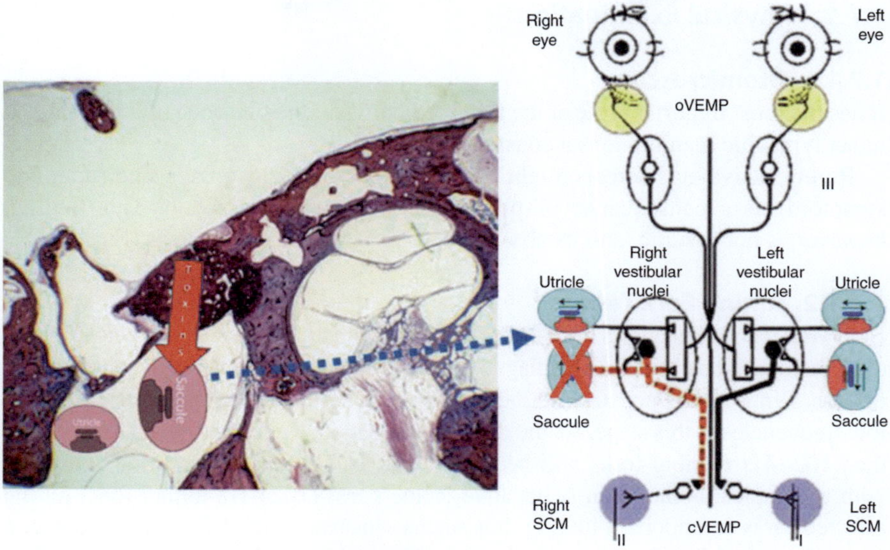

Fig. 1.13 A case of right ear otosclerosis. Otolith damage in otosclerosis appears more at the saccule than at the utricle, the saccule lying closer to the footplate than the utricle and the released toxins (red arrow) might affect the saccule easier and earlier before the utricle as shown by different VEMP studies; cVEMP is affected on the right side while oVEMP is preserved

Enzyme release from the remodeling bone affects the homeostasis of the perilymph and endolymph through the vascular labyrinth barrier structures in the inner ear leading to an endolymphatic hydrops, most frequently a saccular hydrops (Fig. 1.13) [69]. Very rarely the hydrops could be due to a direct invasion of the vestibular aqueduct by the otosclerotic focus.

Many reports have described [70, 71] the relationship between endolymphatic hydrops and otosclerosis. Paparella and Chasin reported about otosclerosis patients with typical signs and symptoms of Meniere's disease [72]. Shea et al. revealed endolymphatic hydrops in five patients with otosclerosis using electrocochleography [71–73]. Human temporal bone studies revealed the coexistence of endolymphatic hydrops in patients with otosclerotic focus [71, 74, 75]. Seo et al. reported that patients with cochleo-saccular hydrops revealed by VEMP did not complain of any recurrent vertigo but of recurrent short-lasting dysequilibrium [76].

1.7 Clinical Evaluation

Clinical diagnosis of stapes fixation is based on the case history of progressive hearing loss, tinnitus, dizziness, paracusis, familial history, etc., normal otoscopic findings, negative Rinne's test, conductive and/or mixed hearing loss, type-As tympanogram, and increased middle ear resonance frequency (>1100 Hz) measured by multifrequency tympanometry.

1.7.1 Physical Examination

1.7.1.1 Otomicroscopy

It has the most important role at the first medical visit: the presence of a normal and intact tympanic membrane is a constant finding.

Rarely, active otosclerosis might be associated with Schwartze's sign (flamingo symptom) as a consequence of promontory hypervascularization. This finding, however, is not specific, and its absence does not exclude otosclerosis (Fig. 1.14).

1.7.1.2 Tuning Fork Tests

Both Weber and Rinne tests must be performed: when tuning fork tests are not in favor of a conductive hearing loss, the diagnosis must be reviewed. In the early stages of the disease, Rinne test is negative at 256-Hz only, because hearing loss affects only the low frequencies at this stage. As the disease progresses, Rinne tests using the 512 and then 1024-Hz tunning forks will become negative. The results are to be correlated with a complete audiogram. A negative Rinne's test (1024 Hz tuning fork) on the affected ear is an important finding. It is such a sensitive method that a stapes surgeon can make a decision for surgical intervention based on this finding. However, indication for stapes surgery is generally based on 25–30 dB ABG on pure tone audiometry (PTA) and clinico-radiological correlations (see Sect. 10.2.3.).

1.7.2 Audiological Testing

Complete audiological evaluation serves as the basis for the diagnosis of otosclerosis. Subjective or objective audiological examinations, however, are not specific for otosclerosis (see Sect. 10.2.3).

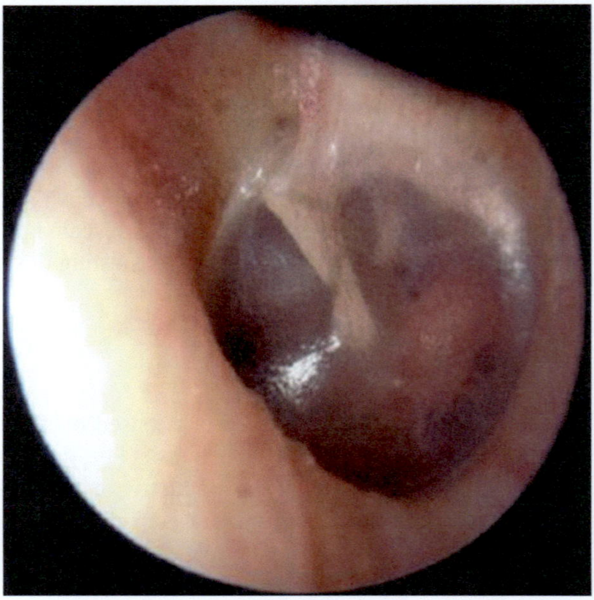

Fig. 1.14 Left ear Schwartze's sign

1.7.2.1 Pure Tone Audiometry

This is the most fundamental test that should be performed in any patient presenting with impairment in hearing. However it should be remembered that it is a subjective test and the results can vary from laboratory to laboratory. Nonetheless it is the single most necessary test that needs to be performed. PTA must be done accurately and always requires adequate masking with a white noise.

I) Air Conduction: The primary acoustic consequence of otosclerosis in its early stages is the increase in the stiffness reactance component of the total middle ear impedance. This results in a reduction of transmission efficiency for low frequencies as seen in elevated thresholds. In the early stages, a gradually progressive low-frequency conductive hearing loss is first seen. Initially, patients may be unaware of such a hearing impairment until it crosses the 25dB range. The hearing loss may be confined to frequencies below 1000Hz. The footplate with partial mobility maintains the capacity for the transmission of the high frequencies and thus high frequencies thresholds are typically unaffected at this stage. This characteristic rising audiogram configuration has been referred to as the "stiffness tilt".

As the footplate becomes completely fixed and the otosclerotic focus proliferates, a mass effect is added to the audiogram. The low-frequency hearing loss doesn't increase and appears to stabilize. However, the hearing loss progresses in the high frequencies and there is a gradual widening of the air-bone gap. The audiogram configuration now changes to a flat pattern from the upward sloping pattern that it had in the early stages.

In the absence of cochlear involvement, the pure conductive hearing loss produced by the complete stapes fixation is limited to 40 dB to 50 dB with a maximum air-bone gap across the frequency range.

In cochlear otosclerosis, air conduction thresholds continue to worsen and the loss starts to become mixed or sensorineural, with the high frequencies becoming severely affected. The typical pattern of cochlear otosclerosis in the early stages is the "cookie bite"pattern where the greatest degree of hearing loss occurs in the mid-frequency hearing range and is characteristically a mixed hearing loss [77].

Tinnitus is usually present in a large percentage of patients. If the tinnitus is severe, it may interfere with the patients ability to respond reliably to pure tone testing. Usage of pulsed or warbled tones may help the patient to identify tinnitus from pure tone test stimuli when being tested.

II) Bone Conduction: Bone conduction is especially useful when testing patients suffering from otosclerosis. It reveals characteristics that are typical of otosclerosis and determines the amount of cochlear reserve in each ear. Further, bone conduction helps to identify if stapedial or cochlear otosclerosis is present. This, in turn, helps the surgeon to decide which ear should be operated and to predict the optimum postoperative results.

Stapes fixation is usually associated with the presence of Carhart's notch which is characterized by elevation of bone conduction thresholds of approximately 5 dB at 500 Hz, 10 dB at 1000 Hz, 15 dB at 2000 Hz and 5 dB at 4000 Hz (Fig. 1.15). Carhart's notch is in fact an audiological artifact; it is not a true representation of cochlear reserve and usually disappears after a successful stapes surgery. Carhart's notch phenomenon occurs because not all of the sound waves applied to the cranium by the bone vibrator reach the cochlea through the osseous route only. A variety of pathways

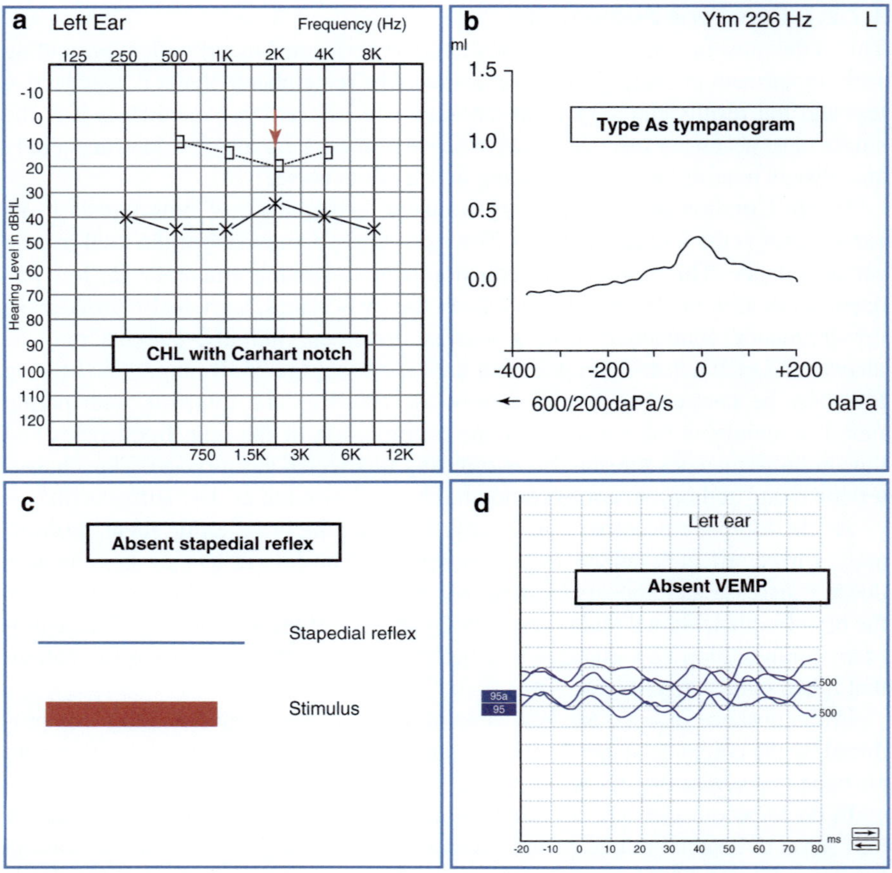

Fig. 1.15 Typical audiological studies in a patient with otosclerosis. (**a**) audiogram with conductive hearing loss and Carhart notch (red arrow). (**b**) As type tympanogram. (**c**) absent stapedial reflex. (**d**) absent VEMP response

of bone conduction exist and may be summarized as follows: bone to cochlea, bone to middle ear to cochlea, and bone to external canal to middle ear to cochlea [78–80]. As 2 kHz is the normal resonance frequency of human ossicles, the bone to middle ear to cochlea pathway is very prominent at this frequency. A bone vibrator with 2 kHz frequency applied to the cranium reaches the cochlea through the bone to cochlea and through the bone to middle ear to stapes to the cochlea pathways. A fixed stapes will attenuate the second pathway and will prevent part of the bone vibrator energy from reaching the cochlea; this will be reflected by an elevated bone-conduction threshold at this frequency. This BC level will be restored to normal after stapes surgery. Despite the fact that Carhart notch is frequently observed in otosclerosis, it is not specific for otosclerosis and it can be seen in other middle ear diseases.

If the air conduction and bone conduction levels are roughly parallel, the elevated bone conduction thresholds probably represent a true sensorineural hearing loss. Sensorineural hearing losses are most commonly associated with basal turn involvement and are invariably present with endosteal layer involvement.

Word recognition scores or speech discrimination is usually normal unless there is a significant sensorineural component; in such case, a speech discrimination test is recommended in order to exclude or to confirm roll-over recruitment phenomenon. Speech audiometry is also a mandatory examination if hearing deteriorates after stapes surgery in order to adequately fit a hearing aid.

1.7.2.2 Tympanometry and Multifrequency Tympanometry

Tympanometry measures the peak pressure and peak-compensated static admittance of the middle ear at the eardrum. As the stapes is ankylosed in otosclerosis, the lateral end of the ossicular chain may still be quite mobile. Therefore, otosclerosis may only slightly reduce the admittance, resulting in either a shallow tympanogram (type As), or a normal tympanogram (type A).

During standard tympanometry a low frequency probe of 226 Hz is commonly used.

Multi-frequency tympanometry provides more accurate and detailed information about the middle ear dynamics than standard tympanometry.

Multi-frequency tympanometry is based on the analysis of tympanograms at a wide range of frequencies between 226 and 2000 Hz. The resonant frequency (RF) is described as the frequency at which both middle ear stiffness and admittance are equal. Multi-frequency tympanometry can be a useful tool to predict the diagnosis of various middle ear pathologies preoperatively, as changes in mass and/or stiffness of the mechano-acoustic system of the middle ear are found to affect the resonant frequency.

Otosclerosis increases in the stiffness of the middle-ear system, raising its resonant frequency. This can be quantified using multi-frequency tympanometry. Thus, a high resonant-frequency pathology such as otosclerosis can be differentiated from low resonant-frequency pathologies such as ossicular discontinuity.

1.7.2.3 Stapedial Reflex

Stapedial reflex testing should be part of the standard audiometric evaluation in patients with conductive hearing loss. Since clinical otosclerosis partially or totally fixates the stapes, the muscular effect is modulated. Typically, at the beginning of disease, the acoustic reflex may show diphasic pattern (on-off phenomenon). The diphasic pattern reflex is characterized by brief increases in compliance that occur at the onset and at the termination of the stimulus when the probe is in the affected ear. In early stages of the disease where the anterior footplate is fixed to the oval window, the elasticity of the involved footplate and crura allows the posterior portion of the footplate to move, in response to contraction of the stapedius muscle, independent of the anterior portion of the footplate, creating the onset compliance change. The elasticity of the footplate returns to its resting position where it remains until the pull of the tendon of the stapedius is relaxed allowing another brief change in compliance at the offset of the signal [81]. Later, when the stapes has become totally fixed, then stapedius muscle contraction does not significantly decrease the admittance and no change in compliance due to sound stimulus can be seen. In advanced stage of the disease, the stapedial reflex is absent.

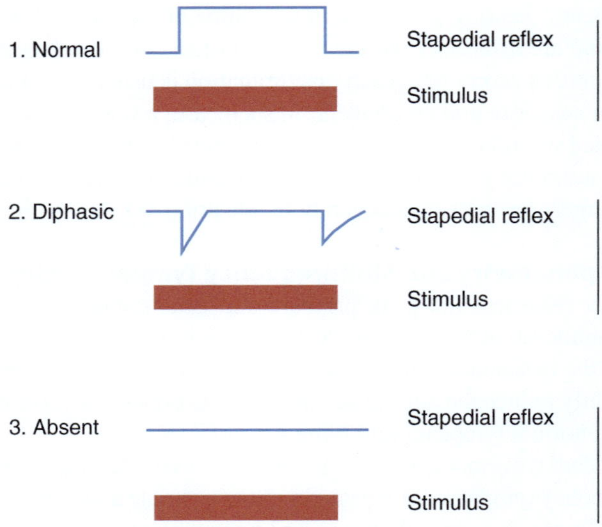

Fig. 1.16 Stapedial reflex patterns

In conclusion, two distinct patterns of abnormal stapedial reflexes are seen in otosclerosis. If the stapes is firmly fixed, no reflexes can be elicited from the affected ear. If footplate mobility has decreased but it is not yet completely fixed, nearly all patients will show a biphasic response, the so-called on-off effect (Fig. 1.16).

1.7.2.4 Laser Doppler Vibrometry

Laser-Doppler Vibrometry (LDV) is a method that uses multiple frequencies for testing middle ear dynamics. In LDV, the vibration of the tympanic membrane is evaluated with the aid of a Laser. This method has shown promising results for distinguishing stapes ankylosis, superior semicircular canal dehiscence, malleus fixation and partial or total ossicular interruption [82, 83]. LDV's clinical applicability is evident, but it has not yet established itself as a standard diagnostic test: it is expensive and normative data are not yet well established for all ear diseases [84].

1.8 CT-Imaging

Currently conventional high resolution computed tomography (HRCT) represents the gold standard for otosclerosis imaging. A high sensitivity of 91% was already stated by Shin in 2001 (Shin [85]), raised up to 95% in further studies [86], whereas specificity reached 99%. All technical conditions to obtain a HRCT of good quality with very thin cuts are explained in the addendum (see Chapter 11).

Preliminary results with Cone Beam-CT (**CBCT**) have been positive to detect mostly active otosclerotic foci [87], *however the sensitivity of CBCT for inactive foci (sclerotic phase) seems to be low* [88, 89]. Nevertheless CBCT is becoming

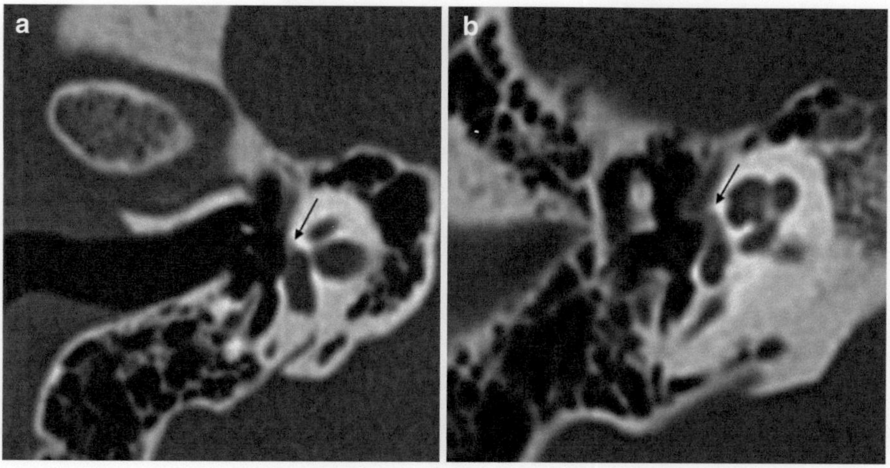

Fig. 1.17 Axial CT-images of the right ear of two different patients with typical foci of otosclerosis in the fissula ante fenestram (AF): (**a**) Small hypodense focus (arrow) < 1 mm; (**b**) large hypodense focus > 1 mm (arrow). Both foci are well delineated due to their important hypodensity

valuable as an additional imaging tool in otosclerosis for the disease follow up and the postoperative evaluation of the prosthesis conditions; the HRCT remains the initial imaging modality for otosclerosis assessment.

1.8.1 Fenestral Otosclerosis

1.8.1.1 Oval Window

The Ante Fenestral Focus (AF)

A hypodense focus situated anterior to the vestibule in the fissula ante fenestram, more or less extending to the footplate, is diagnostic for otosclerosis (Fig. 1.17).

The Size of the Focus

Several studies failed to find a correlation between the size of the otosclerotic focus on CT and the threshold of the conductive hearing loss [89]. Even a very small focus can be associated to a large air bone gap (Fig. 1.18), while a large ante-fenestral focus may not leave any hearing impairment (Fig. 1.19).

The Density of the Focus

The sensitivity of CT scan for histologically active otosclerosis is of 100% when the focus is markedly hypodense compared to the surrounding bone. In contrary, histologically inactive forms are visualized only in about 60% of the cases [90]. They could have densities rather similar to the normal neighboring bone (Fig. 1.20); this may explain cases of clinical otosclerosis and false negative CT.

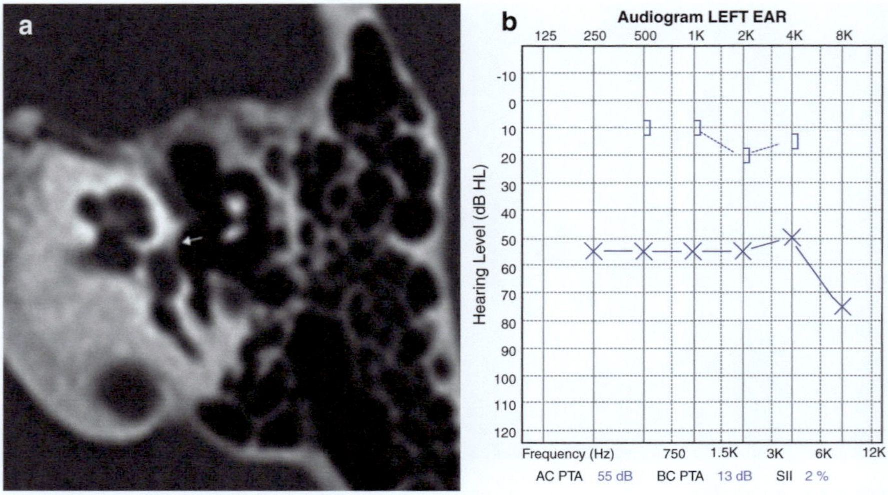

Fig. 1.18 (**a**) axial CT-image of the left ear: very small AF-focus (arrow), no otosclerotic focus found elsewhere (**b**) audiogram of the left ear: 55 dB CHL

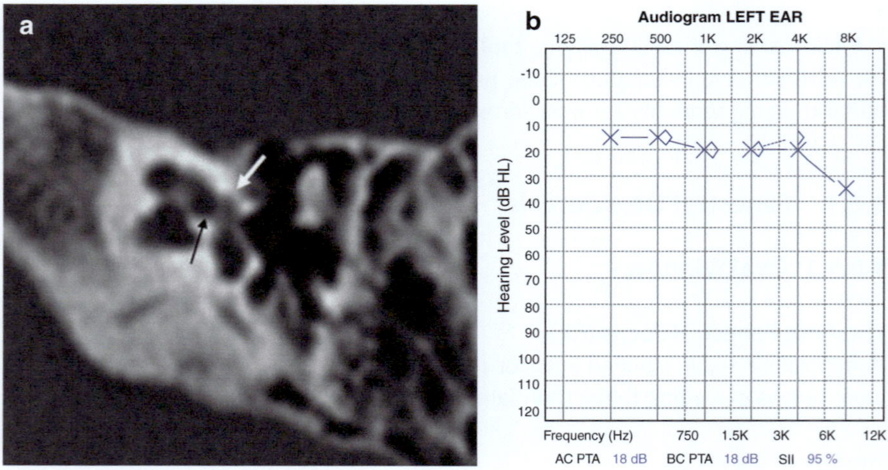

Fig. 1.19 (**a**) axial CT-image of the left ear: large very hypodense focus (white arrow) measured with a density of 680 UH, coming in close contact with the endosteum of the cochlea (black arrow) (**b**) audiogram almost normal

Therefore the measurement of the density of the AF on the CT image may be helpful in some doubtful cases of otosclerosis: it is stated that density values inferior to the cut off value of 2.187 UH are diagnostic for an antefenestral focus of otospongioses [91]. Further study confirmed the significant differences between the density of the otosclerotic foci and the one of the otic capsule bone, when density measurement of the two different sites is done by CT-histograms [91].

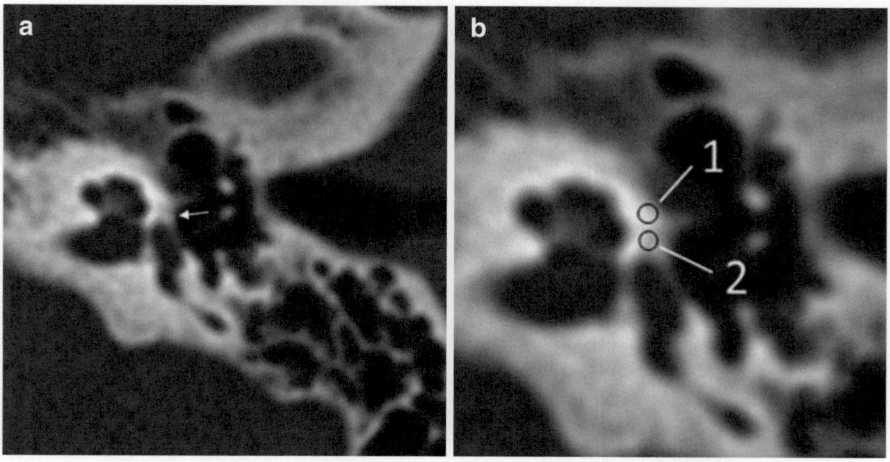

Fig. 1.20 Axial CT-images of the left ear with a small ante-fenestral focus that is merely hypodense: (**a**) the otosclerotic focus (arrow) is difficult to distinguish visually from the surrounding bone (**b**) but density measurements show a significant difference between the otic capsule density (circle 1 = 2607 ± 63 UH) and the otosclerotic focus (circle 2 =1803 ± 109 UH)

Clinico-Radiologic Correlations

The CT density of an otosclerotic focus establishes the maturation phase of the disease. The more the focus is sclerotic, the more the acoustic sound energy is shunted to the temporal bone through the dense focus instead of entering into the cochlea itself [92].

Assessment of the Footplate

The footplate is a very thin structure that is easily superimposed by the adjacent borders of the oval window. Taking into account the partial volume effects between the OW border and the footplate, a cut off value of ***0.7 mm*** was established to represent a pathologic thickening of the footplate [93]. The SAP reconstruction plan (see addendum) along the stapes plane represents the whole stapes on one solely "key" image. In this plan, the footplate thickness is not any more affected by the partial volume effects and its normal thickness is found to range ***between 0.1 and 0.4 mm***.

Clinico-Radiologic Correlations

Clinical and audiological tests cannot predict the thickness of the footplate. Knowing in advance the thickness of the footplate is a valuable issue for the preoperative planning and counseling. CT-Imaging can determine the footplate thickness being normal (Fig. 1.21a), moderately thickened (Fig. 1.21b) or even obliterative (above 0.8–0.9 mm). Moreover, in the obliterating forms, CT can demonstrate, if there is a remaining unaffected part of the footplate (Fig. 1.22a) or if it is fully obliterated rendering the oval window difficult to localize (Fig. 1.22b). Such information is very instructive as for the preoperative workup.

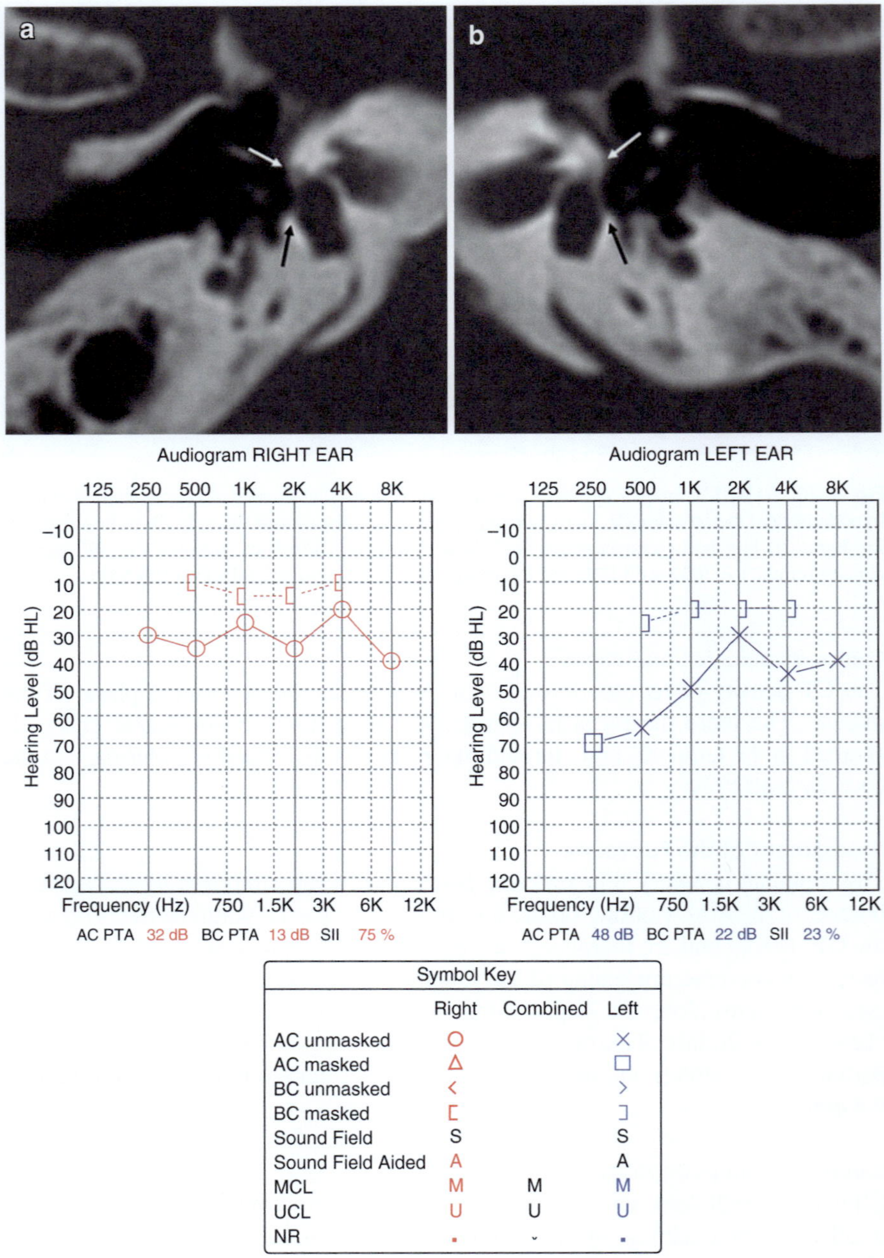

Fig. 1.21 Patient with bilateral CHL, (**a**) Right axial CT-image: thin footplate (black arrow), small hypodense AF-focus (white arrow) (1100 UH) (**b**) Left axial CT-image: thick footplate (black arrow), dense AF Focus (white arrow) (1600 UH) (**c**) corresponding pure tone right and left audiogram: 32 dB HL with a gap of 15 dB on the right side, 55 dB HL with a gap of 27 dB on the left side

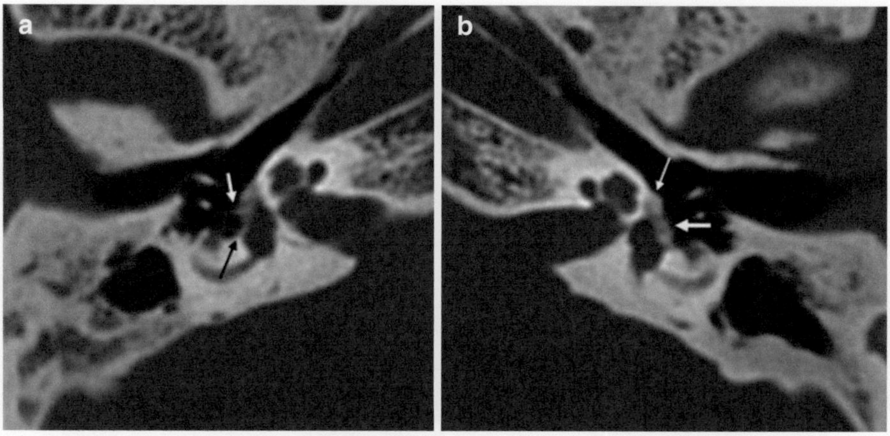

Fig. 1.22 (**a**) Axial CT-image of a right ear: otosclerotic ante fenestral focus encasing the anterior crus of the stapes (white arrow) and obliterating the anterior part of the footplate with a thickness > 1 mm, the posterior part of the footplate is slightly dense (black arrow) (**b**) axial CT-image of the left ear of the same patient: otosclerotic ante fenestral focus (thin white arrow) in continuity with an obliterative otosclerosis involving the entire footplate (thick white arrow)

Table 1.1 Round window otosclerosis staging

Stage	CT-Finding
RW 1	Otosclerotic focus on the inferior border of the RW
RW 2	Otosclerotic focus of a part of the RW
RW 3	Otosclerotic thickening of the whole round window, but air remaining in the RW recess
RW 4	Complete otosclerotic obliteration of the RW and the recess
RW 5	Complete otosclerotic obliteration of the RW and the recess in the context of FAO

1.8.1.2 Round Window Otosclerosis

A clinico-radiologic classification of different stages of round window otosclerosis correlated to preoperative and postoperative hearing results was recently established by the authors [60] (Table 1.1).

The relative clinical study based on this classification stated that:

- Stage RW1 or RW2 otosclerosis do not have any negative impact on the hearing outcome after stapes surgery (Fig. 1.23).
- Stage RW3 otosclerosis (Fig. 1.24a) has a relative impact on the stapedotomy result: only a partial closure of the ABG was obtained after stapedotomy
- Stage RW4 otosclerosis: stapedotomy not only fails to close the ABG (Fig. 1.24b) but also may be associated to a postoperative deterioration of the bone conduction.

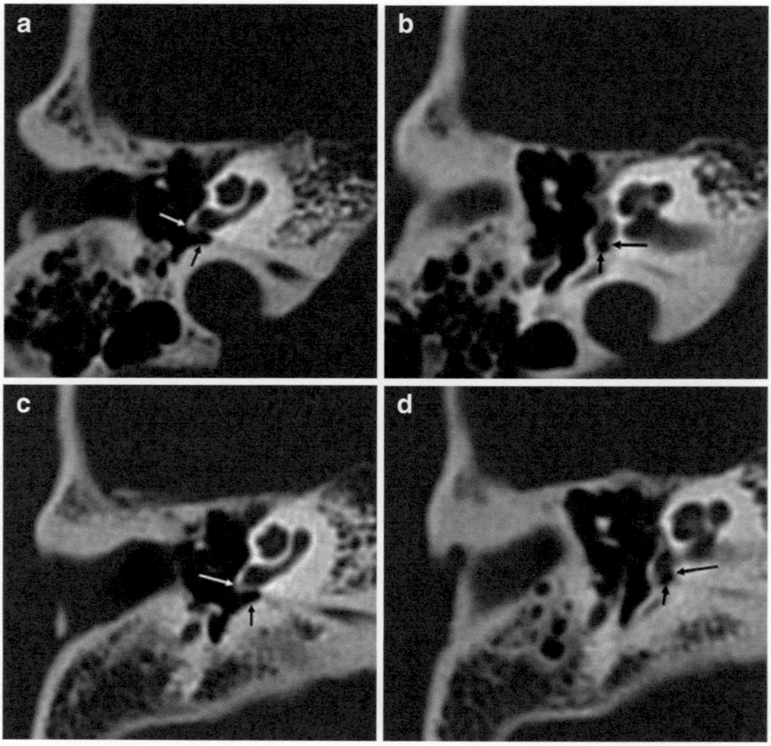

Fig. 1.23 Axial CT-images with otosclerosis on the round window. ***RW1***(**a**) and (**b**): successive cuts in caudocranial direction (**a**) otosclerotic focus on the lateral border of the RW (*white arrow*), persistent air in the recess (*small black arrow*), (**b**) very thin round window membrane (*long black arrow*), persistant air in the recess (*short black arrow*). ***RW2*** (**c**) and (**d**) successive cuts in caudocranial direction: (**c**) otosclerotic focus on the entire inferior RW (*white arrow*) but normal RW membrane (*long black arrow*) in (**d**), slightly above (**c**). Persistent air in the recess (*small black arrow*)

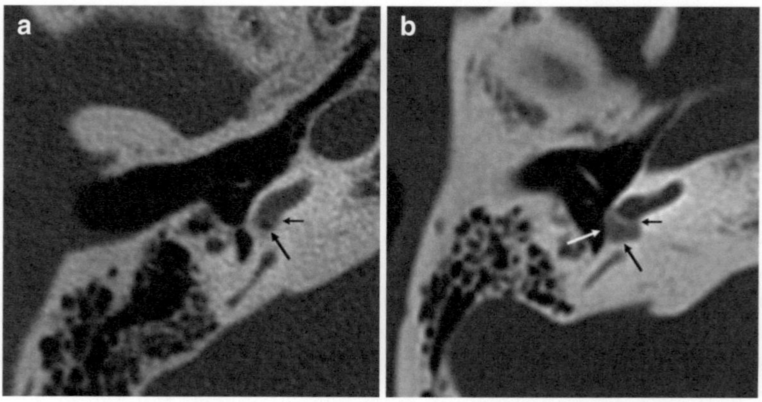

Fig. 1.24 Axial CT-images on right ears of different patients with round window otosclerosis: (**a**) ***RW3***: otosclerotic focus on the round window (*small arrow*), with persistent air in the round window recess (*long arrow*) (**b**) ***RW4***: Obliterative otosclerosis of the round window membrane (*small arrow*) and the entire recess (*long arrows*)

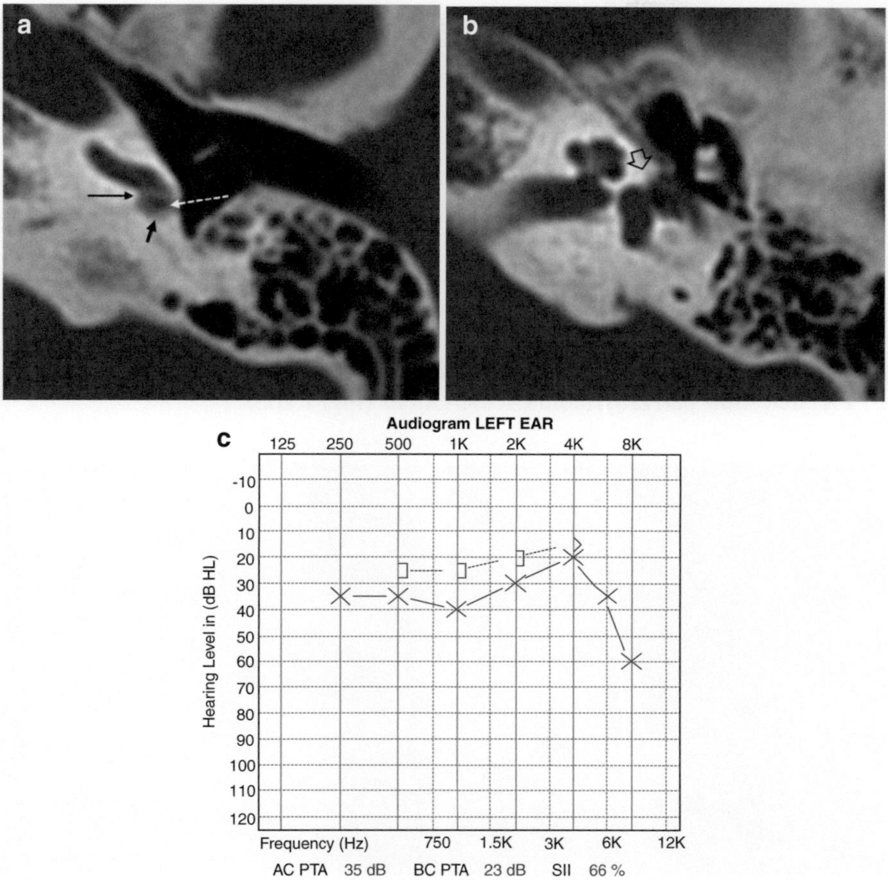

Fig. 1.25 Axial CT-images with left ear RW otosclerosis (RW3): (**a**) RW focus (*long black arrow*), otosclerosis surrounding the recess of the RW (small arrow), persistent air in the RW recess (*dashed arrow*), (**b**) normal footplate with absence of any ante fenestral focus (*empty arrow*), or other localizations of the disease in the otic capsule, (**c**) audiogram: slight hearing impact

Since audiometry and otoendoscopy are unable to assess correctly the degree of RW invasion by otosclerosis and knowing about its impact on hearing outcome after stapedotomy, CT-Imaging is essential for an adequate evaluation of round window otosclerosis before proceeding to surgery.

Rarely, round window otosclerosis is found as an isolated localisation (0.85% according to Veillon) [93] (Fig. 1.25).

1.8.2 Retrofenestral Otosclerosis

Retrofenestral otosclerosis may be suspected by an audiological evaluation but only CT-Scan can determine the different sites of retrofenstral disease invasions such as:

- extension of the AF focus by contiguity to the endosteum of the cochlea (Fig. 1.26a),
- other peri-cochlear foci surrounding the cochlea (Fig. 1.26b)
- fusion of foci into a complete hypodense rim (Fig. 1.26c).
- foci far from the cochlear endosteum (Fig. 1.26b, c),
- foci that encroach the different turns of the cochlea (Fig. 1.26d).
- foci that show peri labyrinthine localisations (Fig. 1.26b)

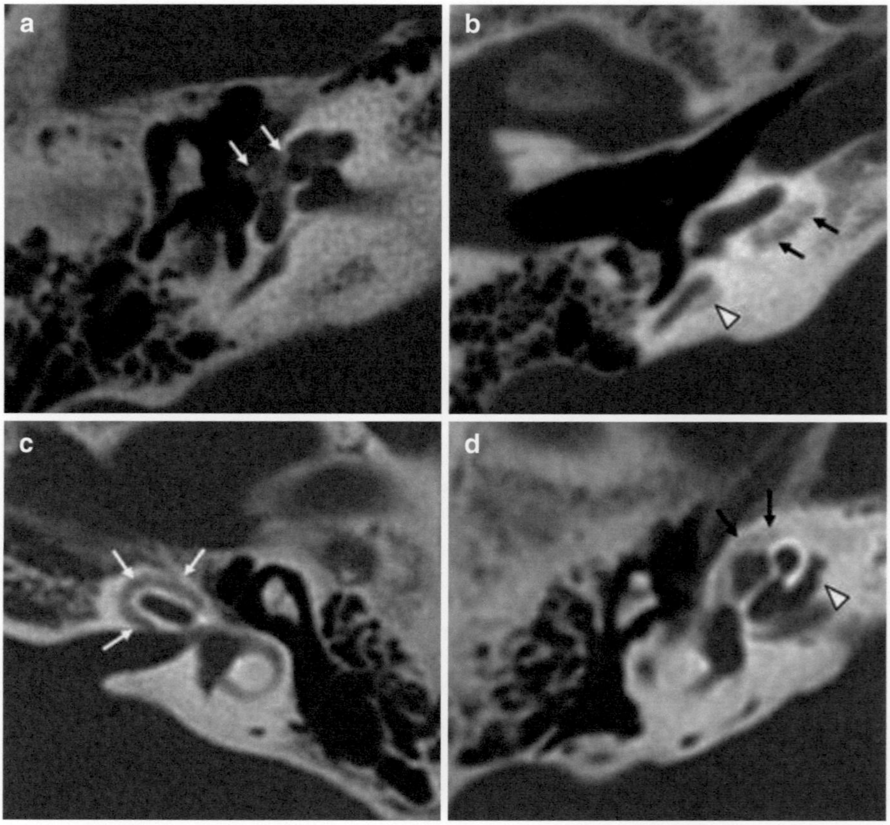

Fig. 1.26 Different sites of invasion of retrofenestral otosclerosis (**a**) large antefenestral focus (white arrows) extended into close contact with the cochlea (**b**) large peri-cochlear focus around the basal turn of the cochlea (black arrows), without a direct contact to the endosteum; small peri-labyrinthine otosclerotic focus posterior to the inferior limb of the PSCC (arrow head) (**c**) extended hypodense otosclerotic rim around the cochlea (white arrows), no contact to the endosteum (**d**) peri-cochlear foci in close contact with the endosteum of the apical cochlea (black arrows), large hypodense focus in continuity with the anterior wall of the IAC (arrowhead)

1.8.2.1 Clinico-Radiological Correlations

Otosclerotic involvement of the cochlear endosteum could be associated with elevated bone conduction (BC) thresholds. The SNHL component could be due to a hyalinization of the spiral ligament adjacent to the active endosteal focus. The otosclerotic focus may start immediately from the medial aspect of the footplate to develop inside the vestibule proximal to the saccule, causing dizziness (Fig. 1.27).

1.8.2.2 Cochlear Otosclerosis

Cochlear otosclerosis is a form of otosclerosis that invades solely the cochlear endosteum. CT shows pericochlear otosclerotic foci, but with the absence of an ante fenestral focus. The clinical manifestation is a pure sensorineural hearing loss. Cochlear otosclerosis is rare; still it has to be considered in the differential diagnosis of SNHL cases (Fig. 1.28).

1.8.3 Doubtful or Negative CT with a Clinical Diagnosis of Typical Otosclerosis

Occasionally, CT fails to demonstrate evidence of typical images of otosclerosis; however in such circumstances few indirect imaging findings, described below, could be considered as diagnostic hints for otosclerosis.

1.8.3.1 Triangular Thickening of the Insertion of the Anterior Stapes Crura to the Footplate

CT images of a thickened insertion of the anterior crus of the stapes (Fig. 1.29) without any lesion found elsewhere in the otic capsule could indicate an otosclerosis

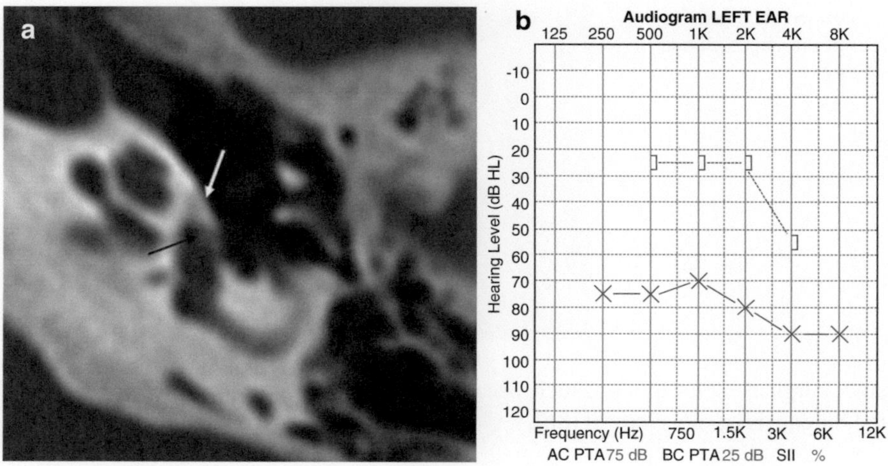

Fig. 1.27 (**a**) A large slightly hypodense antefenestral focus (white arrow) compared to the otic capsule, extended to the anterior part of the footplate and inside the vestibule (black arrow). (**b**) Audiogram showing a large air-bone gap and high frequencies SNHL (note that no peri-cochlear foci were seen elsewhere)

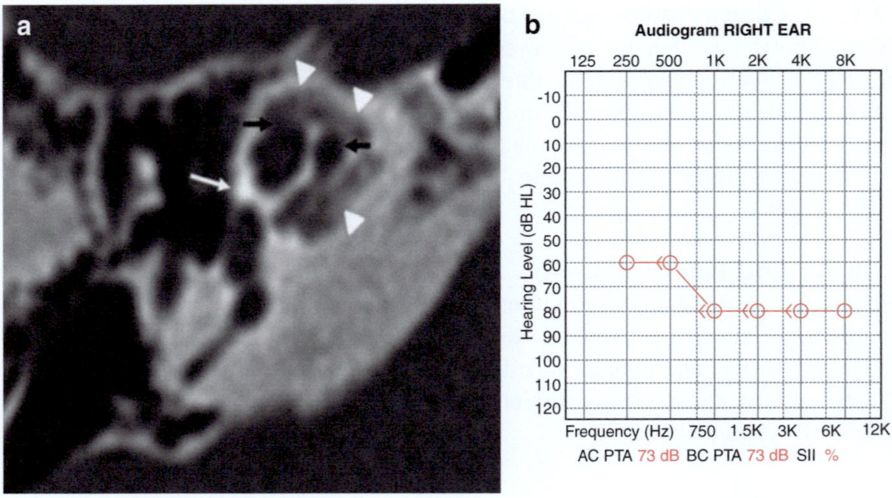

Fig. 1.28 A case of cochlear otosclerosis: (**a**) the axial CT-image of the right ear shows large peri-cochlear otosclerotic foci (white arrow heads) that come into close contact with the endosteum of the cochlea (black arrows). Note the absence of any involvement of the footplate nor the fissula ante fenestram (white arrow). (**b**) the audiogram shows a pure SNHL

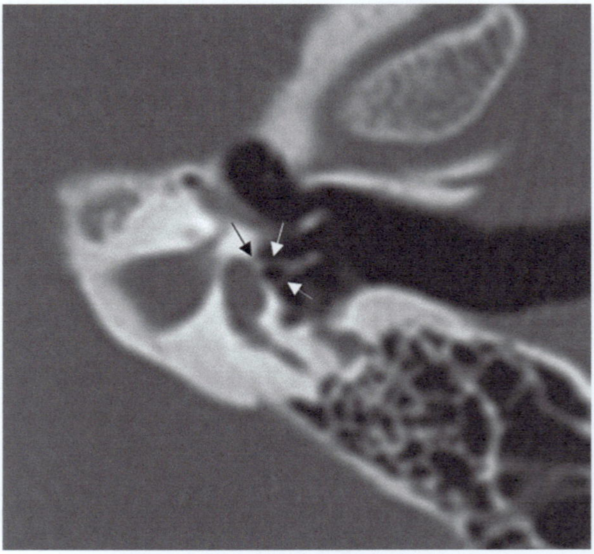

Fig. 1.29 Axial CT-image of the stapes: the anterior crus of the stapes (white arrow) shows a triangular thickening (black arrow) at its insertion on the footplate — no other CT finding elsewhere in favour of otosclerosis. Posterior crus of the stapes (dotted arrow)

since surgical explorations of such disease presentation has confirmed per-operatively the diagnosis of otosclerosis [86].

1.8.3.2 Hypodensity at the Anterior Wall of the IAC ("Diverticulum" or "Nipple Sign")

A small condensation image like a diverticulum found at the anterior border of the internal auditory canal is often associated with otosclerosis and can be specific of the disease in about 93% of cases [94]. It is also called the "Nipple sign". This

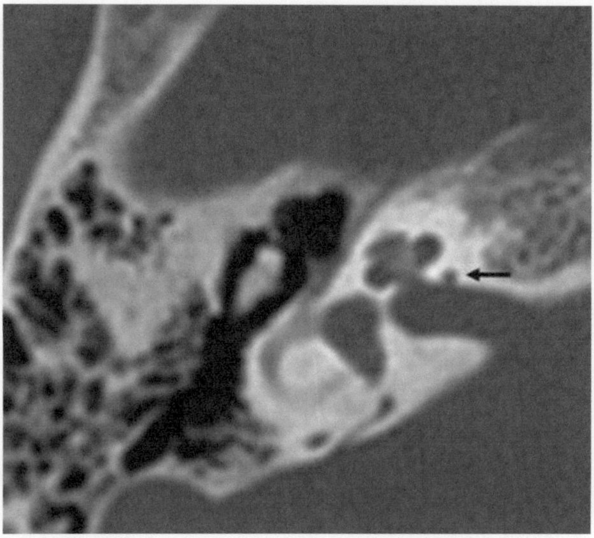

Fig. 1.30 Axial CT-image of the right ear of a patient with bilateral CHL: round hypodensity (diverticulum, "nipple sign") in front of the IAC (arrow)

imaging sign (Fig. 1.30) is significantly more encountered in infra radiologic and pauci radiologic cases of otosclerosis than in a normal cohort.

1.8.3.3 Negative CT in Otosclerosis; Infra-Radiologic Otosclerosis

In a small percentage of patients with clinical diagnosis of otosclerosis, the CT-Scan does not demonstrate any radiologic finding suggestive of otosclerosis or pathology able to explain the complaint of conductive hearing loss. However, during surgical exploration of 40% of these cases, the diagnosis of otosclerosis was confirmed [95]. This is an indication that few patients may have an "infra radiological" otosclerosis and the definitive diagnosis would be confirmed only during surgical exploration.

1.8.4 Radiologic Classifications of Otosclerosis

Different scanographic classifications of otosclerosis have been proposed. The classifications of Symons and Fannings in 2005 [96] concerned especially candidates with far advanced otosclerosis before cochlear implant indications. They emphasize mostly on the different degrees of involvement of the cochlear endosteum. However since the fenestral forms of otosclerosis are by far the most frequent presentation, the classification proposed by Veillon becomes more useful in regard to otology practice. Veillon classification [97] divides fenestral otosclerosis extension into three grades and indicates any peri-cochlear focus as a grade IV (See Table 1.2).

However, advances in the scanographic analyses of otosclerotic foci in different localizations, along with their potential impact on the hearing and consequently on the surgical outcomes, made every proposed classification of otosclerosis unable to categorize adequately the multiple extensions in one satisfactory grading system.

Table 1.2 Classification of Veillon

Type	Description
Ia	Isolated thickening of the footplate hypodensity
Ib	Isolated anterior fenestral hypodensity <1 mm (AFH)
II	Isolated anterior fenestral hypodensity >1 mm (AFH)
III	Anterior fenestral hypodensity >1 mm, which extends to the endosteum of cochlea
IVa	Hypodense foci in the entire middle layer of the otic capsule: Peri-cochlear hypodensity (PH), internal auditory canal hypodensity (IACH)
IVb	Involvement of the entire otic capsule including the vestibule and semicircular canals

Table 1.3 "Methodological CT-imaging table for otosclerosis"

Fenestral			
Ante fenestral (AF)	Normal Density > 2200 UH	Focus Density: ______UH	
Footplate (SAP) thickening	Anterior border	Posterior border	Entirely
Footplate thickness (standard OM plan)	Normal ≤ 0.5 mm	Moderately thickened 0.6–0.9 mm	Obliterated ≥ 1 mm
Footplate thickness (SAP)	Normal 0–0.4 mm	Moderately thickened 0.5–0.8 mm	Obliterated ≥ 0.9 mm
Round window	RW 1 + 2	RW 3	RW 4
Retrofenestral			
Ante fenestral (AF)	No AF	AF with cochl. contact	
Pericochlear Foci	No cochlear contact	With cochlear contact	
Intracochlear Calcif	Basal Turn	Middle and Apical Turn	
Initial/Subtle Findings			
Several sites	Footplate thickness ______mm	Thickened (triangular) insertion of the ant. crus	IAC focus

Therefore it would be more appropriate to describe systematically the main sites of the disease invasions according to a "*Methodological CT-Imaging Table for Otosclerosis*" (Table 1.3) used as follows:

The **antefenestral focus** is evaluated for its density, the **footplate invasion** is described as anteriorly, or posteriorly or globally thickened. The **footplate thickness** is evaluated, relative to the used standard acquisition plan or more appropriate the SAP "stapes axial plan". The **round window** must be analyzed according to the classification described above. The **retrofenestral foci** consist essentially of peri cochlear foci, that have different impacts if they are at distance or in contact with the endosteum of the cochlea. **Intracochlear calcifications** are very important to be indicated, especially if cochlear implantation is planned. Finally, also the **doubtful manifestations** such a doubtful footplate thickness, a thickened anterior insertion of the anterior stapedial crus or an IAC focus are to be mentioned.

1.8.5 Anatomic Abnormalities: Impact on the Surgical Access to the Stapes

1.8.5.1 Narrow Oval Window Niche

A narrow oval niche could be congenital or due to an otosclerotic growth block (Fig. 1.31). The assessment of this region is essential because a narrow oval window niche may be responsible for technical conflicts during the stapedotomy. A study in

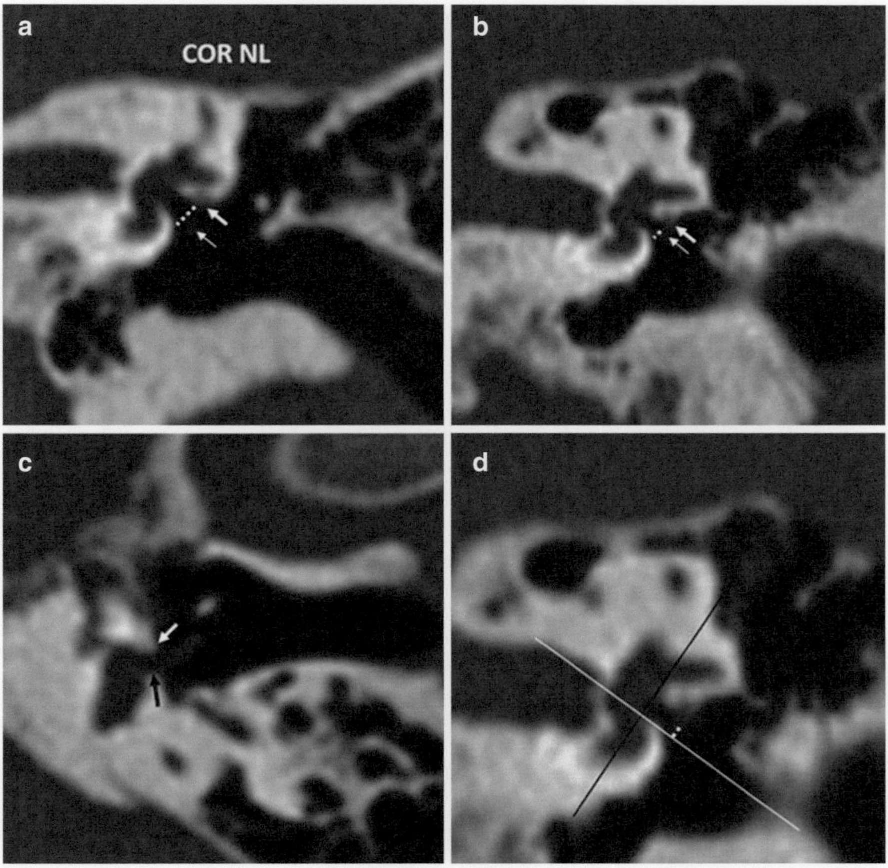

Fig. 1.31 (**a**) coronal CT-image of a left ear with a normal oval window niche height (dashed line), notice the large space between the head of the stapes (thin arrow) and the facial nerve (thick arrow) (**b**) Coronal reconstruction on a left ear: reduced height of the oval window niche (dashed line), see the close relation between head of the stapes (thin arrow) and the facial nerve (thick arrow) (**c**) axial CT-image of the same ear as in (**b**): large anterior otosclerotic focus (white arrow), and advanced posterior border of the OW niche (black arrow) narrowing the antero-posterior diameter of the OW niche (**d**) measurement of the OW niche height: drawing a line (black line) parallel to the footplate, drawing perpendicular to the black line a line along the inferior border of the oval niche (white line), establish the distance between the inferior border of the facial nerve and the white line (dashed line)

2013 established a preoperative measurement of the height of the oval window niche, parallel to the line along the footplate, extended from the inferior limit of the facial nerve to the inferior border of the oval niche, and found that the height of narrow niches varied between 0.7 and 1.3 mm [98]. Another recent study stated that the discomfort of the surgeon in approaching the oval niche starts when the width is of ***1.1 mm*** and less, measured on coronal CT-images, with a sensibility of 71% and a specificity of 84% [99].

1.8.5.2 Overhanging Second Portion of the Facial Nerve

A prolapse of the facial nerve covering the oval niche (Fig. 1.32a) may render the access to the footplate difficult or becoming a risk of a possible nerve injury during a stapedotomy. Also it can decrease the mobility of the stapes by direct contact (Fig. 1.32b).

1.8.5.3 Persistent Stapedial Artery

Rarely (less than 0.02–0.05% in surgical series) [100], a stapedial artery may persist as a 1.5–2 mm branch of the petrous internal carotid (Figs.1.33 and 1.34). It may be found during surgery and compromise the stapedotomy. As the scanographic study is usually done without intravenous injection of iodine contrast, the persistent stapedial artery may be visualized as a nonspecific condensation image on the footplate or it may be easily overlooked or mistaken for an otosclerotic focus of the footplate (Fig. 1.35a, b).

Therefore, when suspected, the *foramen spinosum* has to be looked for and if absent (Fig. 1.35c) on CT, this is a precious indirect sign to suspect such abnormality [101] and complete the exam by injection.

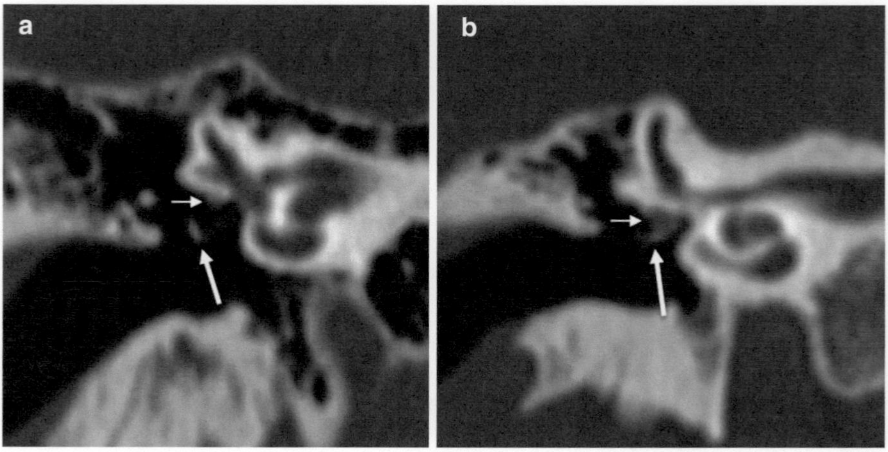

Fig. 1.32 Coronal CT-images of the oval niche and the facial nerve (**a**) prolapsed facial nerve (arrow) out of the canal, but still at distance from the stapes (long arrow) (**b**) overhanging of the facial nerve (short arrow) in contact with the stapes (long arrow)

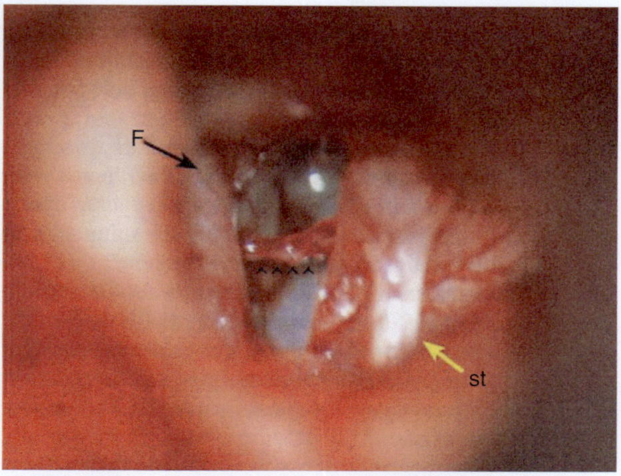

Fig. 1.33 Right middle ear exploration showing persistent stapedial artery (black arrowheads) passing above the footplate; *F* facial nerve, *st* stapedial tendon

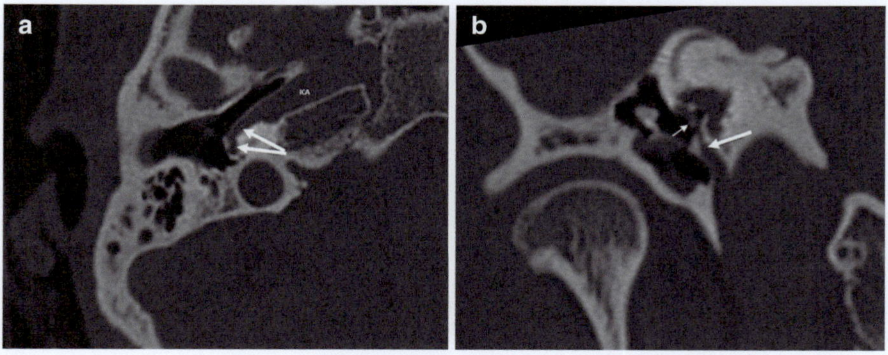

Fig. 1.34 CT scan of a patient with a persistent stapedial artery. (**a**) Axial CT of the temporal bone showing the aberrant stapedial artery (*white arrows*) arising from the junction between the vertical and horizontal segments of the intra-petrous internal carotid artery (ICA). (**b**) Coronal CT scan of the temporal bone showing the aberrant arterial trajectory through the promontory (*thick white arrow*) and in front of the oval window (*thin small arrow*) *courtesy Dr. Sanjuan*

1.9 Primary Stapes Surgery

Stapedotomy is the most fascinating surgery in otology. Although still the crown jewel of otology, stapes surgery is no longer performed with the breadth and wealth of experience once enjoyed; the "golden era" of otologic surgery has passed. Over the last 50 years, there has been a decline in the number of stapes surgeries performed, with the depletion of backlogged older otosclerotic patients partly to blame. With the vanishing numbers of these surgeries has come the loss of the broader technical proficiency enjoyed by those who trained during the earlier era.

Nowadays fewer and fewer ears suitable for stapes surgery are available for teaching; so senior residents finish their training with little hands-on experience performing

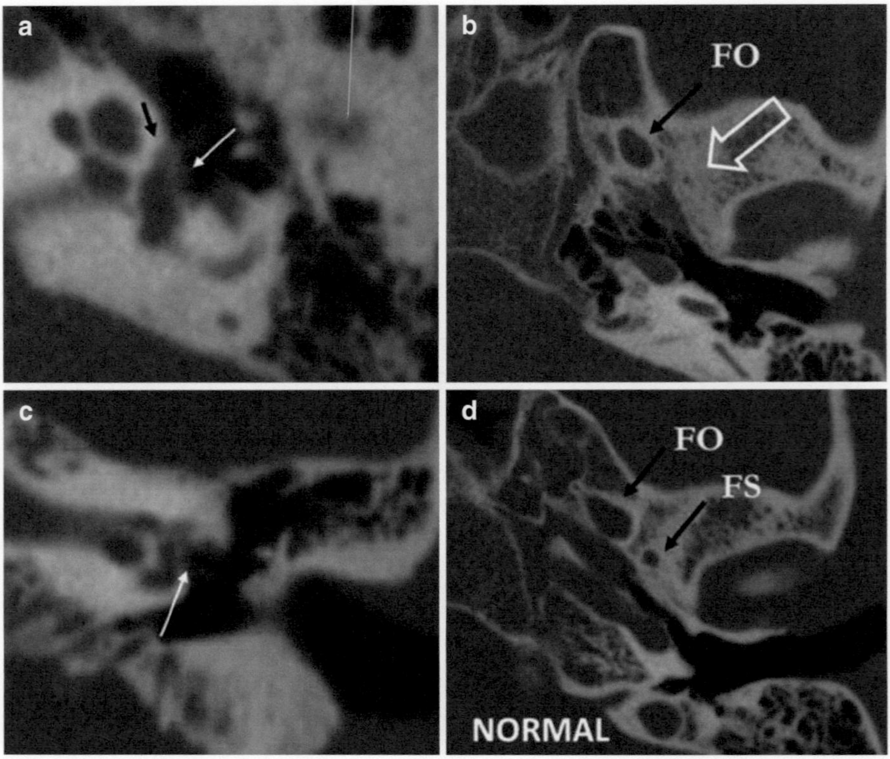

Fig. 1.35 (**a**) axial CT-image of the left ear: typical otosclerosis of the fissula ante fenestram (black arrow), a rounded isodense structure in close contact with the footplate (white arrow) is not specific, but raises the suspicion of a persistent stapedial artery (**b**) coronal CT-image of the same ear: atypical round soft tissue formation along the oval window niche (**c**) absent foramen spinosum at the skull base (empty arrow), (**d**) comparison with a normal image of the skull base: *FO* foramen ovale, *FS* foramen spinosum

this technically demanding surgery. Not uncommonly, as they may encounter only a few potential stapes cases yearly, they may feel compelled to refer these either to those with a larger otologic practice or to specific centers of excellence.

1.9.1 Biomechanics of Stapes Surgery

In humans, the rigidity of the annular ligament represents almost 90% of the impedance of the middle ear, especially at low frequencies. This annular ligament, therefore, dominates the transmission of sound at speech frequencies in the normal middle ear in humans. The collagen fibers of the annular ligament determine the amplitude of the stapedial footplate vibration in response to low-frequency acoustic stimulation [102]. The sound pressure at the entrance of the cochlea is directly proportional to the volume velocity of the stapes footplate, which in turn, corresponds to the volume of the liquid that is displaced by the vibration of the stapes footplate.

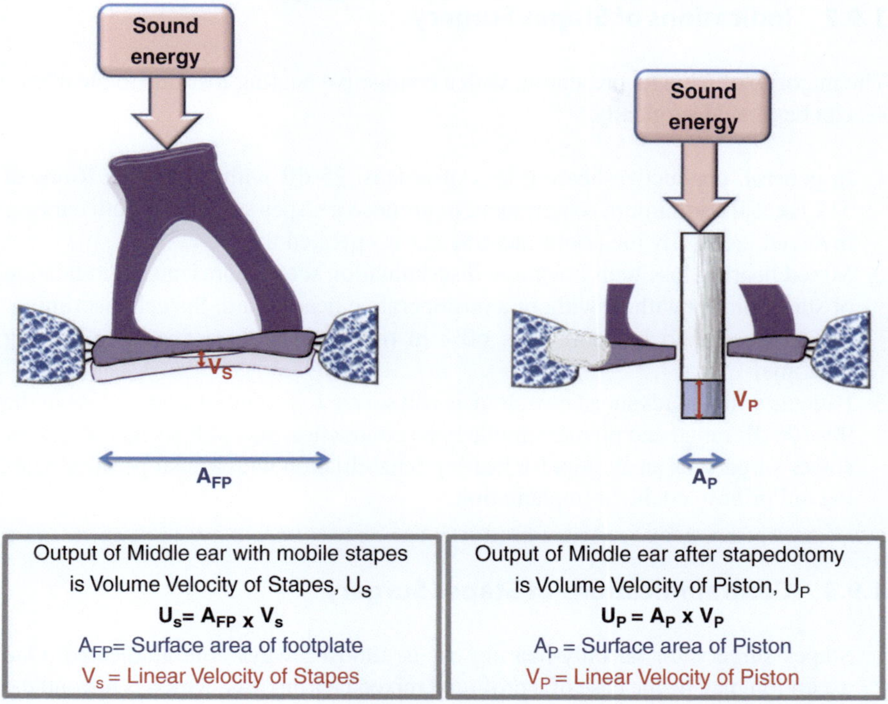

Fig. 1.36 Biomechanics of stapedotomy (Modified from Otology and Neurotology 24:548–559 © 2003, Otology & Neurotology, Inc. Biomechanics of Stapesplasty: A Review. Karl-Bernd Hüttenbrink)

The output of the middle ear can be quantified by the "volume velocity" of the stapes footplate. Volume velocity can be defined as the product of stapes linear velocity and the area of the stapes footplate [102, 103].

The stapes footplate has an area of approximately 3.2 mm^2. This exerts vibrations with amplitudes of only a few nanometers for displacement of a large amount of fluid to transmit sound pressure into the cochlea at physiologic sound pressures.

Following stapedotomy, the annular ligament effect is canceled and the piston will have increased linear velocity. At the same time, the effective vibrating area is reduced to the area where the prosthesis has been inserted. A stapes prosthesis, with its smaller contact area (32 mm^2 area of footplate vs. 0.28 mm^2 area of fenestra in a 0.6 mm stapes prosthesis), can vibrate with much larger amplitude at equivalent sound pressures. Compensation takes place because the increased linear velocity of the smaller piston compensates for the decrease in the surface area [102]. (Fig. 1.36)

Animal experiments suggest that the maximal vibrational amplitude of the sound-transmitting structures is attained at a piston with a diameter less than 0.4 mm, and volume velocity will decrease with smaller diameters [104]. Nevertheless, pistons with sufficiently large diameter of 0.4 mm and above should have similar sound transmission properties to normal middle ear, if the vibrational capacity of the middle ear structures is unrestricted.

1.9.2 Indications of Stapes Surgery

The majority of patients presenting with a conductive hearing loss due to otosclerosis can be treated surgically.

1. In general, conductive hearing loss of at least 25 dB with a negative Rinne at 512 Hz is the minimum requirement to propose a stapes surgery. If both ears are involved, generally the poorer hearing ear is operated first.
2. Mixed hearing loss with favorable discrimination score represents an indication of stapedotomy with or without a postoperative hearing aid. Speech discrimination score should be more than 60% in order to obtain a favorable hearing outcome.
3. Patients with far advanced otosclerosis and severe to profound hearing loss in the 90–100 dB range and no measurable bone conduction may still be candidates for stapes surgery, as an attempt for hearing rehabilitation with a postoperative hearing aid prior to cochlear implantation.

1.9.3 Contraindications of Stapes Surgery

1. Stapes surgery for an only-hearing ear is almost always contraindicated. One exception may be the case of a profound mixed hearing loss, which is beyond the level of benefit of a conventional hearing aid. Such a patient would be candidate for stapes surgery as an attempt prior to cochlear implant rehabilitation.
2. Stapes surgery is contraindicated in cases of chronic otitis media or chronic otitis externa.
3. Stapes surgery should be postponed in the presence of vertigo with a clinical evidence of labyrinthine hydrops.
4. Stapes surgery is contraindicated in case of unfavorable systemic medical conditions.
5. Relative contraindication for patients above 70 years old: there is a 40% chance of worsening the discrimination, also a greater risk for perilymphatic fistula complication because of poor wound healing in elderly.
6. During pregnancy.

1.9.4 Informed Consent

All informations about the disease progress, the surgical technique and its inherent complications must be discussed with the patient. The communication with the patient must be clear, avoiding inducing a feeling of fear of the surgery.

Patient must understand that:

- Stapes surgery can close the air-bone gap but it cannot control the disease itself or its fate: the disease is unpredictable and could be evolutive.

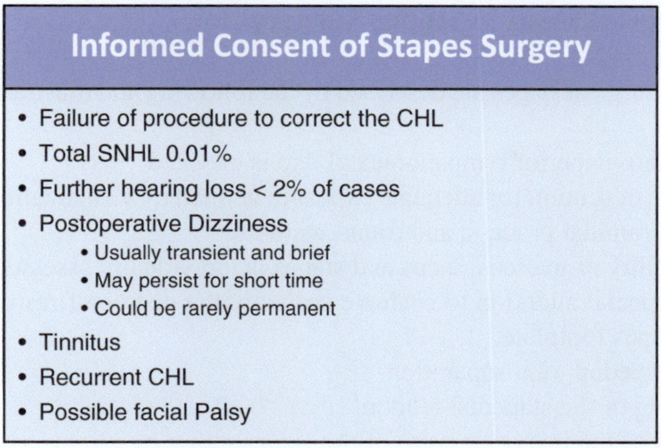

Fig. 1.37 Informed consent of stapes surgery

- There are potential benefits of hearing aids.
- There are the following potential risks (Fig. 1.37): failure of the surgery, post-op SNHL either partial or complete, vestibular dysfunction, disturbance in taste, development of a perilymphatic fistula, eardrum perforation, exceptional risk of facial nerve injury… However, such risks have significantly decreased nowadays and became very rare in experienced hands.

1.9.5 Anesthesia in Stapes Surgery

Primary stapes surgery can be performed under either general or local anesthesia.

General anesthesia provides assurance of an absolute control of head motion, prevention of pain or vomiting. General anesthesia is more comfortable for the patient, the surgeon, and the training environment and more suitable for cases of revision stapes surgery. However, a statistically significant increased risk of immediate dead ear following stapes surgery done under general anesthesia has been reported [105].

Local anesthesia with sedation is safer; it prevents general anesthetic complications and is associated with less bleeding than general anesthesia. Intraoperative improvement in hearing can be tested under local anesthesia. There is a belief that the patient's ability to report intraoperative vertigo may help the surgeon to avoid injury to the saccule. Local anesthesia technique requires a cooperative patient and collaboration of the surgical team.

Nevertheless, a recent systematic review of 257 studies by Wegner et al. showed no difference in post-op air-bone gap closure and postoperative vertigo either the surgery was done under local or general anesthesia [105].

1.9.6 Surgical Steps in Stapes Surgery

The different surgical stapes are described by the following and illustrated in Fig.1.38.

1. The postero-superior tympanomeatal flap is elevated
2. Curetting of scutum for adequate exposure defined by visualization of the facial nerve, pyramidal process, and round window.
3. The mobility of malleus, incus and stapes is individually assessed. Some cases require special attention to evaluate correctly the degree of restricted mobility of the stapes footplate.
4. Incudostapedial joint separation.
5. Sectioning of the stapedial tendon.
6. Removal of the posterior crura of the stapes either by microscissor, microdrill or laser.
7. The footplate became visible; the next step is down fracture and removal of the remaining stapes superstructure, during this step the surgeon must keep an eye on the footplate not to dislocate.
8. Mensuration of the distance from the incus to the footplate.
9. Fenestration of the footplate either by perforator, microdrill, or laser. The optimal site for the fenestration opening is at the posterior half of the footplate.
10. Insertion of the piston in the fenestration and crimping it to the incus. The prosthesis should extend into the vestibule for at least 0.25 mm. The suitable penetration of the prosthesis in the vestibule is generally obtained with a prosthesis length of 4.5 mm.
11. The prosthesis must move freely within the fenestra. This can be assessed by gently elevating the manubrium of the malleus while watching the motion of the prosthesis.

1.9.7 Microscopic Versus Endoscopic Stapes Surgery

Endoscopic stapes surgery offers many benefits such as good visualization, and easy accessibility to the stapes, posterior and anterior crus, oval window niche, and facial nerve. Removal of the scutum and manipulation of the chorda tympani nerve are less frequent with the endoscopic technique. The hole in the footplate is better appreciated by the trainees. Nevertheless endoscopic surgery does not achieve better results than surgery done under microscope. One hand surgery and longer initial operative times and a steep learning curve are the principal reasons that make most ear surgeons reluctant to switch to endoscopic stapes surgery [106]. It is important to remember that much heat from the endoscope placed near the open vestibule could be harmful with possible sensorineural damage [107].

Endoscopic stapes surgery:

Advantages include decreased scutum removal and reduced chorda tympani manipulation and injury.

Disadvantages include the loss of stereopsis, the potential risk of thermal injury to the inner ear resulting in sensorineural hearing loss and vestibular dysfunction

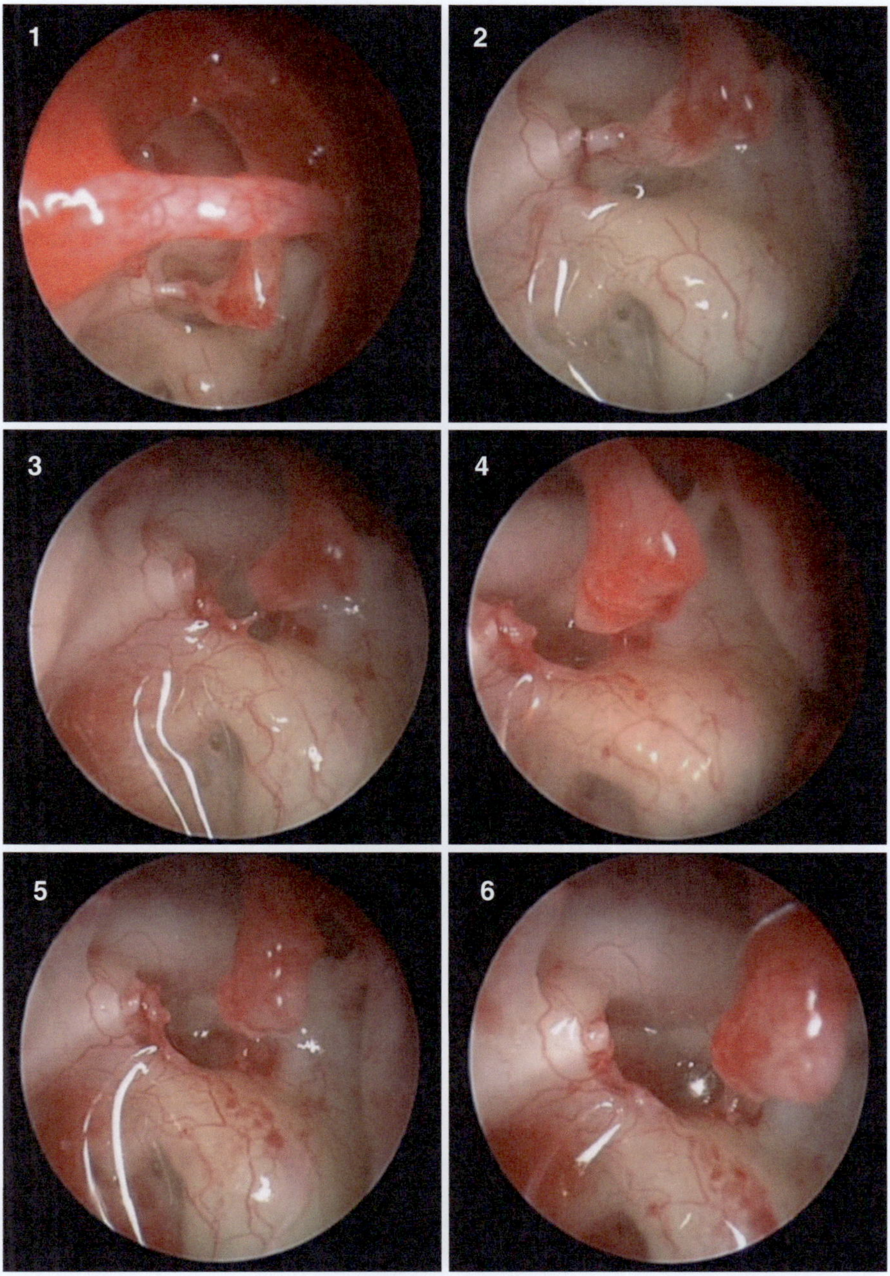

Fig. 1.38 Classical steps of a stapedotomy in a right ear: 1: elevation of tympanomeatal flap and curetting of scutum for adequate exposure defined by visualization of the facial nerve, pyramidal process, and round window 2: Mensuration from medial aspect of the incus to the footplate, incudo-stapedial joint separation, and sectioning of the stapedial tendon. 3 and 4: drilling of the posterior crura of the stapes and the footplate became visible; the next step is down- fracture of the remaining stapes superstructure, during this step the surgeon must keep an eye on the footplate not to dislocate. 5: fenestration of the footplate. 6: insertion of the piston in the fenestration and crimping it to the incus

secondary to the proximity of the light source; the least temperature elevation was found with the LED light source with a 3-mm endoscope [92].

1.9.8 Stapedectomy Versus Stapedotomy

After a long era of debates, nowadays stapedotomy is the consensus procedure because of less trauma to the inner ear. Stapedotomy offers lesser risk of migration of the prosthesis and secondary postoperative perilymphatic fistula. Stapedotomy gave better gain of high-frequency and better postoperative speech discrimination scores [108–112]. Stapedectomy, in turn, may give better gain at the lower frequencies [112, 113]. However, most studies have demonstrated good short- and/or long-term hearing results, without statistically significant differences between both [114–117] procedures. Comparaison of outcomes after stapedectomy versus stapedotomy is done in Table 1.4.

1.9.9 Laser in Stapes Surgery

The laser was introduced in middle-ear surgery by Escudero et al., in 1979, when the argon laser was used in a tympanoplasty operation [118]. In the same year, Palva was the first surgeon to use Laser for the perforation of the footplate [119]. Perkins subsequently reported 11 argon laser stapedectomies with good clinical results [120]. Nowadays Laser is used in stapes surgery to divide the stapedius tendon, divide the anterior and posterior crura, and perforate the footplate [121] (Fig. 1.39).

Evidence based data showed that the use of laser in otosclerosis surgery decreases the risk of postoperative SNHL because it traumatizes less the inner ear; also it offers better control for hemostasis. Still there is no difference in postoperative vertigo rate and air-bone gap closure when compared with standard techniques [122].

Table 1.4 Stapedectomy versus stapedotomy; CHL: conductive hearing loss

Outcome	Stapedotomy	Stapedectomy
Hearing outcome	Good hearing results over all the frequencies	Good hearing results at the speech frequencies
	Better gain at higher frequencies	Better gain at lower frequencies
	Better postoperative speech discrimination scores	Poorer high-frequency hearing (4–8 kHz)
Tinnitus outcome	High rate of tinnitus suppression	High rate of tinnitus suppression
Development of vertigo	Very low risk of vertigo	Higher risk of vertigo
Floating footplate	Less risk for floating footplate	Higher risk for floating footplate
Perilymphatic fistula	Zero	4%
Prosthesis migration	Less incidence of prosthesis migration	Increased potential for prosthesis migration
	Less fixation of prosthesis by scar tissue	
Recurrent CHL	4%	12%

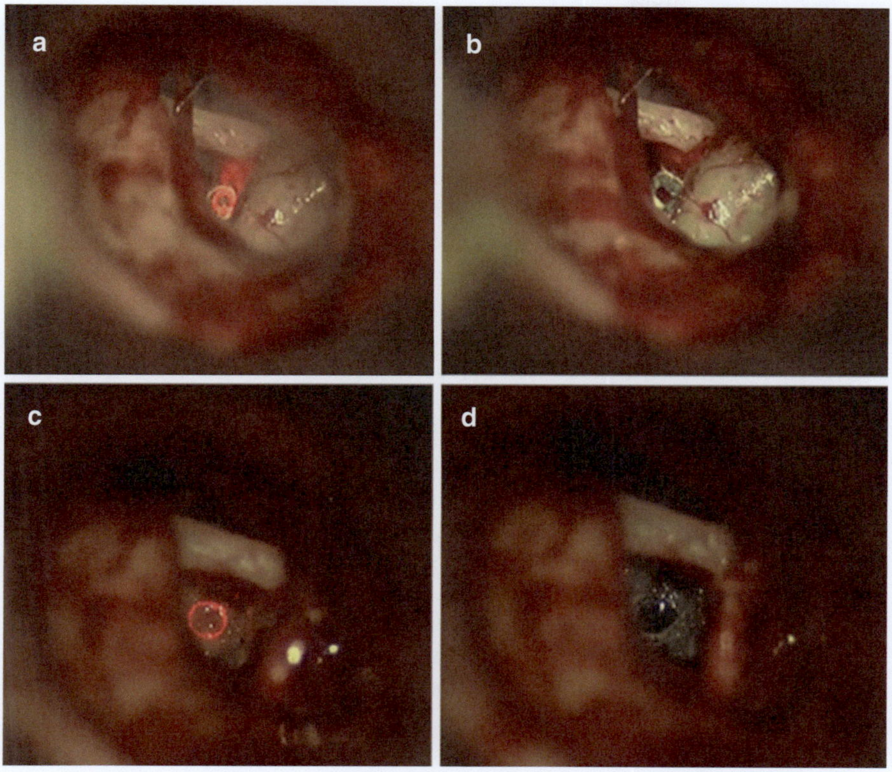

Fig. 1.39 CO_2 laser stapedotomy in a right ear, (**a**) Vaporisation of the stapedial tendon using a CO_2 laser: (**b**) Vaporisation of the posterior crura using a CO_2 laser, (**c**) fenestration of the footplate using SurgiTouch scanner system (Lumenis); (**d**) a calibrated fenestration of the footplate of 0.8 mm was done without touching it

Advantages of the use of Laser are:

1. *Haemostatic properties especially in secondary stapes surgery*
2. *Increased precision that exceeds by far other handheld instruments*
3. *Reduced risk of a floating footplate or losing footplate fragments into the vestibule*
4. *No excessive perilymph mobilization by the ability to create a precise fenestrum in the footplate thus minimizing the risk of acoustic trauma*
5. *Can fenestrate a relatively mobile footplate without the risk of depression of the footplate into the vestibule, which is an inherent risk of other fenestration techniques.*

The ideal laser in stapes surgery should not penetrate deeply into the perilymph (risk of heating) and should have good water absorption, equating to high bone ablation efficiency. Until now still there is no ideal laser for stapes surgery. Although each of the lasers differs in terms of wavelength, absorption characteristics and delivery. Clinically, there is little evidence to support the use of one laser over another, although the surgeon may wish to use the laser which is more readily available at hand.

Visible lasers (Argon and KTP), especially the argon laser, have an excellent optical precision and have the advantage of reaching targets that are partially obscured by other structures, however, these lasers pass easily through the perilymph and may reach and damage the utricle and saccule. The one shot pulsed CO_2 laser is most elegant and it has the advantage that energy is absorbed by water, but it is somehow cumbersome because of its increased working distance and it cannot be used in a narrow oval window niche. It has less focus and decreased microscopic light. It has a greater risk of heating the perilymph. Table 1.5 summarizes the advantages and disadvantages of each laser, that are shown in Fig. 1.40.

Laser stapedotomy minus prosthesis:
In cases of blue footplate and limited otosclerosis fixation of its anterior part, Silverstein and coworkers [123] described the laser stapedotomy minus prosthesis (laser STAMP) operation which consists in mobilizing and isolating the posterior crus and posterior segment of the footplate. Argon laser was used to vaporize the anterior crus via an endoprobe. Laser was also used to divide the anterior and posterior segments of the footplate, leaving a 0.5-mm gap (in laser stapedioplasty, a prototype Argon laser endoscope was used to provide visualization as well as instrumentation in the small surgical field). None of the patients who had undergone the laser STAMP procedure developed hyperacusis, possibly due to the preservation of the stapedius tendon and hence the acoustic reflex. Additionally, the laser STAMP procedure demonstrated statistically significant improvement in the 6 to 8 kHz range compared with laser stapedotomy. Follow up demonstrated stable hearing

Table 1.5 Advantages and disadvantages of different types of laser used in stapes surgery; (see Fig. 1.40)

Laser	Advantages	Disadvantages
Argon	Short wavelength (**514** nm) Visible light Delivered by fibreoptic handpiece Well absorbed by hemoglobin Good hemostasis	Not well absorbed by bone Higher penetration of radiation Potential danger to inner ear structures
KTP	Short wavelength (**532** nm) Visible light Delivered by fiberoptic handpiece Well absorbed by hemoglobin Good hemostasis	Not well absorbed by bone Higher penetration of radiation Potential danger to inner ear structures
Er:YAG	Strong bone absorption Minimal penetration to surrounding tissues Less risk of inner ear trauma	Potential risk of acoustic trauma Poor hemostasis
CO_2	Long wavelength (**10,000** nm) Strong bone absorption Minimal penetration to surrounding tissues Less risk of inner ear trauma Available with fiberoptic micro-handpiece	Invisible, requires aiming beam (red helium-neon) Readily absorbed by perilymph and collagen Risk of heating of perilymph Previously only available with micromanipulator

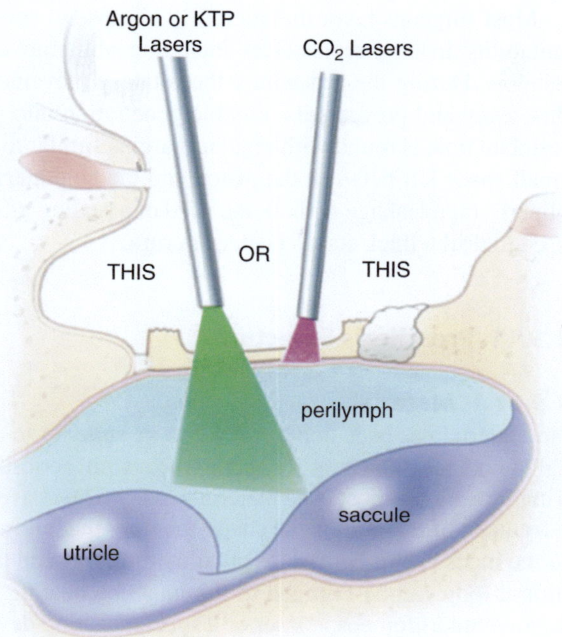

Fig. 1.40 Visual spectrum laser (e. g. Argon or KTP) (green bundle) passes through the perilymph and may reach the utricle and saccule. CO_2 laser is not visible to the human eye, is shown in color for demonstration. CO_2 laser energy is absorbed by the perilymph thus possible heating side effect

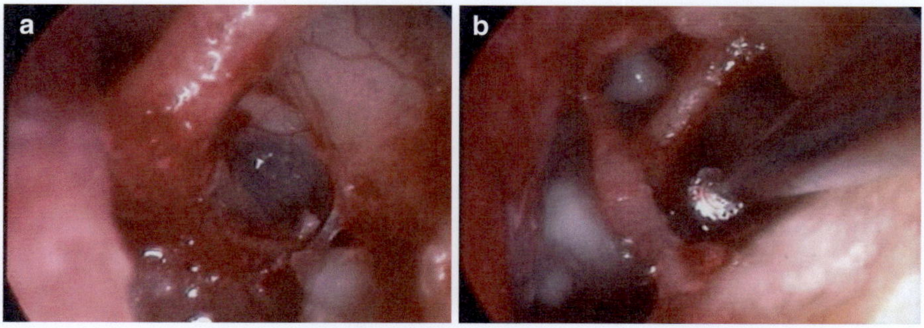

Fig. 1.41 Left ear stapedectomy using microdrill. (**a**) after removing of stapes superstructure, the footplate is fully exposed; (**b**) a microdrill with diamond burr is used to open the footplate

gain and very low percentage of refixation in a selected group of patients. It could be used in 45% to 50% of all cases of otosclerosis cases requiring surgery.

1.9.10 Micro-Drill in Stapedotomy

The microdrill is an elegant and safe tool that is used for footplate fenestration during stapedotomy. The microdrill is a small electric motor with small diamond burrs from 0.5 to 1 mm size; it has low noise intensity and low torque and thus, it is a safe tool for footplate fenestration, without causing acoustic trauma, when used for few seconds [124, 125] (Fig. 1.41).

Most surgeons favor the microdrill because of several advantages, especially its suitability in all circonstances including obliterative otosclerosis or narrow oval window. During the procedure, the rotatory movement of the drill takes the bone dust away and prevents its possible penetration into the vestibule. In all cases, the resultant hole is round with regular margins similar to a piston shaft. There is a very small space left between the piston and the hole margin decreasing the probability of perilymph leakage without the need of a sealing graft. The microdrill may also be used to drill a thick stapes posterior crura.

1.9.11 Prosthesis Selection

1.9.11.1 Material

No material has been demonstrated to be superior to another in terms of audiological outcomes which is in accordance with acoustic models [103]. Teflon and Titanium are the most used materials today. They have a good biocompatibility. One advantage of titanium is the shape-memory that allows the use of a clip attachment to the incus [126]. Nitinol® is an alloy of nickel and titanium. Teflon pistons with a nitinol loop can be crimped to the incus by heating the loop with bipolar current bayonet microforceps, a laser or a special heating device.

Only titanium, platinum and plastic prosthesis are compatible with MRI.

1.9.11.2 Length

The length of the prosthesis should be of 0.5 mm longer than the distance measured between the footplate and the medial edge of the long process of the incus. In cases when the prosthesis will require bending to enter perpendicularly into the fenestra, an additional 0.25 mm should be added.

On the preoperative CT scan, the distance between the inner surface of the long process of the incus and the lateral surface of the footplate can be measured, when the stapes axial plan (SAP) is obtained by several reconstructions (see Chapter 11 and Fig. 1.42).

1.9.11.3 Diameter

In general, a larger diameter gives better hearing improvement, but the risk of inner trauma increases with larger diameters. A middle ear mechanics study reported a better performance with 0.6 mm compared to 0.4 and 0.8 mm prosthesis diameter [103]. Systematic review and meta analysis showed that 0.6 mm pistons are significantly superior to 0.4 mm pistons in closing the ABG especially at low and mid frequencies [127]. A significantly superior performance of 0.4-mm pistons was reported in the higher frequencies as compared with 0.6-mm pistons [128–130]. Nevertheless the consensus is that a 0.6 mm piston seems to be the most suitable size for most cases. The 0.4 mm piston is reserved to a narrow OW recess or facial nerve prolapse.

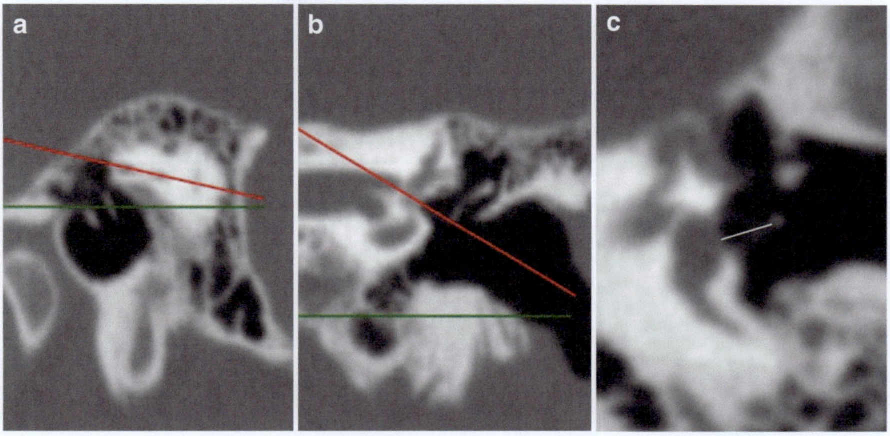

Fig. 1.42 Multiplanar reconstructions on a left ear to establish the distance between the outer surface of the footplate and the inner surface of the long process of the incus (**a**) red reference line along the LSCC arch → standard axial plan (**b**) red reference line along the stapes axis → stapes plan (**c**) measurement from the inner side of the long process of the incus to the outer surface of the footplate (here 3.94 mm)

1.9.11.4 Crimping of the Prosthesis

Solid attachment with a firm crimping of the prosthesis to the long process of the incus is a dominant factor for effective energy transmission. In the absence of a firm crimping, a hearing loss of up to 25 dB may occur [131]. A prosthesis with elastic clips and loops with shape-memory helps fixation of the prosthesis to the incus without the need for crimping. A recent meta-analysis of 22 studies by Bance et al. showed that the heat crimping piston (smart piston) has superior acoustic outcome than the forceps crimping piston (Schuknecht piston), which is still better than clipping pistons (soft clip) [132]. The so-called "smart" prosthesis gives the best acoustic outcome because of its best crimping procedure with the least trauma to the incus (in contrast to clipping or crimping). It is made of the metal nitinol that can be crimped by heat activation of the open loop. It has the advantage not to require mechanical crimping, and a very secure crimp can be accomplished either by heating the wire with a laser burst or by small bipolar forceps. However there has been some concern that one component of this metal alloy is nickel, which may not be highly biocompatible. The most frequently used prosthesis are represented in Fig. 1.43.

1.9.12 Oval Window Sealing

A careful sealing of the inner ear seems clearly indicated in case of a partial or total stapedectomy. Adipose tissue or a thin vein has offered a good protection to the vestibule. In contrary, sealing materials are not necessary in a stapedotomy

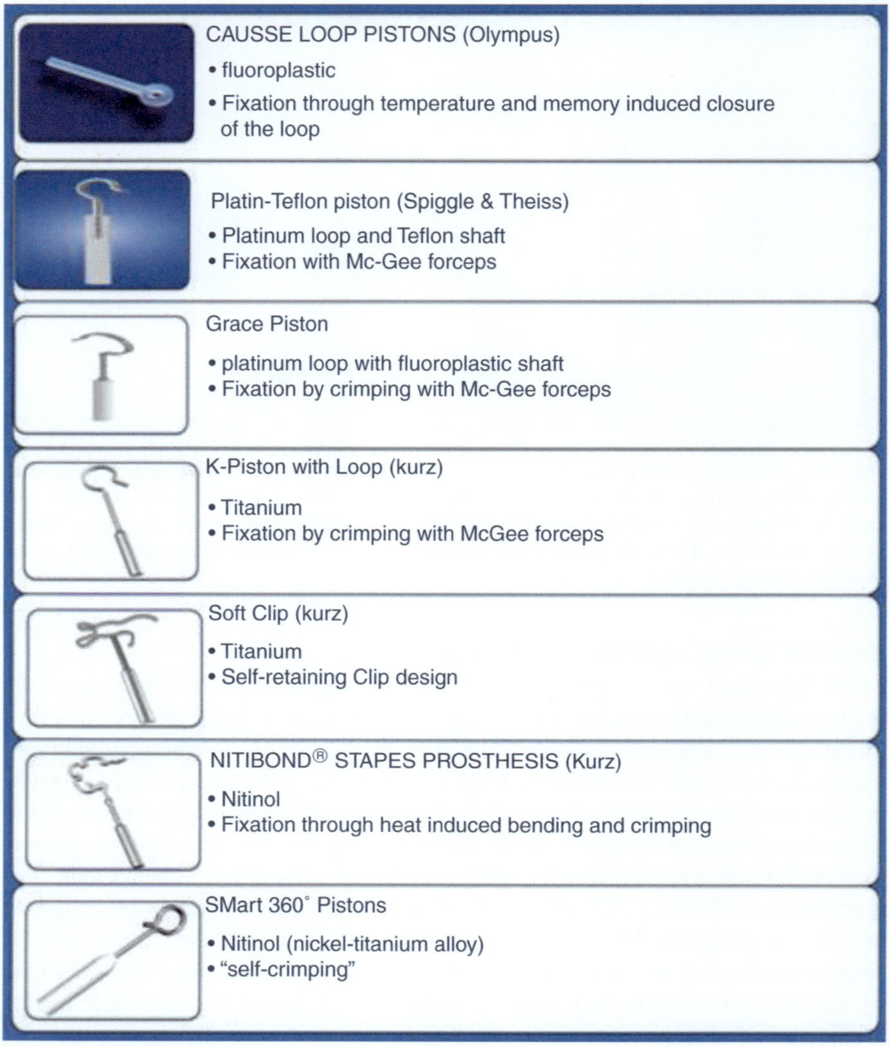

Fig. 1.43 Most common prosthesis in current use for stapes surgery

procedure with calibrated fenestration, unless if the patient is at risk for recurrent middle ear barotraumas (divers and pilots).

1.9.13 Stapedial Tendon Preservation

Although not commonly done, stapedial muscle preservation is intended to maintain the blood supply of the lenticular process of the incus which may reduce the risk of incus necrosis. Another theoretical advantage of stapedial muscle preservation is to maintain the stapedial reflex which reduces hyperacusis and offers better discrimination in noisy environment.

1.9.14 Surgical Treatment of Bilateral Otosclerosis (Contralateral Stapedectomy)

Otosclerosis is bilateral in 60–70% of patients [69]. The consensus is to operate first the worst hearing ear. The indication to operate the second ear is still controversial. The risk of SNHL (3.4%) [133] and a vestibular deficit [134] are postoperative issues of high clinical concern that persist even for years after surgery; nevertheless the advantage of a second ear surgery remains the recovery of a binaural hearing which offers an accurate sound localization and better discrimination in a noisy environment.

Despite the absence of a consensus about the delay between the first ear and a second ear intervention, the installation of advanced operative tools and techniques succeeded to decrease dramatically the risk of complications, facilitating the decision to operate on both ears in shorter time with more confidence [116, 117, 135]. However a minimal delay of 6 months should be practiced.

1.9.15 Intraoperative Challenges in Stapes Surgery

Careful evaluation of a preoperative CT scan may enable the surgeon to be better prepared to face intraoperative challenges such the following:

1.9.15.1 Malleus Ankylosis

The incidence of malleus fixation in association with otosclerosis is reportedly between 1% and 10% [136–139]. Malleus fixation may stem from ossification of the superior and anterior suspensory ligaments, leading to attachment of the head to the anterior wall of the epitympanum [140]. It may follow a congenital anomaly [141] or chronic infection of the ear [142]. It has also been suggested that otosclerotic bones have a high incidence of anterior mallear ligament hyalinization [143, 144]. It is routine during any stapedectomy procedure that all ossicles be individually palpated for mobility. Palpation of the malleus by delicate displacement is a routine step in the procedure before addressing the stapes. Malleus ankylosis may be congenital or acquired and be obscured from visualization because of its location in the epitympanum. Unrecognized ossicular fixation may be responsible for failure to close the air-bone gap postoperatively. A preoperative CT is valuable to detect the pathology (see Sect 10.4.2.) and thus influence the preoperative counseling of the patient in regard to the corresponding surgical technique and the reduced postoperative hearing recovery. When the malleus head is ankylosed to the wall or the roof of the epitympanum, incus and head of the malleus should be removed, and reconstruction should be done with a malleus attachment prosthesis. When the anterior malleal ligament is calcified, there is no major impact on hearing loss and stapedotomy could be proceeded.

1.9.15.2 High Jugular Bulb

A laterally located jugular bulb may come into juxtaposition with the tympanic annulus and is easily vulnerable to injury during elevation of the tympanomeatal flap inferiorly. The preoperative CT scan predicts such abnormality (Fig 1.44) to

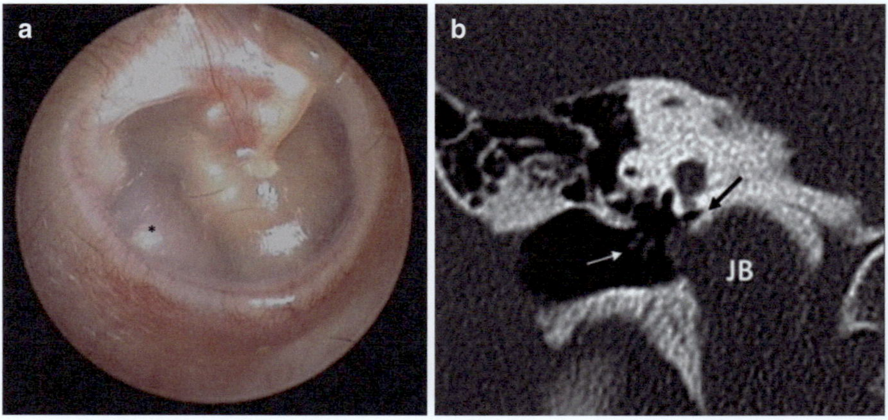

Fig. 1.44 (**a**) Right ear otoscopic image of the typical bluish appearance of the prominent high jugular bulb (asterix) visible through the tympanic membrane (**b**) coronal CT-reconstruction of a right ear, showing a prominent jugular bulb (JB), protruding into the hypotympanic cavity up to the level of the round window recess (*black arrow*). Tympanic aerator (*white arrow*) inserted through a thin tympanic membrane

alert the surgeon to be cautious. An incidental tear of the jugular bulb results in profuse bleeding which can be controlled by hemostatic packing.

1.9.15.3 Overhanging Facial Nerve

Overhanging facial nerve occurs in approximately 9% of stapes procedures. The operation could be completed by using a small fine pick or a small burr to create a fenestra through the well visualized inferior aspect of the footplate (Figs. 1.45 and 1.46). *Laser fenestration should be avoided in these cases because of the risk of facial nerve injury*.

Despite a good hearing, recovery an intermittent facial palsy was reported after stapes surgery in such cases, when the prosthesis came into contact with the overhanging facial nerve. When the facial nerve covers the large part of the footplate, a stapedotomy should not be attempted and the patient should be referred for a hearing aid.

1.9.15.4 Floating or Depressed Footplate

A floating footplate may occur in ears with a slight stapes fixation; it results from the mechanical pressure applied to the stapes footplate. Cases of clinical diagnosis of otosclerosis with negative preoperative CT-SCAN findings must alert the surgeon of the possibility of such an event. The use of Laser prevents this complication.

A thick footplate with marginal fixation will require careful pressure with the drill to avoid a floating footplate. When floating happens, several maneuvers can be attempted to capture the depressed footplate. The technique for safe removal of the floating footplate, avoiding subluxation, is insertion of a small hook into the cleft between the margin of the footplate and the oval window. Rotation of the hook 90° can bring it under the edge of the footplate for extraction by tilting. If this cannot be accomplished, then a 1-mm drill hole is made just outside the stapedio-vestibular

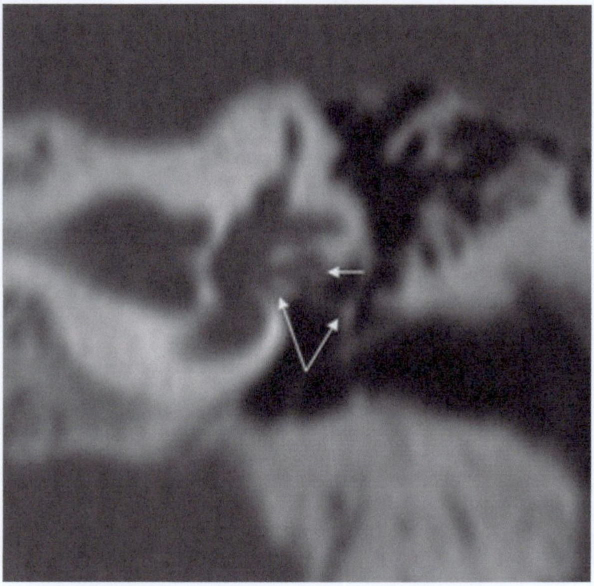

Fig. 1.45 Coronal CT-image of a left ear: stapes prosthesis (*joined arrows*) introduced into the oval niche inferior to the overhanging facial nerve (*arrow*)

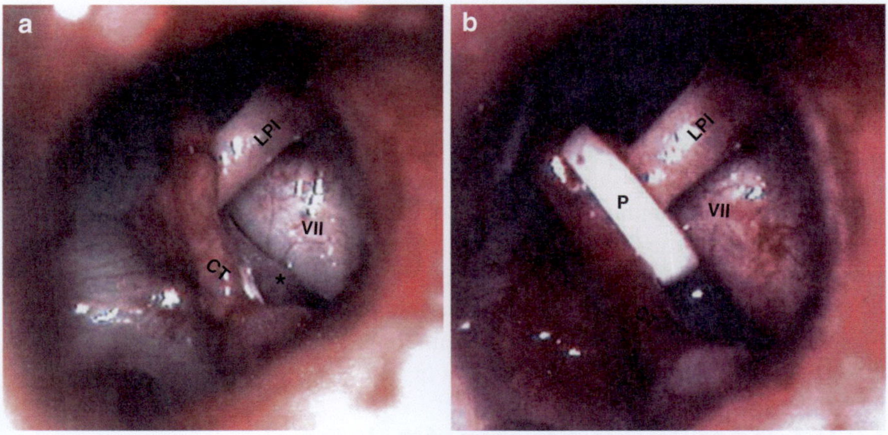

Fig. 1.46 Left ear stapes surgery challenged by overhanging facial nerve (VII) that is lying on the crura of the stapes (* in **a**) and narrowing significantly the oval window niche. (**b**) Fenestration was achieved with a 0.5 mm burr and a 0.4 piston (P) was inserted without contact with the VII. *LPI* long process of incus, *CT* chorda tympani

joint for insertion of a small hook to lift the footplate; this technique must be carefully decided and performed with great caution to avoid vestibular trauma. In case of a floating footplate, depression of the footplate into the vestibule has to be avoided, where it cannot be retrieved. If this occurs, then the depressed footplate should be left in the vestibule, the oval window be covered by a fascia, and a shorter-than-required prosthesis be inserted in the oval window; followed 6 months later by a revision surgery if the hearing is not adequate (Fig. 1.47).

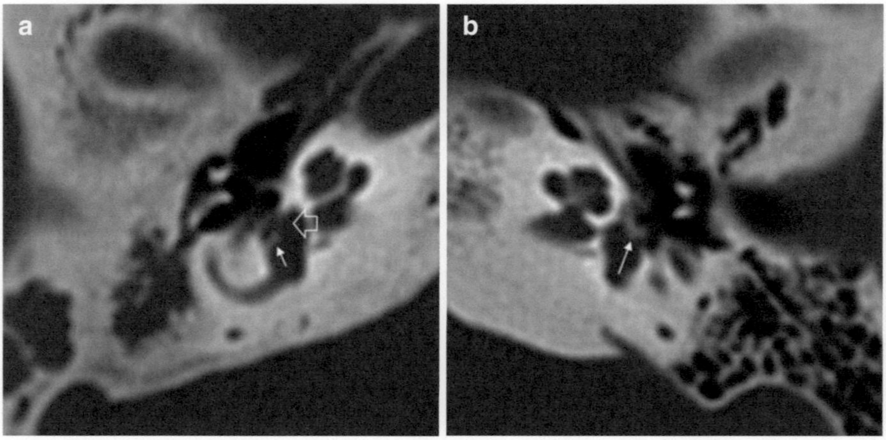

Fig. 1.47 Footplate incidents in two different patients (**a**) right axial CT-image: the posterior half of the footplate has fallen into the vestibule (white arrow), the middle part of the footplate is partially missing (empty arrow) (**b**) left axial CT-image: the anterior part of the footplate is in place, moderately angulated with the middle portion of the footplate, that is fragmented (long arrow)

1.9.15.5 Obliterative Otosclerosis of the Oval Window

In obliterative otosclerosis, the stapes footplate is greatly thickened and diffusely replaced by a massive otosclerotic deposit that fills the oval window niche. The incidence of obliterative otosclerosis varies from 4 to 13% of all otosclerotic patients that are surgically treated [145–147].

A large stapedotomy opening is the procedure of choice in these patients [148]. The size of the opening should be large enough to prevent a lateral contact of the piston with the surrounding bone (Figs. 1.48 and 1.49). Surgery requires saucerization of the bone in the OW niche with a diamond burr drill of 1 mm to convert the posterior part of the obliterative footplate to a blue footplate with visualization of the vestibule. Complete fenestration is then accomplished with a 0.7 mm diamond burr. Mensuration of the distance between the incus and vestibule is done prior to the fenestration step. Laser is not efficient in such cases.

1.9.15.6 Incidental Disarticulation of the Incus

Disarticulation or a subluxation of the incus can occur during curettage, while separating the incudostapedial joint or during clipping of the prosthesis on the incus. This can be avoided by preserving the anterior crus of the stapes till the end or by the use of laser during the procedure. The initial maneuver is to replace the incus into its anatomical position, relying on healing of the ligaments to retain it. However, if the dislocation is severe, and the incus does not retain its relocated position, then malleus attachment for the prosthesis is the most reliable solution for a satisfactory result.

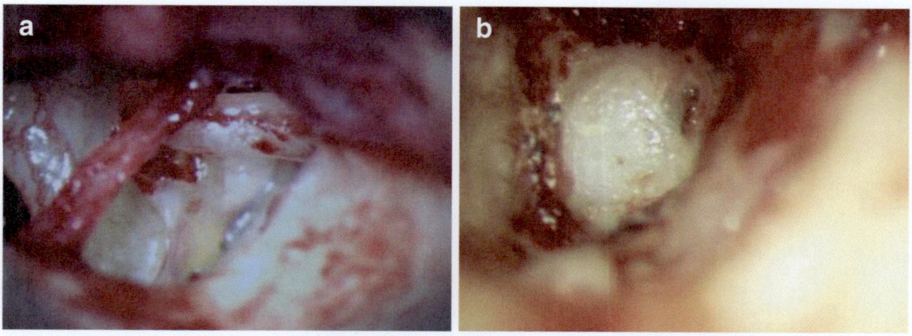

Fig. 1.48 (**a**) Left middle ear with obliterative otosclerosis. (**b**) at higher magnification, drilling out for obliterative otosclerosis was done, anterior crus still visible

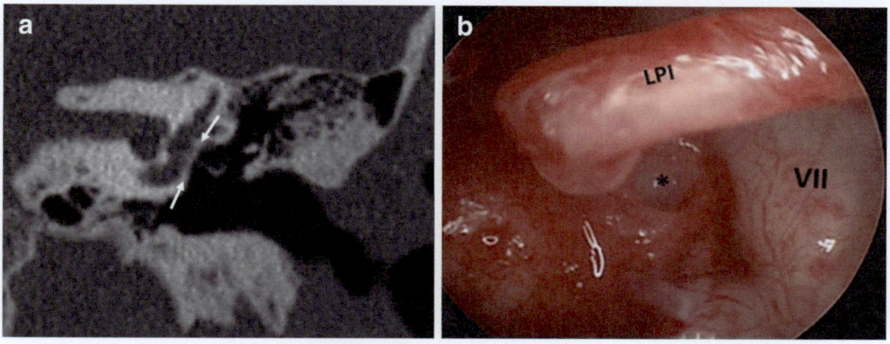

Fig. 1.49 A case of left obliterative otosclerosis. (**a**) Coronal CT reconstruction showing a complete obliteration of the oval niche (between the two arrows). (**b**) during surgical intervention, microdrill was used to open the footplate, more than 1 mm of depth has been drilled in the footplate (*) and still the footplate was not perforated. VII: facial nerve, LPI: long process of incus

1.9.15.7 Round Window Otosclerosis

As described above, round window otosclerosis is not rare; it has different degrees of involvement and can have a negative impact on the surgical results when ignored. Intraoperatively it is very difficult to assess the severity of RW otosclerosis even with the use of angled endoscopes (Fig. 1.50). In no case should the bone around the round window niche be drilled out, as it is prone to regeneration, and the procedure may violate the round window membrane, causing sensorineural hearing loss.

The surgeon should always rely on a preoperative CT scan to assess the degree of involvement of the RW. In cases of complete obliteration (Stages RW-IV or RW-V), stapedotomy is not recommended and the patient should be rehabilitated by a hearing aid.

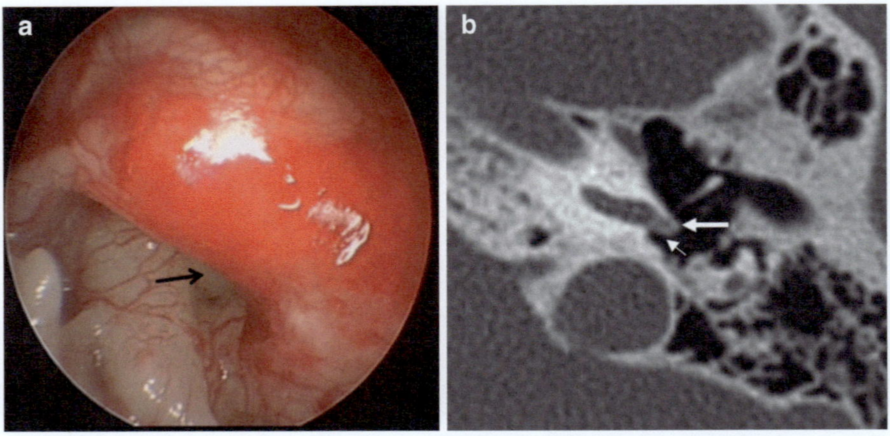

Fig. 1.50 A case of otosclerosis with RW-III otosclerosis. (**a**) During surgery, otosclerosis could be identified in the round window niche (black arrow), a complete evaluation of the round window niche and round window membrane and the degree of the otosclerosis involvement cannot be fully assessed even with the use of HD angled endoscopes. The preoperative CT-Scan (**b**) is a must to determine correctly the stage of the round window otosclerosis. Round window niche (thin arrow), large otosclerotic focus on the inferior edge of the round window (thick arrow)

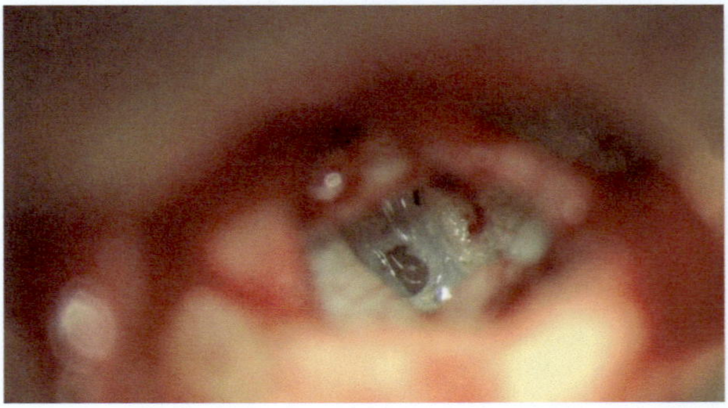

Fig. 1.51 Gusher after footplate fenestration during stapedotomy in a right ear (Courtesy of Dr. Robert Vincent)

1.9.15.8 Perilymph Gushers and Oozers

Occasionally, fenestration of the footplate results in the free flow of fluid from the vestibule into the middle ear (Fig. 1.51). A constant but persistent trickle of fluid that wells up through the fenestrum is often called a "perilymph oozer" and is usually due to a large vestibular aqueduct. A heavy fluid flow from the oval window under pressure after opening the OW is called Gusher. A perilymph gusher is very rare (<0.05%) and occurs as a result of a defect in the cribrosa area of the internal auditory canal. Gusher is treated with soft tissue plugging and prosthesis to maintain the soft tissue sealer in place. Oozers require a perichondrium or vein seal.

1.9.15.9 Persistent Stapedial Artery

At surgery, often a remnant of the stapedial artery can be encountered as a small vessel that crosses the footplate, that can be easily coagulated with the laser; this is

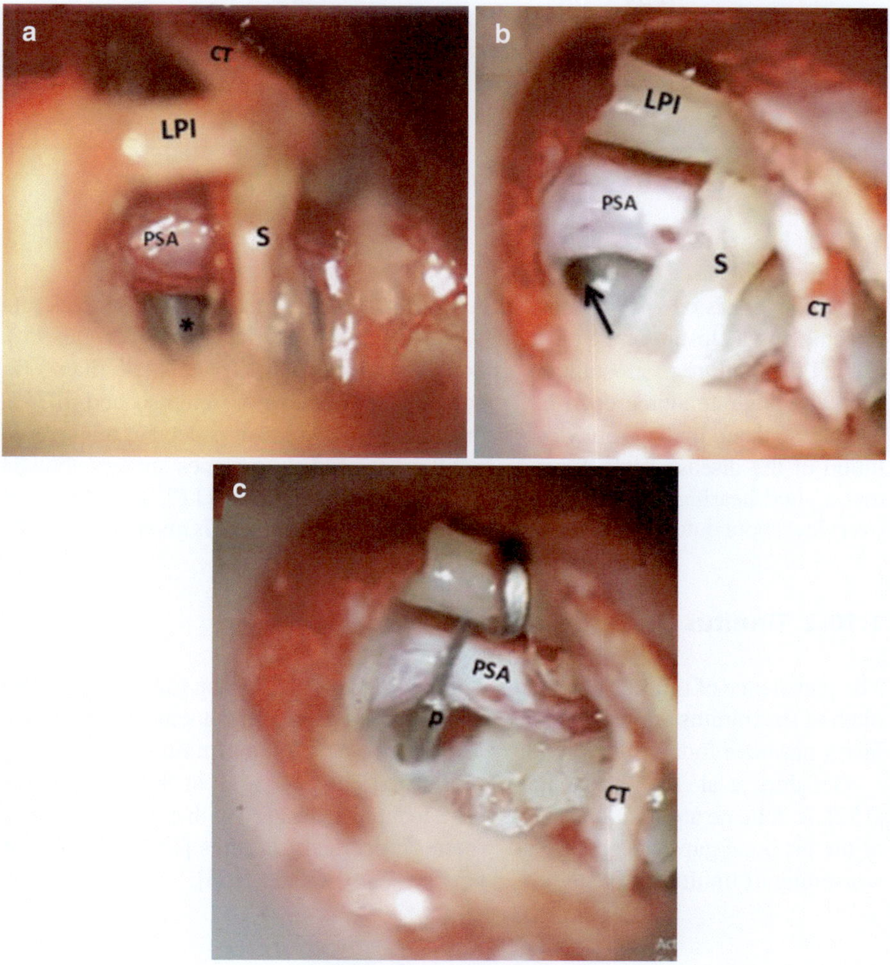

Fig. 1.52 Right ear otosclerosis with persistent stapedial artery (PSA). (**a**) the posterior half of the footplate is visible (*) and could be accessible for fenestration. (**b**) fenestration was done in the footplate (black arrow) using microdrill. (**c**) a titanium prosthesis (*P*) was inserted in the fenestration. *LPI* long process of incus, *CT* chorda tympani, *S* stapes (Courtesy of Dr. Sree Ram Murthy)

not a persistent stapedial artery. A true persistent stapedial artery may be found in 1 out of 5000 cases and in some cases it may nearly fill the footplate area [100]. As it is a very rare finding, and its imaging aspect on the routinely non injected CT is rather non-specific, it is usually discovered peroperatively. A persistent stapedial artery cannot be safely coagulated. In most cases, the procedure should be aborted. In very rare occasions, if the posterior half of the footplate is visible and could be easily approached, an extremely cautious stapedotomy could be attempted (Fig. 1.52). Titanium prosthesis is preferable because it transmits less the pulsations of the artery. It remains that in cases of large stapedial artery obscuring the whole footplate, the stapedotomy procedure must be aborted. On a preoperative CT scan, the absence of the foramen spinosum at the skull base should alert the radiologist and otologist about this anomaly (see Fig. 1.35).

1.10 Results of a Primary Stapes Surgery

1.10.1 Hearing Outcome

Stapes surgery is one of the most successful surgeries in medicine, the success rate of achieving a closure of the air-bone gap (AB-gap) to less than 10 dB is about 95% [135, 149]. Failure of closing the air-bone gap to less than 10 dB is less than 5 %, however, this rate increases to 12% in cases of obliterative otosclerosis and to 35% when associated malleus ankylosis is present. Long-term results depend on the evolution of the disease itself. Long-term follow-up studies of stapes surgery showed that a good hearing was maintained in 75% of operated cases [117, 135, 150]. An overview about outcome and complications of the stapes surgery is given in Fig. 1.53.

1.10.2 Tinnitus Outcome

The prevalence of tinnitus in patients with otosclerosis is 65–92% [62, 63, 151]. The pitch of the tinnitus does not predict its postoperative outcome: not any preoperative factor has been found to predict the postoperative outcome of tinnitus.

Gersdorf et al. found that tinnitus disappears or decreases in 80% of patients [152]. A delicate atraumatic small fenestra technique surgery with complete closure of the air-bone gap is necessary for a better outcome of tinnitus [153]. The risk of worsening of tinnitus after surgery is between 5–10% [152, 153].

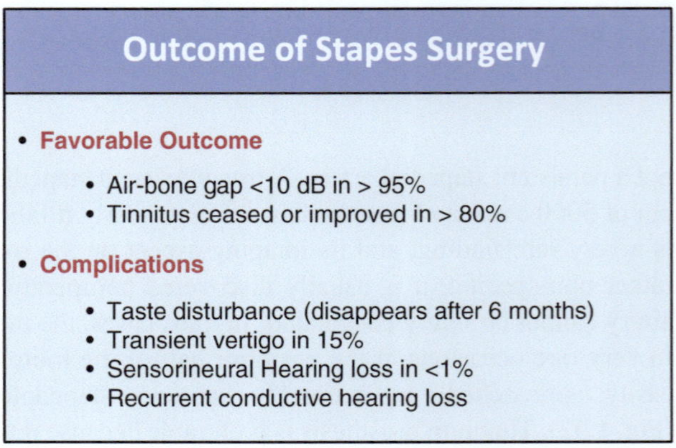

Fig. 1.53 Outcome of stapes surgery

1.10.3 Complications of Stapes Surgery

1.10.3.1 Taste Disturbances

The chorda tympani nerve (CTN) is within the operative field and it is usually necessary to manipulate it in order to achieve free access to the oval window.

Patients with an injury to the CTN present with symptoms of a metallic or sweet taste and numbness or tingling of the tongue. Usually, these symptoms are transient and resolve in 3–6 months.

The incidence of taste disturbance after stapes surgery is high (61.9%), whereas the majority (94.8%) recovers within 1 year [154].

More severe surgical nerve trauma caused more disturbance, implying that the nerve should be handled carefully during surgery. If the CTN was transected, the symptoms are more severe and long-lasting. Half of the patients with CTN cut will have mild to moderate symptoms for more than six months [155]. The Greater Superficial Petrosal Nerve may ensure the compensation process in the remaining half of patients. Therefore, it is our recommendation that, where possible, the chorda be preserved.

However when present, taste disturbances must be taken into consideration during the counseling for a contralateral stapes surgery.

1.10.3.2 Dizziness or Vertigo

The normal healing response to stapedectomy involves a low level serofibrinous labyrinthitis. As a result, most patients will report some degree of dizziness, especially with rapid head movements, immediately following the procedure. This dizziness will usually clear in the first few postoperative days. In 12–45% of patients, postoperative vestibular symptoms occur after total stapedectomy in relation to the opening duration of the vestibule during the surgery and the various surgical manoeuvers (labyrinthine insult). Stapedotomy reduces drastically the postoperative dizziness. Usually, these symptoms resolve after 3–6 days and the use of corticosteroids is helpful [156, 157].

When vertigo is present and c-VEMP arising from the saccule are not decreased after the surgery, this indicates that the function of the saccule is preserved or not been seriously affected [158, 159]. VOG is an effective method to evaluate vestibular organ irritation or real injury.

A heating effect of Laser or the installation of a long piston can cause vestibular problems because of the proximity of the stapedial footplate to the otolithic organs [160].

Persistent vertigo may be due to a depressed footplate fragment into the vestibule or simply because of a long prosthesis. Long lasting vertigo implies a surgical exploration to rule out perilymphatic fistula.

1.10.3.3 Sensorineural Hearing Loss

The most worrisome complication of stapes surgery is SNHL. The overall incidence, in the hands of experienced surgeons, is less than 1% [161]. Post-stapedotomy SNHL can occur immediately or weeks to months following the procedure. SNHL that occurs in the early postoperative period can be attributed to the surgical trauma.

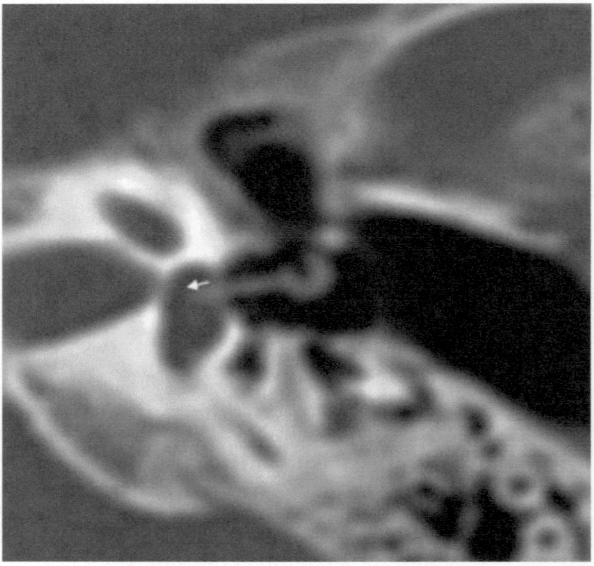

Fig. 1.54 Reconstructed CT-Image along the piston of the stapes prosthesis with excess of intravestibular penetration (arrow)

High frequency hearing loss above 4000 Hz is likely related to acoustic trauma caused by excessive manipulation of either the footplate or the prosthesis. Steroids are very helpful in the early stages.

In Vincents' report (2006) of 3050 stapedotomies performed between 1991 and 2004, SNHL was seen in 0.5% of the patients (13/2525 patients); there were two dead ears (0.07%) and a SNHL of 15–55 dB in the others [135].

Surgical management for postoperative SNHL is recommended as soon as the etiological diagnosis is made:

- A suspected perilymphatic fistula: the diagnosis is mostly clinical.
- A very long prosthesis penetrating deeply in the vestibule: CT is helpful (Fig. 1.54).
- A granuloma formation: the diagnosis is mostly clinical.

Despite a good surgical management, the recovery of a post-stapedotomy SNHL is always difficult to obtain.

1.10.3.4 Perilymphatic Fistula

In a perilymph fistula (PLF), fluid leaks from the inner ear, leading to a disturbance of the cochlear and vestibular function.

Some leakage always occurs during stapedectomy, and if this persists, the fistula is referred to as a ***primary fistula***. The larger the space around the prosthesis in the fenestra, the greater the incidence for nonhealing of this space and leakage of perilymph.

If perilymph leakage occurs after the oval window has been successfully sealed for a period of time, it is called a ***secondary fistula***. Classical symptoms of PLF

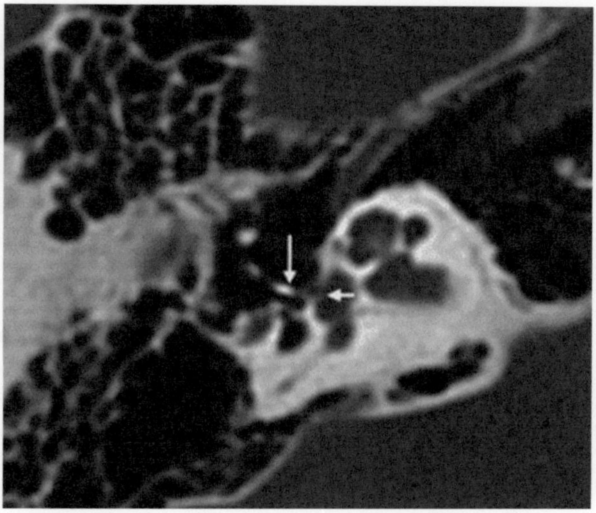

Fig. 1.55 Axial CT image of a right ear: the prosthesis (long arrow) is displaced outside the oval window. The central persistent opening of the footplate is well visualized (short arrow) suggestive of perilymphatic fistula in the clinical context

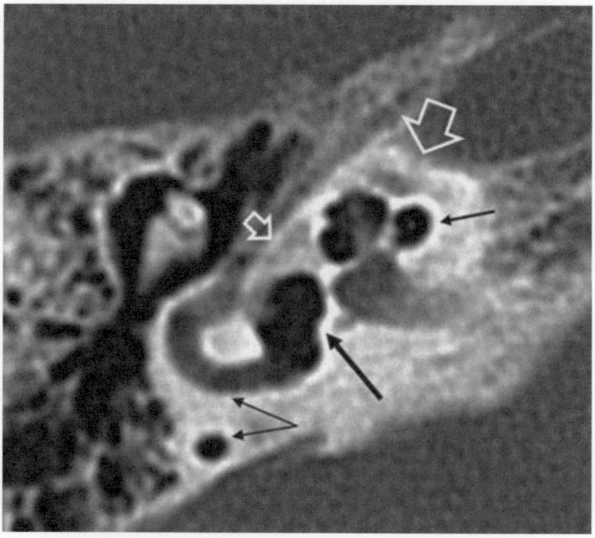

Fig. 1.56 Axial CT-image of the right ear: the whole labyrinth is filled with air: the cochlea (thin black arrow), the vestibule (thick black arrow), the semicircular canals (V shaped arrows). Extended otosclerotic foci: antefenestral (small empty arrow), pericochlear (large empty arrow)

are a fluctuating SNHL, episodic unsteadiness, and tinnitus. The diagnosis should be suspected in patients who have a positive fistula test or in whom Hallpike positional testing results in a vertigo and nystagmus with the affected ear in a down position.

In most cases, secondary fistulas are associated to prosthesis dislocation. CT scan and the very promising CBCT are the methods of choice to assess the prosthesis displacement: it can show the residual opening of the footplate and the situation of the prosthesis outside the oval window opening (Fig. 1.55). Later on, a pneumolabyrinth could occur (Fig. 1.56).

Explorative tympanotomy is indicated when a perilymph fistula is suspected. When demonstrated during revision, a new correct prosthesis placement along with an adequate sealing with a connective tissue of the oval window are performed.

1.10.3.5 Reparative Granuloma

A reparative granuloma results from exuberant inflammatory reactive granulation tissues in response to surgery and the inadvertent inclusion of a foreign body (Gloves powder, Gelfoam, Prosthesis). The incidence of reparative granuloma has been estimated to be 0.1% after stapedectomy and 0.07% after stapedotomy [162].

If a granuloma invades the vestibulum, symptoms of vertigo, hearing loss, and tinnitus appear within 7–15 days after an uneventful surgery and an unremarkable immediate postoperative period. The tympanic membrane may show a reddish discoloration in the postero-superior quadrant. The audiogram reveals typically a mixed or pure sensorineural hearing loss that affects mostly and severely the high frequencies. CT-scan shows hazy condensation images around the prosthesis and filling the oval window niche (Fig. 1.57). The overall outcome of such devastating process depends of its early diagnosis and its treatment. Unfortunately most cases result in a permanent sensorineural hearing loss.

1.10.3.6 Facial Palsy

An *immediate* post-stapedectomy facial palsy is due to excessive infiltration of local anesthetics at the time of surgery and usually remits within few hours. *Delayed Facial Paralysis* occurs 5–16 days post-stapedectomy and results most probably from activation of a herpes virus or varicella zoster virus as seen in Bell's palsy.

1.10.3.7 Otitis Media

Acute otitis media in the early postoperative period is very rare and it is worrisome. The patients are at high risk to develop sensorineural hearing loss, suppurative labyrinthitis and meningitis. Patients should be admitted to the hospital for agressive IV antibiotherapy with corticotherapy and removal of the packing.

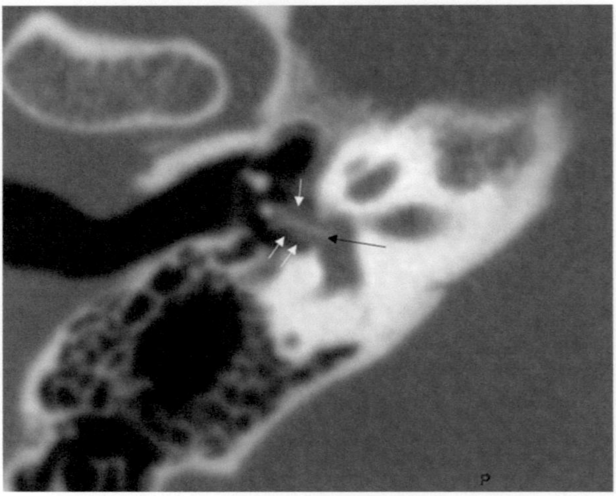

Fig. 1.57 Axial CT-image of a right ear: stapes prosthesis in place (black arrow). The piston is surrounded by hazy condensations (white arrows) corresponding to the proliferative inflammatory tissue of the granuloma.

1.10.3.8 Post-Stapedotomy Retraction Pocket and Cholesteatoma

Tympanic Membrane Retraction Pocket formation is uncommon after stapedotomy (1%, Ozgirgin, [163]), (Fig. 1.58). It is secondary to a dysventilation syndrome. It may be facilitated by a too large curettage of the bony tympanic ring in its posterosuperior part increasing the area of weakness of this part of the tympanic membrane.

The retraction pocket epithelium should be completely and totally excised. The middle ear cavity should be freed from any epithelial rests and perichondrium/cartilage strips and myringoplasty be done. Because opening the vestibule in the presence of a cholesteatoma is fraught with the risk of SNHL and dizziness, it is preferable to avoid this complication and it is mandatory to stage stapes surgery.

Stapedectomy should be avoided in patients with poor tubal function.

If for some reason this is required, consideration should be given to reinforce the atticotomy defect with cartilage.

1.10.4 Failure in Stapes Surgery

Failure in stapes surgery could be immediate when the patient does not recover his hearing right after his surgery; or delayed when after a good recovery of hearing the conductive deafness recurs again.

A methodologic review and work up to elicit the etiological diagnosis of the persistent or recurrent conductive hearing loss after adequate stapedotomy is mandatory.

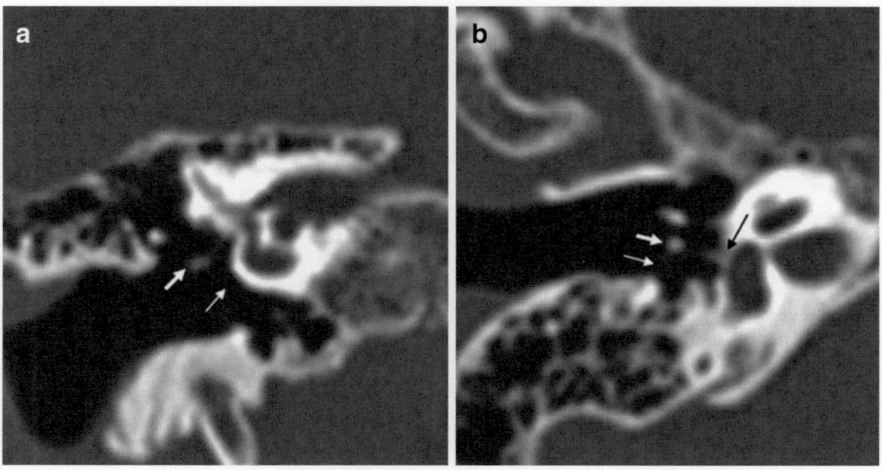

Fig. 1.58 Right ear, (**a**) coronal and (**b**) axial view showing the retracted very thin tympanic membrane (thin arrows) on the distal end of the incus in close contact to the prosthesis (thick arrow); in (**b**) see the distal prosthesis (black arrow) inserted into the footplate level but not reaching the vestibule

1. A postoperative residual conductive hearing loss of more than 15 dB is mostly due to surgical pitfalls.
2. Recurrent conductive hearing loss could be due to different causes, that are represented in Fig. 1.59. CT is helpful to give a probable diagnosis before a revision is decided; it may show the following [164]:
   (a) Resorptive osteitis of the incus at the site of the prosthesis attachment (Sect. 1.10.4.1.)
   (b) The prosthesis lying on a footplate fragment or abutting the bony margin of the oval window rather than centered in the fenestration (Sect. 1.10.4.2)
   (c) Insufficient opening of the footplate during the primary surgery or new bone formation around the prosthesis (Sect. 1.10.4.3)
   (d) Evolutive round window otosclerosis (Sect. 1.10.4.4)

1.10.4.1 Resorptive Osteitis of the Incus

Incus necrosis manifests clinically by a recurrent conductive hearing loss long time after a successful surgery and closure of the air-bone gap. Regardless of the type of prosthesis, causes of incus necrosis include pressure necrosis due to over crimping, loose crimp, or damage to the mucosa cover of the incus, which is presumed to provide anastomotic blood supply to the incus (Fig. 1.60). A solid and constant contact of the vibrating prosthesis on a fixed residual footplate is also suspected as a possible mechanism behind incus necrosis [165].

Migration of the loose prosthesis after incus necrosis can be demonstrated by the CT-Scan showing the prosthesis completely detached and lying on the floor of the cavity (Fig. 1.61a) or exteriorized through the tympanic membrane, possibly covered by granulation tissue (Fig. 1.61b). It could also fall deeper in the vestibule with symptoms of vertigo or unsteadiness.

Stapes Surgery Failure

- **Persistent Conductive Hearing Loss**
  - Missed malleus ankylosis
  - Missed third window
  - Short prosthesis or small diameter
  - Prosthesis abutting fenestration margin
  - Round window otosclerosis
- **Recurrent Conductive Hearing Loss**
  - Resorptive osteitis of the incus
  - Prosthesis displacement
  - New bone formation in the oval window
  - Obliteration of the round window by otosclerosis

Fig. 1.59 Causes of stapes surgery failure

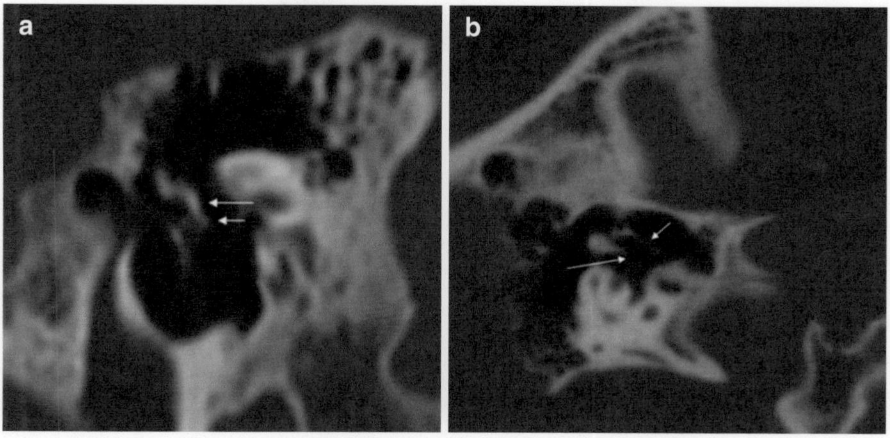

Fig. 1.60 (**a**) Reconstruction perpendicular to the long process of the incus (long arrow), that is amputated above the wire of the prosthesis (short arrow) (**b**) Reconstruction along the axis of the long process of the incus, showing the missing end of the long process (long arrow), manubrium of the malleus (short arrow)

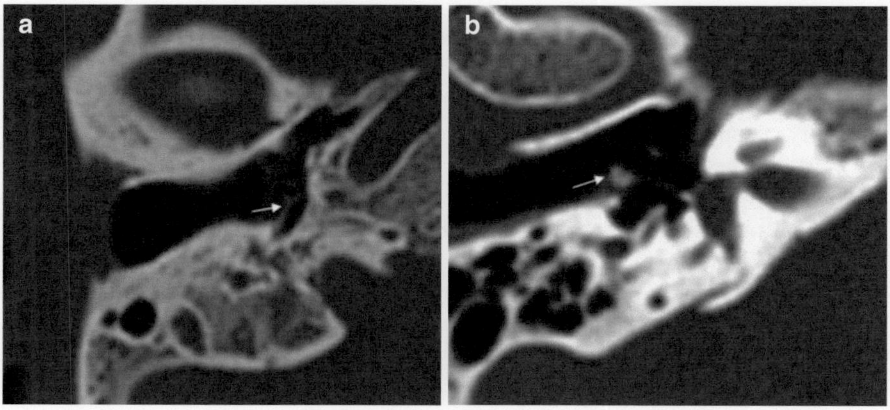

Fig. 1.61 (**a**) Axial CT-image of a right ear: a completely displaced prosthesis lying on the floor of the ME cavity (arrow) (**b**) axial CT-image of a right ear with a lateralized prosthesis that has migrated through the tympanic membrane, the hook is visible in the EAC (white arrow)

1.10.4.2 Misplaced Prosthesis

A prosthesis abutting the bony margin of the oval window or lying on the residual footplate (prosthesis migration and contact with footplate fragments) could be the cause of failure of hearing recovery.

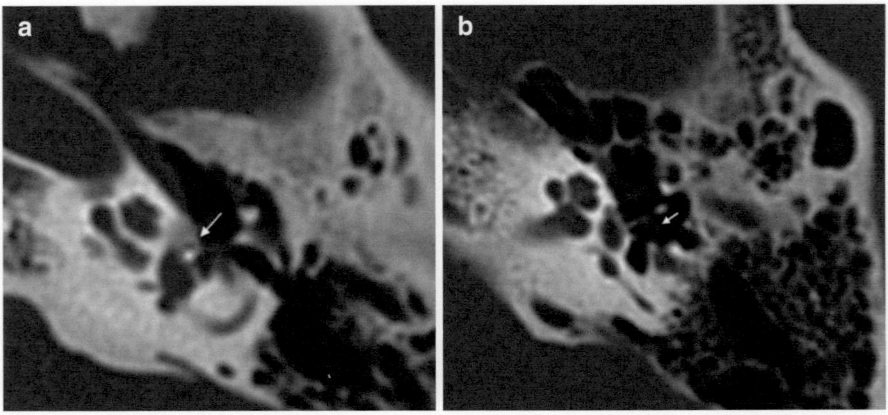

Fig. 1.62 Axial CT-Image of different left ears: (**a**) Prosthesis anteriorly displaced, abutting the anterior border of the OW (arrow) (**b**) Thick fibrotic band (white arrow) retracting and fixing the prosthesis piston

The mechanism causing prosthesis migration was found to be:

- A contraction of the sealing material with lifting of the prosthesis from the fenestration (Fig. 1.62a),
- Contraction from adhesions (Fig. 1.62b),
- Faulty crimping of the incus,
- Short prosthesis [166].

1.10.4.3 Insufficient Opening or a New Bone Formation in the Oval Window

New bone formation at the oval window occurs especially when a drill has been used to open a densely obliterated oval window niche. To avoid such situation, the fenestration should be comfortably larger than the piston prosthesis to prevent a possible postoperative new bone formation from abutting the prosthesis. In some cases the so-called new bone formation or recurrence of otosclerosis is in fact due to originally an insufficient size of stapodotomy opening during the primary surgery (Figs. 1.63 and 1.64).

1.10.4.4 Progressive Obliteration of the Round Window by Otosclerosis

Stapedotomy offers a relatively good outcome in stage RW3, but long after a successful stapedotomy, a recurrent hearing loss may be the case if the disease process at the RW continues its progress to reach an obliterative stage (RW4 or more). In such cases a preoperative CT scan would preclude unnecessary revision procedures.

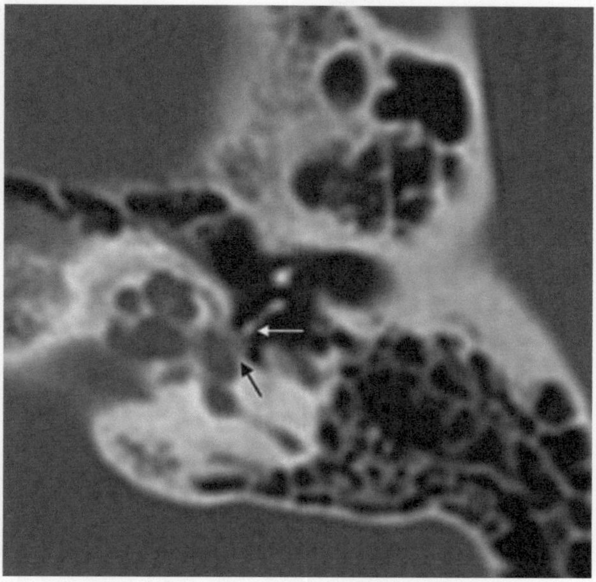

Fig. 1.63 Axial CT-image of a left ear, showing a footplate extremely thickened by otosclerotic material (black arrow), the distal prosthesis piston (white arrow) far away from the vestibule

1.11 Revision of Stapes Surgery

Despite constant improvement in managing otosclerosis, revision stapes surgeries are needed not infrequently and can present a technical challenge. Revision surgeries are most frequently needed due to the late failure of initially successful stapes surgeries. During a 20-year period of observation, at least 10 to 20% of stapedectomy patients would have a revision for further conductive hearing losses [166, 167].

Prosthesis displacement is the most common reason for stapes surgery failure; incus erosion is the second most common reason.

Very rarely, the indication for revision surgery is persistent vertigo, either immediate or delayed.

Admittedly, although primary otosclerotic surgery may be technically demanding, revision stapes procedures are often some of the most challenging otology cases to be encountered. In revision surgeries, the ABG was closed to within 10 dB in 63 percent of the cases.

The decision to undergo a revision stapes surgery must be judged in relation to: the value of the residual ABG, the bone conduction threshold, speech discrimination score, status of the contralateral ear, and postoperative risk of deterioration. Thus a revision stapedotomy requires a complete work up and a very good counseling.

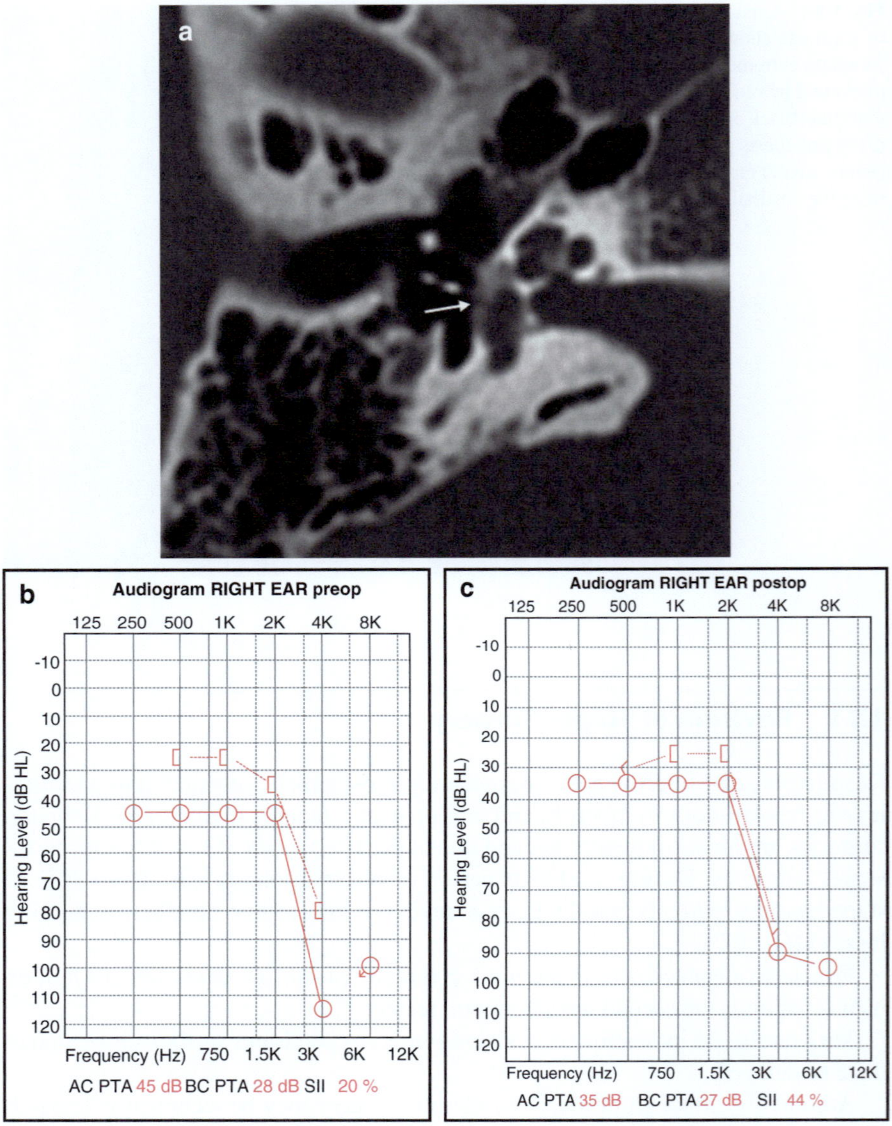

Fig. 1.64 (**a**) Axial CT-image of the right ear: a very small opening (white arrow) is left after retraction of the prosthesis on an obliterative footplate. (**b**) audiogram showing preoperative gap. (**c**) audiogram 7 months postop revision: closure of the gap

1.11.1 Persistent Vertigo and Prosthesis Penetrating Too Long Inside the Vestibule

In some cases of persistent severe vertigo, patients become more interested to be relieved from vertigo than to improve the hearing.

A long intravestibular prosthesis must be removed carefully from the vestibule, keeping in mind the probability of intra-vestibular adhesions with the possible risk of SNHL and a possible secondary vestibular deficit. Then a shorter prosthesis should be replaced through the same oval window opening. In the majority of such revision procedures, Laser is appreciated for better surgical performance [166].

1.11.2 Recurrent Conductive Hearing Loss with Prosthesis Situated Out of the Oval Window

1.11.2.1 Short Prosthesis, Incus Intact

The most common cause of a post-stapedotomy conductive hearing loss leading to a revision is the prosthesis migration out of the oval window [165, 167, 168]. The prosthesis displacement is mostly due to a short prosthesis with adhesions or a faulty crimping [165] (Figs. 1.62 and 1.63). Prior to revision surgery, a CT scan could show if the long process of the incus is intact. In such case, a sufficient opening of the footplate must be insured after an adequate measurement of the distance between the medial aspect of the incus and the footplate (see Fig. 1.42). The prosthesis placement should be achieved with a good penetration into the vestibule and well crimped on the incus. The stability and the good function of the ossicular system must be verified by manipulation of the manubrium. This procedure could be performed under local anesthesia in order to check the hearing recovery at the end of the procedure.

1.11.2.2 Incus Necrosis

Recurrent conductive hearing loss could be the result of a shortened incus by necrosis. CT-Imaging could demonstrate its status (Fig. 1.60).

Incus necrosis could be managed as follow:

1. Malleo-vestibular reconstruction: This surgery is not as easy to perform as it could be described but when successfully done it provides a stable long term reconstruction. The malleo-stapedial prosthesis is mostly a custom made wire and fat: 5.5–6 mm of length, correctly attached to the neck of the malleus, partially curved to become perpendicular to the oval window opening. It must penetrate sufficiently at least 0.5 mm deep into the oval window in order to compensate the stronger mechanics of the malleus.
2. Reconstruction of the incus with cement is simple and efficient but long term results are not predictable. Long term stability and resistance of the cement reconstruction under the persisting movement effect of the prosthesis has to be demonstrated (Fig. 1.65).

1.11.2.3 Secondary Obliterative Otosclerosis

Progressive obliteration of the oval window may be the cause of recurrent conductive hearing loss. This is encountered mostly in juvenile otosclerosis when the disease continues its progress to strangulate the prosthesis or following an excessive drilling during the primary surgery. Such revision surgery consists of a larger drilling around the prosthesis to deliver it and replace it with extreme care after insuring

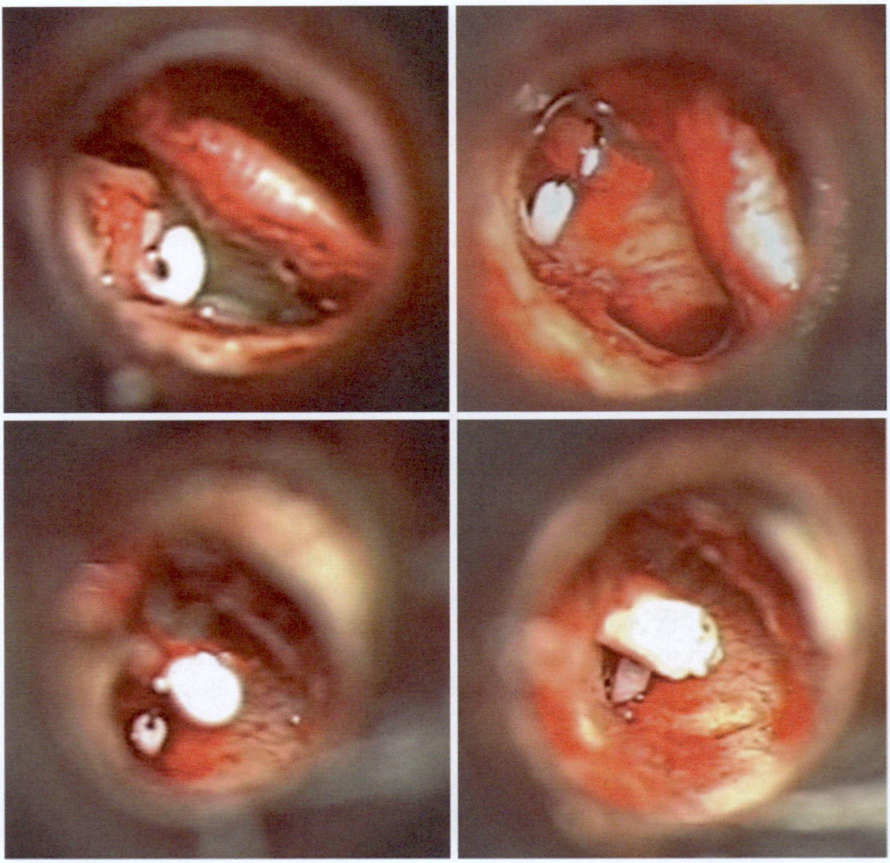

Fig. 1.65 Right ear revision stapedectomy showing incus necrosis and displacement of the piston. A new piston was replaced and the missed part of incus was reconstructed by bone cement

a sufficient oval window opening. This surgery must be decided cautiously because of the disease aggressive evolution, revision surgery carries risk of rapid hearing loss recurrence and inner damage.

1.12 Conservative Treatment of Hearing Loss in Otosclerosis

1.12.1 Hearing Aid

Hearing aid should always be discussed and offered to the patient before stapes surgery. Occasionally there are patients who do not select surgical management as a solution for their hearing loss and choose amplification. Additionally, because of some unforeseen circumstances, patients' hearing does not improve or even worsen after stapes surgery and patients are advised to use hearing aids. Hearing loss after successful stapes surgery can also later deteriorate because of sensorineural involvement and patients are advised to use hearing aids as well.

Most of today's hearing aids are digital and have the ability of super computation and signal processing. The employment of wireless technology, such as Bluetooth, has enabled users to stream their telephone conversation and music or news to their hearing aids reducing the stigma of hearing aid use.

Otologists should encourage their patients to use hearing aids and emphasize the role of neuroplasticity and enhancement of auditory function for the impaired hearing.

1.12.2 BAHA

BAHA or Middle ear implants [169, 170] would be a solution to rehabilitate otosclerosis patients with conductive or mixed hearing loss that could not fit with conventional hearing aid.

1.12.3 Medical Treatment

Despite several studies regarding a possible therapeutic effect of substances that may suppress bone remodeling in the temporal bone, still there is no curative medical therapy for otosclerosis. Otologists may consider prescribing medication therapy in patients with signs of greater activity, such as presence of Schwartze sign, onset or worsening of tinnitus and/or vertigo, and progressive deterioration of the sensorineural component of hearing. Medication may also be introduced, with evidence in the imaging studies of demineralization foci that involve the endosteum, even in the absence of hearing loss, with the purpose to inactivate the otospongiotic lesions and prevent future hearing loss. Options for the medical treatment of otosclerosis include sodium fluoride and bisphosphonates.

1.12.3.1 Sodium Fluoride

Sodium fluoride acts by changing an active otospongiotic lesion to an inactive otosclerotic lesion. This conversion of otospongiosis to mature sclerosis occurs as a result of reduced enzyme activity derived from otospongiosis and from diminished rate of osteoblast-induced bone remodeling.

1.12.3.2 Bisphosphonates

Bisphosphonates have replaced the sodium fluoride in the treatment of osteodystrophy, such as Paget disease, osteogenesis imperfecta, and osteoporosis, because of their improved antiresorptive properties and a higher affinity with bone tissue. Following this line of therapy, bisphosphonates have begun to be used to treat otosclerosis. These drugs interact with osteoclast metabolism to induce osteoclast apoptosis, therefore inhibiting bone resorption. By that same mechanism, the production of toxic enzymes secondary to abnormal bone metabolism is reduced.

1.13 Juvenile Otosclerosis

Juvenile otosclerosis is the rare onset of otosclerosis in childhood and adolescence and should be distinguished from congenital stapes fixation. The most important characteristics of juvenile otosclerosis in children is the progressive nature of a conductive hearing loss associated to a positive family history, in contrary to the congenital stapes ankylosis with its stable non-progressive conductive deafness (Fig. 1.66).

It is important to differentiate preoperatively between otosclerosis and congenital stapes fixation, because the postoperative results in congenital stapedial fixation tend to be inferior. Juvenile otosclerosis is associated with a higher incidence of simultaneous malleus fixation which was found in 6% of children compared to 1% in adults otosclerosis [171].

Surgeons may choose to postpone surgical treatment of juvenile otosclerosis until the children become old enough to participate in the ethics of counseling around the age of 10–12 years.

The results of primary stapedotomy in children with otosclerosis are comparable to the results of primary stapedotomy in adult patients. Success percentages are high, with an air-bone gap closure to within 10 dB in 93% of stapedotomies and air-bone gap closure within 20 dB in 98% of stapedotomies [172–175].

Juvenile otosclerosis has a tendency to progress rapidly to the obliterative form. Moreover after stapedotomy and primary successful closure of the air-bone gap, the

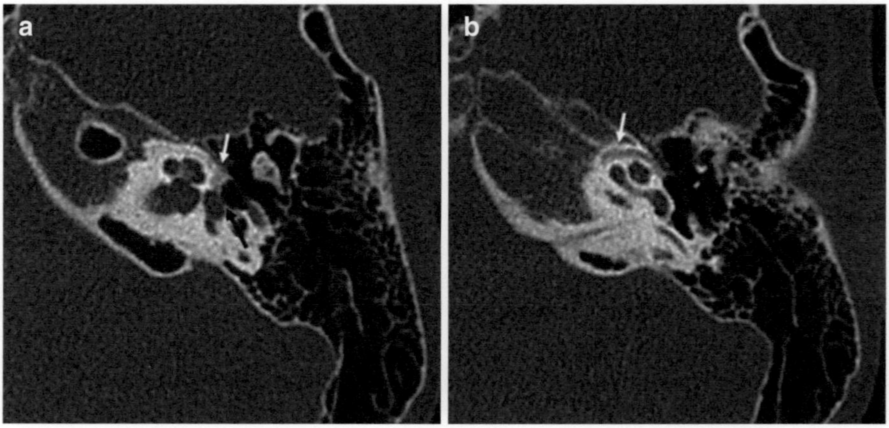

Fig. 1.66 Eight years- old girl with bilateral conductive hearing loss. Axial CT-images show: (**a**) a typical focus of prevestibular otosclerosis (*white arrow*), the footplate is thin (*black arrow*) (**b**) a typical pericochlear hypodense manifestation of otosclerosis (*arrow*), not coming into direct contact with the endosteum of the cochlea

disease may progress rapidly postoperatively to strangulate and immobilize the prosthesis, with resultant recurrent hearing loss, in a short period of time more rapidly than in adults. In such case a CT scan is helpful to decide a revision stapedotomy through a good counseling with the child and parents.

1.14 Far Advanced Otosclerosis

The term "*far-advanced otosclerosis*" was introduced by House and Sheehy in1961 to describe a clinical otosclerosis with an *air conduction level of 85 dB or greater* and non-measurable bone conduction levels [176]. Its incidence is about 1% of clinical otosclerosis. Lurato et al. proposed even the term *very far-advanced otosclerosis* for otosclerotic patients with non-measurable air and bone conduction thresholds on a standard clinical audiometer resulting in a blank audiogram (Fig. 1.67) [177].

In far advanced otosclerosis, several pericochlear foci may manifest as a "cavitating otosclerosis", (Fig. 1.68), as recently reported [178]. However, the pathophysiology of the formation of these cavities in the foci of pericochlear otosclerosis is not yet understood. Cavitating otosclerosis could be the cause of a third window phenomenon, CSF gusher during stapes surgery or cochlear implantaion, or lead to an electrode misplacement in cochlear implantation. Moreover, cochlear implant could be of limited benefit in cavitating otosclerosis due to diffusion of the electric signal away from the modiolus in the dimineralized and cavitatory otic capsule. In addition, it could be associated to an increased risk of complications such as facial stimulation, CSF leak, and electrode misplacement [178].

1.14.1 CT Imaging in Far Advanced Otosclerosis

As described above, the diagnosis of far advanced or even very far advanced otosclerosis is based on the audiometric parameters. However, high-resolution CT Imaging (Fig. 1.69) is a complementary tool that may show extended foci of

Clues to Diagnosis of Far Advanced Otosclerosis

- Positive family history of otosclerosis
- Onset of deafness in early childhood
- Gradual and fast progressive hearing loss
- Satisfied with hearing aid despite the important HL
- Schwartze sign could be found
- Response to 512 Hz tuning fork placed on the mastoid despite the blank audiogram

Fig. 1.67 Clues to diagnosis of far advanced otosclerosis

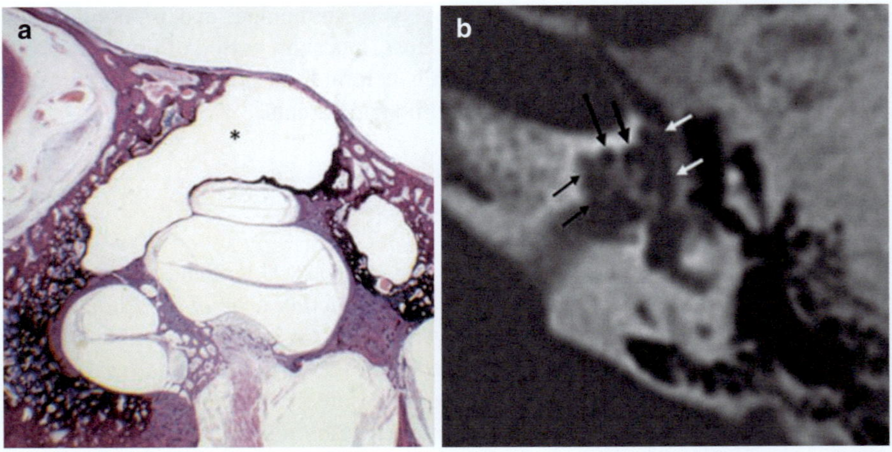

Fig. 1.68 (**a**) Histologic aspect of a cavitating otosclerosis focus (*) anterior to the cochlea and anterior to the stapes (**b**) axial CT-view of a left ear, showing a large hypodense rim of otosclerosis (white arrows) in close contact with the 2nd and apical turns of the cochlea (thick black arrows) and large otosclerotic hypodense focus (thin black arrows) in very close contact with the basal turn of the cochlea. The very low "water like" density of the foci on the CT-Scan is corresponding to the histological aspect of cavitations

otosclerosis which may correlate with the clinical presentations. CT may rule out a pure cochlear otosclerosis.

If cochlear implant is planned, CT-Imaging may indicate the presence of very low density foci around the cochlea that could represent a possible cavitating form (Fig. 1.68). CT-imaging may predict several surgical difficulties especially in advanced round window otosclerosis, when the otosclerotic foci cover extensively the whole round window region (Fig. 1.69a) rendering the surgical approach difficult, or calcifications are demonstrated of the round window or more extended behind the round window along the turns of the cochlea (Fig. 1.69b–d), that may represent a considerable difficulty to insert the implant deeply enough.

1.14.2 Management of Far Advanced Otosclerosis

A major controversy remains in the management of these patients. The treatment options include:

1. Stapes surgery as first option followed by Hearing Aid
2. Cochlear implant as first option versus stapedotomy.
3. Cochlear implant for cases of failure of improvement by previous measures

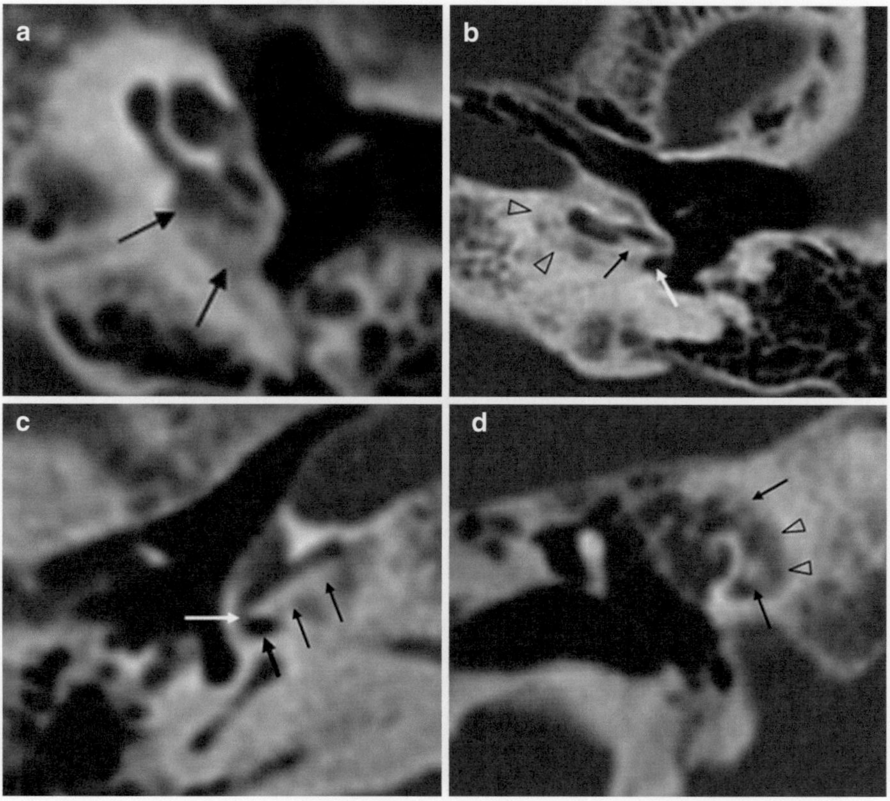

Fig. 1.69 Extensive otosclerotic foci (**a**) axial CT-image of a left ear: huge otosclerotic foci (black arrows) occupying the whole round window recess and the neighboring structures, all anatomic landmarks to reach the round window have disappeared (**b**) axial CT image of a left ear, showing a well aerated RW recess (white arrow), a complete calcification of the proximal part of the scala tympani behind the round window membrane (black arrow), diffuse otosclerotic foci around the basal turn of the cochlea (arrowheads), (**c**) axial CT image of a right ear: the scala tympani (black arrows) is completely calcified, the round window (white arrow) is well delineated by a well aerated recess (thick black arrow) (**d**) coronal CT-image of a right ear, the cochlea shows spotty calcifications (black arrows) at several points of the cochlea turns in addition to an extensive pericochlear otosclerotic rim (arrowheads), that is not delimitable from the cochlea

1.14.2.1 Stapedotomy in Far Advanced Otosclerosis

Some patients with far advanced otosclerosis may benefit from stapes surgery in achieving a level of hearing that can be rehabilitated with a powerful hearing aid.

In 1996, Glasscock et al. showed that stapedectomy was effective in 60% of patients with far-advanced otosclerosis [179]. However it is clear that it is very hard to predict the outcome of a stapedotomy in patients with severe to profound mixed hearing loss [180–182]. There is higher risk of failure of stapedotomy among patients with very far advanced otosclerosis with non measurable air and bone conduction thresholds and 0% discrimination where the chances of stapedotomy success do not exceed 30% [183].

Despite the fact that stapedotomy outcome is unpredictable in FAO, it should be attempted before considering CI. Acoustic stimulation through hearing aids, when effective, provides better overall sound quality [180].

In Far Advanced Otosclerosis, stapedotomy, when successful, may offer several important advantages over cochlear implant: It is less expensive and less complex. After stapedotomy, only a fitting with a hearing aid is required, whereas CI is followed by an intensive rehabilitation program. The quality of the sound is more natural after stapedotomy/hearing aid and the appreciation of music seems to be better perceived.

It is of interest to consider that the classical standard criteria for measuring the success of a stapedotomy in fenestral otosclerosis (closure of the air-bone gap to 10 dB or less) are not applicable for patients with FAO, because in the latter bone conduction levels are often not measurable even postoperatively. Although several criteria have been proposed for a correct definition of the success of stapedectomy in FAO: the more accurate definition of stapedotomy success in FAO is considered when the Word Recognition Score (WRS) greater than 50% is achieved with a well-fitted ipsilateral hearing aid [182–186]. When obtained, these results exclude the patient from the range of cochlear implant candidacy. If the first stapedotomy was successful, a consecutive contralateral stapedotomy can offer the benefits of binaural rehabilitation [180].

Nevertheless when a unilateral stapedotomy followed by hearing aid does not give a satisfactory outcome as defined above, a contralateral stapedotomy can be performed before proceeding to cochlear implantation.

In case a stapedectomy/hearing aid fails to help these patients, as explained above, they remain good candidates for cochlear implants [61]. The challenge in FAO rehabilitation is to know preoperatively which patients will not benefit from acoustic stimulation (even with bilateral stapedotomy) so to proceed directly to cochlear implantation [187–189].

1.14.2.2 Cochlear Implant in Far Advanced Otosclerosis

During the last decades, numerous studies have evaluated CI as a treatment for patients affected by FAO [96, 190, 191]. Although there is an evidence of reduction of neural tissue in patients with advanced otosclerosis, implanted patients with advanced otosclerosis present excellent discrimination; this is due to the memory of language in post lingual adults. Patients with FAO demonstrate mean Speech Recognition Scores of 54–75% after CI [96, 192–194].

However, CI is not without difficulties and sometimes disappointing:

- Otosclerotic bone formation around the round window requires extra drilling. Intracochlear osteoneogenesis might result in a difficult or only partial electrode insertion with frustrating results.

- Pericochlear confluent otospongiosis lesions around the cochlea (cavitating otosclerosis) could disperse the current easily, acting as a shunt away from the modiolus, and cause lesser pitch and timber definition [96, 190, 191]. This leads to a poor music appreciation, poor melody perception, and worse discrimination in loud environments [195].
- Non-Auditory stimulations were reported to be more common in patients with FAO after cochlear implantation, these include: facial nerve stimulation, pain in the ear from tympanic plexus stimulation, and dizziness from stimulation of vestibular structures.
- Even after a successful implantation, the rehabilitation of patients with otosclerosis is challenging because progressive otosclerotic changes in the cochlea can affect the performance of the implant. Reprogramming with higher stimulus levels might be required to obtain auditory responses [196].
- It remains that Cochlear Implants are financially costful and not easily available in all countries.

Moreover patients with bilateral FAO who previously have received a unilateral CI may still benefit from a contralateral stapedotomy because this can restore binaural hearing by means of bimodal stimulation [197] .

Conclusion

For multiple reasons, otosclerosis implies nowadays correct investigation measures before any designed therapeutical approach. CT-Imaging represents, together with the advanced audiometric tests, an indispensable preoperative work up and must provide the adequate medical and medico legal documentation. Stapes surgery in otosclerosis represents the most successful functional middle ear surgery with more than 95% of positive results. In contrary, failure of the surgery is very frustrating for the patient as well as for the surgeon. In addition to the required surgical expertise, the improved technique and better available prosthesis, the postoperative results are expected to be now of excellent outcome with less unfavorable events than before. It remains that stapedotomy is not the end point of the management of otosclerosis, but the disease needs a long term follow up to recognize its unpredictable dynamic evolution.

Advances in implant surgery may answer positively some of the frustrating and dramatic situations in otosclerotic patients especially in far advanced otosclerosis.

More advances in genetic research and secondary clinical therapeutical applications are awaited for better control of the disease.

References

1. Politzer A. Über primäre Erkrankung der knöchernen Labyrinthkapsel. Z Ohrenheilkd. 1894;25:309.
2. Politzer A. Diseases of the ear. London: Bailliere; 1909.

3. Schuknecht HF, Barber W. Histologic variants in otosclerosis. Laryngoscope. 1985;95:1307-17.
4. Shambaugh GE. Fenestration operation for otosclerosis. Acta Otolaryngol Suppl. 1949;79:1–15.
5. Arnold W, Friedmann I. Presence of viral specific antigens (measles, rubella) around the active otosclerotic focus. Ann Otol Rhinol Laryngol. 1987;66:167–71.
6. Konigsmark BW, Gorlin RJ. Genetic and metabolic deafness. Philadelphia, PA: W.B. Saunders; 1976.
7. Guild SR. Histologic otosclerosis. Ann Otol Rhinol Laryngol. 1944;53:246–67.
8. Schuknecht HF, Kirchner JC. Cochlear otosclerosis: fact or fantasy. ? Laryngoscope. 1974;84:766–82.
9. Engström H. On the frequency of otosclerosis. Acta Otolaryngol. 1939;27:608–14.
10. Weber M. Otosklerose und Umbau der Labyrinthkapsel. Leipzig: Poeschel and Trepte; 1935.
11. Jørgensen MB, Kristensen HK. Activity of otosclerosis assessed histologically. J Laryngol Otol. 1967;81:911–4.
12. Hueb MM, Goycoolea MV, Paparella MM, Oliveira JA. Otosclerosis: the University of Minnesota temporal bone collection. Otolaryngol Head Neck Surg. 1991;105:396–405.
13. Yagi T. Incidence and characteristics of otosclerosis in the Japanese population. Auris Nasus Larynx. 2002;29:257–60.
14. Ohtani I, Baba Y, Suzuki T, Suzuki C, Kano M, Deka RC. Why is otosclerosis of low prevalence in Japanese? Otol Neurotol. 2003;24:377–81.
15. Kapur YP, Patt AJ. Otosclerosis in South India. Acta Otolaryngol. 1966;61:353–60.
16. Jahn AF, Vernick D. Otosclerosis: diagnosis and treatment. SIPAC. Am Acad Otolaryngol Head Neck Surg. 1986:12–20.
17. Jørgensen MB, Kristensen KH. Frequency of histologic otosclerosis. Ann Otol Rhinol Laryngol. 1967;76:83–8.
18. Altmann F, Glasgold A, Macduff JP. The incidence of otosclerosis as related to race and sex. Ann Otol Rhinol Laryngol. 1967;76:377–92.
19. Tshifularo MI, Joseph CA. Otosclerosis among south African indigenous blacks. East Afr Med J. 2005;82:223–5.
20. Davenport C, Milles B, Frink L. The genetic factor in otosclerosis. Arch Otolaryngol. 1933;17:135–70.
21. Cawthorne T. Otosclerosis. J Laryngol Otol. 1955;69:437–56.
22. Morrison AW. Genetic factors in otosclerosis. Ann R Coll Surg Eng. 1967;41:202–37.
23. Hall JG. Otosclerosis in Norway. A geographical and genetical study. Acta Otolaryngol Suppl. 1974;324:1–20.
24. Pearson RD, Kurland LT, Cody DTR. Incidence of diagnosed clinical otosclerosis. Arch Otolaryngol. 1974;99:288–91.
25. Gapany-Gapanavicius B. Otosclerosis: genetics and surgical rehabilitation. New York: Halsted Press; 1975.
26. Cawthorne T. Otosclerosis. J Laryngol Otol. 1955;9:437–56.
27. Uzicanin A, Eggers R, Webb E, Harris B, Durrheim D, Ogunbanjo G, Isaacs V, Hawkridge A, Biellik R, Strebel P. Impact of the 1996–1997 supplementary measles vaccination campaigns in South Africa. Int J Epidemiol. 2002;31:968–76.
28. Lippy WH, Berenholz LP, Burkey JM. Otosclerosis in the 1960s, 1970s, 1980s, and 1990s. Laryngoscope. 1999;109:1307–9.
29. Kos CM. Stapedectomy—experiences with drill-out and vein plug prosthesis. Laryngoscope. 1970;80:1272–80.
30. Declau F, van de Heyning P. Genetics of otosclerosis: state of the art. In Martini A, Stephens S (Eds.), Hereditary deafness. London: Willey, 1996, pp 221–231.
31. Zehnder AF, Kristiansen AG, Adams JC, Kujawa SG, Merchant SN, McKenna MJ. Osteoprotegrin knockout mouse demonstrate abnormal remodeling of the otic capsule and progressive hearing loss. Laryngoscope. 2006;116:201–6.
32. Kanzaki S, Ito M, Takada Y, Ogawa K, Matsuo K. Resorption of auditory ossicles and hearing loss in mice lacking osteoprotegerin. Bone. 2006;39:414–9.
33. Hirose S, Li M, Kojima T, de Freitas PH, Ubaidus S, Oda K, et al. A histological assessment on the distribution of osteocytic lacunar canalicular system using silver staining. J Bone Miner Metab. 2007;25:374–82.

34. McKenna MJ, Mills BG, Galey FR, Linthicum FH Jr. Filamentous structures morphologically similar to viral nucleocapsids in otosclerotic lesions in two patients. Am J Otol. 1986;7:25–8.
35. Arnold W, Altermatt HJ, Kraft R, Pfaltz CR. Otosclerosis. A paramyxovirus-induced inflammatory reaction. HNO. 1989;37:236–41.
36. Niedermeyer HP, Gantumur T, Neubert WJ, Arnold W. Measles virus and otosclerosis. Adv Otorhinolaryngol. 2007;65:86–92.
37. Horner KC. The effect of sex hormones on bone metabolism of the otic capsule—an overview. Hear Res. 2009;252:56–60.
38. Sørensen MS, Jørgensen MB, Bretlau P. Drift barriers in the postcartilaginous development of the mammalian otic capsule. Eur Arch Otorhinolaryngol. 1992;249:56–61.
39. Iyer PV, Gristwood RE. Histopathology of the stapes in otosclerosis. Pathology. 1984;16:30–8.
40. Thys M, Schrauwen I, Vanderstraeten K, Dieltjens N, Fransen E, Ealy M, Cremers CW, van de Heyning P, Vincent R, Offeciers E, Smith RH, van Camp G. Detection of rare nonsynonymous variants in TGFB1 in otosclerosis patients. Ann Hum Genet. 2009;73:171–5.
41. Ealy ML. Otosclerosis – identifying genetic contributions to a complex hearing disorder. PhD thesis, University of Iowa; 2011.
42. McKenna MJ, Kristiansen AG, Tropitzsch AS. Similar COLA1 expression in fibroblasts from some patients with clinical otosclerosis and those with type I osteogenesis imperfecta. Ann Otol Rhinol Laryngol. 2002;111:184–9.
43. Moumoulidis I, Axon P, Baguley D, Reid EA. Review on the genetics of otosclerosis. Clin Otolaryngol. 2007;32:239–47.
44. Markou K, Goudakos J. An overview of the etiology of otosclerosis. Eur Arch Otorhinolaryngol. 2009;266:25–35.
45. Sabitha R, Ramalingam R, Ramalingam KK, Sivakumaran TA, Ramesh A. Genetics of otosclerosis. J Laryngol Otol. 1997;111:109–12.
46. Ealy M, Chen W, Ryu GY, Yoon JG, Welling DB, Hansen M, Madan A, Smith RJ. Gene expression analysis of human otosclerotic stapedial footplates. Hear Res. 2008;240:80–6.
47. Thys M, Van Camp G. Genetics of otosclerosis. Otol Neurotol. 2009;30(8):1021–32.
48. Arnold W, Niedermeyer HP, Lehn N, Neubert W, Höfler H. Measles virus in otosclerosis and the specific immune response of the inner ear. Acta Otolaryngol. 1996;116(5):705–9.
49. Karosi T, Jókay I, Kónya J, Petkó M, Szabó LZ, Sziklai I. Expression of measles virus receptors in otosclerotic, non-otosclerotic and in normal stapes footplates. Eur Arch Otorhinolaryngol. 2007;264:607–13.
50. Vrabec JT, Coker NJ. Stapes surgery in the United States. Otol Neurotol. 2004;25:465–9.
51. Arnold W, Busch R, Arnold A, Ritsher B, Neiss A, Niedermeyer HP. The influence of measles vaccination on the incidence of otosclerosis in Germany. Eur Arch Otorhinolaryngol. 2007;264:741–8.
52. Niedermeyer HP, Arnold W. Otosclerosis: a measles virus associated inflammatory disease. Acta Otolaryngol. 1995;115:300–3.
53. Lolov SR, Encheva VI, Kyurkchiev SD, Edrev GE, Kehayov IR. Antimeasles immunoglobulin G in sera of patients with otosclerosis is lower than that in healthy people. Otol Neurotol. 2001;22:766–70.
54. Precechtel A. Determination of the effect of pregnancy on the activation of otosclerosis. Acta Otolaryngol. 1967;63:121–7.
55. Gristwood RE, Venables WN. Pregnancy and otosclerosis. Clin Otolaryngol Allied Sci. 1983;8:205–10.
56. Grayeli AB, Sterkers O, Roulleau P, Elbaz P, Ferrary E, Silve C. Parathyroid hormone-parathyroid hormone-related peptide receptor expression and function in otosclerosis. Am J Phys. 1999;277:1005–12.
57. Yoo TJ. Etiopathogenesis of otosclerosis: a hypothesis. Ann Otol Rhinol Laryngol. 1984;93:28–33.
58. Cureoglu S, Schachern PA, Ferlito A, Rinaldo A, Tsuprun V, Paparella MM. Otosclerosis: etiopathogenesis and histopathology. Am J Otolaryngol. 2006;27(5):334–40.
59. Valvassori GE. Imaging of otosclerosis. Otolaryngol Clin N Am. 1993;26:359–71.
60. Mansour S, Nicolas K, Ahmad HH. Round window otosclerosis: radiologic classification and clinical correlations. Otol Neurotol. 2011;32:384–92.

61. van Loon MC, Merkus P, Smit CF, Smits C, Witte BI, Hensen EF. Stapedotomy in cochlear implant candidates with far advanced otosclerosis: a systematic review of the literature and meta-analysis. Otol Neurotol. 2014;35(10):1707–14.
62. Gristwood RE, Venables WN. Otosclerosis and chronic tinnitus. Ann Otol Rhinol Laryngol. 2003;112:398–403.
63. Szymański W, Gołabek R. Mills effect of stapedectomy on subjective tinnitus. J Laryngol Otol. 2003;117:261–4.
64. Tsai BS, Sweetow RW, Cheung SW. Audiometric asymmetry and tinnitus laterality. Laryngoscope. 2012;122:1148Y53.
65. Causse JB, Vincent R. Poor vibration of inner ear fluids as a cause of low tone tinnitus. Am J Otol. 1995;16:701–2.
66. Hulk J, Jongkees LBW. Vestibular examination in cases of otosclerosis. J Laryngol Otol Rhinol. 1950;64:126.
67. Sando I, Hemenway WG, Miller DR, Black FO. Vestibular pathology in otosclerosis temporal bone histopathological report. Laryngoscope. 1974;84:593Y605.
68. Pauw BK, Pollak AM, Fisch U. Utricle, saccule, and cochlear duct in relation to stapedotomy. A histologic human temporal bone study. Ann Otol Rhinol Laryngol. 1991;100:966Y70.
69. Menger DJ, Tange RA. The aetiology of otosclerosis: a review of the literature. Clin Otolaryngol Allied Sci. 2003;28:112–20.
70. Yoon TH, Paparella MM, Schachern PA. Otosclerosis involving the vestibular aqueduct and Meniere's disease. Otolaryngol Head and Neck Surg. 1990;103(1):107–13.
71. Black FO, Sando I, Hildyard VH, Hemenway WG. Bilateral multiple otosclerotic foci and endolymphatic hydrops. Ann Otol Rhinol Laryngol. 1969;78:1062–73.
72. Paparella MM, Chasin WD. Otosclerosis and vertigo. J Laryngol Otol. 1966;80:511–9.
73. Shea JJ, Ge X, Orchik DJ. Endolymphatic hydrops associated with otosclerosis. Am J Otol. 1994;15:348–57.
74. Johnsson LG, Hawkins JE, Rouse RC, Linthicum FH. Cochlear and otoconial abnormalities in capsular otosclerosis with hydrops. Ann Otol Rhinol Laryngol. 1982;91:3–15.
75. Liston SL, Paparella MM, Mancini F, Anderson JH. Otosclerosis and endolymphatic hydrops. Laryngoscope. 1984;94:1003–7.
76. Seo T, Node M, Miyamoto A, Yukimasa A, Terada T, Sakagami M. Three cases of cochleosaccular endolymphatic hydrops without vertigo revealed by furosemide-loading vestibular evoked myogenic potential test. Otol Neurotol. 2003;24:807–11.
77. Hannley MT. Audiologic characteristics of the patient with otosclerosis. Otolaryngol Clin North Am. 1993;26(3):373–87.
78. Tondorf JA. New concept of bone conduction. Arch Otolaryngol. 1968;87:595–600.
79. Freeman S, Sichel JY, Sohmer H. Bone conduction experiments in animals—evidence for a non-osseous mechanism. Hear Res. 2000;146:72–80.
80. Sohmer H, Freeman S, Geal-Dor M, et al. Bone conduction experiments in humans-a fluid pathway from bone to ear. Hear Res. 2000;146:81–8.
81. Bel J, Causse J, Michaux P, Cézard R, Canut Y, Tapon J. Mechanical explanation of the on-off effect (diphasic impedance change) in otospongiosis. Audiology. 1976;15(2):128–40.
82. Huber AM, Schwab C, Linder T, Stoeckli SJ, Ferrazzini M, Dillier N, Fisch U. Evaluation of ear drum laser Doppler interferometry as a diagnostic tool. Laryngoscope. 2001;111:501–7.
83. Rosowski JJ, Mehta RP, Merchant SN. Diagnostic utility of laser-Doppler vibrometry in conductive hearing loss with normal tympanic membrane. Otol Neurotol. 2003;24:165–75.
84. Jakob A, Bornitz M, Kuhlisch E, Zahnert T. New aspects in the clinical diagnosis of otosclerosis using laser doppler vibrometry. Otol Neurotol. 2009;30:1049Y1057.
85. Shin YJ, Deguine O, Cognard C, Sévely A, Manelfe C, Fraysse B. Reliability of CT scan in the diagnosis of conductive hearing loss with normal tympanic membrane. Rev Laryngol Otol Rhinol (Bord). 2001;122(2):81–4.
86. Lagleyre S, Sorrentino T, Calmels MN, Shin YJ, Escudé B, Deguine O, Fraysse B. Reliability of high-resolution CT scan in diagnosis of otosclerosis. Otol Neurotol. 2009;30(8):1152–9.

87. Ariadna M, Cozma S, Murariu O, Radulescu L, Haba MSC, Vreme RM, Haba D, Iasi/RO. ECR 2017 Diagnostic value of CBCT in otosclerosis Poster No 2283; 2017.
88. Redfors YD, Gröndahl HG, Hellgren J, Lindfors N, Nilsson I, Möller C. Otosclerosis: anatomy and pathology in the temporal bone assessed by multi-slice and cone-beam CT. Otol Neurotol. 2012;33(6):922–7.
89. Révész P, Liktor B, Liktor B, Sziklai I, Gerlinger I, Karosi T. Comparative analysis of preoperative diagnostic values of HRCT and CBCT in patients with histologically diagnosed otosclerotic stapes footplates. Eur Arch Otorhinolaryngol. 2016;273(1):63–72.
90. Kawase S, Naganawa S, Sone M, Ikeda M, Ishigaki T. Relationship between CT densitometry with a slice thickness of 0.5 mm and audiometry in otosclerosis. Eur Radiol. 2006;16:1367–73.
91. Yamashita K, Yoshiura T, Hiwatashi A, Togao O, Kikuchi K, Inoguchi T, Kumazawa S, Honda H. The radiological diagnosis of fenestral otosclerosis: the utility of histogram analysis using multidetector row CT. Eur Arch Otorhinolaryngol. 2014;271(12):3277–82.
92. Magnan J, Bremond G, Chays A, et al. Otosclerosis surgery: identical results for different techniques. Why? pp. 217–22. Édited by Sacristan T, Alvarez-Vicent J, Antoli-Candela F. Proceedings of XIV world congress of ORL Madrid, 1990 Kugler& Ghedini Publications. Amsterdam, Berkeley, Milano Density measurements reflect the progress of the disease process.
93. Veillon F, Stierle JL, Dussaix J, et al. Otosclerosis imaging: matching clinical and imaging data. J Radiol. 2006;87:1756–64.
94. Craighero F, Van Driessche V, Van Dinther J, Offeciers EF, De Foer B, Verstraete K, Casselman JW. Valeur de l'hypodensité préméatique interne (HPMI) dans l'otospongiose. JFR. 2011.
95. Dudau C, Salim F, Jiang D, Connor ST. Diagnostic efficacy and therapeutic impact of computed tomography in the evaluation of clinically suspected otosclerosis. Eur Radiol. 2017;27(3):1195–201.
96. Marshall AH, Fanning N, Symons S, Shipp D, Chen JM, Nedzelski JM. Cochlear implantation in cochlear otosclerosis. Laryngoscope. 2005;115:1728–33.
97. Veillon F, Casselman JV, Meriot P, Cahen-Riehm S, Sick H. Imagerie de l'oreille et de l'os temporal. Paris: Medecine Sciences Publications; 2013.
98. Ukkola-Pons E, Ayache D, Pons Y, Ratajczak M, Nioche C, Williams M. Oval window niche height: quantitative evaluation with CT before stapes surgery for otosclerosis. AJNR Am J Neuroradiol. 2013;34:1082–5.
99. Parra C, Trunet S, Granger B, Nguyen Y, Lamas G, Bernardeschi D, Hervochon R, Tankere F. Imaging criteria to predict surgical difficulties during stapes surgery. Otol Neurotol. 2017;38(6):815–21. https://doi.org/10.1097/MAO.0000000000001417.
100. Mansour S, Magnan J, Haidar H, et al. Comprehensive and clinical anatomy of the middle ear. Berlin/Heidelberg: Springer; 2013. p. 68–71.
101. Sugimoto H, Ito M, Hatano M, Yoshizaki T. Persistent stapedial artery with stapes ankylosis. Auris Nasus Larynx. 2014;41(6):582–5.
102. Hüttenbrink K-B. Biomechanics of middle ear reconstruction. Laryngol Rhinol Otol. 2000;79(Suppl 2):23–51.
103. Rosowski JJ, Merchant SN. Mechanical and acoustic analysis of middle ear reconstruction. Am J Otol. 1995;16:486–97.
104. Dancer A, Franke R. Biomechanics of the middle ear [in French]. Rev Laryngol Otol Rhinol. 1995;116:5–12.
105. Wegner I, Bittermann AJ, Zinsmeester MM, van der Heijden GJ, Grolman W. Local versus general anesthesia in stapes surgery for otosclerosis: a systematic reviewof the evidence. Otolaryngol Head Neck Surg. 2013;149(3):360–5.
106. Iannella G, Magliulo G. Endoscopic versus microscopic approach in stapes surgery: are operative times and learning curve important for making the choice? Otol Neurotol. 2016;37(9):1350–7.

107. Dundar R, Bulut H, Güler OK, Yükkaldiran A, Demirtaş Y, Iynen I, Bozkuş F, Kulduk E. Oval window temperature changes in an endoscopic Stapedectomy. J Craniofac Surg. 2015;26(5):1704–8.
108. Fisch U. Stapedotomy versus stapedectomy. Otol Neurotol. 2009;30(8):1166–7.
109. Bailey HA Jr, Pappas JJ, Graham SS. Small fenestra stapedectomy technique: reducing risk and improving hearing. Otolaryngol Head Neck Surg. 1983;91:516–20.
110. Cremers CW, Beusen JM, Huygen PL. Hearing gain after stapedotomy, partial platinectomy, or total stapedectomy for otosclerosis. Ann Otol Rhinol Laryngol. 1991;100:959–61.
111. Spandow O, Soderberg O, Bohlin L. Long-term results in otosclerotic patients operated by stapedectomy and stapedotomy. Scand Audiol. 2000;29:186–90.
112. Kos MI, Montandon PB, Guyot JP. Short- and long-term results of stapedotomy and stapedectomy with a Teflon-wire piston prosthesis. Ann Otol Rhinol Laryngol. 2001;110:907–11.
113. Persson P, Harder H, Magnuson B. Hearing results in otosclerosis surgery after partial stapedectomy, total stapedectomy and stapedotomy. Acta Otolaryngol. 1997;117:94–9.
114. Fisch U. Stapedectomy versus stapedectomy. Am J Otol. 1982;4:112–7.
115. Esquivel CR, Mamikoglu B, Wiet RJ. Long-term results of small fenestra stapedectomy compared with large fenestra technique. Laryngoscope. 2002;112:1338–41.
116. House HP, Hansen MR, Al Dakhail AAA, House JW. Stapedectomy versus stapedotomy: comparison of results with long-term follow-up. Laryngoscope. 2002;112:2046–50.
117. Aarnisalo AA, Vasama J-P, Hopsu E, Ramsay H. Long-term hearing results after stapes surgery. A 20-year follow-up. Otol Neurotol. 2003;24:567–71.
118. Escudero LH, Castro AO, Drummond M, et al. Argon laser in human tympanoplasty. Arch Otolaryngol. 1979;105:252–3.
119. Palva T. Argon laser in otosclerosis surgery. Acta Otolaryngol. 1979;104:153–7.
120. Perkins RC. Laser stapedotomy for otosclerosis. Laryngoscope. 1980;90:228–41.
121. Young E, Mitchell-Innes A, Jindal M. Lasers in stapes surgery: a review. J Laryngol Otol. 2015;129(7):627–33.
122. Wegner I, Kamalski DM, Tange RA, Vincent R, Stegeman I, van der Heijden GJ, Grolman W. Laser versus conventional fenestration in stapedotomy for otosclerosis: a systematic review. Laryngoscope. 2014;124(7):1687–93.
123. Silverstein H. Laser stapedotomy minus prosthesis (laser STAMP): a minimally invasive procedure. Am J Otol. 1998;19:277–82.
124. Yavuz H, Caylakli F, Ozer F, Ozluoglu LN. Reliability of microdrill stapedotomy: comparison with pick stapedotomy. Otol Neurotol. 2007;28(8):998–1001.
125. Gjuric M. Microdrill versus perforator for stapedotomy. Clin Otolaryngol Allied Sci. 1990;15:411Y3.
126. Wengen DF. A new self-retaining titanium clip stapes prosthesis. Adv Otorhinolaryngol. 2007;65:184–9.
127. Laske RD, Röösli C, Chatzimichalis MV, Sim JH, Huber AM. The influence of prosthesis diameter in stapes surgery: a meta-analysis and systematic review of the literature. Otol Neurotol. 2011;32(4):520–8.
128. Mann W, Beck C. Functional results of stapes surgery. Laryngol Rhinol Otol (Stuttg). 1983;62:387Y90.
129. Teig E, Lindeman HH. Stapedotomy piston diameter: is bigger better? Otorhinolaryngol Nova. 1999;9:253Y7.
130. Böheim K, Nahler A, Schlögel H, Filzmoser P. Ergebnisse mit Goldpistons bei der Stapedektomie mit kleiner Fensterung. Otorhinolaryngol Nova. 1997;7:235Y40.
131. Huber AM, Ma F, Felix H, Linder T. Stapes prosthesis attachment: the effect of crimping on sound transfer in otosclerosis surgery. Laryngoscope. 2003;113:853–8.
132. Wegner I, Swartz JE, Bance ML, Grolman W. A systematic review of the effect of different crimping techniques in stapes surgery for otosclerosis. Laryngoscope. 2016; 126(5):1207–17.
133. Ludman H, Grant H. The case against bilateral stapedectomy, and problems of postoperative follow-up from the King's college hospital series. J Laryngol Otol. 1973;87:833–43.

134. Smyth GDL, Kerr AG, Singh KP. Second ear stapedectomy-a continued controversy. J Laryngol Otol. 1975;89:1047–56.
135. Vincent R, Sperling NM, Oates J, Jindal M. Surgical findings and long-term hearing results in 3050 Stapedotomies for primary otosclerosis: a prospective study with the otology-neurotology database. Otol Neurotol. 2006;27:S25–47.
136. Powers WH, Sheehy JL, House HP. The fixed malleus head. A report of 35 cases. Arch Otolaryngol. 1967;85:177–81.
137. Lippy WH, Schuring AG, Ziv M. Stapedectomy for otosclerosis with malleus fixation. Arch Otolaryngol. 1978;104:388–9.
138. Causse J, Causse JB. Eighteen-year report on stapedectomy. I: Problems of stapedial fixation. Clin Otolaryngol 1980;5:49-59.
139. Covell WP, Feinmesser M. Further studies on the pathology of ossicles in otosclerosis. Laryngoscope. 1959;69:164-73.
140. Moon CN Jr, Hahn MJ. Primary malleus fixation: diagnosis and treatment. Laryngoscope 1981;91:1298-307.
141. House HP. Diagnostic aspects of congenital ossicular fixation. Trans Am Acad Ophthalmol Otolaryngol. 1956;60:787–90.
142. Hilding DA. Postinflammatory fixation of the malleus. Its surgical correction. Arch Otolaryngol. 1965;81:17–9.
143. Nandapalan V, Pollak A, Langner A, et al. The anterior and superior malleal ligaments in otosclerosis: a histopathologic observation. Otol Neurotol. 2002;23:854–61.
144. Huber A, Koike T, Wada H, et al. Fixation of the anterior mallear ligament: diagnosis and consequences for hearing results in stapes surgery. Ann Otol Rhinol Laryngol. 2003;112:348–55.
145. Obliterative Otosclerosis. Tympanoplasty, mastoidectomy, and stapes surgery, by Ugo Fisch et al., Thieme, 2008.
146. Ayache D, Sleiman J, Plouin-Gaudon I, Klap P, Elbaz P. Obliterative otosclerosis. J Laryngol Otol. 1999;113(6):512–4.
147. Amedee RG, Lewis ML Jr. Obliterative otosclerosis. Laryngoscope. 1987;97(8 Pt 1):922–4.
148. Gierek T, Witkowska M, Zbrowska-Bielska D, Klimczak-Gołab L. Analysis of results of stapedotomy in patients with obliterative otosclerosis. Otolaryngol Pol. 2006;60(3):377–83.
149. Shea JJ Jr. Forty years of stapes surgery. Am J Otol. 1998;19:52–5.
150. Karhuketo TS, Lundmark J, Vanhatalo J, Rautiainen M, Sipilä M. Stapes surgery: a 32-year follow-up. ORL. 2007;69:322–6.
151. Oliveira CA. How does stapes surgery influence severe disabling tinnitus in otosclerosis patients? Adv Otorhinolaryngol. 2007;65:343–7.
152. Gersdorff M, Nouwen J, Gilain C, Decat M, Betsch C. Tinnitus and otsclerosis. Eur Arch Otorhinolaryngol. 2000;257:314–6.
153. Ayache D, Earally F, Elbaz P. Characteristic and postoperative course of tinnitus in otosclerosis. Otol Neurotol. 2003;24:48–51.
154. Berling Holm K, Knutsson J, Strömbäck K, Danckwardt Lillieström N, Papatziamos G, Rosenblad A, Von Unge M. Taste disturbance after stapes surgery: an evaluation of frequency, severity, duration, and quality-of-life. Acta Otolaryngol. 2017;137(1):39–43.
155. Mahendran S, Hogg R, Robinson JM. To divide or manipulate the chorda tympani in stapedotomy. Eur Arch Otorhinolaryngol. 2005;262:482–7.
156. Birch L, Elbrond O. Stapedectomy and vertigo. Clin Otolaryngol. 1985;10:217–23.
157. Wang ZM, Chi FL, Dai CF. Modified stapes prosthesis to limit postoperative vertigo. Otolaryngol Head Neck Surg. 2005;132:50–4.
158. Singbartl F, Basta D, Seidl RO, Ernst A, Todt I. Perioperative recordings of vestibularevoked myogenic potentials in otosclerosis. Otol Neurotol. 2006;27:1070–3.
159. Stapleton E, Mills R, Tham C. Sacculo-collic response in otosclerosis and following successful stapes surgery. J Laryngol Otol. 2008;122:347–50.
160. Mansour S, Magnan J, Haidar H, et al. Comprehensive and clinical anatomy of the middle ear. Berlin/Heidelberg: Springer; 2013. p. 49–81.
161. Glasscock ME III, Storper IS, Haynes DS, Bohrer PS. Twenty-five years of experience with stapedectomy. Laryngoscope. 1995;105:899–904.

162. Seicshnaydre MA, Sismanis A, Hughes GB. Update of reparative granuloma: survey of the American Otological Society and the American Neurotology Society. Am J Otol. 1994;15:155–60.
163. Ozgirgin N. The problems encountered during stapes surgery and their solutions. Balkan J Otol Neuro-Otol. 2004;4(1):23–7.
164. Nadol JB Jr. Histopathology of residual and recurrent conductive hearing loss after stapedectomy. Otol Neurotol. 2001;22(2):162–9.
165. Lesinski GS. Causes of conductive hearing loss after stapedectomy or stapedotomy: a prospective study of 279 consecutive surgical revision. Otol Neurotol. 2002;23:281–8.
166. Lippy WH, Battista RA, Berenholz L, Schuring AG, Burkey JM. Twenty-year review of revision stapedectomy. Otol Neurotol. 2003;24:560–6.
167. Meyer TA, Lambert PR. Primary and revision stapedectomy in elderly patients. Curr Opin Otolaryngol Head Neck Surg. 2004;12:387–92.
168. Sheehy JL, Nelson RA, House HP. Revision stapedectomy: a review of 258 cases. Laryngoscope. 1981;91:43–51.
169. Venail F, Lavieille JP, Meller R, Deveze A, Tardivet L, Magnan J. New perspectives for middle ear implants: first results in otosclerosis with mixed hearing loss. Laryngoscope. 2007;117(3):552–5.
170. Martin C, Deveze A, Richard C, Lefebvre PP, Decat M, Ibañez LG, Truy E, Mom T, Lavieille JP, Magnan J, Dubreuil C, Tringali S. European results with totally implantable carina placed on the round window: 2-year follow-up. Otol Neurotol. 2009;30(8):1196–203.
171. Vincent R, Sperling NM, Oates J, Jindal M. Surgical findings and longterm hearing results in 3,050 stapedotomies for primary otosclerosis: a prospective study with the otology–neurotology database. Otol Neurotol. 2006;27:S25–47.
172. Vincent R, Wegner I, Vonck BM, Bittermann AJ, Kamalski DM, Grolman W. Primary stapedotomy in children with otosclerosis: a prospective study of 41 consecutive cases. Laryngoscope. 2016;126(2):442–6.
173. An YS, Lee KS. The surgical results of stapes fixation in children. Int J Pediatr Otorhinolaryngol. 2014;78:55–9.
174. Bachor E, Just T, Wright CG, Pau HW, Karmody CS. Fixation of the stapes footplate in children: a clinical and temporal bone histopathologic study. Otol Neurotol. 2005;26:866–73.
175. Carlson ML, van Abel KM, Pelosi S, et al. Outcomes comparing primary pediatric stapedectomy for congenital stapes footplate fixation and juvenile otosclerosis. Otol Neurotol. 2013;34:816–20.
176. House HP, Sheehy JL. Stapes surgery: selection of the patient. Ann Otol Rhinol Laryngol. 1961;70:1062–8.
177. Lurato S, Ettorre GC, Onofri M, Davidson C. Very faradvanced otosclerosis. Am J Otol. 1992;13:4827.
178. Makarem AO, Hoang TA, Lo WW, Linthicum FH Jr, Fayad JN. Cavitating otosclerosis: clinical, radiologic, and histopathologic correlations. Otol Neurotol. 2010;31(3):381–4.
179. Glasscock ME, Storper IS, Bigelow DC. Management of far advanced otosclerosis in the era of cochlear implantation. Otol Neurotol. 2001;22:471–4.
180. Berrettini S, Burdo S, Forli F, et al. Far advanced otosclerosis: stapes surgery or cochlear implantation? J Otolaryngol. 2004;33:165–71.
181. Glasscock ME, Storper IS, Haynes DS, Bohrer PS. Stapedectomy in profound cochlear loss. Laryngoscope. 1996;106:831–3.
182. Khalifa A, El-Guindy A, Erfan F. Stapedectomy for far-advanced otosclerosis. J Laryngol Otol. 1998;112:158–60.
183. Kabbara B, Gauche C, Calmels MN, Lepage B, Escude B, Deguine O, Fraysse B, Marx M. Decisive criteria between stapedotomy and cochlear implantation in patients with far advanced otosclerosis. Otol Neurotol. 2015;36(3):e73–8.
184. Shea PF, Ge X, Shea JJ Jr. Stapedectomy for far-advanced otosclerosis. Am J Otol. 1999;20:4259.
185. Lippy WH, Burkey JM, Arkis PN. Word recognition score changes after stapedectomy for far advanced otosclerosis. Am J Otol. 1998;19:568.

186. Frattali MA, Sataloff RT. Far-advanced otosclerosis. Ann Otol Rhinol Laryngol. 1993;102:4337.
187. Rotteveel LJ, Proops DW, Ramsden RT, et al. Cochlear implantation in 53 patients with otosclerosis: demographics, computed tomographic scanning, surgery, and complications. Otol Neurotol. 2004;25:943–52.
188. Ramsden R, Rotteveel L, Proops D, et al. Cochlear implantation in otosclerotic deafness. Adv Otorhinolaryngol. 2007;65:328–34.
189. Cureoglu S, Baylan MY, Paparella MM. Cochlear otosclerosis. Curr Opin Otolaryngol Head Neck Surg. 2010;18:357–62.
190. Rama-Lopez J, Cervera-Paz FJ, Manrique M. Cochlear implantation of patients with far-advanced otosclerosis. Otol Neurotol. 2006;27:153–8.
191. Semaan MT, Gehani NC, Tummala N, et al. Cochlear implantation outcomes in patients with far advanced otosclerosis. Am J Otolaryngol. 2012;33:608–14.
192. Abdurehim Y, Lehmann A, Zeitouni AG. Stapedotomy vs cochlear implantation for advanced otosclerosis: systematic review and meta-analysis. Otolaryngol Head Neck Surg. 2016;155(5):764–70.
193. Quaranta N, Bartoli R, Lopriore A, Fernandez-Vega S, Giagnotti F, Quaranta A. Cochlear implantation in otosclerosis. Otol Neurotol. 2005;26:983–7.
194. Sainz M, Garcia-Valdecasas J, Ballesteros JM. Complications and pitfalls of cochlear implantation in otosclerosis: a 6-year follow-up cohort study. Otol Neurotol. 2009;30:1044–8.
195. Drennan WR, Rubinstein JT. Music perception in cochlear implant users and its relationship with psychophysical capabilities. J Rehabil Res Dev. 2008;45:779–89.
196. Toung JS, Zwolan T, Spooner TR, Telian SA. Late failure of cochlear implantation resulting from advanced cochlear otosclerosis: surgical and programming challenges. Otol Neurotol. 2004;25:723–6.
197. Ching TY, Incerti P, Hill M. Binaural benefits for adults who use hearing aids and cochlear implants in opposite ears. Ear Hear. 2004;25:9–21.

Acute Otitis Media and Acute Coalescent Mastoiditis

2

Contents

S. Mansour et al., *Middle Ear Diseases*,
https://doi.org/10.1007/978-3-319-72962-6_2

2.1 Introduction

Otitis media (OM) comprises a wide spectrum of diseases that include acute otitis media (AOM), recurrent acute otitis media (rAOM), otitis media with effusion (OME), chronic otitis media with effusion (COME) and chronic suppurative otitis media (CSOM) [1–3].

AOM is an acute inflammation and infection of the middle ear caused by bacteria and/or viruses. In general, it is a childhood disease that manifests as a rapid onset of fever and otalgia [1, 2, 4]; if the child has ≥3 episodes of AOM in the preceding 6 months, or ≥4 episodes in the preceding 12 months, he should be considered to have rAOM [1, 5, 6]. Patients who have more than six episodes in the first 6 years of life are called otitis "prone" [7]. The presence of fluid in the middle ear with absence of acute signs and symptoms of infection and inflammation is defined as OME, and if the fluid persisted more than 3 months, it is considered as COME [1]. CSOM is defined as an ear discharge with tympanic membrane (TM) perforation for more than 3 months [1].

This chapter will scope on AOM and its complications, mainly acute and coalescent mastoiditis.

2.2 Epidemiology

AOM is the second most common reason for a family physician's visit and the most common reason for prescribing antimicrobial drugs. It accounts for 10–15% of all childhood medical visits.

AOM has an incidence rate of 10.8/100 people per year [8]. *70% of children manifest at least one episode of AOM even in developed countries.* Males have a higher incidence of AOM [1, 9].

AOM has a peak incidence at the age of 6–11 months [1, 9]; 59% of children will have one episode of AOM and 30% will have two episodes or more by the age of 2 [1]. **rAOM** resolve spontaneously when the child gets older, often at 3–4 years of age. AOM incidence rate drops rapidly after the age of 5 years.

2.3 Pathogenesis

AOM has multiple risk factors (host factors, environmental, microbiological and genetic factors) that interact with each other and make the patient more susceptible to become affected by AOM [10–12].

AOM is related to upper respiratory infections (URTI): More than 90% of AOM episodes develop after ***URTI*** [1, 7]; one of three children will develop AOM after URTI [12]. URTI causes nasopharyngitis which affects Eustachian tube function, and induces a negative pressure in the middle ear with secondary suction of the nasopharyngeal secretions inside the middle ear. This explains why aspirates of AOM can show bacteria like *Streptococcus pneumoniae, Haemophilus influenzae and Moraxella catarrhalis* [2, 9], which are commensal to the nasopharynx [13]. This mechanism is exaggerated by bottle-feeding, pacifier use, and other sucking behaviors. The initial course of the disease is thought to be of viral origin followed by superimposed bacterial infections [2, 12]. Many viruses have been implicated as causative agents which are found in 90% of AOM cases, such as the rhinovirus, coronavirus, enterovirus, respiratory syncytial virus (RSV), parainfluenza type 1, 2 or 3, influenza A or B, and adenovirus [1, 2, 7, 8, 14]. Among all of these, RSV is believed to have the most frequent association with AOM [12]. These viruses are thought to increase the adherence of the bacteria to the epithelium so enhancing bacterial colonization [12, 14], however, there is a rising evidence that viruses alone can cause AOM without bacterial superinfection in 10–15% of cases, a point that should be kept in mind while treating AOM with antibiotics [12, 14].

Genetics play an important role in the susceptibility of an individual to AOM [1, 2, 9, 11, 12]: When comparing genetic to environmental risk factors, genetic predisposition with a specific genotype was found to be a stronger risk factor than the socioeconomic status. Positive family history of otitis media is a strong risk factor for developing AOM and other forms of otitis media.

Native American Maori or Australian Aborigine populations have more prevalence of AOM as compared to the white population [1]. One cohort study showed that heritability is found in 38.5% in rAOM [11]. Some investigators have linked this susceptibility to inherited poor ET function [2]. Other investigators found that specific polymorphisms of some cytokines have been correlated to the susceptibility of an individual to AOM and to the severity of the disease as well [10, 12]. IL-1s, IL-6 and TNFα have been found in nasopharyngeal secretions during URTI and increased levels of IL-1s are linked to the transition to AOM [12]. TNFα-308 polymorphisms are associated with AOM that follows URTI. In addition, some rAOM patients were found to have TNFα-308 and IL-6-174 polymorphisms [12]. Genes for Fcg-receptor IIa (FcgRIIa), IL-10, CD14, toll-like receptor 4 (TLR4), surfactant, and interferon gamma (IFNg) are believed to be responsible for an AOM risk [11].

The importance of environmental factors must not be underestimated in the pathogenesis of AOM; **Paternal smoking** is one of otitis media major risk factors [1, 3, 8–10]. Passive smoking causes mucosal inflammation, goblet cells hyperplasia and an increase in the production of mucus, all together impairs mucosal mucociliary clearance and increases bacterial colonization by enhancing the bacterial binding to respiratory epithelium [1, 10]. Children of mothers who smoked during pregnancy and stopped after delivery still have a higher incidence of AOM [10].

Some studies found a role of gastroesophageal reflux disease (GERD) [1, 15]; ***GERD*** is found in 62.9% of patient with rAOM. In fact, pepsin/pepsinogen can be found in the middle ear in 85.3% of otitis media patients that could be explained by the reflux; however a cause and effect relationship could not be established [15].

There are **other** risk factors that are related to AOM, like prematurity [9], young age [1, 8], day care attendance [3, 9, 10], increased number of siblings, dummy use [1, 9], autumn and winter seasons [1], craniofacial anomalies [8], asthma [3] and atopy [3, 8] (Fig. 2.1).

An epidemiological survey from Denmark [16] stated that the following factors were predictive of early AOM and rAOM: male gender, prematurity, parity (number of pregnancies the mother has had), maternal age, maternal self-estimated health, maternal intake of penicillin during pregnancy, and termination of breastfeeding before the child was 6 months old (Fig. 2.1).

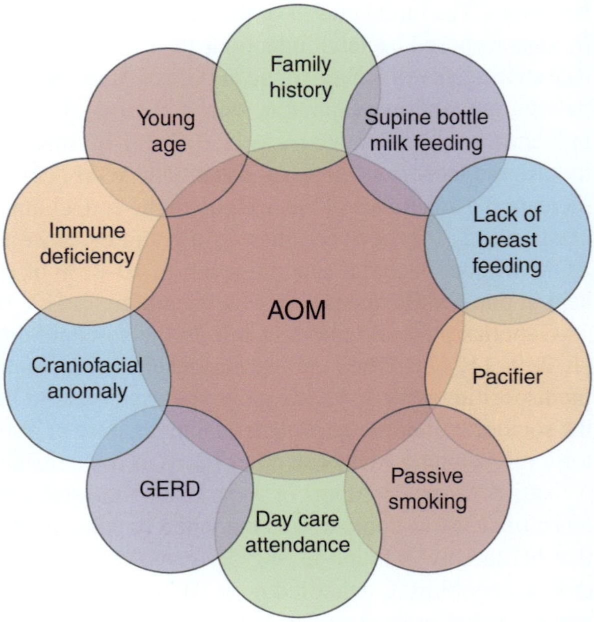

Fig. 2.1 Interactive predisposing factors of acute otitis media

2.4 Microbiology

AOM is usually a complication of an acute viral upper respiratory infection. The most common bacterial pathogens associated with the diagnosis of AOM are: *Streptococcus pneumoniae, Haemophilus influenzae and Moraxella catarrhalis* [3, 17, 18].

Streptococcus pneumoniae is the most common, found in 35–45% [3, 18]. Patients infected with this microorganism tend to have more severe disease [3, 13]. The serotypes responsible have been changed after the introduction of pneumococcal 7-valent conjugate vaccine (PCV-7) [3].

Haemophilus influenza has become more common after PCV-7 vaccine [3]. It is related to bilateral disease, recurrent cases, and conjunctivitis with the so called "otitis-conjunctivitis syndrome" [3, 13, 17].

Moraxella catarrhalis is found in 10–20% of cases [17], 100% are beta lactamase producers [17].

All of the above pathogens have the ability to form biofilms [13], which are thought to be responsible for the resistance to antimicrobial therapy [13].

Group A Streptococcus, Group B Streptococcus, Staphylococcus aureus and gram-negative bacilli are other bacteria that can be encountered in approximately 15% of cases [3]. A first episode of bacterial infection with invasive strains (like invasive strains of *Streptococcus pneumoniae*) can lead to mucosal changes which make the ear more susceptible to acquire the disease by less virulent strains [19].

Approximately 5% of ears have multiple pathogens. In approximately 20–30% of ears with clinical AOM [20], *no bacterial pathogen was identified by tympanocentesis.*

Respiratory viruses including RSV, rhinovirus, adenovirus, influenza virus, parainfluenza virus, and CMV are isolated from the cultures of approximately 20% of middle ear samples, half of them have bacterial/viral co-infections [20].

In cases of simultaneous infection with pathogenic viruses and bacteria, antibiotic response appears to be inferior to that of children that have only a bacterial infection, and microbiologic failure can occur despite clear in vitro sensitivity to the used antibiotic. Consequently, a second course of antibiotics can effectively clear the bacteria after the immune system has cleared up the viral infection.

2.5 Clinical Manifestations

2.5.1 Symptomatology

AOM has typically a short history of onset; it is commonly associated with fever, otalgia, ear pulling, irritability, lethargy, anorexia, and vomiting.

Earache *is one of the most common and distressing symptoms of AOM.*

Ear pulling is not specific as only 10% of ear pullers will have AOM.

These symptoms alone lack sensitivity and specificity; the diagnosis of AOM must rely on otoscopy findings.

Immunosuppressed patients, particularly those undergoing chemotherapy, may not manifest the typical acute inflammatory symptoms whereas systemic sepsis and middle ear effusion might be the only indicators of AOM.

2.5.2 Examination

Performed under ideal conditions, otomicroscopy with adequate visualization of the eardrum (cleaning the ear canal is most often required) allows proper diagnosis of AOM (Fig. 2.2). Non-cooperative children usually need to be restrained. Diagnosis may be difficult in very young children but it is important to accurately do so. A first episode of AOM before 6 months of age is likely to lead to recurrence of AOM, and subsequently, significant periods of OME with diminished hearing and delayed speech.

The common otoscopic findings of AOM are:

- **Hyperemic** and hypervascularized tympanic membrane. Early AOM may be diagnosed by inflammation which is seen along the handle of malleus and in the superior pole of the tympanic membrane.
- **Bulging** tympanic membrane is the only specific sign for AOM. In the absence of a bulging ear drum but with clinical suspicion of AOM, pneumatic otoscopy is necessary to differentiate AOM from myringitis.
- **Purulent effusion** behind a bulging tympanic membrane.
- When the process advances, a **perforation** of the tympanic membrane may occur, which allows spontaneous drainage of pus from middle ear and the patient would generally experience rapid relief of the pain and fever. Nowadays, it is not unusual that the otologist sees the patient at this stage. During otoscopic examination, a yellowish pulsatile discharge is seen oozing through pinpoint perforation.
- **The discharge** is initially purulent, though it may be thin and watery or bloody; pulsation of the otorrhea is common. Otorrhea from an acute perforation normally lasts 1–2 days before spontaneous healing occurs. Otorrhea may persist if the perforation is accompanied by mucosal swelling or polypoid changes.

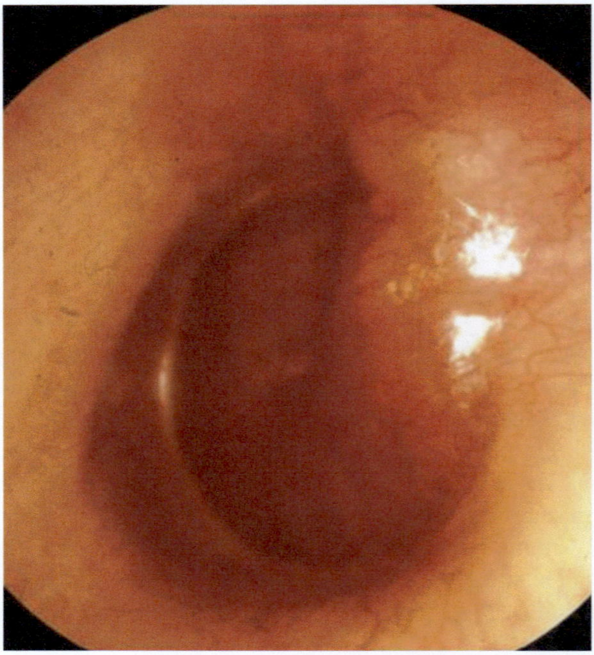

Fig. 2.2 Left ear acute otitis media with bulging of the hyperemic tympanic membrane and yellowish effusion in the middle ear cavity

2.6 Diagnosis

The diagnosis of AOM requires the presence of inflammation and pus in the middle ear, and acute onset of symptoms and sign of ear infection, i.e., earache, fever, irritability, poor feeding or vomiting, often associated with cough and rhinitis.

Diagnosis of acute otitis media (AOM) requires

1. Symptoms of fever, otalgia, or irritability in young children
2. Bulging of the tympanic membrane
3. Erythema and hypervascularisation

Pneumatic otoscopy in AOM is very painful and must be avoided.

Otomicroscopy and ***otoendoscopy*** are helpful to differentiate AOM from *acute bullous myringitis* and other differential diagnosis (Fig. 2.3).

Tympanometry is helpful but must still be used in conjunction with compatible history.

Tympanocentesis: Tympanocentesis is considered as the gold standard therapy in AOM; especially after failure of second course of antibiotics, the aspirate provides material for the culture to direct antibiotherapy [4, 7].

Laboratory studies: Not needed for the diagnosis. However one study by Pichichero and Almudevar indicated that the presence of AOM caused by non-typeable *H. influenzae*, as well as the disease's cure, can be determined from serum levels of S100A12 protein and interleukin-10 (IL-10) [21].

Imaging studies: Radiologic studies are generally unnecessary in uncomplicated AOM. Role of CT-Scan or MRI in the diagnosis of complications will be presented in a dedicated chapter (see Chap. 9).

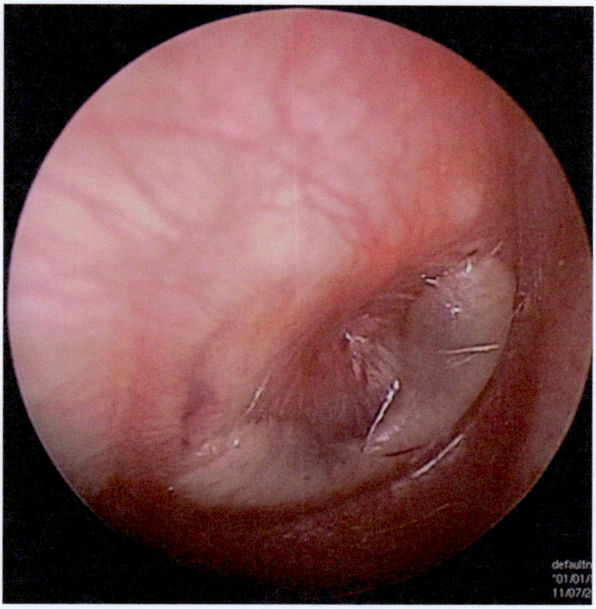

Fig. 2.3 Right ear otoscopy in a child presented with ear pain and fever showing bullous myringitis

2.7 Differential Diagnosis of AOM

- ***Myringitis*** - inflammation of the tympanic membrane. This is usually associated with viral infections of the upper respiratory tract.
- ***Acute bullous myringitis***, (rare) - caused by *Mycoplasma pneumonia*, and causes severe localized otalgia without systemic symptoms and without middle ear effusion. The bullae or blebs may contain serous or hemorrhagic fluid and pain is relieved by puncturing the bleb without opening the eardrum (Fig. 2.3).
- Otitis externa, rare in children, usually occurs after swimming and is associated with severe pain and tragal tenderness. The child is usually afebrile with good general condition.
- Dental pain
- Acute viral pharyngitis

2.8 Management of AOM

2.8.1 General Concepts

1. *Routine use of antibiotics, especially in children 2 years and older, is not indicated because of the high rate of spontaneous resolution. Watchful waiting for 48 to 72 hours before initiating antibiotic therapy if symptoms are manageable with analgesics.*
2. *The goals of antibiotic treatment of AOM are to:*
   - *Produce fast clinical cure*
   - *Prevent complications*
   - *Eradicate bacteria from middle ear and thus reduce recurrence rate*

3. *The most important factor is not to prescribe antibiotics for inappropriate diagnosis of AOM. Inappropriate use of antibiotics have caused adverse effects and increased antibiotic resistance.*
4. *S. pneumonia has the lowest spontaneous resolution rate and is associated with more serious complications, it is essential to ensure optimal coverage for this organism.*
5. *Observation alone is not suitable for high-risk or vulnerable populations such as indigenous children in remote settings or those with cleft palate, Down syndrome or immunodeficiency syndromes* [2]
6. *Children younger than 6 months of age with AOM must be treated with antibiotics without the initial observational waiting time.*
7. *Oral antibiotic treatment of a first AOM episode occurring during infancy does not affect the number of AOM recurrences.*
8. *Persistent otitis media infections can arise from the failure to completely eradicate the original bacterial infection, the presence of biofilms, or intracellular bacterial infection of the middle ear mucosal cells, particularly mucus-secreting cells* [22].

2.8.2 Guidelines

- Every nation has its own guidelines of therapy recommendations, there is no universal guidelines. In general, guidelines are more applied by the young generation of physicians than by the older ones.
- Most guidelines use the same diagnostic criteria, and propose *watchful waiting* in mild-moderate scenarios
- *The routine prescription of antibiotics for AOM ranges from 31% in the Netherlands to 98% in the USA and Australia.*
- *Current American Academy of Pediatrics Guidelines for the treatment of AOM recommend:*
  - *that antibiotics should be used in children aged over 6 months when unilateral or bilateral AOM is severe (moderate to severe otalgia, otalgia lasting at least 48 h, temperature 39 °C)* [23].
  - *Antibiotics should also be prescribed if AOM is not severe but bilateral in a child aged 6–23 months.*
  - *In the case of non-severe unilateral AOM in a child aged 6–23 months, or non-severe unilateral/bilateral AOM in a child aged 24 months or older, antibiotics may be prescribed or observation offered; if observation is chosen, a mechanism should be in place to give antibiotics if symptoms do not improve in 48–72 h.*
- ***For rAOM****, insertion of ventilation tubes should be considered if rAOM is associated with a persistent middle ear effusion between AOM attacks* [24]
- *No prophylactic antibiotics for rAOM*

2.8.3 Choice of Antibiotics

(a) ***Amoxicillin*** *is the first-line agent for the treatment of acute otitis media in children* [5–7]*; as most S. pneumoniae and H. influenzae are still susceptible* [9]. *If* *severe signs and symptoms persisted more than 2–3 days of amoxicillin use, then antibiotics should be changed to amoxicillin-clavulanate, or second generation or third generation cephalosporin* [5].

(b) *If there is a recent history of amoxicillin use in the last 30 days, in recurrent cases or if the patient has conjunctivitis, then Beta lactamase coverage should be added* [5, 7]. *Cefdinir, cefuroxime and ceftriaxone should be considered in case of penicillin allergy* [5], *macrolides can be used in allergic cases as well* [5, 9].

2.8.4 The Duration of Antibiotherapy

The duration of antibiotherapy *is for 10 days for children below 2 years and 5–7 days for older children* [5–7]. *Children who present with perforation of the tympanic membrane should receive 10 days of antibiotic therapy.*

Antibiotherapy of 10 Days Duration

1. ***< 24 months old***
2. ***Perforated eardrum***
3. ***Recurrent AOM***
4. ***Failure of first line agents***

Clinicians should reevaluate a child whose symptoms have worsened or that did not respond to the initial antibiotic treatment within 48–72 h and change the treatment.

It is not indicated to give antihistamine, decongestants or corticosteroids [2, 6].

2.8.5 Tympanocentesis

Few days after the start of the therapy, when the medical treatment is ineffective and the purulent effusion is under pressure, tympanocentesis is the solution because it permits an efficient drainage and immediate relief of symptoms and allows identification of the causative bacteria and its sensitivity. Also it is found that tube insertion reduces the recurrence rates of AOM [6, 7, 9], and improves the quality of life of children in terms of hearing and speech [5]. Actually one of the main factors behind the rAOM is the lack of good control of the first episode of AOM when the ear is left with an important residual middle ear effusion.

Tympanocentesis should be performed in the following AOM patients [25]:

- Patients in whom adequate antimicrobial treatment has failed to control the infection
- Patients who have a complication that requires a culture for adequate therapy
- Neonates younger than 6 weeks (more likely to have an unusual invasive pathogen)
- Patients who are immunosuppressed or immunocompromised

2.8.6 Anti-GERD

No sufficient data is present about using anti-reflux in rAOM [15] but some studies found that controlling GERD by anti-reflux medication can decrease rAOM and tympanostomy tube insertion rates.

2.8.7 Follow up

Normally the symptoms of AOM should resolve within 72 hours of initiating antibiotic treatment. However, middle ear effusion may persist for up to 1 month in 50% and up to 3 months in 25% of patients despite bacteriological cure. Therefore, persistence of middle ear fluid after full course of antibiotic therapy for AOM is not an indication for continued antimicrobial therapy. Follow up should be done after 4–8 weeks for uncomplicated cases of AOM to look for persistent middle ear effusion [6] (See Chap. 3). In general, AOM is a symptomatic disease and screening is not indicated [8].

2.9 Prevention of Recurrent AOM

Recurrent otitis media (rAOM) is defined as 3 or more episodes of AOM over the preceding 6 months, or 4 or more episodes in the last year. Under these circumstance, prevention of further attacks is desirable. Modification of risk factors, when possible, are of benefit. Breast feeding has a protective effect at least for the first 6 months and preferentially to be continued for the first year [5]. Elimination of smoking from the environment and avoidance of pacifiers have been shown to help reduce the recurrence of AOM. Vaccinations are other preventive measures [3, 5, 7, 26]. PCV7 has been shown to decrease AOM rates and tympanostomy tube placement for recurrent diseases [26] and is more effective if given during infancy [6]. It can prevent the early episodes of the disease and prevent the mucosal changes, that make the ear more susceptible to infection by other *S. pneumoniae* serotypes, that are not covered by PCV [19]. Some studies found that Live Attenuated Influenza Vaccine (LAIV) has decreased the incidence of AOM by 12.4%, if given between 6 and 71 months of age [7], but others found influenza vaccine is not effective in preventing AOM [6]. The American Academy of Pediatrics recommends administration of pneumococcal conjugate vaccine and influenza vaccine for all children [5].

Despite promising results, there is still a real concern about the long-term benefit from vaccination. A recent study has highlighted concerns regarding the increasing incidence of AOM-related complications. Following the introduction of vaccinations, AOM-related complications, including mastoiditis and other intracranial complications, diminished considerably, however, they returned to pre-vaccination levels after a few years [27]. Antibiotic prophylaxis has only minimal effects on recurrent otitis media, decreasing recurrence by approximately one episode per year. Antibiotic prophylaxis is no longer recommended in the management of rAOM.

As the child grows older, the incidence of recurrence declines.

2.10 Acute Otitis Media in Adult

AOM in adult is:

Much less common than in children: the incidence in adults is widely quoted as 0.25% per year.

- Mostly bacteria and mainly *Haemophilus Influenzae* is the dominating germ; *S. pneumoniae* is less involved since vaccination
- Otalgia is a more common presenting symptom and may occur without fever or hearing loss and may be the only presenting feature.
- Complications are rare

Immediate antibiotic prescription to an adult with AOM:

- To patients who are systemically unwell but do not require admission.
- To those at high risk of complications because of significant heart, lung, kidney, diabetes, liver or neuromuscular disease, or to those who are immunocompromised.

2.11 Complications of Acute Otitis Media

Tympanic membrane perforation occurs in 7% of the cases and tends to heal in 98% of cases in the first 1–2 weeks [7]. Other complications and sequelae of AOM are important causes of preventable hearing loss, particularly in developing countries. ***Meningitis*** (pneumococcal origin of AOM is the most important pathogen linked to meningitis [7]), facial ***palsy and coalescent mastoiditis***. Also systemic complications could occur such as bacteremia, septic arthritis, or bacterial endocarditis.

2.11.1 Facial Paralysis

Incidence: *Nowadays, facial paralysis is a very uncommon complication of AOM with an estimated incidence of 0.005%; it was not so rare in the pre-antibiotic era* [28].

Mechanism of facial paralysis: It is thought that facial paralysis in AOM is caused by spread of infection under pressure from the middle ear cavity into the facial nerve sheath with resultant intrafallopian inflammatory edema and consequent ischemia and neuropraxia. Presumably this occurs either through [1] preexistent bony dehiscences [2], physiologic canaliculi between the middle ear and the Fallopian canal, or [3] vascular connections between the Fallopian canal and the mastoid air cells.

Site of involvement: the exact site of the inflammatory involvement causing facial palsy in AOM is difficult to determine, but through the topographic tests it was observed that the site of involvement is infrageniculate in 90% of cases and suprageniculate in 10% [29].

Treatment: it is a consensus among most otologists that the conservative approach for facial palsy in AOM is the most appropriate one: it consists of *antibiotherapy and myringotomy with tube placement; steroids may be added.* In certain cases when the facial recovery is delayed and the patient keeps a grade VI paralysis after 3 weeks of treatment, imaging is indicated to rule out associated pathologies.

Unlike in CSOM, facial palsy in AOM presents, in most cases, an excellent prognosis with the adequate treatment.

2.12 Acute Coalescent Mastoiditis in Children

Acute coalescent mastoiditis is the most common suppurative complication of AOM in young children.

In many cases, this may be the presenting complaint of children with AOM. Early diagnosis and adequate treatment of this condition are essential to avoid fatal complications. In the era of antibiotics, coalescent mastoiditis has an incidence of <1% in patients with AOM [30]. The incidence and the clinical picture of mastoiditis have changed greatly with the advent of antibiotics when reliance on antibiotics alone leads to less vigilance in diagnostic and therapeutic interventions; "this has led to a generation of ENT specialists and pediatricians trained in an atmosphere of complacency in the treatment of AOM; recently, a delay is noted in the recognition of mastoiditis and its related intracranial complications in children and in the initiation of the appropriate therapy" [31].

Despite the use of advanced imaging modalities, antibiotics, and microsurgical procedures, the resulting mortality of intracranial otogenic complications in acute coalescent mastoiditis remains of approximately 10% [32].

2.12.1 Definitions

Acute mastoiditis is subdivided according to the pathologic stage:

- **Acute mastoiditis with periostitis** (also called incipient mastoiditis) is defined by the presence of purulent material only in the mastoid cavity.
- **Acute coalescent mastoiditis** (also called "acute mastoid osteitis") ***is defined by the acute form of destruction of the thin bony septae between mastoid air cells***. It may be followed by the formation of abscess cavities and the dissipation of pus into adjacent areas.
- **Masked mastoiditis** (also called subacute mastoiditis) refers to a low-grade, subacute, but persistent infection in the middle ear and mastoid with destruction of the bony septae between air cells. It occurs in patients with persistent middle ear effusion or recurrent episodes of AOM without sufficient antimicrobial therapy.

2.12.2 Pathogenesis

The clinical course of AOM is often short and self limited because of the host's immune system defense, the infection-resistant nature of the mucosal linings, and the susceptibility of the major organisms to oral antibiotics.

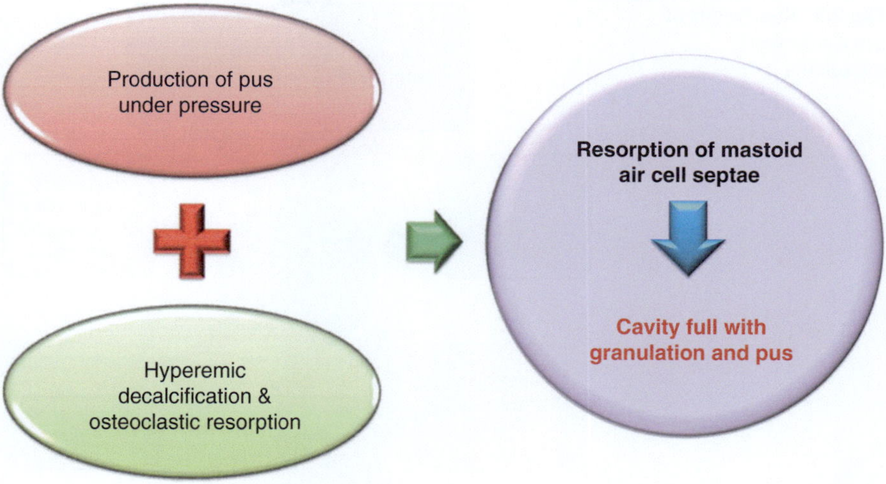

Fig. 2.4 Pathogenesis of coalescent mastoiditis

Approximately 1–5% of untreated or inadequately treated patients with AOM may experience complications. Prior to these complications, alarming signs and symptoms may appear: severe earache and/or headache; vertigo; chills and fever; and meningeal symptoms or signs [33].

Acute coalescent mastoiditis is a rare complication of severe AOM. During an episode of severe AOM, the mucosa in the epitympanum becomes hyperplastic, it blocks the aditus ad antrum leading to entrapment of purulent material within the mastoid air cells. As pus and granulations accumulate under pressure, mastoid air cells bony septation become subjected to pressure and osteitic necrosis; small air cells coalesce into larger ones by bony septation necrosis with a resultant *coalescence of mastoid air cells* called "acute coalescent mastoiditis" (Fig. 2.4).

Essentially, coalescent mastoiditis is an empyema of the temporal bone. Pus may leave the area of coalescence by direct extension, thrombophlebitis, or through preformed bony pathways. If the outer cortical bone is violated a postauricular, subperiosteal abscess is formed, causing an ear protrusion downward and outward. However, if the inner cortical table is violated, an intracranial complication can occur: sigmoid sinus thrombosis, meningitis, epidural or subdural abscess, or brain abscess.

Subperiosteal abscess is seen in nearly 50% of patients diagnosed with coalescent mastoiditis [34–37]. If not recognized at its early stage, the coalescent mastoiditis could be the cause of fatal intracranial complications. The incidence of intracranial complications has been reported between 6.8% and 23% when acute mastoiditis is diagnosed [38, 39] (see Chap. 9).

2.12.3 Risk Factors

As with most infectious processes, host and microbial factors have to be considered when evaluating acute mastoiditis (Fig. 2.5).

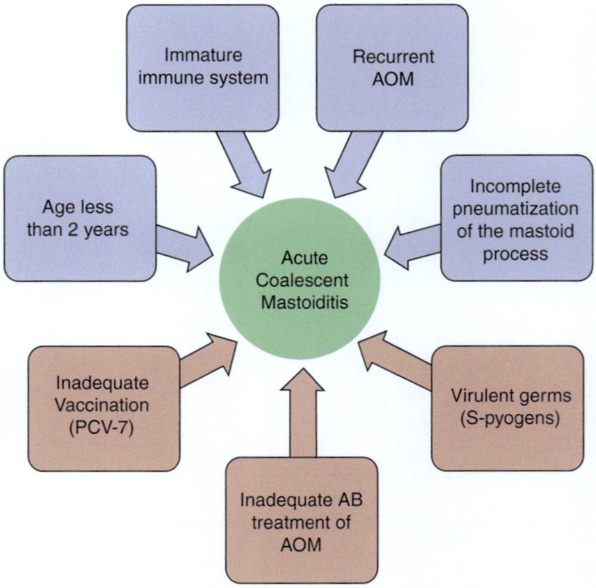

Fig. 2.5 Risk factors of acute coalescent mastoiditis

2.12.3.1 Host Factors

Age < 2 years: Most children presenting with acute coalescent mastoiditis are younger than 2 years of age and have little history of otitis media. At this age, the immune system is relatively immature, particularly with regard to its ability to respond to challenges from polysaccharide antigens.

Incomplete mastoid pneumatization: Mastoid antrum is the only mastoid air cell present at birth. Mastoid pneumatization starts shortly after birth, but it is not active during the first two years of life. After the age of 2 years, mastoid pneumatization becomes very active and is almost complete at the age of 10 years. The antrum and the mastoid air cells are lined with respiratory epithelium that becomes oedematous due to inflammation and infection. Non-pneumatized mastoid is more prone to coalescent mastoiditis because the narrow aditus ad antrum can be easily blocked by inflammatory epitympanic mucosa during an episode of severe AOM.

Other host factors, such **autism spectrum disorders**, have shown an increased likelihood of developing middle ear infections and more than two-fold greater predisposition for coalescent mastoiditis [40].

2.12.3.2 Microbial Factors

The most common etiologic agent causing mastoiditis is *Streptococcus pneumoniae*, followed by *Haemophilus influenzae* and group A *Streptococcus pyogenes* (GAS). Each of these bacteria has invasive forms and is recovered most often from children presenting with acute mastoiditis.

Reported pathogens in mastoiditis include the following [41–60]

- *Streptococcus pneumoniae*—Most frequently isolated pathogen in acute mastoiditis, prevalence is approximately 25%
- *Group A beta-hemolytic streptococci*

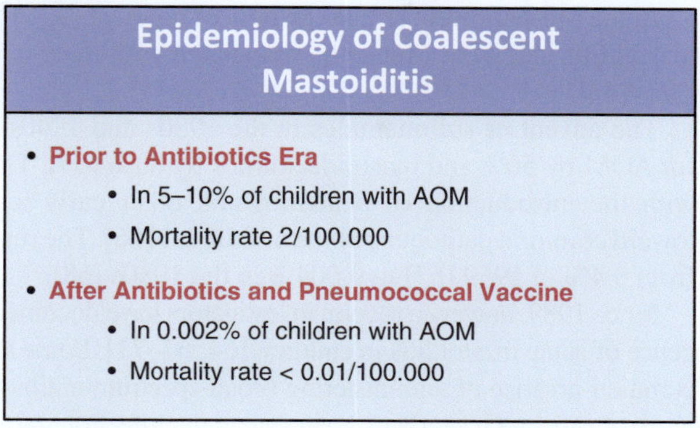

Fig. 2.6 Epidemiology of acute coalescent mastoiditis

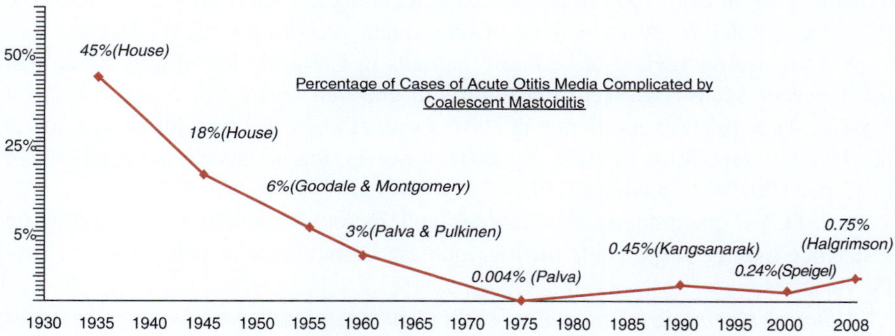

Fig. 2.7 The evolution of incidence of acute coalescent mastoiditis over time

- *Staphylococcus aureus*
- *Streptococcus pyogenes*
- *Haemophilus influenzae*

Several case series show that 33–81% of patients diagnosed with acute coalescent mastoiditis had been treated with appropriate first-line agents for AOM prior to development of mastoiditis, suggesting that antibiotics administered for AOM treatment do not eliminate the risk of developing this complication [61].

2.12.4 Epidemiology (Figs. 2.6 and 2.7)

Today, the estimated incidence of coalescent mastoiditis is less than 0.01% of AOM [55].

Acute mastoiditis is a disease of the very young. Most patients present younger than the age of 2 years, with a median age of 12 months. However, it can occur in persons of any age. Some fear that untreated otitis media increases the risk of acute mastoiditis and is the cause of higher incidences in developing countries and very young children [62, 63].

In the pre-antibiotic era, up to 20% of cases of AOM were complicated by acute mastoiditis and were frequently associated with more severe intracranial complications [64].

The advent of sulfonamides in the 1930s and 1940s decreased hospitalizations for AOM by 50% and mastoidectomies by 80% [65]. This reduction was amplified with the introduction of penicillin and other early antibiotic regimens directed toward common pathogens of the middle ear [66]. The reported incidences decreased from 0.4% in 1959 [67] to 0.004% in the 1980s [68].

Since 1989, however, several investigators have documented an epidemiologic resurgence of acute mastoiditis in children [64, 67–71]. Some studies have incriminated the common practice of administering broad-spectrum antibiotics in increasing the prevalence of resistant bacteria that can spread the infection into the mastoid bone [72–76].

The incidence of acute mastoiditis in children <2 years of age exhibited a dynamic pattern from 1999 to 2008: a significant decline early after introduction of PCV-7 was followed by an increase in subsequent years to pre-PCV-7 levels.

A retrospective review of pediatric patients in Colorado found that the annual incidence of acute coalescent mastoiditis in children under age 2 years dropped from 11.0 per 100,000 population in 2001, a year after PCV-7 was introduced, to 4.5 per 100,000 population in 2003. By 2008, however, the incidence had again raised to 12 per 100,000 population [77].

Non-PCV-7 pneumococcal serotypes and increased pneumococcal antibiotic resistance may be responsible for this increase in incidence in comparison to pre-PCV-7 rates.

Although becoming less common, coalescent mastoiditis remains even nowadays a subject of first interest and concern for pediatricians and otolaryngologists.

2.12.5 Clinical Features

Approximately 40% of children with acute mastoiditis had a positive history of previous AOM, and 50% of patients having coalescent mastoiditis had received antibiotics before presentation. However, the absence of AOM (current or recent) does not exclude the diagnosis of coalescent mastoiditis because it may take place very rapidly during the onset of an AOM episode.

The diagnosis of acute mastoiditis is usually made clinically in children with characteristic findings. The most frequent diagnostic criteria include (Figs. 2.8 and 2.9):

1. Irritability and lethargy
2. Fever
3. Otalgia
4. Postauricular erythema, tenderness, swelling, fluctuance, or mass
5. Protrusion of the auricle
6. Oedema and sagging of the posterosuperior wall of the external auditory canal
7. Nipplelike protrusion of the central tympanic membrane, usually oozing pus

Fig. 2.8 Main clinical features of acute coalescent mastoiditis

Clinical Features of Acute Coalescent Mastoiditis

- **Symptoms**
  - Earache
  - Fever
  - Ear discharge: profuse and purulent
- **Signs**
  - Mastoid tenderness
  - Sagging of the postero-superior meatal wall
  - Swelling, redness and bulging over the mastoid

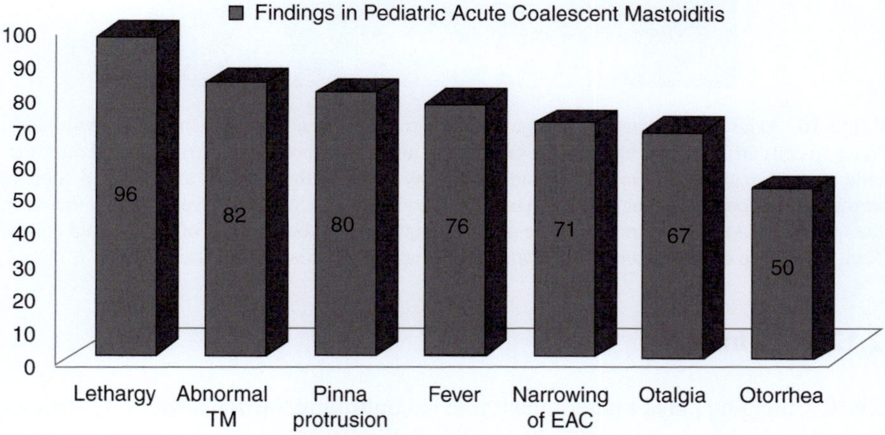

Fig. 2.9 Signs and symptoms of acute coalescent mastoiditis in order of frequency: Lethargy/malaise (96%); Abnormal tympanic membrane (82%); Postauricular erythema, postauricular tenderness, and/or protrusion of the pinna (80%); Fever (76%); Narrowing of the external auditory canal (71%); Ear pain (67%); Otorrhea (50%)

Fever is a nonspecific sign but it is sensitive and may be predictive of complications or the need for surgical intervention. High-spiking "picket-fence" fever may be indicative of sigmoid sinus thrombophlebitis.

Examination of the tympanic membrane: Tympanic membrane findings consistent with AOM (e.g., bulging, marked erythema or acute perforation with purulent otorrhea in the absence of otitis externa) are often present.

A normal-appearing tympanic membrane usually (but not invariably) excludes mastoiditis.

Laboratory Features: The peripheral white blood cell count in children with acute coalescent mastoiditis is usually elevated, often with a left shift. The erythrocyte sedimentation rate and C-reactive protein are also elevated.

Immunologic evaluation may be warranted in children with recurrent episodes of AOM leading to mastoiditis.

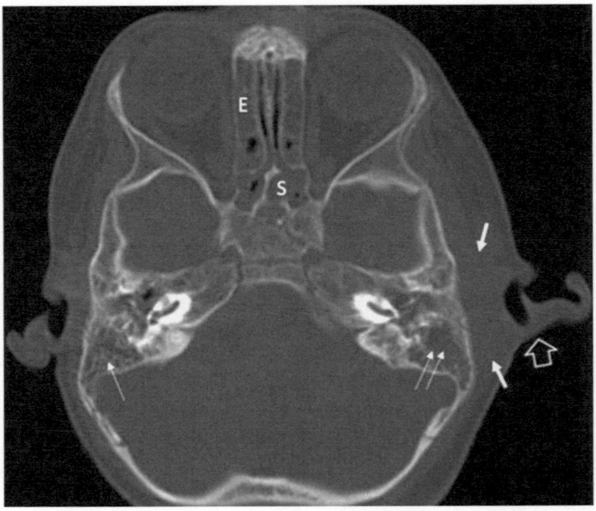

Fig. 2.10 Axial non injected CT-image of a 2 y-o boy with acute otitis media on both sides. Mastoid cells are opacified on the right side (single arrow), the bony septa are preserved: non specific sign of mastoiditis. On the left side, the bony septa of the mastoid are resorbed (double arrow): sign of coalescent mastoiditis. Associated large retroauricular soft tissue swelling (between the white arrows) with protrusion of the auricle (empty arrow), but no lysis of the mastoid cortex. Note the diffuse condensation of the ethmoidal (E) and sphenoidal (S) sinusses

2.12.6 CT-Imaging

The CT Imaging plays a determinant role in confirming the diagnosis and in orienting plans for management. CT allows differentiation between a mere condensation of the mastoid system in common acute purulent otitis media and disruption of the intercellular bone septa that is indicative for coalescent mastoiditis. Also CT-Scan may confirm the diagnosis in children without characteristic clinical findings.

CT findings in children with acute coalescent mastoiditis include the following:

1. *Fluid and/or mucosal thickening in the middle ear and mastoid condensation images*: this is a nonspecific finding that occurs early in the course; it is often seen in children with AOM with mastoiditis and may even be observed as an incidental finding in asymptomatic children.
2. *Loss of definition of the bony septae that define the mastoid air cells*: this finding is diagnostic of coalescent mastoiditis (Fig. 2.10).
3. *Destruction or irregularity of the mastoid cortex* (Fig. 2.11).
4. *Periosteal thickening, disruption of the periosteum, subperiosteal abscess* (Figs. 2.10 and 2.11).

In case of suspected complications, CT has preferentially to be done with contrast injection or should be followed by MRI, dependent on age and compliance of the patient.

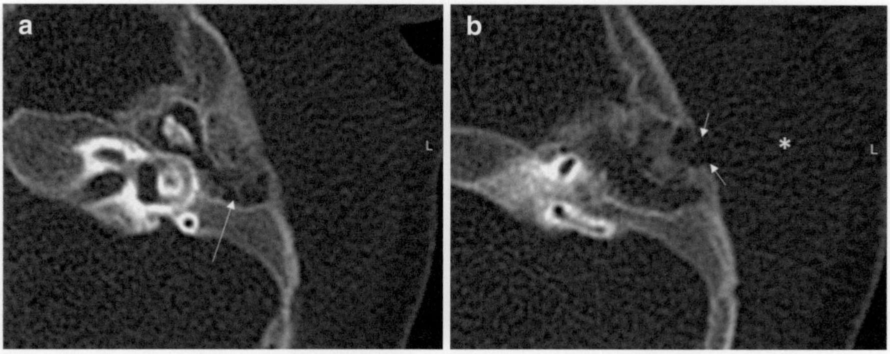

Fig. 2.11 Axial non injected CT-image of another 1½ year child, with acute otitis media and retroauricular swelling. (**a**) The mastoid is not well developed, atticoantral and mastoid cell condensations. (**b**) destruction of the mastoid cortex (between the two arrows) and a voluminous extratemporal soft tissue thickening (*): subperiosteal abscess

2.12.7 Differential Diagnosis

The differential diagnosis of acute coalescent mastoiditis includes other causes of postauricular inflammation or swelling:

- **Periauricular cellulitis related to otitis externa**: This is a common mimicker of mastoiditis. Severe pain over the tragus and pinna differentiates this entity from mastoiditis.
- **Perichondritis of the auricle**: Characterized by swelling and erythema of the pinna and may spread to the periosteum of the postauricular area. In contrast to acute mastoiditis, the postauricular crease is preserved, and the tympanic membrane appears normal.
- **Tumoral**: Benign and malignant tumors of the mastoid bone (e.g., aneurysmal bone cyst, acute lymphocytic leukemia, Langerhans cell histiocytosis) may have clinical features similar to mastoiditis.

2.12.8 Complications

Complications of coalescent mastoiditis are related to the spread of infection from the middle ear or mastoid to contiguous structures. In some cases, the complication is the presenting complaint.

In most case series, the rate of complications is approximately 10–20% (range 7–60%) [41, 42, 46, 47, 57, 58, 78, 79]. In a multicenter study, *S. pyogenes* was associated with the highest rate of complications at presentation (50%) and *S. aureus* with the highest rate of complications during hospitalization (31%) [42].

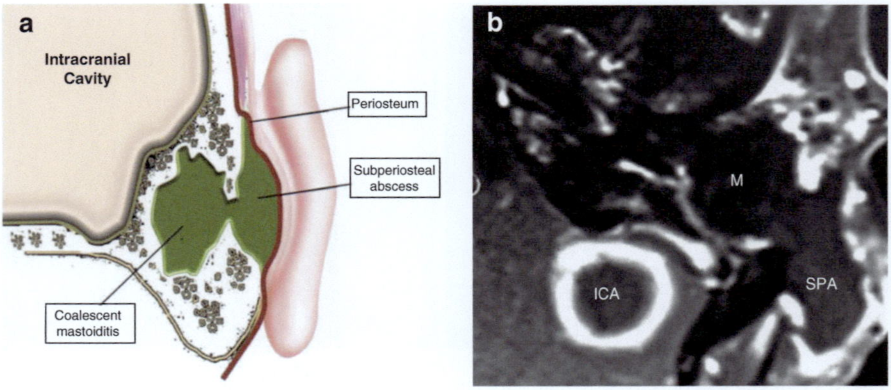

Fig. 2.12 Coalescent mastoditis with subperiosteal abscess (**a**) schematic drawing (**b**) T1 weighted MRI image after i.v. injection of gadolinium showing the coalescent mastoiditis (M) with exteriorisation of the purulent material in the subperiosteal space (SPA) through a large cortical defect. An intracerebral abscess (ICA) is another concomitant complication in this case

2.12.8.1 Extracranial Complications of Acute Coalescent Mastoiditis Include (See also Chap. 9)

Subperiosteal Abscess—(Fig. 2.12)

Signs of subperiosteal abscess include erythema, fluctuance, and a tender mass overlying the mastoid bone. Subperiosteal abscess occurs in about 50% of cases of acute mastoiditis [79].

Facial Nerve Palsy

Facial nerve palsy can result from infectious neuritis or inflammatory compression of the facial nerve as it traverses the temporal bone.

Labyrinthitis

Clinical features of labyrinthitis include tinnitus, hearing loss, nausea, vomiting, dizziness, vertigo, and nystagmus. Labyrinthtitis is caused by spread of bacteria from the middle ear to the labyrinthine space through the round window membrane. More often the involvement of the labyrinth is a reaction to bacterial exotoxins rather than bacterial invasion. This so-called otogenic labyrinthitis is unilateral in contrast to meningogenic labyrinthitis which is usually bilateral. MRI is the study of choice and shows that the endo- and perilymphatic spaces are filled with purulent material (Fig. 2.13a). The inner ear enhances on the T1-weighted images performed after gadolinium injection (Fig. 2.13b).

Petrous apicitis

Infection in the mastoid may spread to other parts of the skull, resulting in osteomyelitis. Osteomyelitis of the petrous apex may be associated with facial nerve palsy or Gradenigo syndrome (i.e., otorrhea, retro-orbital pain, ipsilateral abducens [sixth cranial nerve] palsy, and possibly other cranial nerve deficits).

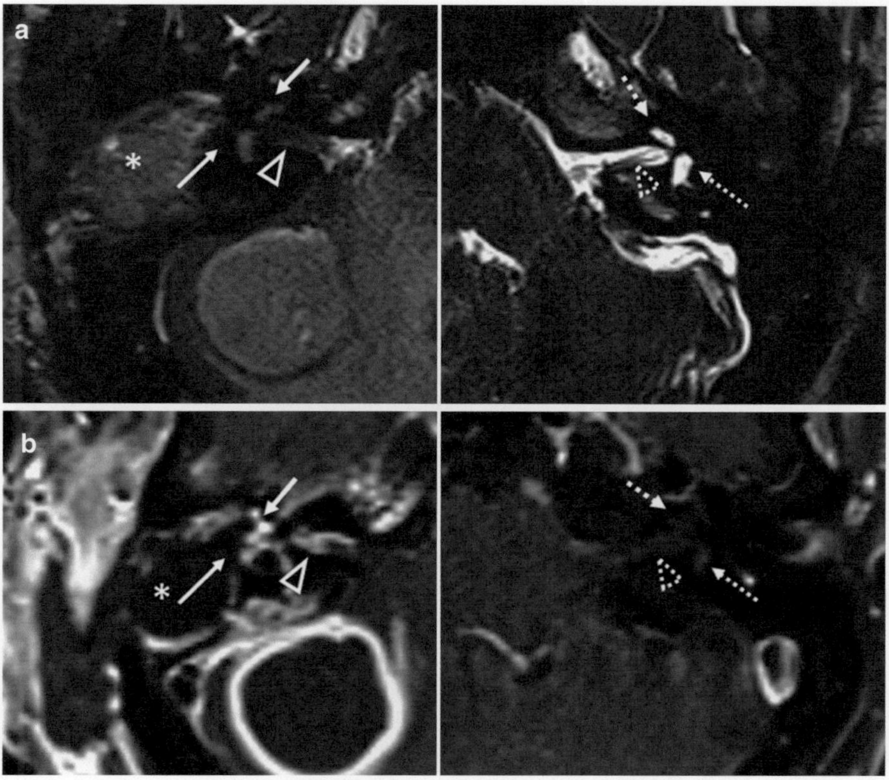

Fig. 2.13 Axial IRM images of a coalescent mastoiditis complicated by labyrinthitis (**a**) T2 weighted axial image showing purulent material in the mastoid as being slightly hyperintense (*). The endolymphatic/perilymphatic spaces of the cochlea (short arrow) and the semicircular canals (long arrow) are hypointens, as the content of the IAC (white empty arrowhead) in comparison to the normal left side with hyperintense fluid in the cochlea (short dashed arrow), the semicircular canals (long dashed arrow) and the IAC (dashed arrowhead). (**b**) on T1 weighted image post Gd and fatsat, the purulent material in the mastoid does not show any enhancement (*), but the whole right labyrinth shows an important contrast uptake, also the ICA, in comparison to the normal left side (same annotations for the different anatomic structures as in (**a**)

Bezold abscess

A Bezold abscess is a neck abscess located in the sheath of the sternocleidomastoid muscle. Clinical features of Bezold abscess include swelling and tenderness below the mastoid process and under the sternocleidomastoid muscle.

2.12.8.2 Intracranial Complications of Acute Coalescent Mastoiditis

Intracranial complications occurs in about 6% to 23% of cases with coalescent mastoiditis [38, 39, 79]. Altered mental status, neurologic deficits including cranial nerve palsy, high fever, neck stiffness, seizures, and severe headache should be concerning for intracranial disease.

Meningitis

Temporal Lobe or Cerebellar Abscess

Increasing temporoparietal headache, near the affected ear, is often the only indication of otogenic brain abscess formation [33] (See Figs. 9.17–9.20, Sect. 9.9).

Epidural or Subdural Abscess

Although rarely seen, among all intracranial complications of middle ear disease, epidural abscess formation is the most common [80] (See Fig. 9.19, Sect. 9.9).

Venous Sinus Thrombosis

Sinus thrombosis is the least frequent one [81]. Sigmoid sinus thrombosis has become increasingly uncommon, whereas in the pre-antibiotic era this complication was mortal in over 90% of the cases [81, 82].

Patients may present with otorrhea, otalgia, neck pain, fever, and chills [83]. But often presenting signs and symptoms are subtle or nonspecific and not in proportion to the magnitude of the problem, leading to a common delay in diagnosis [84, 85]. Consequently, a high index of suspicion is actually required to make the diagnosis [81, 82].

Imaging studies should be performed in all coalescent mastoiditis patients with pain or vertigo that is not rapidly resolving after appropriate antibiotic treatment [82] (See Figs. 9.14 and 9.15, Sect. 9.9). The therapeutic strategy is a point of debate, and ranges from internal jugular vein ligation, anticoagulation therapy, to the administration of less conventional antibiotic therapy [86].

2.12.9 Management

2.12.9.1 General Concept

The treatment of acute coalescent mastoiditis depends upon the stage and presence or absence of complications.

- ***Antimicrobial therapy and drainage of the middle ear and mastoid are the cornerstones of therapy for coalescent mastoiditis.***
- ***The rates of mastoidectomy*** in treatment of acute coalescent mastoiditis vary greatly in the range between 9 and 88%, as is reported in the literature [62]
- ***Antimicrobial therapy alone*** may fail to prevent the development of complications of acute coalescent mastoiditis. In a series of 223 patients, 8.5% developed complications during antimicrobial therapy [42].
- The use of single, high-dose intravenous (IV) steroids is warranted to decrease mucosal swelling and promote natural drainage through the aditus ad antrum into the middle ear.

Mastoidectomy may be warranted if one or more of the following are present

  – Postauricular fluctuant, mass, or swelling (suggesting subperiosteal abscess)
  – Cervical fluctuance (i.e., Bezold abscess).

- Imaging studies with evidence of rim-enhancing fluid collection, mastoid air cell coalescence, cortical bone erosion, or intracranial involvement.
- High-spiking "picket-fence" fever (may indicate sigmoid sinus thrombophlebitis)
- Neurologic signs (e.g., facial weakness, meningeal signs, focal deficits, altered level of consciousness, seizures); consultation by a neurosurgeon is also indicated.

2.12.9.2 Management of Uncomplicated Coalescent Mastoiditis

Uncomplicated acute coalescent mastoiditis is treated with intravenous (IV) antimicrobial therapy and myringotomy with placement of a tympanostomy tube

Numerous patients with uncomplicated mastoiditis respond well to conservative treatment. Unfortunately, we are still not able to predict which patient will have a poor response or which will develop severe complications.

Patients should be monitored daily for clinical response. If there is no clinical improvement in 48 h, mastoidectomy should be done.

2.12.9.3 Management of Complicated Mastoiditis

Acute coalescent mastoiditis with extracranial or intracranial complications is usually treated with IV antibiotics, myringotomy with placement of a tympanostomy tube, and mastoidectomy.

When a subperiosteal abscess is noted at presentation, *some otologists favor postauricular aspiration as the initial procedure* [87].

2.12.9.4 Antimicrobial Therapy

Because of the diversity of causative organisms in acute coalescent mastoiditis and the growing resistance of bacteria to the various antibiotics, all means to obtain a sample for culture and sensitivity prior to antibiotic treatment should be taken.

Empiric antimicrobial therapy for children with acute mastoiditis without a history of recurrent AOM or recent antibiotic administration should provide coverage for the most frequent bacterial pathogens: *S. pneumoniae* (including multiply resistant *S. pneumoniae*), *S. pyogenes*, and *S. aureus* (including methicillin-resistant *S. aureus*).

In a child with either no previous history of AOM or a history of a remote episode (i.e., >6 months before), empiric antimicrobial therapy with *vancomycin* alone (60 mg/kg per day divided every 6 h with a maximum dose of 4 gm/day) should be started until microbiologic results are available.

For children with a history of recurrent AOM (most recent episode within 6 months) or recent antibiotic use, adequate coverage for gram-positive and gram-negative pathogens usually entails combination therapy. Antibiotics active against *P. aeruginosa* should be included in the empiric regimen.

Upon diagnosis of the acute mastoiditis, initial antimicrobial is given intravenously. The patient can be switched to oral antibiotics when improved clinically and culture sensitivity days and oral antibiotics to complete a 4 weeks course.

2.12.9.5 Surgical Treatment

Early drainage interrupts the pathologic process and prevents complications [42].

Myringotomy

Myringotomy permits drainage of the mastoid if the aditus ad antrum is not blocked. Tympanostomy tubes permit drainage over a longer duration. Postoperatively, antibiotic/steroid drops are used to keep the tube patent and to reduce middle ear swelling. Antibiotic/steroid drops are continued until the otorrhea ceases.

Mastoidectomy

Mastoidectomy is performed to remove the mastoid infection, open the aditus ad antrum, and provide external drainage. Indications for mastoidectomy may include:

- Computed tomography evidence of coalescent mastoiditis (regardless of other clinical features)
- Subperiosteal abscess
- Other suppurative complications of acute mastoiditis
- Progression or persistence of fever, ear pain, postauricular swelling, or drainage despite parenteral antimicrobial therapy and tympanocentesis/myringotomy

2.12.9.6 Treatment Response

The response to treatment of acute mastoiditis is monitored through serial examination of the postauricular region, the external auditory canal, and the tympanic membrane and through measurement of inflammatory markers (WBC count and CRP).

In patients with acute mastoiditis, the above signs and symptoms should start to improve 48 hours after tympanocentesis/myringotomy and initiation of adequate antimicrobial therapy. Mastoidectomy is indicated in children who do not demonstrate adequate treatment response after 48 h. In this condition, imaging control of the temporal bone with intravenous contrast is indicated preoperatively.

2.12.9.7 Prevention

Early and adequate treatment of AOM reduces the risk of developing mastoiditis. Early recognition of the coalescent mastoiditis and its prompt treatment will decrease the risk of developing complications of mastoiditis.

2.12.10 Summary of Acute Coalescent Mastoiditis

Acute coalescent mastoiditis is a complication of AOM in which purulent material accumulates within the mastoid cavity. As the pressure increases, the bony septae between the mastoid air cells may be destroyed (coalescent mastoiditis), abscess cavities may form, and the purulent material may progress into adjacent areas.

Characteristic features of coalescent mastoiditis include postauricular abnormalities (tenderness, erythema, swelling, fluctuance, mass and protrusion) of the auricle; most patients also have fever and ear pain.

The diagnosis of acute coalescent mastoiditis is usually made clinically in children with characteristic examination findings. Imaging is necessary to confirm the diagnosis and evaluate suspected complications.

Treatment requires empiric antimicrobial therapy and drainage of pus from the middle ear and mastoid cavity.

Conclusion

AOM remains a common pathology for children even in developed countries. Its accurate diagnosis is simple and relies on adequate otoscopy. In nowadays practice, presumptive or confused diagnosis is inacceptable. The correct evaluation of the middle ear under perfect conditions during the presenting episode must be the rule. Antibiotics and paracentesis are the valuable means of treatment.

Strict follow up when the child becomes asymptomatic is of the utmost importance in order to evaluate residual effusions, avoid recurrences, complications and sequelae. For these objectives, the positive collaboration between family physicians, pediatrics and otologists is a major disciplinary measure to implement for a better outcome.

References

1. Bhutta MF. Epidemiology and pathogenesis of otitis media: construction of a phenotype landscape. Audiol Neurootol. 2014;19(3):210–23. https://doi.org/10.1159/000358549. Epub 2014 May 10. Review
2. Morris PS, Leach AJ. Acute and chronic otitis media. Pediatr Clin N Am. 2009;56(6):1383–99. https://doi.org/10.1016/j.pcl.2009.09.007. Review
3. Cunningham M, Guardiani E, Kim HJ, Brook I. Otitis media. Future Microbiol. 2012;7(6):733–53. https://doi.org/10.2217/fmb.12.38. Review
4. Pichichero ME. Acute otitis media: Part I. Improving diagnostic accuracy. Am Fam Physician. 2000;61(7):2051–6. Review
5. Siddiq S, Grainger J. The diagnosis and management of acute otitis media: American Academy of Pediatrics Guidelines 2013. Arch Dis Child Educ Pract Ed. 2015;100(4):193–7.
6. Wasson JD, Yung MW. Evidence-based management of otitis media: a 5S model approach. J Laryngol Otol. 2015;129(2):112–9.
7. Thomas JP, Berner R, Zahnert T, Dazert S. Acute otitis media – a structured approach. Dtsch Arztebl Int. 2014;111(9):151–9.
8. Schilder AG, Chonmaitree T, Cripps AW, Rosenfeld RM, Casselbrant ML, Haggard MP, Venekamp RP. Otitis media. Nat Rev Dis Primers. 2016;2:16063.
9. Atkinson H, Wallis S, Coatesworth AP. Acute otitis media. Postgrad Med. 2015;127(4):386–90. https://doi.org/10.1080/00325481.2015.1028872. Review
10. McCormick DP, Grady JJ, Diego A, Matalon R, Revai K, Patel JA, Han Y, Chonmaitree T. Acute otitis media severity: association with cytokine genepolymorphisms and other risk factors. Int J Pediatr Otorhinolaryngol. 2011;75(5):708–12.

11. Hafrén L, Kentala E, Järvinen TM, Leinonen E, Onkamo P, Kere J, Mattila PS. Genetic background and the risk of otitis media. Int J Pediatr Otorhinolaryngol. 2012;76(1):41–4.
12. Nokso-Koivisto J, Marom T, Chonmaitree T. Importance of viruses in acute otitis media. Curr Opin Pediatr. 2015;27(1):110–5.
13. Vergison A. Microbiology of otitis media: a moving target. Vaccine. 2008;26(Suppl 7):G5–10. https://doi.org/10.1016/j.vaccine.2008.11.006. Review
14. Heikkinen T, Chonmaitree T. Importance of respiratory viruses in acute otitis media. Clin Microbiol Rev. 2003;16(2):230–41. Review
15. Miura MS, Mascaro M, Rosenfeld RM. Association between otitis media and gastroesophageal reflux: a systematic review. Otolaryngol Head Neck Surg. 2012;146(3):345–52.
16. Kørvel-Hanquist A, Koch A, Niclasen J, Dammeye J, Lous J, Olsen SF, et al. Risk factors of early otitis media in the Danish National Birth Cohort. PLoS One. 2016;11(11):e0166465.
17. Gould JM, Matz PS. Otitis media. Pediatr Rev. 2010;31(3):102–16. Review
18. Ngo CC, Massa HM, Thornton RB, Cripps AW. Predominant bacteria detected from the middle ear fluid of children experiencing otitis media: a systematic review. PLoS One. 2016;11(3):e0150949.
19. Dagan R, Pelton S, Bakaletz L, Cohen R. Prevention of early episodes of otitismedia by pneumococcal vaccines might reduce progression to complex disease. Lancet Infect Dis. 2016;16(4):480–92.
20. Shawabka MA, Haidar H, Larem A, Aboul-Mahmood Z, Alsaadi A, et al. Acute otitis media- an update. J Otolaryngol ENT Res. 2017;8(2):00252.
21. Pichichero ME, Almudevar A. Serum cytokine biomarkers accurately predict presence of acute otitis media infection and recovery caused by Haemophilus influenzae. Int J Pediatr Otorhinolaryngol. 2016;83:200–4.
22. Massa HM, Cripps AW, Lehmann D. Otitis media: viruses, bacteria, biofilms and vaccines. Med J Aust. 2009;191(9 Suppl):S44.
23. American Academy of Pediatrics Subcommittee on Management of Acute Otitis Media. Diagnosis and management of acute otitis media. Pediatrics. 2004;113(5):1451–65.
24. Rosenfeld RM, Schwartz SR, Pynnonen MA, Tunkel DE, Hussey HM, Fichera JS, Grimes AM, Hackell JM, Harrison MF, Haskell H, Haynes DS, Kim TW, Lafreniere DC, LeBlanc K, Mackey WL, Netterville JL, Pipan ME, Raol NP, Schellhase KG. Clinical practice guideline: tympanostomy tubes in children. Otolaryngol Head Neck Surg. 2013;149(1 Suppl):S1–35.
25. Donaldson JD. Acute otitis media workup. In: Meyers AD, editor. Drugs & diseases, Otolaryngology and facial plastic surgery; 2017.
26. Levi JR, Brody RM, McKee-Cole K, Pribitkin E, O'Reilly R. Complementary and alternative medicine for pediatric otitis media. Int J Pediatr Otorhinolaryngol. 2013;77(6):926–31.
27. Daniel M, Gautam S, Scrivener TA, Meller C, Levin B, Curotta JJ. What effect has pneumococcal vaccination had on acute mastoiditis? Laryngol Otol. 2013;127(Suppl 1):S30–4.
28. Gaio E, Marioni G, de Filippis C, Tregnaghi A, Caltran S, Staffieri A. Facial nerve paralysis secondary to acute otitis media in infants and children. J Paediatr Child Health. 2004;40(8):483–6.
29. Yonamine FK, Tuma J, Silva RF, Soares MC, Testa JR. Facial paralysis associated with acute otitis media. Braz J Otorhinolaryngol. 2009;75(2):228–30.
30. Piegel JH, Lustig LR, Lee KC, Murr AH, Schindler RA. Contemporary presentation and management of a spectrum of mastoid abscesses. Laryngoscope. 1998;108(6):822–8.
31. Kuczkowski J, Mikaszewski B. Intracranial complications of acute and chronic mastoiditis: report of two cases in children. Int J Pediatr Otorhinolaryngol. 2001;60(3):227–37.
32. Kaftan H, Draf W. Intracranial otogenic complications: inspite of therapeutic progress still a serious problem. Laryngorhinootologie. 2000;79(10):609–15.
33. Dobben GD, Raofi B, Mafee MF, Kamel A, Mercurio S. Otogenic intracranial inflammations: role of magnetic resonance imaging. Top Magn Reson Imaging. 2000;11(2):76–86.
34. Glynn F, Osman L, Colreavy M, et al. Acute mastoiditis in children: Presentation and long term consequences. J Laryngol Otol. 2008;122(3):233–7., http://dx.doi.org/S0022215107009929 [pii].
35. Psarommatis I, Giannakopoulos P, Theodorou E, et al: Mastoid subperiosteal abscess in children: Drainage or mastoidectomy? J Laryngol Otol 126(12):1204-1208, http://dx.doi.org/10.1017/S0022215 112002332, 2012

36. Zevallos JP, Vrabec JT, Williamson RA, et al. Advanced pediatric mastoiditis with and without intracranial complications. Laryngoscope. 2009;119(8):1610–5., https://doi.org/10.1002/lary.20259.
37. http://dx.doi.org/S0165-5876(00)00425-0
38. http://dx.doi.org/S0165-5876(00)00283-4
39. Luntz M, Keren G, Nusem S, et al. Acute mastoiditis—revisited. Ear Nose Throat J. 1994;73(9):648–54.
40. Adams DJ, Susi A, Erdie-Lalena CR, Gorman G, Hisle-Gorman E, Rajnik M, Elrod M, Nylund CM. Otitis media and related complications among children with autism spectrum disorders. J Autism Dev Disord. 2016;46(5):1636–42. (ISSN: 1573-3432)
41. Geva A, Oestreicher-Kedem Y, Fishman G, et al. Conservative management of acute mastoiditis in children. Int J Pediatr Otorhinolaryngol. 2008;72:629.
42. Luntz M, Brodsky A, Nusem S, et al. Acute mastoiditis – the antibiotic era: a multicenter study. Int J Pediatr Otorhinolaryngol. 2001;57:1.
43. Katz A, Leibovitz E, Greenberg D, et al. Acute mastoiditis in Southern Israel: a twelve year retrospective study (1990 through 2001). Pediatr Infect Dis J. 2003;22:878.
44. Thorne MC, Chewaproug L, Elden LM. Suppurative complications of acute otitis media: changes in frequency over time. Arch Otolaryngol Head Neck Surg. 2009;135:638.
45. Benito MB, Gorricho BP. Acute mastoiditis: increase in the incidence and complications. Int J Pediatr Otorhinolaryngol. 2007;71:1007.
46. Bilavsky E, Yarden-Bilavsky H, Samra Z, et al. Clinical, laboratory, and microbiological differences between children with simple or complicated mastoiditis. Int J Pediatr Otorhinolaryngol. 2009;73:1270.
47. Oestreicher-Kedem Y, Raveh E, Kornreich L, et al. Complications of mastoiditis in children at the onset of a new millennium. Ann Otol Rhinol Laryngol. 2005;114:147.
48. Palma S, Fiumana E, Borgonzoni M, et al. Acute mastoiditis in children: the "Ferrara" experience. Int J Pediatr Otorhinolaryngol. 2007;71:1663.
49. Ruiz Díaz AI, del Castillo Martín F, Bilbao Garitagoitia A, et al. Acute mastoiditis: an increasing entity. An Esp Pediatr. 2002;57:427.
50. Roddy MG, Glazier SS, Agrawal D. Pediatric mastoiditis in the pneumococcal conjugate vaccine era: symptom duration guides empiric antimicrobial therapy. Pediatr Emerg Care. 2007;23:779.
51. Ho D, Rotenberg BW, Berkowitz RG. The relationship between acute mastoiditis and antibiotic use for acute otitis media in children. Arch Otolaryngol Head Neck Surg. 2008;134:45.
52. Mustafa A, Debry CH, Wiorowski M, et al. Treatment of acute mastoiditis: report of 31 cases over a ten year period. Rev Laryngol Otol Rhinol (Bord). 2004;125:165.
53. Baljosevic I, Mircetic N, Subarevic V, Markovic G. Acute mastoiditis in infants. Eur Arch Otorhinolaryngol. 2006;263:906.
54. Heslop A, Ovesen T. Severe acute middle ear infections: microbiology and treatment. Int J Pediatr Otorhinolaryngol. 2006;70:1811.
55. Nussinovitch M, Yoeli R, Elishkevitz K, Varsano I. Acute mastoiditis in children: epidemiologic, clinical, microbiologic, and therapeutic aspects over past years. Clin Pediatr (Phila). 2004;43:261–7. (ISSN: 0009-9228)
56. Ongkasuwan J, Valdez TA, Hulten KG, et al. Pneumococcal mastoiditis in children and the emergence of multidrug-resistant serotype 19A isolates. Pediatrics. 2008;122:34.
57. Stähelin-Massik J, Podvinec M, Jakscha J, et al. Mastoiditis in children: a prospective, observational study comparing clinical presentation, microbiology, computed tomography, surgical findings and histology. Eur J Pediatr. 2008;167:541.
58. Groth A, Enoksson F, Hultcrantz M, et al. Acute mastoiditis in children aged 0–16 years – a national study of 678 cases in Sweden comparing different age groups. Int J Pediatr Otorhinolaryngol. 2012;76:1494.
59. Anthonsen K, Høstmark K, Hansen S, et al. Acute mastoiditis in children: a 10-year retrospective and validated multicenter study. Pediatr Infect Dis J. 2013;32:436.
60. Ghadersohi S, Young NM, Smith-Bronstein V, et al. Management of acute complicated mastoiditis at an urban, tertiary care pediatric hospital. Laryngoscope. 2017;127(10):2321–7.

61. Lieberthal AS, Carroll AE, Chonmaitree T. The diagnosis and management of acute otitis media. Pediatrics. 2013;131:e964–99.
62. Psarommatis IM, Voudouris C, Douros K, Giannakopoulos P, Bairamis T, Carabinos C. Algorithmic management of pediatric acute mastoiditis. Int J Pediatr Otorhinolaryngol. 2012;76(6):791–6. (ISSN: 1872-8464)
63. Palma S, Bovo R, Benatti A, Aimoni C, Rosignoli M, Libanore M, Martini A. Mastoiditis in adults: a 19-year retrospective study. Eur Arch Otorhinolaryngol. 2014;271(5):925–31. (ISSN: 1434-4726)
64. Spratley J, Silveira H, Alvarez I, PaisClemente M. Acute mastoiditis in children. Review of the current status. Int J Pediatr Otolaryngol. 2000;56:33–40.
65. House HP. Otitis media; a comparative study of the results obtained in therapy before and after the introduction of the sulfonamide compounds. Arch Otolaryngol. 1946;43:371–8.
66. Goldstein NA, Casselbrant ML, Bluestone CD, et al. Intratemporal complications of acute otitis media in infants and children. Otolaryngol Head Neck Surg. 1998;119(5):444–54., http://dx.doi.org/S019459989 8003507 [pii].
67. Palva T, Pulkkinen K. Mastoiditis. J Laryngol Otol. 1959;73:573–88.
68. Lund FH. Acute and latent mastoiditis. J Laryngol Otol. 1989;103:1158–60.
69. Hoppe JE, Koster S, Bootz F, Neithammer D. Acute mastoiditis—relevant once again. Infection. 1994;22:178–82.
70. Ghaffar FA, Wordemann M, McCracken GH Jr. Acute mastoiditis in children: a seventeen-year experience in Dallas. Texas Pediatr Infect Dis J. 2001;20:376–80.
71. Dhooge IJ, Alberts FW, Van Cauwenberge PB. Intratemporal and intracranial complications of acute suppurative otitis media in children: renewed interest. Int J Pediatr Otorhinolaryngol. 1999;49:S109–14.
72. Antonelli PJ, Dhanani N, Giannoni CM, Kubilis PS. Impact of resistant pneumococcus on rates of acute mastoiditis. Otolaryngol Head Neck Surg. 1999;121:190–4.
73. Gliklich RE, Eavey RD, Iannuzzi RA, Camacho AE. A contemporary analysis of acute mastoiditis. Arch Otolaryngol Head Neck Surg. 1996;122:135–9.
74. Mathews TJ, Oliver SP. Bacteriology of mastoiditis. A five-year experience at Groote Schuur Hospital. J Laryngol Otol. 1988;102:397–8.
75. Meyerhoff WL, Gates GA, Montalbo PJ. Pseudomonas mastoiditis. Laryngoscope. 1977;87:483–92.
76. Ostfeld E, Rubinstein E. Acute gramnegative bacilliary infections of middle ear and mastoid. Ann Otol Rhinol Laryngol. 1980;89:33–6.
77. Halgrimson WR, Chan KH, Abzug MJ, Perkins JN, Carosone-Link P, Simões EA. Incidence of acute mastoiditis in Colorado children in the pneumococcal conjugate vaccine era. Pediatr Infect Dis J. 2014;33(5):453–7. (ISSN: 1532-0987)
78. Pang LH, Barakate MS, Havas TE. Mastoiditis in a paediatric population: a review of 11 years experience in management. Int J Pediatr Otorhinolaryngol. 2009;73:1520.
79. van den Aardweg MT, Rovers MM, de Ru JA, et al. A systematic review of diagnostic criteria for acute mastoiditis in children. Otol Neurotol. 2008;29:751.
80. Bizakis JG, Velegrakis GA, Papadakis CE, Karampekios SK, Helidonis ES. The silent epidural abscess as a complication of acute otitis media in children. Int J Pediatr Otorhinolaryngol. 1998;45(2):163–6.
81. Rocha JL, Kondo W, Gracia CM, Baptista MI, Büchele G, da Cunha CA, Martins LT. Central venous sinus thrombosis following mastoiditis: report of 4 cases and literature review. Braz J Infect Dis. 2000;4(6):307–12.
82. Keogh IJ, Hone SW, Colreavy M, Gaffney R. Sigmoid sinus thrombosis: an old foe revisited. Ir Med J. 2001;94(4):117–8.
83. See KC, Leong JL, Tan HK. Otogenic lateral sinus thrombosis – a case report. Ann Acad Med Singap. 2000;29(6):753–6.
84. Fritsch MH, Miyamoto RT, Wood TL. Sigmoid sinus thrombosis diagnosis by contrasted MRI scanning. Otolaryngol Head Neck Surg. 1990;103(3):451–6.

85. Ram B, Meiklejohn DJ, Nunez DA, Murray A, Watson HG. Combined risk factors contributing to cerebral venous thrombosis in a young woman. J Laryngol Otol. 2001;115(4):307–10.
86. Dallari S, Zaccarelli SC, Sintini M, Gatti G, Balli R. Acute mastoiditis with complications: a report of two cases. Acta Otorhinolaryngol Belg. 1997;51(2):113–8.
87. Lahav J, Handzel O, Gertler R, et al. Postauricular needle aspiration of subperiosteal abscess in acute mastoiditis. Ann Otol Rhinol Laryngol. 2005;114:323.
88. Nitsche MP, Carreño M. Antibiotics for acute otitis media in children. Medwave. 2015;15(Suppl 2):e6295. https://doi.org/10.5867/medwave.2015.6295.
89. Venekamp RP, Sanders SL, Glasziou PP, Del Mar CB, Rovers MM. Antibiotics for acute otitis media in children. Cochrane Database Syst Rev. 2015;6:CD000219.

Otitis Media with Effusion

3

Contents

S. Mansour et al., *Middle Ear Diseases*,
https://doi.org/10.1007/978-3-319-72962-6_3

3.1 Introduction

Otitis media with effusion (OME), eloquently described by Politzer under the name of "Otitis Catarrhalis" in 1884, is also called serous otitis media, seromucous otitis media, exudative otitis media, nonsuppurative otitis media or "glue ear". It is an inflammatory middle ear disease, defined by the presence of fluid in the middle ear behind an intact tympanic membrane without signs and symptoms of an acute infection. It is called chronic OME, if effusion persists for 3 months or longer.

The term "glue ear" is reserved for cases in which the effusion in the middle ear became thick and glue-like, also called mucoid otitis media.

OME is a consequence of inflammation of the middle ear mucosa that occurs before or after an episode of acute otitis media (AOM); but it may also occur in the absence of AOM. OME is the most common cause of hearing impairment in children potentially causing language delays, learning and behavioral problems.

3.2 Epidemiology

Following an acute otitis media episode, an effusion is formed in the middle ear and may persist for weeks to months after the acute symptoms have resolved [1, 2]. OME is common among apparently asymptomatic young children; 90% of children had at least one episode of OME by the age of 4 years [3]. The prevalence ranges from 10 to 17% among children younger than 4 years old, and then decreases to 3 to 4% between 6 and 8 years old [3–5]. At any given time, 5% of children aged 2–4 years experience hearing loss due to a middle ear effusion that lasts 3 months or longer (chronic OME).

Some findings suggest that males may have a slightly higher incidence of the disease. OME is more common in winter than in summer [6]. The decline in tympanostomy tube insertion rates among children following universal immunization with pneumococcal conjugate vaccine suggests that the current prevalence of OME may have declined from the prevaccine era.

3.3 Predisposing Factors

Family history of otitis media, milk bottle feeding (as opposed to breastfeeding), daycare attendance, atopy and adenoidal hypertrophy, exposure to tobacco smoke, and low socioeconomic level are important risk factors for the development of acute otitis media (AOM) and otitis media with effusion (OME) [1, 4, 6–8]. Children with a cleft palate are particularly prone to have chronic OME.

The factors promoting the persistence of middle ear effusion in patients with AOM remain insufficiently defined.

3.4 Pathogenesis

There is a general agreement that OME is the result of middle ear global dysventilation which is an imbalance between gas gain through ET ventilation and gas loss through mastoid mucosal gas diffusion (see sect. 7.3). Global middle ear dysventilation leads to a "gas deficiency" status of the middle ear which is the hallmark of OME.

The controversy in pathogenesis of OME exists in the mechanism that "gas deficiency" can lead to effusion. Two theories exist:

1. Gas deficiency builds negative pressure in the middle ear which creates a vaccum effect and leads to passive transudation of fluid into middle ear (**The Ex Vacuo theory**).
2. Gas deficiency leads to middle ear hypoxia which leads to hypoxia-induced mucosal inflammation with resultant active exudation of fluid into the middle ear (**Inflammatory theory**).

3.4.1 The Ex Vacuo Theory of the Eustachian Tube

Long time and largely popularized by Politzer, the ex vacuo theory prevails: a blockage of the Eustachian tube, by adenoid hypertrophy or tubal mucosa oedema, induces middle ear vacuum status resulting in transudation of the mucosa and effusion.

The chain of events would be:

ET obstruction → negative pressure → absorption and/or diffusion of nitrogen and oxygen into the middle ear mucosal cells → transudate from the mucosa → development of a flora of bacteria.

However, there are several arguments opposed to the ex vacuo theory:

(a) In fact, the ET plays a minor role in regulating the ME pressure as the opening duration of ET is very brief (200 ms) and the frequency of openings is only every 1–2 min (a total of 3–4 min a day, allowing only a small volume of gas to pass through the ET, around *1 mL a day*). Such amount represents about *10% of the total volume of the ME cleft*. Under normal conditions, the intermittent openings of ET supply the middle ear with sufficient amount of gas to compensate which was lost from the middle ear by normal mucosal gas exchange; but ET cannot assume the excessive needs during a mucosal inflammatory condition of ME, where mucosal gas exchange becomes intense and results in extra absorption and loss of gas from the ME. This inability of the ET is named "ET dysfunction". This does not imply an intrinsic ET pathology or ET responsibility: [9];

(b) In pathological conditions, the ME pressure values are either atmospheric or a few millimeters below, which is not sufficient to produce a transudate [10].
(c) Biochemical analysis of the effusion shows to be an active exudate rather than a passive transudate
(d) Eustachian tube endoscopy during chronic otitis media have never shown abnormal narrowing or obstruction of the tube lumen [11]
(e) It has been demonstrated that ME pressure depends mainly on gas exchange between mucosal blood supplies and ME cavity [12]
(f) Thus the "ex vacuo" mechanical theory does not take into account the inflammatory process of the ME mucosa with the resulting metaplasia, mucin production and hypersecretion.

3.4.2 The Inflammatory Theory

OME is an inflammatory middle ear pathology that results from a variety of inciting events that converge on a common pathway of inflammation, then mucosal metaplasia and effusion.

Middle ear global dysventilation leads to gaz deficit and secondary hypoxia in the middle ear. In addition, during episodes of acute otitis media, the large amount of inflammatory cells and the hyperplasia of the mucosa participate to the consumption of O_2, leading to hypoxia. Hypoxia induces response of stress from cells trying to reduce their metabolism to save O_2. Cellular responses to hypoxia are central to the pathophysiology of OME. Gene expression profile changes significantly when cells are exposed to hypoxia. Hypoxia inducible factor (HIF) is a pivotal transcription factor induced under hypoxia which transactivates target genes such as vascular endothelial growth factor (VEGF). VEGF acts to induce angiogenesis, increases vascular permeability and recruitment of neutrophils and macrophages and may therefore contribute to OME by the accumulation of exudate fluid and inflammatory cells within the middle ear (see Fig. 3.3 and Sect. 3.6.3). In vivo, rats with Eustachian tube blockage showed otitis media with development of effusion and elevated expression of HIF-1α, VEGF, IL-1β, and TNF-α [13]). In addition, inflammation itself creates hypoxia due to increased metabolic activity outpacing the availability of oxygen in the middle ear. There is a strong cross talk between hypoxia and inflammation: Hypoxia induces inflammatory response and inflammation can cause hypoxic stress and further inflammation.

Hypoxia → Inflammation → Hypoxia → Inflammation

Inflammation stimulates the activation of EGF, IL-13, IL-10 IL-1β and TNF-α to induce middle ear mucosal hyperplasia and metaplasia into mucin secreting mucosa with differentiation of basal cells of the epithelium into goblet cells, responsible for the secretion of mucin and of a viscous effusion (see Fig. 3.2).

Infection/Inflammation (TNF-α) → Mucosal Hyperplasia (EGF + IL-13) → ciliated cells metaplasia to goblet cells (IL-10 IL-1β and TNF-α) → persistent mucosal overproduction of mucin (IL-10).

Also poor clearance of middle ear fluid [14, 15] is incriminated in the effusion persistence once the inflammation has resolved. Poor clearance is due to ciliary dysfunction, mucosal edema, hyperviscosity of the effusion and, possibly, an unfavorable pressure gradient.

In addition, genetic predisposition [16, 17], allergies [18–24], and gastroesophageal reflux [25] may contribute to the pathogenesis of OME.

3.5 Risk Factors of OME

Several factors are associated with increased risk of OME (Fig. 3.1).

3.5.1 Age

The incidence of OME decreases steadily with age. This is likely reflective of an increased maturity of the Eustachian tube and the immune system and completion of childhood vaccinations. A decrease of OME is also observed as the anatomy of the

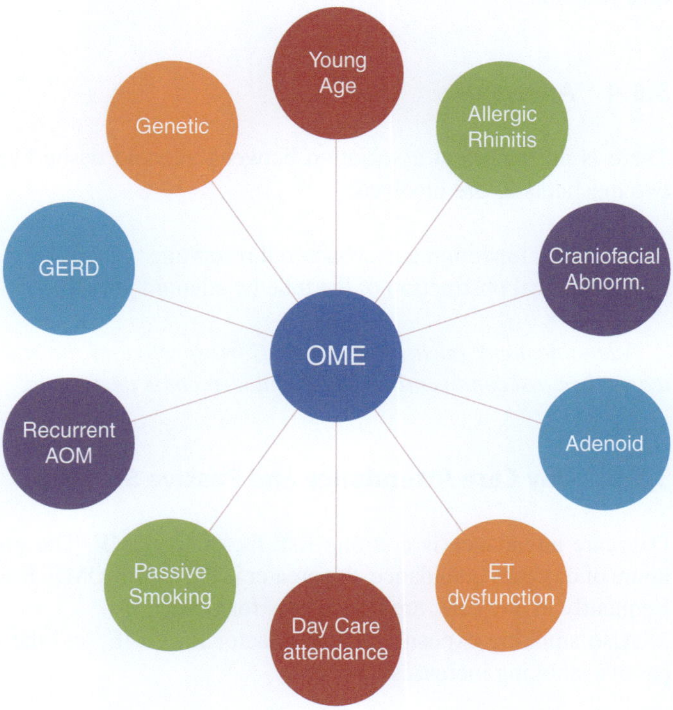

Fig. 3.1 Risk factors associated with OME

Eustachian tube changes with age related craniofacial maturation. Although less common than in children, OME can occur in adults, usually developing after a severe upper respiratory tract infection such as sinusitis, severe allergy, or rapid changes in atmospheric pressure (barotrauma) after a plane flight or a scuba diving.

3.5.2 Eustachian Tube Anatomy

Premature floppy tube and horizontal orientation of the tube are well known risk factors for OME, allowing direct entry of bacteria from the nasopharynx into the middle ear.

3.5.3 Craniofacial Abnormalities

Studies of patients born with craniofacial abnormalities provide evidence to the role of Eustachian Tube (ET) maturation in the pathogenesis of OME. Histological studies of ET tissue from children born with cleft lip or palate show evidence of immaturity of the cartilaginous tissue of the tube, which may explain the higher propensity towards infection in those children. There is higher incidence of OME in children with uncorrected cleft palate than in normal children. However, when the cleft is corrected, OME is reduced, possibly because it allows improved Eustachian tube function.

3.5.4 Adenoids

There is an important association between adenoid tissue hyperplasia and OME: two mechanisms are involved:

1. Adenoids functioning as a bacterial reservoir.
2. Mechanical obstruction of the tube by adenoid growth.

Adenoidectomy must be performed, irrespective of the size of the adenoids, at least when a second ventilation tube placement is performed.

3.5.5 Day Care Attendance and Passive Smoking

Day care attendance is a strong risk factor for OME. The greater the number of hours of day care attendance, the greater is the risk of OME. Frequent colds, trapped frequently in day care, are risk factors for OME.

Also smoking exposure is a risk factor for OME, and the risk associated with passive smoking increases with age.

3.5.6 Recurrent Middle Ear Infections

The effusion of OME is not sterile. Multiple studies have revealed that the same type of bacteria is present in otitis media with effusion as in acute otitis media. The only difference with the pathogens in OME compared to AOM is that in the first the frequency of *S pneumoniae* is not as high, and *H influenzae* and *M catarrhalis* are moderately more common. Haemophilus influenzae was isolated predominantly from serous effusions and Staphylococcus epidermidis predominantly from mucoid samples [26]. Moreover it is concluded that endotoxin may be one of the important factors in the pathogenesis of onset of OME, as well as in the delayed recovery from OME in children: 83% of mucoid MEE from children contained endotoxin, compared with 41% of serous MEE [27].

3.5.7 Biofilms

Biofilms appear to play an important role in the pathogenesis of OME: chronic OME is the result of a bacterial biofilm forming directly on the mucosal surface of the middle ear [28].

In order to prevent the evolution of the disease into a chronic stage, understanding the mechanisms implicated in OME development in response to bacteria, and how their interaction evolves into chronic OME, is needed. The innate immune system plays a central role in OME: after having crossed the eventual innate immune barriers in the middle ear, bacteria reach the middle ear epithelium, and adhere to its cells, using adherence molecules of variable nature depending on the bacteria types. Adherence of a great number of bacteria to the epithelium cells of the ME is followed by the creation of an extracellular matrix and biofilm formation. The growth of bacteria in biofilms gives them the ability to hide from the immune system of the host (see Sect. 6.6.1).

It is possible that biofilms are a defense mechanism offering to bacteria a niche to protect themselves from a hostile inflammatory environment, waiting that immune responses decrease in order to better infect the host.

3.5.8 Allergic Rhinitis

There are many epidemiologic, and therapeutic evidences showing that allergic rhinitis contributes to the pathogenesis of OME. In fact, allergic rhinitis reduces the immune competencies of the mucosal immune system of the upper respiratory tract and makes the middle ear more prone to infection. In addition, mucosal oedema present in allergic rhinitis, impairs the function of the ET.

Persistent middle-ear effusion (MEE) was found for 2 months or longer in children with atopic manifestations more than in those that were non-allergic.

Early introduction of cow's milk is also a risk factor for OME.

3.5.9 Gastroesophageal Reflux

Gastroesophageal reflux is also hypothesized to contribute to OME, but causality has not been proven. In a systematic review of 15 studies of gastroesophageal or laryngopharyngeal reflux and otitis media, the prevalence of gastroesophageal reflux appeared to be increased in children with OME compared with the overall prevalence in children. In several of the included studies, pepsin/pepsinogen was detected in the middle ear fluid of the majority of children; however the mean concentration varied widely [25].

3.5.10 Genetic Predisposition

It is well known that having siblings, in whom tympanostomy tube placement has been performed, is an important risk factor for OME. The strongest evidence of a genetic susceptibility to OME was shown in studies involving twins and triplets. In the prospective twins and triplets Pittsburgh study, where monthly monitoring of the middle ear was done, the estimated heritability of otitis media at the 2-year endpoint was 0.79 in girls and 0.64 in boys [29]. The correlation between twins for the proportion of time with MEE was significantly higher in the monozygotic than in the dizygotic twins. The estimated heritability of the proportion of time with MEE in the first 5 years of life is 72% [30].

As otitis media is a multifactorial disease in humans, it is not probable that one unique gene is the cause of otitis media. The first linkage study was performed by Daly et al. [31] that provided evidence of linkage of COME to 10q26.3 and to 19q13.43. Another study was conducted at Pittsburgh and showed a significant linkage peak on chromosome 17q12, and in 10q22.3 [32].

Potential therapeutic targets are the genes regulating mucin expression, mucus production and host response to bacteria in the middle ear [33]. The identification of the susceptibility genes to otitis media could improve the knowledge of the otitis media physiopathology and provide the development of molecular diagnostic methods that could be used to establish the risk for otitis media of a specific child and perhaps modify the follow-up and the treatment according to this established risk.

3.6 Molecular Biology of OME

Serous effusions contain proteins similar to the blood, so it is suggested that serous fluids are the result of a passive transudation of blood components in the middle ear due to a negative pressure in the middle ear, likely because of the Eustachian tube blockage [34, 35]. Serous effusions do not contain mucins and are not viscous. Serous effusions are believed to have better prognosis.

In chronic OME (mucoid or "Glue ear") ME effusions are exsudative, highly viscous and contain a high content of mucins. Mucoid effusion is the result of an active production of mucin. Mucoid effusions are difficult to clear spontaneously from the middle ear.

3.6.1 Role of Inflammation

Analysis of middle ear effusions demonstrated high concentrations of a panel of pro-inflammatory cytokines and inflammatory cells which is a proof that OME is an inflammatory disease.

Inflammation seems to appear at the early stages of OME development when the middle ear is trying to react against middle ear hypoxia or trying to fight the infection and it persists until more chronic stages even when the bacteria count becomes lower.

The chronic stages of OME also show a diversity of cytokines in high concentration in the middle ear, suggesting the persistence of inflammation phenomenon despite the near absence of pathogens. The reduced muco-ciliary clearance of the metaplastic mucin secreting middle ear mucosa might limit the efficiency of the clearance of killed pathogens; thus keeping bacterial antigens and cytokines in the middle ear that still stimulate the immune responses.

Some defects in cytokine production, dependent on genetic and environmental influence, might also explain why children tend to be prone to recurrent and persistent OME. Cytokines exhibit strong effects that, if not balanced, can lead to a disproportionate immune response. *IL-8 and IL-10 were detected in higher concentrations in mucoid effusions compared to serous ones.*

In addition, many immune cells are found in ME effusion such lymphocytes and granulocytes as neutrophils, basophils, and eosinophils and phagocytic cells as macrophages and dendritic cells. These immune cells are supposed to come from the nasopharynx [36].

3.6.2 Mucous Cell Metaplasia and Mucin Production

Upregulation of mucin expression has been found to be induced by both microbial and host-derived factors, including OM pathogens, cytokines, and growth factors. Otitis media pathogens not only activate host positive signaling pathways but also suppress inhibitory signaling pathways to upregulate mucin expression (*Interleukin-10 induces mucin overproduction*). The production of these inflammatory mediators, along with the production of VEGF, causes an increase in the vascular permeability and leads to the formation of MEE. In mucoid otitis media, the middle ear effusions are characterized by the presence of mucoid glycoproteins. Mucins are produced at later stages of OME course by goblet cells of the middle ear epithelium and mucus glands. Several factors play a role in the remodeling of the epithelium of the middle ear:

As mentioned above, infection of the Middle Ear results in pro-inflammatory mediator expression; mainly IL-10 IL-1β and TNF-α induce middle ear metaplasia and hyperplasia as well as effusion production containing mucins (Fig. 3.2).

Therefore much work is needed in this particular area for identification of effective agents to stop mucous cell metaplasia/hyperplasia in OM [37].

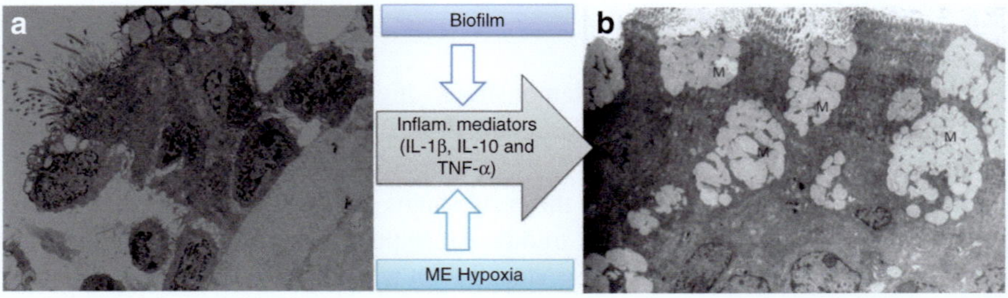

Fig. 3.2 In chronic secretory otitis media, the normal cuboidal ME epithelium (**a**) undergoes a progressive metaplasia and transition to a columnar ciliated epithelium with numerous secretory goblet cells (**b**). Inflammation damages the epithelium and paralyzes ciliary motility especially in "Glue Ear"

3.6.3 Role of Hypoxia

During otitis media, the large amount of inflammatory cells and the hyperplasia of the mucosa participate to the consumption of O_2, leading to hypoxia. In addition, the ET is often blocked by oedema and secretions increasing the hypoxia. Middle ear hypoxia induces the formation of:

- The transcription factor hypoxia inducible factor 1α **(HIF-1α)** and
- The secreted protein vascular endothelial growth factor **(VEGF)** [38].

Hypoxia inducible factor (HIF) is a pivotal transcription factor induced under hypoxia which transactivates target genes such as vascular endothelial growth factor (VEGF). VEGF acts to induce angiogenesis, increases vascular permeability and recruitment of neutrophils and macrophages and may therefore contribute to OME by the accumulation of exudate fluid and inflammatory cells within the middle ear. This results in mucosal inflammation and perpetuates the vicious circle of the inflammatory process in the middle ear epithelium between Inflammation and Hypoxia (Fig. 3.3) [38].

3.6.4 Aquaporins

Aquaporins (AQPs) facilitate water movement within specific organs, allowing water to move along the osmotic gradient. Aquaporins appear to be involved in the water balance of the middle ear. The expression of various AQP has been reported in the tissues and cell linings of the tubotympanum. Recent researches showed that a specific aquaporin, aquaporin 5 (AQP5), regulates gel-forming mucin expression and may influence middle ear effusion viscosity by altering its mucin composition." [39].

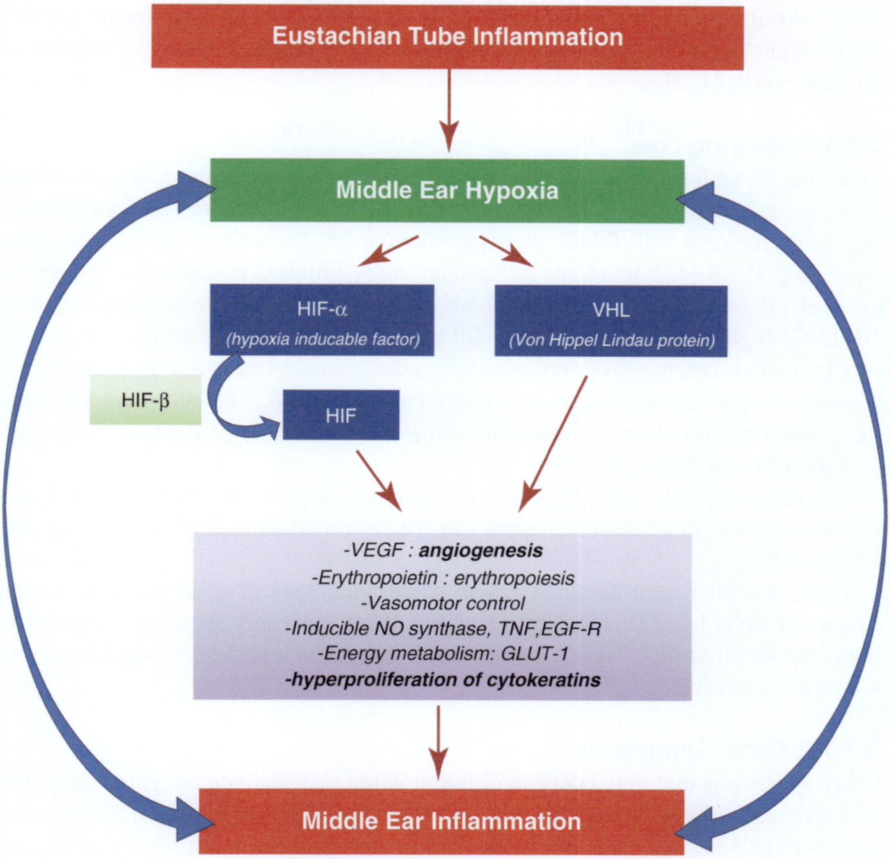

Fig. 3.3 The chain of events that leads from Eustachian tube dysfunction and hypoxia to the development of middle ear inflammation

3.7 Clinical Features and Diagnosis

3.7.1 Symptomatology

Clinical signs of acute infection are, by definition, absent in patients with otitis media with effusion (OME). In the majority of patients, OME is transient. When patients are symptomatic, the predominant symptom is hearing loss. The hearing loss typically is mild and fluctuating [40]. It may be detected during school hearing screening or audiology screening [41]. Although the hearing loss is usually mild, some children with OME present with parental concerns about hearing, language development, behavior, or school performance [8, 40, 41]. OME also may be detected during ENT consultation after an episode of acute otitis media (AOM) [41]; middle ear effusion often persists for weeks to months following resolution of the acute otitis [1, 2].

3.7.1.1 Hearing Loss

Otitis media with effusion (OME) is the leading cause of hearing loss in children. Conductive hearing loss occurs whenever fluid fills the middle ear. The average hearing levels for ears with OME often measures at 25 dB, with about 20% of cases exceeding 35 dB [42]. In a large prospective study, children younger than 3 years of age with bilateral middle ear effusion had hearing thresholds that were approximately 10–15 dB higher than similarly aged children without middle ear effusion [43].

Conductive hearing loss may adversely affect binaural processing, sound localization, and speech perception in a noisy background [42, 44–48]. Children who have prolonged middle ear effusion have lower scores on tests of speech, language, and cognitive abilities [49–51].

The impact of mild conductive hearing loss associated with persistent middle ear effusion is likely to be more significant in children with an underlying hearing disability [52, 53].

OME has also been associated with some temporary or even permanent high frequency SNH loss. This is due to passage of inflammatory mediators, present in high concentration in OME, from the middle ear to the inner ear through the round window membrane.

3.7.1.2 Other Symptoms

Other symptoms that may occur in children with OME include ear pain, sleep disturbance, ear fullness feeling, tinnitus, or balance problems [41, 54–60]. Young children with balance problems may present with disequilibrium, falling, stumbling, or clumsiness [55–58]. These symptoms are nonspecific; other causes should be considered and evaluated before being attributed to OME.

3.7.2 Otoscopic Findings

Diagnosis of OME requires a careful visualization of the tympanic membrane which may be of difficult access during otoscopy especially in young children with narrow and oblique external ear canals, or obstruction by cerumen debris.

1. An air-fluid level may be present behind the tympanic membrane and it is the most suggestive finding but not the most frequent (Figs. 3.4 and 3.5);
2. Amber-colored eardrum by middle ear fluid is common, although the fluid may be colorless with a gray or translucent tympanic membrane (Fig. 3.6)
3. In the "Glue ear" cases, the most common otoscopic finding is opacification (the light is not reflected) of the tympanic membrane, which may appear dull, yellow and retracted (Fig. 3.7)
4. Often and due to the retraction of the eardrum, the handle of malleus looks shorter and horizontal with a prominent short process.

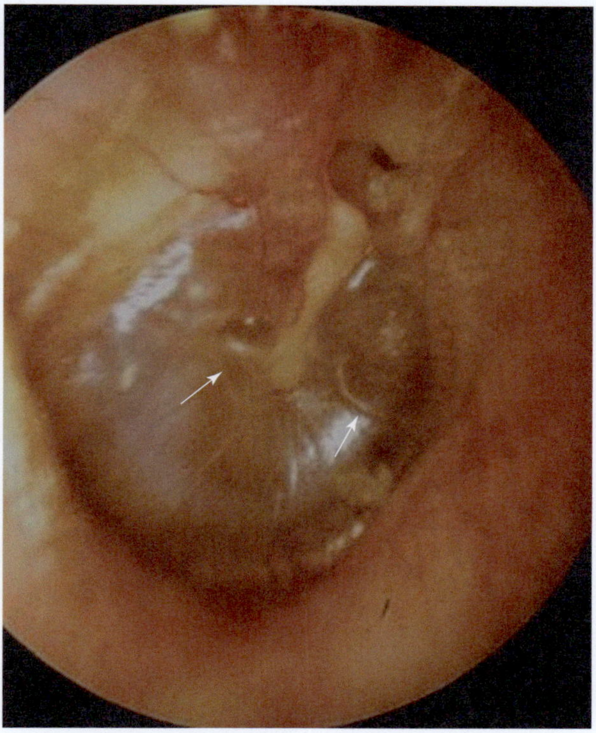

Fig. 3.4 Right ear otomicroscopy: retrotympanic air fluid level (*arrows*)

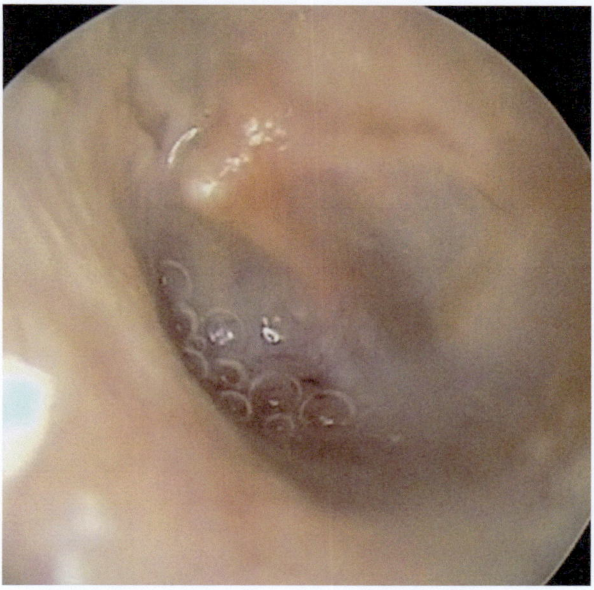

Fig. 3.5 Left ear with serous effusion. After Valsalva maneuver, air bubbles appeared anteriorly

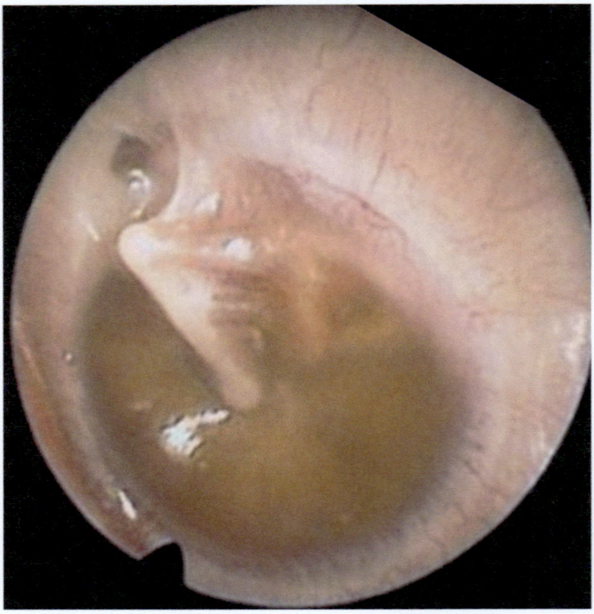

Fig. 3.6 Left ear with abundant serous effusion

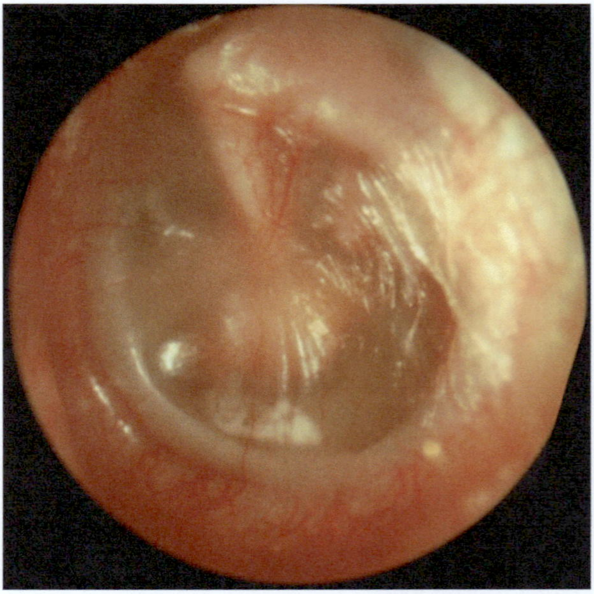

Fig. 3.7 Left ear with mucoid effusion and retracted drum

3.7.3 Pneumatic Otoscopy

Pneumatic otoscopy shows an impaired mobility of the tympanic membrane when a positive pressure is applied; however, some movement may be apparent when negative pressure is applied initially to the tympanic membrane. In children tympanic membrane mobility test is not easy to perform [61].

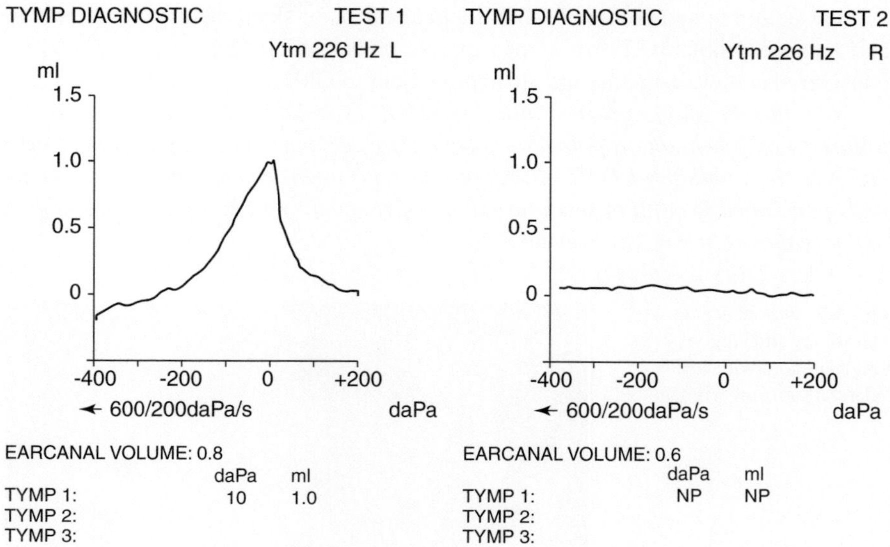

Fig. 3.8 Patient with a normal left ear and a right glue ear; Tympanometry showing curve type A in the left ear and type B in the right ear

3.7.4 Tympanometry

1. Tympanometry is the most useful of all tests in diagnosing OME. Studies have shown a higher rate of sensitivity and specificity, both around 90%.
   - Tympanometry is a cost-effective adjunct to physical examination
   - Tympanometry is an objective test not requiring active cooperation from the patient and therefore can be done whatever the age
   - Tympanometry helps the clinician to rule out middle ear effusion (MEE) for what appears to be an immobile tympanic membrane on pneumatic otoscopy.
   - A flat curved (type B) tympanometry is quasi pathognomonic of OME when otoscopic examination is doubtful (Fig. 3.8).

3.7.5 Hearing Assessment

Hearing assessment is recommended at the time of diagnosis of OME for children who are at risk for speech, language, or learning disorders; otherwise audiometry is obtained if OME has persisted for ≥3 months (i.e., chronic OME).

3.8 Differential Diagnosis of OME

Acute otitis media (AOM) is defined by fluid in the middle ear accompanied by acute signs of illness. The presence of pain and bulging of a red tympanic membrane effectively excludes OME.

Less common symptoms of OME include ear pain; sleep disturbance, tinnitus, and balance problems. These symptoms are nonspecific; other causes should be considered and evaluated before attributing them to OME.

Note that the single greatest pitfall in OME, especially when unilateral, is the failure to fully evaluate a potential nasopharyngeal mass in an adult patient who has recurrent unilateral OME. Flexible nasopharyngoscopy should be systematically performed in adult or in unilateral OME (Figs. 3.9 and 3.10). *Imaging studies and possibly even biopsies may be indicated.*

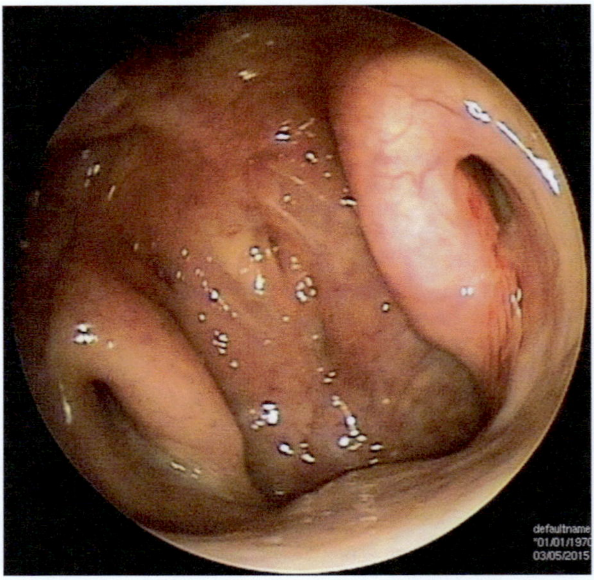

Fig. 3.9 Nasopharyngeal endoscopy showing very small adenoid with free bilateral torus tubaris

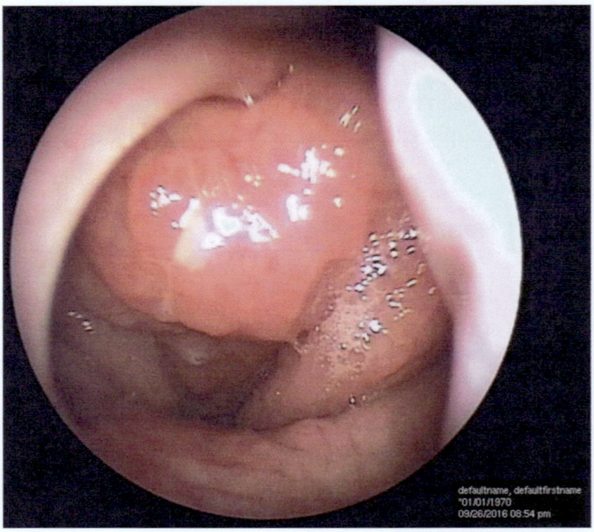

Fig. 3.10 Nasopharyngeal mass compressing the left torus tubaris

The following are conditions that should be considered when evaluating patients with refractory otitis media with effusion:

- Benign nasopharyngeal masses
- Nasopharyngeal carcinoma
- Adenoid hypertrophy
- Congenital defects affecting the Eustachian tube
- Ciliary dyskinesia
- Immunoglobulin G (IgG) subclass deficiencies

3.9 Natural Evolution of OME

Otitis media with effusion usually resolves spontaneously in >85% within 3 months. Approximately 30–40% of children have recurrent episodes. Newly diagnosed OME of unknown duration also usually resolves spontaneously, the episodes are usually cleared within 6 weeks.

When silent inflammation is maintained, neglected OME may evolve to the following pathologies:

- **TM Perforation** is more likely to occur if tympanostomy tubes (TTs) are retained beyond 36 months (40%).The incidence of tympanic membrane perforation for short-term TTs is 1% versus 15% in long term TTs. Drops of AB/steroids in post TT seems to favor persistent perforation
- **Tympanosclerosis**—Tympanosclerosis or myringosclerosis could be encountered after several episodes of middle ear inflammation (OME or AOM). The middle ear could be occasionally involved as well. In most cases, the tympanosclerosis is of no functional importance, but in some cases after a long period of quiescent inflammatory process, the deposits may envelop the ossicles resulting in a conductive hearing loss. (See Chap. 5)
- **Atelectasis, Retraction pocket, Adhesive otitis:**—When the chronic inflammatory process of the ME mucosa with the so called "Eustachian tube dysfunction" persists over a long time (i.e., years) it may result in atelectasis, retraction pockets, or adhesive otitis (See Chap. 4 and 7)
- **Cholesteatoma**—It is common to say that cholesteatomas can occur within the middle ear space after OME. In fact, only less than 1% of neglected OME induce cholesteatoma. (See Chap. 8)

3.10 Treatment of OME

The major goal of treatment of OME is the prevention of language delay or a slow psychodynamic development secondary to hearing loss, which occur over a long period of time. Also treatment of OME aims to avoid silent complications.

3.10.1 Medical Treatment

The use of antibiotics, oral steroids, mucolytics, antihistamines and decongestants in the treatment of OME has not been shown to be of significant clinical benefit. The risk of adverse events which may occur with all medical therapies, outweigh their minor benefit.

Results of small trials have shown that nasal steroids speed the clearance of otitis media with effusion (OME) and prevent its recurrence. A 2011 meta-analysis confirmed these findings [62]. However no evidence exists that nasal steroids has any effect on decreasing potential complications of OME, such as hearing loss and delayed language development. The discovery of hypoxia and HIF–mediated VEGF pathways as playing pivotal role in the development of OME lead us to assume that targeting molecules in HIF–VEGF signaling pathways could have therapeutic potential in the treatment of chronic OME.

3.10.2 Surgical Treatment

- OME of less than 3 months usually resolves spontaneously in >80% of cases. Twenty percent of effusions lasting more than 3 months will have spontaneous resolution 25% after 6 months, and 30% after 1 year [17].
- Absolute benefits of myringotomy with placement of pressure equalization tubes are improved hearing and decreased rates of recurrent acute otitis media (rAOM) episodes. Prolonged aeration of the middle ear has been shown to reverse the mucosal hyperplasia and metaplasia associated to OME.

3.10.2.1 Myringotomy + Transtympanic Tube Insertion (TT)

Myringotomy and tube placement were first proposed by a french physician Bonnafont in 1860. Then Politzer designed a specific device, the Politzer' tube, but the technique has been forgotten until 1954 when Armstrong redescribed the procedure and popularized it.

At present it is the most frequent surgical procedure in pediatric surgery (Fig. 3.11).

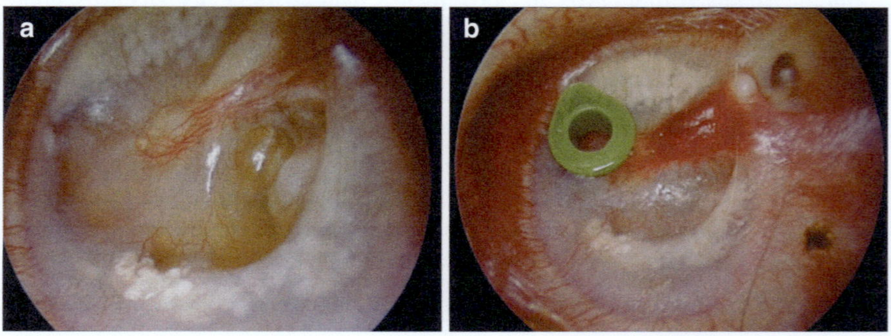

Fig. 3.11 Left glue ear (**a**) treated by myringotomy and grommet insertion (**b**)

3.10.2.2 Transtympanic Tube Insertion Indications

1. Children with persistent middle-ear fluid should not be treated with antihistamines, decongestants, or corticosteroids [63].
2. TT should not be performed in children with a single episode of OME of less than 3 months duration, except in "at-risk" children (recognized HL) [63]
3. Children with chronic OME who do not receive TT should be re-evaluated at 3- to 6-month intervals until the effusion has resolved. If significant hearing loss is detected, or structural abnormalities of the tympanic membrane or middle ear are suspected, TT insertion is recommended [1].
4. TT may be performed in children with unilateral or bilateral OME of less than 3 months duration if they also have symptoms that are attributable to OME, such as balance disturbance, poor school performance, behavioral issues, ear discomfort [63],
5. Children with bilateral chronic OME of less than 3 months duration and documented hearing loss should be offered TT [63]
6. Certain changes in the tympanic membrane (retractions) may mandate pressure equalization tube insertion despite normal hearing
7. For patients with hearing loss and OME, a loss of 30 dB or greater is an indication for pressure equalization tube insertion.

3.10.2.3 Tympanostomy Tube Types

The ideal TT would be the one which is easy to insert with a predictable time to extrusion and not associated to complications.

- Short term tubes (Armstrong, Shepard grommets, Teflon Reuter Bobine) last anywhere from 6 to 24 months and are indicated for most children who undergo initial TT placement [64, 65].
- The so called long-term tubes are generally reserved in cases, that have required multiple sets of TTs due to failure of resolution of disease after too short acting TT placement.
- Modified Goode T-tubes, butterfly, Triune, and Paparella II are the most commonly used long-acting TT designs. These tubes can last for years (Fig. 3.12).

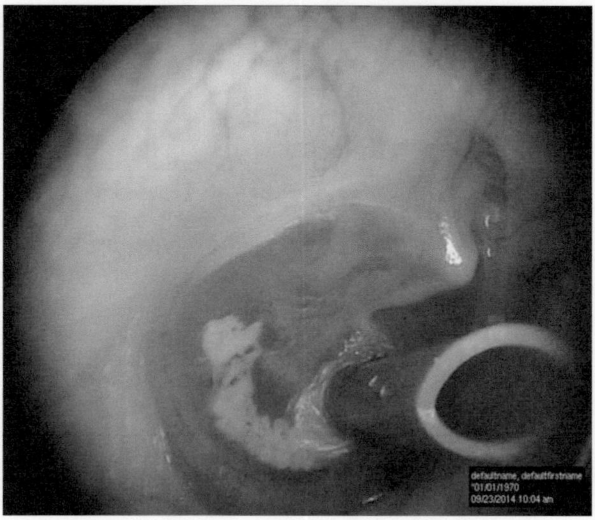

Fig. 3.12 Right ear with T-tube since more than 2 years

3.10.2.4 Tympanostomy Tube Positioning

TT is placed in the antero-inferior quadrant of the tympanic membrane.

Tube positioning in the tympanic membrane has been studied in relation to its effect on duration of action [66]. More recent investigations have shown no difference in the time to extrusion between tubes placed in the anterior-inferior and anterior-superior quadrants [67–69].

Placement in the posterior quadrant was associated with significantly earlier tube extrusion, mainly due to keratin migration patterns of the squamous layer of the TM [70].

- The most important factors affecting the duration of tube retention seem to be principally related to the tube properties, including the length, diameter, and flanges of the tube [71].
- Also subcutaneous, sub-annulus TT placement was described and is suggested for a longer duration of the tube; nevertheless closure with debris of such permanent tube renders it often nonfunctional.

3.10.2.5 Role of Adenoidectomy

Enlarged adenoids may prevent resolution of MEE by physical obstruction of the ET orifice in the nasopharynx. The adenoids have long been thought to serve as a reservoir for pathogens that can cause inflammation, thus disturbing ET function. This is why some otologists believe that children adenoidectomy is beneficial regardless of their size.

Removal of a potential source of inflammation and infection at the Eustachian tube creates a smooth nasopharyngeal mucosa, which decreases the colonization of bacteria that can occur in the crypts of adenoid tissue [72].

Adenoidectomy appears beneficial in reducing the risk of developing additional ME disease (from 20 to 7%) that would require surgery, there are very exceptional risks to include adenoidectomy along with placement of TTs: such the possibility of bleeding, infection, and velopharyngeal insufficiency.

Obviously, children who have symptoms of nasal obstruction or recurrent rhinorrhea at the time of their initial tube placement should be considered for adenoidectomy [73].

3.10.2.6 Long-Term Monitoring Post- TT

Patients who underwent TT undergo the following postoperative visits:

- Post-op 1 week
- Before and after summer time or swimming activities
- Then every 4 months
- Visit in case of otorrhea
- Removal if not exteriorized post-18–24 months, at least after one winter season.
- Before removal, ET function should be assessed before the indication of tube removal
- Control of hearing and speech
- Speech development several months after tube extrusion

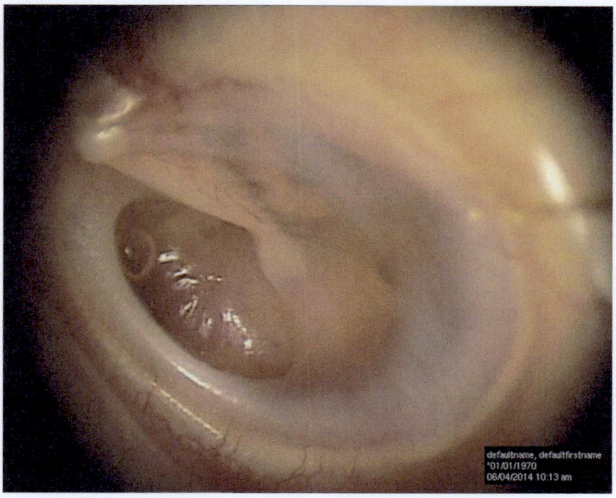

Fig. 3.13 Anterior TM focal atrophy and shallow retraction pocket with recurrence of OME after grommet extrusion

3.10.2.7 Complications of TT

Complications or sequelae of TTs themselves are common but transient (i.e., otorrhea) or do not generally affect function (i.e., tympanosclerosis, focal atrophy, shallow retraction pocket) (Fig. 3.13).

Sometimes, tubes extrude too soon or get occluded, making them nonfunctional. The most problematic, but rare, complications are residual tympanic membrane perforations and iatrogenic cholesteatoma.

Short-Term Complications

- *Otorrhea*: The most common complication is transient otorrhea, occurring in 15% of patients. In the early postoperative period, 16% of children developed otorrhea, whereas 26% developed otorrhea at any time of the TT being in place. Recurrent or chronic otorrhea were rare, seen in only 7.4 and 3.8% of children, respectively [74].
  - The recently published guidelines recommend prescribing topical antibiotic eardrops, without oral antibiotics, for children with uncomplicated otorrhea [63].
  - Topical antibiotic and/or steroid eardrops placed intraoperatively may help in preventing blockage of TTs and early postoperative otorrhea.
- *Occlusion of the tube*: occlusion of the tube lumen occurs in 7% of ears shortly after placement (Fig. 3.14).
- *Premature extrusion*: in 3.9% of ears.
- *Granulation tissue development*: in 4%, and requires removal of the TT
- *Intrusion into the ME*, may happen in 0.5% of ears because of wrong placement or large eardrum opening and may require ME exploration for removal (Fig. 3.15).

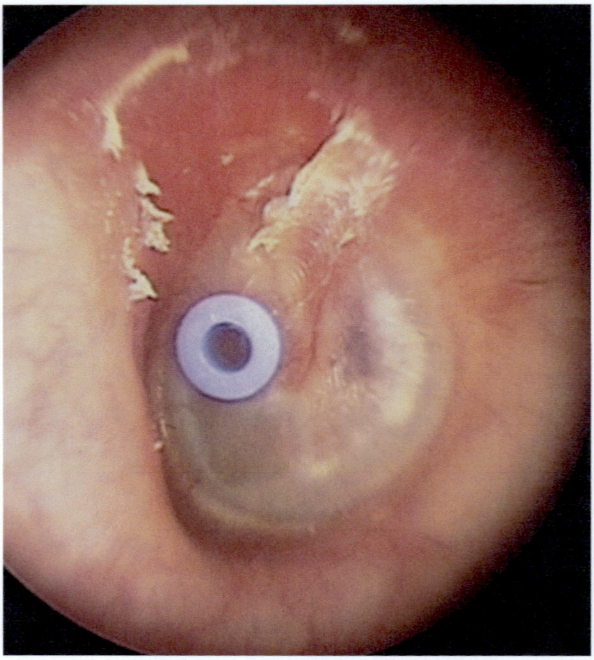

Fig. 3.14 Obstructed grommet by recurrent thick effusion

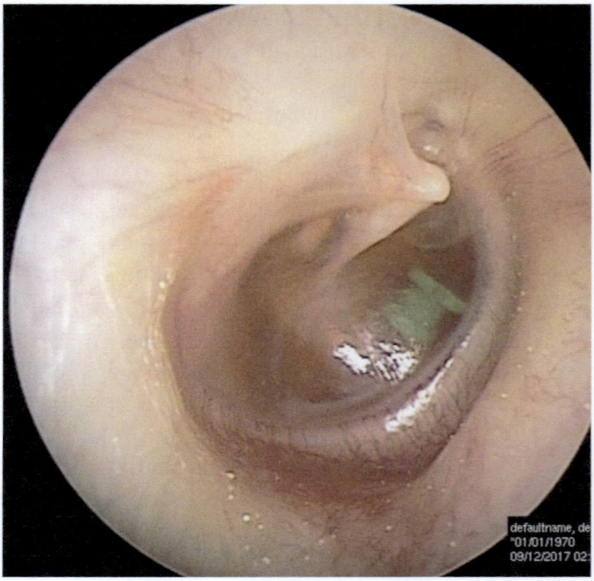

Fig. 3.15 Right ear with intrusion of the grommet into the ME and recurrence of effusion

While not necessarily a complication, water precautions are an issue that must be addressed with TT placement. Multiple studies have shown no benefit of water avoidance or use of earplugs in reducing otorrhea. Children with TT appear to be at minimal, if any, risk for increased otorrhea with water exposure when surface swimming in pools or ocean water [75]. Exposure to soapy water or river/lake water is

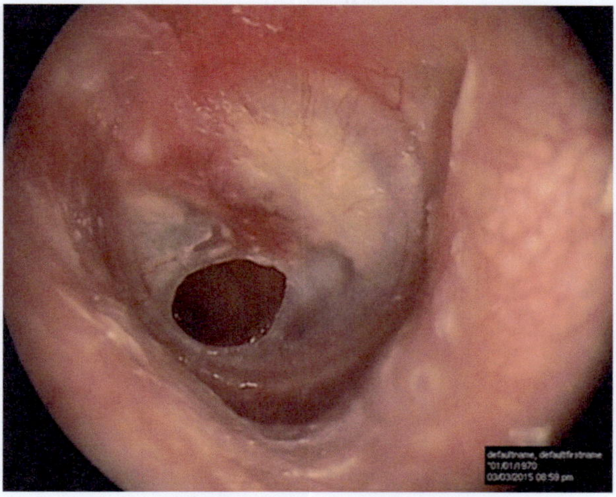

Fig. 3.16 Left ear showing residual antero-inferior tympanic membrane perforation after T-tube removal. Notice the development of myringosclerosis in the posterior part of the drum

controversial; the decreased surface tension and increased bacterial counts may increase the risk of water entering the ME and infection, respectively [76, 77]. Jumping and diving are probably best avoided as the risk of water entering the ME increases with swimming at greater depths.

Long-Term Complications

Long-term complications include TM changes, perforations of the TM, and cholesteatoma.

- *Myringosclerosis*, occurs in approximately 32% of ears after tube extrusion [74]. It is usually limited to the TM and does not cause appreciable hearing loss.
- *Failure of spontaneous tube extrusion*: Beyond 30 months postoperatively, TTs are unlikely to extrude spontaneously [78].
- *Residual Perforation*: Perforation is more likely to occur if TTs are retained beyond 36 months (40%) versus those that are in place for less than 36 months (19%) [79] (Fig. 3.16). The incidence for short-term TTs was 2.2 versus 16.6% in long term TTs [74]. Residual perforation can be easily repaired, after resolution of Eustachian tube dysfunction, by inlay technique using fat or cartilage.
- Rates of cholesteatoma development are higher in patients with long term TTs (1.4%) versus short-term ones (0.5%) [74].

3.10.3 Emerging Technologies (Tuboplasty) in OME Management

A method of improving management of patients with OME is balloon dilation of the ET. It is recommended for patients with long-standing history of COME and multiple TT surgeries.

Although the reported short term results look encouraging, the long term benefit is still doubtful since the pathology of ET dysfunction is a mucosal disease not an

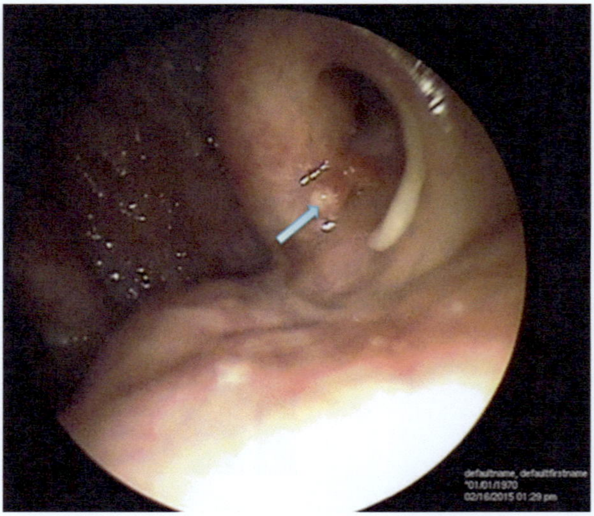

Fig. 3.17 Granuloma in the left Eustachian tube (*blue arrow*) 3 months after tuboplasty

anatomical stenosis to respond to mechanical dilatation. Also post- tuboplasty sequelae, such granulation tissue or long term scarring stenosis, must be considered (Fig. 3.17).

Conclusion

OME is common, it affects 90% of children before 4 years of age. In most of the children, OME are usually asymptomatic and resolve spontaneously, even sometimes unnoticed. OME which persists >3 months (chronic OME) causes conductive hearing loss and may evolve into tympanosclerosis or into a tympanic membrane perforation or retraction pocket in which a cholesteatoma may eventually form. Otitis media with effusion (OME) is the leading cause of hearing loss in children.

Management of children with OME is TT insertion if failure to resolve spontaneously after 3 months with hearing loss or structural changes in the eardrum.

Despite an obvious need for prophylactic measures, genetic engineering or development of highly effective vaccines for OM remain a great challenge for better control of the incidence of OME and recurrent forms. The discovery of hypoxia and HIF–mediated VEGF pathways as playing a pivotal role in the development of OME lead us to assume that targeting molecules in HIF–VEGF signaling pathways could have therapeutic potential in the treatment of chronic OME.

References

1. Teele DW, Klein JO, Rosner BA. Epidemiology of otitis media in children. Ann Otol Rhinol Laryngol Suppl. 1980;89:5.
2. Renko M, Kontiokari T, Jounio-Ervasti K, et al. Disappearance of middle ear effusion in acute otitis media monitored daily with tympanometry. Acta Paediatr. 2006;95:359.
3. Tos M. Epidemiology and natural history of secretory otitis. Am J Otol. 1984;5:459.
4. Casselbrant ML, Brostoff LM, Cantekin EI, et al. Otitis media with effusion in preschool children. Laryngoscope. 1985;95:428.
5. Williamson IG, Dunleavey J, Bain J, Robinson D. The natural history of otitis media with effusion – a three-year study of the incidence and prevalence of abnormal tympanograms in four south west Hampshire infant and first schools. J Laryngol Otol. 1994;108:930.
6. Paradise JL, Rockette HE, Colborn DK, et al. Otitis media in 2253 Pittsburgh-area infants: prevalence and risk factors during the first two years of life. Pediatrics. 1997;99:318.
7. Owen MJ, Baldwin CD, Swank PR, et al. Relation of infant feeding practices, cigarette smoke exposure, and group child care to the onset and duration of otitis media with effusion in the first two years of life. J Pediatr. 1993;123:702.
8. Williamson I. Otitis media with effusion in children. BMJ Clin Evid. 2011;2011. pii: 0502.
9. Hergils L, Magnuson B. Human middle ear gas composition studied by mass spectrometry. Acta Otolaryngol (Stockh). 1990;110:92–9.
10. Buckingham R, Ferre J. Middle ear pressure in Eustachian tube malfunction: manometric studies. Laryngoscope. 1973;83:1585–93.
11. Magnan J, Bremond G, Chays A, et al. In: Sade J, editor. Experience in tubo-tympanic endoscopy in Eustachian tube and middle ear disease. Amsterdam: Kugler and Ghedini Publication; 1991. p. 175–6.
12. Sade J, Ar A. Middle ear and auditory tube: middle ear clearance, gas exchange and pressure regulation. Otolaryngol Head Neck Surg. 1997;116:499–524.
13. Huang Q, et al. Hypoxia-inducible factor and vascular endothelial growth factor pathway for the study of hypoxia in a new model of otitis media with effusion. Audiol Neurootol. 2012;17(6):349–56.
14. Dodson KM, Cohen RS, Rubin BK. Middle ear fluid characteristics in pediatric otitis media with effusion. Int J Pediatr Otorhinolaryngol. 2012;76:1806.
15. Inagaki M, Sakakura Y, Shimizu T, et al. Ultrastructure of mucous blanket in otitis media with effusion. Ann Otol Rhinol Laryngol. 1988;97:313.
16. Rye MS, Warrington NM, Scaman ES, et al. Genome-wide association study to identify the genetic determinants of otitis media susceptibility in childhood. PLoS One. 2012;7:e48215.
17. Hafrén L, Kentala E, Järvinen TM, et al. Genetic background and the risk of otitis media. Int J Pediatr Otorhinolaryngol. 2012;76:41.
18. Alles R, Parikh A, Hawk L, et al. The prevalence of atopic disorders in children with chronic otitis media with effusion. Pediatr Allergy Immunol. 2001;12:102.
19. Hurst DS, Venge P. The impact of atopy on neutrophil activity in middle ear effusion from children and adults with chronic otitis media. Arch Otolaryngol Head Neck Surg. 2002;128:561.
20. Kreiner-Møller E, Chawes BL, Caye-Thomasen P, et al. Allergic rhinitis is associated with otitis media with effusion: a birth cohort study. Clin Exp Allergy. 2012;42:1615.
21. Martines F, Bentivegna D, Maira E, et al. Risk factors for otitis media with effusion: case-control study in Sicilian schoolchildren. Int J Pediatr Otorhinolaryngol. 2011;75:754.
22. Martines F, Bentivegna D, Di Piazza F, et al. The point prevalence of otitis media with effusion among primary school children in western Sicily. Eur Arch Otorhinolaryngol. 2010;267:709.

23. Marseglia GL, Pagella F, Caimmi D, et al. Increased risk of otitis media with effusion in allergic children presenting with adenoiditis. Otolaryngol Head Neck Surg. 2008;138:572.
24. Hurst DS, Amin K, Sevéus L, Venge P. Mast cells and tryptase in the middle ear of children with otitis media with effusion. Int J Pediatr Otorhinolaryngol. 1999;49(Suppl 1):S315.
25. Miura MS, Mascaro M, Rosenfeld RM. Association between otitis media and gastroesophageal reflux: a systematic review. Otolaryngol Head Neck Surg. 2012;146:345.
26. Scott Giebink G, Mills EL, Huff JS, Edelman CK, Weber ML, Juhn SK, Quie PG. The microbiology of serous and Mucoid otitis media. Pediatrics. 1979;63(6):915–9.
27. Iino Y, Kaneko Y, Takasaka T. Endotoxin in middle ear effusions tested with limulus assay. Acta Otolaryngol. 1985;100(1–2):42–50.
28. Ehrlich GD, Veeh R, Wang X, et al. Mucosal biofilm formation on middle-ear mucosa in the chinchilla model of otitis media. JAMA. 2002;287(13):1710–5. https://doi.org/10.1001/jama.287.13.1710. Preliminary Communication April 3, 2002
29. Casselbrant ML, Mandel EM, Fall PA, et al. The heritability of otitis media: a twin and triplet study. JAMA. 1999;282:2125–30.
30. Casselbrant ML, Mandel EM, Rockette HE, et al. The genetic component of middle ear disease in the first 5 years of life. Arch Otolaryngol Head Neck Surg. 2004;130:273–8.
31. Daly KA, Brown WM, Segade F, Bowden DW, Keats B, Lindgren BR, Levine SC, Rich SS. Chronic and recurrent otitis media: a genome scan for susceptibility loci. Am J Hum Genet. 2004;75:988–97.
32. Casselbrant ML, Mandel EM, Jung J, Ferrel RE, Tekely K, Szatkiewicz JP, Ray A, Weeks DE. Otitis media: a genome-wide linkage scan with evidence of susceptibility loci within the 17q12 and 10q22.3 regions. BMC Med Genet. 2009;10:85–94.
33. Li JD, Hermansson A, Ryan AF, Bakaletz LO, Brown SD, Cheeseman MT, Juhn SK, Jung TT, Lim DJ, Lim JH, Lin J, Moon SK, Post JC. Panel 4: recent advances in otitis media in molecular biology, biochemistry, genetics, and animal models. Otolaryngol Head Neck Surg. 2013;148(4 Suppl):E52–63.
34. Yabe R, et al. Gel chromatographic characterization of proteins in mucous and serous middle ear effusions of patients with otitis media in comparison to serum proteins. Eur Arch Otorhinolaryngol. 2008;265(3):293–8.
35. Chung MH, et al. Compositional difference in middle ear effusion: mucous versus serous. Laryngoscope. 2002;112(1):152–5.
36. Mattila PS, et al. Adenoids provide a microenvironment for the generation of CD4(+), CD45RO(+), L-selectin(−), CXCR4(+), CCR5(+) T lymphocytes, a lymphocyte phenotype found in the middle ear effusion. Int Immunol. 2000;12(9):1235–43.
37. Jizhen Lin, et al. Mucin production and mucous cell metaplasia in otitis media. Int J Otolaryngol. 2012 (2012), 745325, 12 page doi:https://doi.org/10.1155/2012/745325.
38. Sekiyama K, et al. The role of vascular endothelial growth factor in pediatric otitis media with effusion. Auris Nasus Larynx. 2011;38(3):319–24.
39. Samuels TL, Yan JC, Khampang P, Dettmar PW, MacKinnon A, Hong W, Johnston N, Papsin BC, Chun RH, McCormick ME, et al. Association of gel-forming mucins and aquaporin gene expression with hearing loss, effusion viscosity, and inflammation in otitis media with effusion. JAMA Otolaryngol Head Neck Surg. 2017;143:810–7.
40. National Institute for Health and Clinical Excellence. Surgical management of otitis media with effusion in children. 2008. www.nice.org.uk/nicemedia/pdf/CG60NICEguideline.pdf. Accessed 8 Nov 2012.
41. Rosenfeld RM, Bluestone CD. Clinical pathway for otitis media with effusion. In: Rosenfeld RM, Bluestone CD, editors. Evidence-based otitis media. 2nd ed. Hamilton, ON: BC Decker Inc; 2003. p. 303.
42. Fria TJ, Cantekin EI, Eichler JA. Hearing acuity of children with otitis media with effusion. Arch Otolaryngol. 1985;111:10.
43. Sabo DL, Paradise JL, Kurs-Lasky M, Smith CG. Hearing levels in infants and young children in relation to testing technique, age group, and the presence or absence of middle-ear effusion. Ear Hear. 2003;24:38.

44. Pillsbury HC, Grose JH, Hall JW 3rd. Otitis media with effusion in children. Binaural hearing before and after corrective surgery. Arch Otolaryngol Head Neck Surg. 1991;117:718.
45. Besing JM, Koehnke J. A test of virtual auditory localization. Ear Hear. 1995;16:220.
46. Gravel JS, Wallace IF. Listening and language at 4 years of age: effects of early otitis media. J Speech Hear Res. 1992;35:588.
47. Schilder AG, Snik AF, Straatman H, van den Broek P. The effect of otitis media with effusion at preschool age on some aspects of auditory perception at school age. Ear Hear. 1994;15:224.
48. Browning GG, Rovers MM, Williamson I, et al. Grommets (ventilation tubes) for hearing loss associated with otitis media with effusion in children. Cochrane Database Syst Rev. 2010;10:CD001801.
49. Klausen O, Møller P, Holmefjord A, et al. Lasting effects of otitis media with effusion on language skills and listening performance. Acta Otolaryngol Suppl. 2000;543:73.
50. Petinou KC, Schwartz RG, Gravel JS, Raphael LJ. A preliminary account of phonological and morphophonological perception in young children with and without otitis media. Int J Lang Commun Disord. 2001;36:21.
51. Bennett KE, Haggard MP, Silva PA, Stewart IA. Behaviour and developmental effects of otitis media with effusion into the teens. Arch Dis Child. 2001;85:91.
52. Roberts JE, Burchinal MR, Zeisel SA. Otitis media in early childhood in relation to children's school-age language and academic skills. Pediatrics. 2002;110:696.
53. Brookhouser PE, Worthington DW, Kelly WJ. Middle ear disease in young children with sensorineural hearing loss. Laryngoscope. 1993;103:371.
54. AHRQ. Evidence-based Practice Center Systematic Review Protocol. Otitis media with effusion: comparative effectiveness of treatments. 2013. http://effectivehealthcare.ahrq.gov/ehc/products/387/1013/OME_AmendedProtocol_20120807.pdf. Accessed 5 Dec 2012.
55. Casselbrant ML, Furman JM, Rubenstein E, Mandel EM. Effect of otitis media on the vestibular system in children. Ann Otol Rhinol Laryngol. 1995;104:620.
56. Orlin MN, Effgen SK, Handler SD. Effect of otitis media with effusion on gross motor ability in preschool-aged children: preliminary findings. Pediatrics. 1997;99:334.
57. Golz A, Angel-Yeger B, Parush S. Evaluation of balance disturbances in children with middle ear effusion. Int J Pediatr Otorhinolaryngol. 1998;43:21.
58. Casselbrant ML, Redfern MS, Furman JM, et al. Visual-induced postural sway in children with and without otitis media. Ann Otol Rhinol Laryngol. 1998;107:401.
59. Abdullah B, Hassan S, Sidek D. Clinical and audiological profiles in children with chronic otitis media with effusion requiring surgical intervention. Malays J Med Sci. 2007;14:22.
60. Karkanevatos A, Lesser TH. Grommet insertion in children: a survey of parental perceptions. J Laryngol Otol. 1998;112:732.
61. Shaikh N, Hoberman A, Rockette HE, Kurs-Lasky M. Development of an algorithm for the diagnosis of otitis media. Acad Pediatr. 2012;12:214.
62. Simpson SA, Lewis R, van der Voort J, Butler CC. Oral or topical nasal steroids for hearing loss associated with otitis media with effusion in children. Cochrane Database Syst Rev. 2011;5:CD001935.
63. Rosenfeld RM, Schwartz SR, Pynnonen MA, Tunkel DE, Hussey HM, Fichera JS, Grimes AM, Hackell JM, Farrison MF, Haskell H, Haynes DS, Kim TW, Lafrenierre DC, Netterville JL, Pipan ME, Raol NP, Schellhase KG. Clinical practice guidelines: tympanostomy tubes in children. Otolaryngol Head Neck Surg. 2013;149(s1):1–35.
64. Lindstrom DR, Reuben B, Jacobson K, Flanary VA, Kerschner JE. Long-term results of Armstrong beveled grommet tympanostomy tubes in children. Laryngoscope. 2004;114(3):490–4.
65. Yaman H, Yilmaz S, Alkan N, Subasi B, Guclu E, Ozturk O. Shepard grommet tympanostomy tube complications in children with chronic otitis media with effusion. Eur Arch Otorhinolaryngol. 2010;267:1221–4.
66. Armstrong BW. Prolonged middle ear ventilation: the right tube in the right place. Ann Otol Rhinol Laryngol. 1983;92(6 Pt 1):582–6.

67. April MM, Portella RR, Orobello PW Jr, Naclerio RM. Tympanostomy tube insertion: anterosuperior vs. anteroinferior quadrant. Otolaryngol Head Neck Surg. 1992;106(3):241–2.
68. Walker P. Ventilation tube duration versus site of placement. Aust N Z J Surg. 1997;67(8):571–2.
69. Hern JD, Jonathan DA. Insertion of ventilation tubes: does the site matter? Clin Otolaryngol Allied Sci. 1999;24(5):424–5.
70. van Baarle PW, Wentges RT. Extrusion of transtympanic ventilating tubes, relative to the site of insertion. ORL J Otorhinolaryngol Relat Spec. 1975;37(1):35–40.
71. Kay DJ. Type of tube to insert. In: Apler C, Bluestone C, Casselbrant M, Dohar J, Mandel E, editors. Advanced therapy of otitis media. 1st ed. Hamilton: BC Decker; 2004. p. 231–7. Print.
72. Chan CL, et al. The microbiome of otitis media with effusion. Laryngoscope. 2016;126:2844–51.
73. Boston M, McCook J, Burke B, Derkay C. Incidence of and risk factors for additional tympanostomy tube insertion in children. Arch Otolaryngol Head Neck Surg. 2003;129:293–6.
74. Kay DJ, Nelson M, Rosenfeld RM. Meta-analysis of tympanostomy tube sequelae. Otolaryngol Head Neck Surg. 2001;124:374–80.
75. Goldstein NA, Mandel EM, Kurs-Lasky M, Rockette HE, Casselbrant ML. Water precautions and tympanostomy tubes: a randomized, controlled trial. Laryngoscope. 2005;115:324–30.
76. Marks NJ, Mills RP. Swimming and grommets. J R Soc Med. 1983;76:23–6.
77. Herbert RL, King GE, Bent JP. Tympanostomy tubes and water exposure: a practical model. Arch Otolaryngol. 1998;124:1118–21.
78. Morris MS. Tympanostomy tubes: types, indications, techniques and complications. Otolaryngol Clin N Am. 1999;32:385–90.
79. Nichols PT, Ramadan HH, Wax MK, Santrock RD. Relationship between tympanic membrane perforations and retained ventilation tubes. Arch Otolaryngol Head Neck Surg. 1998;124:417–9.

Adhesive Otitis Media

4

Contents

4.1 Introduction

Everything is difficult in adhesive otitis media: it is difficult to describe this aspect of chronic otitis media; it is difficult to elucidate its successive and intricate stages; it is difficult to treat.

Many well-known otologists have proposed a definition of this disease. At the end of the XIX century, Von Troeltsch [1] and Politzer [2] wrote a perfect description of the adhesive process. After that, adhesive otitis media fell into obscurity until it was resurrected by the Scandinavian school in the 1950s [3, 4]. Those authors postulated a correlation between serous otitis media and adhesive otitis media; thus adhesive otitis media was included as one of the sequelae of neglected middle ear effusion.

S. Mansour et al., *Middle Ear Diseases*,
https://doi.org/10.1007/978-3-319-72962-6_4

The main feature of adhesive otitis media is the collapse of the entire tympanic membrane, and more specifically its adherence to the medial wall of the middle ear cleft. Consecutively the air space of the middle ear has vanished and the tympano- ossicular system is no longer functional. The lamina propria and the epidermis of the tympanic membrane are very thin and atrophic.

Some times, the collapsed tympanic membrane may lose its self–cleaning potential and possibly become associated with cholesteatoma. In these ears, the epidermal layer of the tympanic membrane shows hyperplasia and hyperkeratosis of its kertanizing stratified squamous epithelium.

Atelectasis, adhesive otitis media and fibro-adhesive otitis media are different forms of retraction of an intact thinned tympanic membrane towards the medial wall of the tympanic cavity (Fig. 4.1):

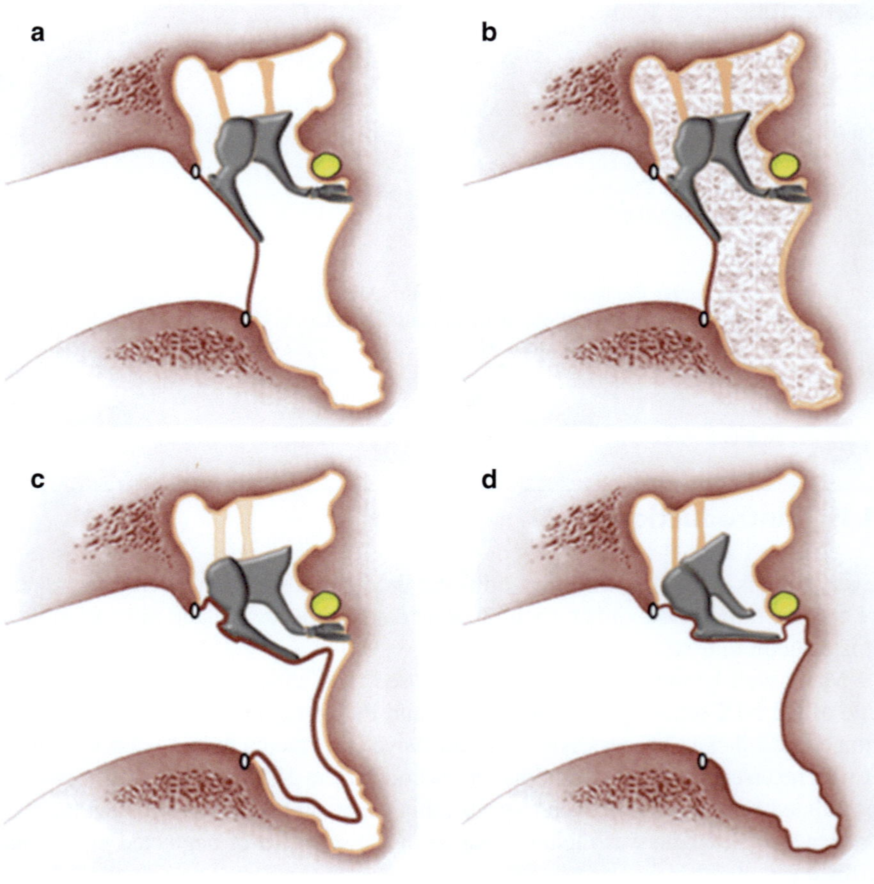

Fig. 4.1 (**a**) normal middle ear, (**b**) fibro-adhesive otitis media; (**c**) atelectasis; (**d**) adhesive otitis media

1. In atelectatic ears, the middle ear space is partially or completely obliterated, but the tympanic membrane is not adherent to the medial wall of the middle ear, and the mucosal lining of the middle ear is still intact.
2. In adhesive otitis media, the tympanic membrane is bound partially or totally to the medial wall of the middle ear by fibrous adhesions without any possibility of reversing the retraction by any reaeration procedure of the middle ear space.

   In cases of partial adhesions, a serous or mucous effusion could be found in the remaining free space of the middle ear. In severely affected ears, the whole area of the middle ear cavity has vanished and the tympano-ossicular system is no longer functional.
3. The form of fibro-adhesive otitis media is characterized by the presence of a dense and extensive fibrous layer filling the middle ear cavity adherent to the tympanic membrane.

Adhesive otitis media accounts for 3–5% of operated chronic otitis media [5, 6]. Adhesive otitis media is frequently bilateral (8–21%) [5], or associated with a contralateral pre-adhesive process. Sometimes it is associated with a contralateral cholesteatoma [7–9]. Cleft palate is associated with an adhesive process in 20% of cases [10, 11].

4.2 Pathogenesis

Adhesive otitis media is a sequela of long standing otitis media with effusion (OME) with Eustachian tube dysfunction [12–19]. Three factors are prerequisites for the development of adhesive otitis media:

- Middle ear negative pressure due to imbalance between Eustachian tube ventilation and mastoid mucosa gaz diffusion (see Sect. 7.3),
- A lack of rigidity of the tympanic membrane,
- Severe middle ear mucosal inflammation and ulceration.

Most patients with chronic OME get cured either spontaneously or after insertion of tympanostomy tubes. Only some patients with neglected chronic OME develop atelectasis of limited degree. Very few cases (2–5%) develop severe atelectasis [7, 20, 21].

Recurrent infection of the middle ear fluid may lead to a progressive necrosis of the lamina propria of the tympanic membrane which becomes atrophic and prone to retraction [7, 15]. Long-standing middle ear global dysventilation due to Eustachian tube dysfunction and mucosal inflammation, leads to a retraction of the whole atrophic TM towards the floor of the tympanic cavity with consequent loss of middle ear space, representing atelectasis.

In some cases of complete atelectasis, a severe inflammatory process, either suppurative or nonsuppurative, provokes mucosal ulcerations, mucosal necrosis, surface breakdown and bone exposure that results in osteitis and periostitis. One of the most common reactions of the mucoperiosteum to injury or severe infection is the production of granulation tissue rich in fibroblasts. These fibroblasts may generate a new fibrous tissue, dense and avascular, as a scar tissue that will form irreversible fibrous adhesions between the under-surface of the atrophic TM and the medial wall of the middle ear [22] (Fig. 4.2).

Since adhesive otitis media is usually the result of several previous episodes of otitis media, any of the mucosal and ossicular residual changes occurring in the chronic otitis media may also be found in adhesive otitis media (e.g. tympanosclerosis (Fig. 4.3), cholesterol granuloma, and/or ossicular erosion).

Once established, the adhesive process is irreversible, hence the need for preventive therapy.

The primary aim of the management should be to prevent the formation of fibrous adhesions during episodes of suppurative ear disease and recurrent mucoid otitis media in childhood. Because the fibrous adhesions that produce this condition are the direct consequence of inflammatory damage to the mucoperiosteum of the middle ear, all middle ear infections should be treated aggressively with full courses of the appropriate antibiotics. Persistent mucoid effusions should be drained.

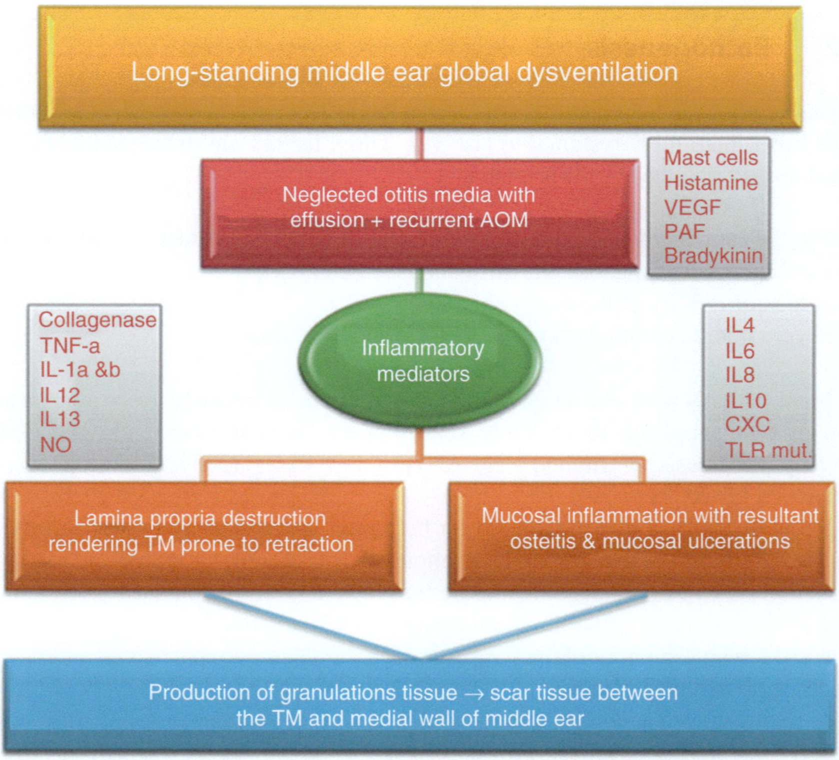

Fig. 4.2 Cascade of events with corresponding inflammatory mediators leading to development of adhesive otitis media

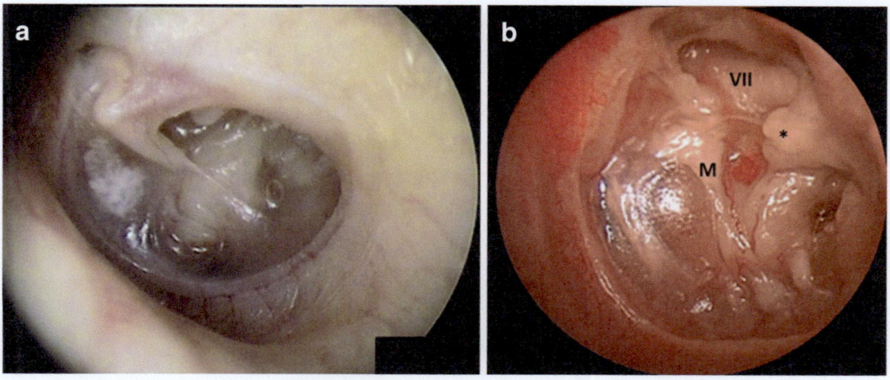

Fig. 4.3 (**a**) Partial adhesive otitis media associated with myringoincudopexy and myringosclerosis in the antero-superior quadrant. (**b**) left ear with adhesive otitis media and tympanosclerotic plaques covering the stapes (*) and around the malleus (M). VII: facial nerve

4.3 Histopathology of Adhesive Otitis Media

The lamina propria of the tympanic membrane is thin, quite atrophic or completely absent in some areas particularly in the central portion of the pars tensa. The lamina propria remains invaded by inflammatory cells, with disorganized and disoriented fibers of collagen. The mucous layer of the eardrum disappeared and is replaced by an inflammatory tissue which induces the adhesion of the epithelial layer of the tympanic membrane to the denuded bone of the promontory.

4.4 Clinical Manifestations

Adhesive otitis media is a silent disease and usually pauci-symptomatic. The most common symptom is an ear blockage because of a negative middle ear pressure. Hearing loss is usually isolated and stable; it could be of insidious onset and progressively worsening over several months or even years.

The audiogram could be normal even in the presence of ossicular erosion due to the adhesion of the drum on the ossicles.

The presence of an aural discharge is an alarming symptom suspecting cholesteatoma formation on the adhesive process. Frequently otorrhea is due to superimposed infections of the peeled epidermal scales accumulated in the fundus of the external ear canal.

Physical examination reveals a global collapse of the tympanic membrane on the ossicles and over the medial wall of the middle ear with failure of resolution of the collapse after Valsalva maneuver (Fig. 4.4).

Unlike the retraction pocket, the entire pars tensa is involved. The eardrum appears very thin, greyish, located in a deeper position with respect to the annulus. It is attached to the medial wall of middle ear cavity and molds intimately the depressions and protrusions of the middle ear cavity. The surface of the eardrum at the level of the tympano malleolar ligaments forms a relief called "clothesline" (Fig. 4.5).

The eardrum molds the promontory along with the elements of the ossicular chain. The handle of the malleus is medialized and the umbo comes sometimes into contact with the promontory. The lateral process of the malleus draws a well-marked projection as a white cone. Behind the handle of the malleus appears the

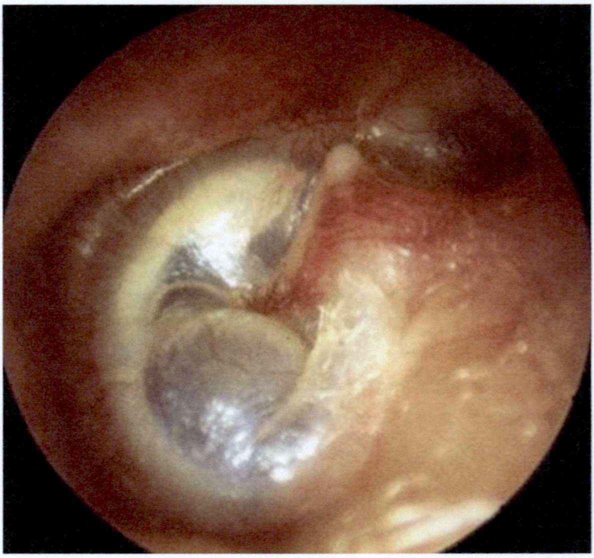

Fig. 4.4 Right ear atelectasis after Valsalva maneuver which brings the major part of the tympanic membrane to its normal position. This finding excludes the diagnosis of adhesive otitis media

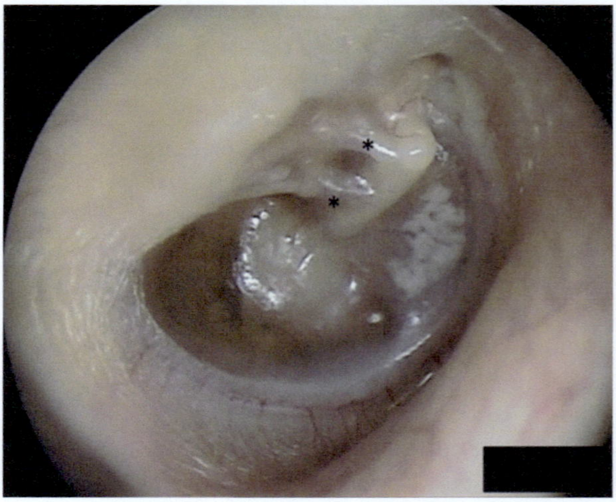

Fig. 4.5 Right ear with adhesive otitis media showing the typical "clothesline" appearance (*)

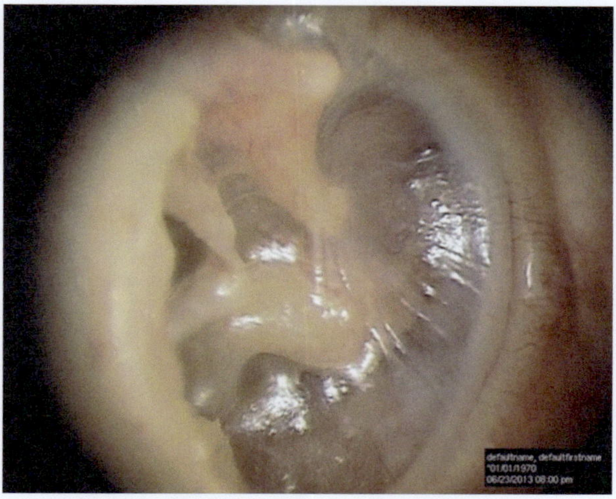

Fig. 4.6 Right ear with adhesive otitis media showing erosion of the incudostapedial joint which is replaced by a fibrous band between the remaining incus and the stapes head. The malleus is medialized

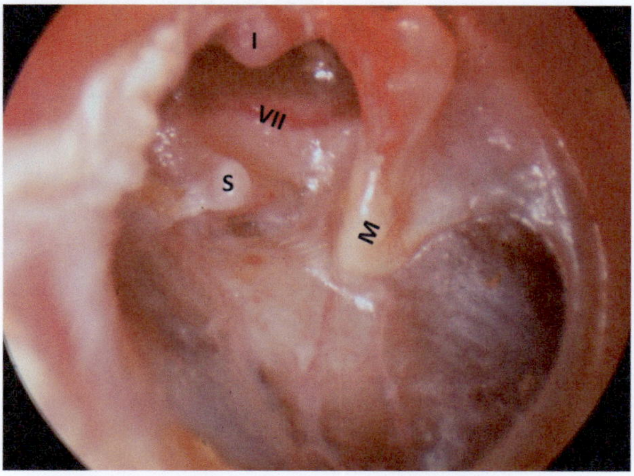

Fig. 4.7 Right ear with adhesive otitis media associated with myringostapediopexy on stapes head (S). Note that the incus (I) is eroded and the drum is adherent to the tympanic segment of the facial nerve (VII) and the ankylosis of the umbo (M) to the promontory

incudostapedial joint which is frequently lysed (Fig. 4.6). The lysis interests mostly the long process of the incus, and the eardrum lines the stapes (Fig. 4.7). If the stapes is eroded, the eardrum covers directly the footplate (Fig. 4.8).

Attempts to mobilize the eardrum, using speculum of Siegle or Valsalva maneuver, always fail.

Audiometry: Generally a conductive hearing loss is demonstrated on audiogram, with an average air-bone gap of 25–50 decibels (dB). Mixed hearing loss can be present in advanced cases of adhesive otitis media and reflects the beginning of a labyrinthine insult. The impedance, not contributive, shows a flat tympanometric curve.

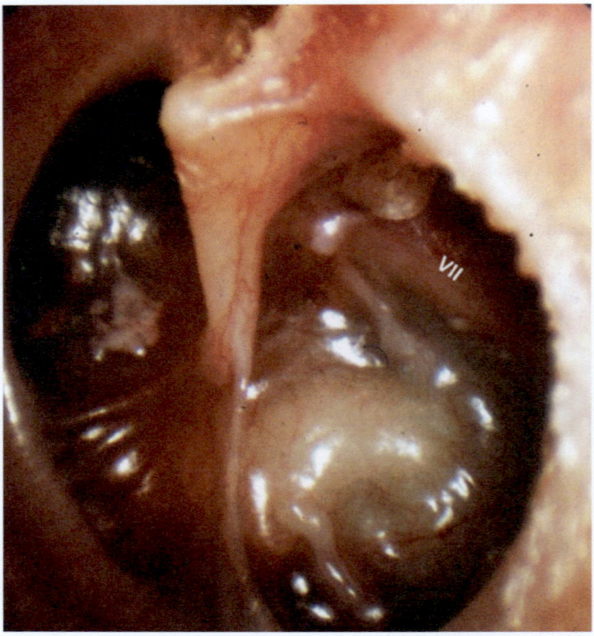

Fig. 4.8 Left ear adhesive otitis media with erosion of the incus and stapes superstructure, the retraced drum lies directly on the footplate and the tympanic segment of the facial nerve (VII). Malleus is medialized and the umbo is in contact with the promontory

4.5 Complications

Recurrent infections, ossicular erosion and progression to cholesteatoma formation, render AdOM a critical ear pathology.

4.5.1 Ossicular Chain Erosion

Adhesion of the retracted tympanic membrane to the ossicles may lead to their resorption which is almost constant in adhesive otitis media. It is found in about 60–80% of cases [7, 23, 24]. This lysis is easily recognized in the otoscopic examination through an atrophic eardrum, molding the ossicular elements.

The commonest ossicular lysis is the erosion of the long process of the incus due to its tenuous blood supply (Figs. 4.6, 4.7 and 4.9) with the result of a natural myringostapediopexy. The stapes is eroded in 25% of cases (Figs. 4.8 and 4.10) [23–25].

The malleus handle is driven medially by the retracted tympanic membrane to the medial wall of the middle ear cavity, due to the unopposed tensor tympani muscle contraction. The otoscopic examination reveals a malleus handle in a horizontal position, pressed against the promontory (Figs. 4.6, 4.7 and 4.8).

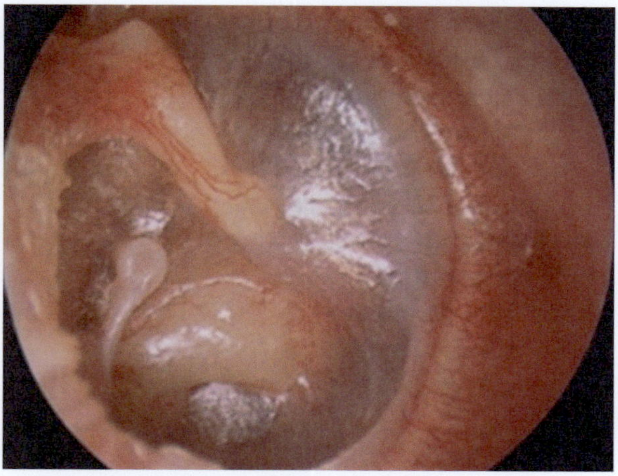

Fig. 4.9 Right ear adhesive otitis media with erosion of the incus and resultant myringostapediopexy

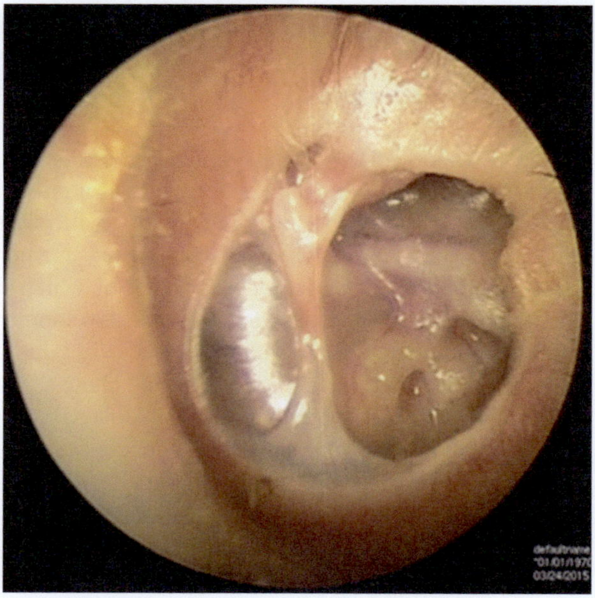

Fig. 4.10 Left ear adhesive otitis media with malleus, medialization, erosion of the incus and stapes superstructure

In a study series published by one of the authors [26], ossicular chain erosion was present in 55% of operated ears. The incus was the most affected ossicle (55%) (Figs. 4.6, 4.7 and 4.9), followed by stapes (21.8%) (Figs. 4.8 and 4.10). Malleus was found to be resilient to erosion; however, it was medialized toward the promontory in all cases and eroded in 12.7% of cases (Fig. 4.11).

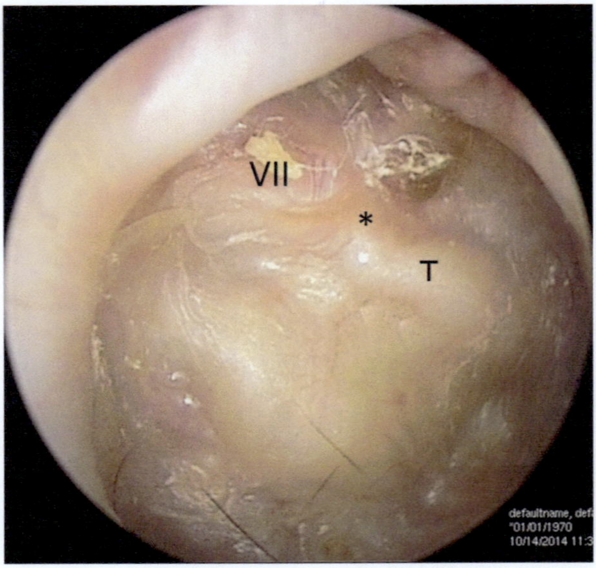

Fig. 4.11 Right ear complete adhesive otitis media with erosion of all the ossicles. *VII* facial nerve; *T* tensor tympani muscle; * cochleariform process

4.5.2 Cholesteatoma

Adhesive otitis media with epithelialization of the middle ear cavity wall leaves a scarred middle ear with debris cover which is almost stable, but it must be distinguished from active lesions evolving readily to a cholesteatoma. In such cases, continuous adhesive retraction of the tympanic membrane into the attic or the retrotympanum may lead to deep pockets in which desquamated keratin debris would be retained. This leads later on to the development of a cholesteatoma which manifests clinically by a recurrent otorrhea.

Association of adhesive otitis media and cholesteatoma is not exceptional: 25% as reported by one of the authors [5, 27]. However, more recently, this association has been found by one of the authors to be less frequent: only 8.3% (5/60 ears) [26] (Figs. 4.12, 4.13 and 4.14). Cholesteatoma formation must be distinguished from secondary superinfections of peeled epidermal debris accumulated in the fundus of ear canal which is poorly ventilated.

The presence of recurrent infections and aural discharge in adhesive otitis media is an important symptom indicating cholesteatoma formation. However, frequent otorrhea could be due to superimposed infections of the peeled epidermal scales accumulating in the fundus of the poorly ventilated external ear canal, as opposed to cholesteatoma (Fig. 4.15).

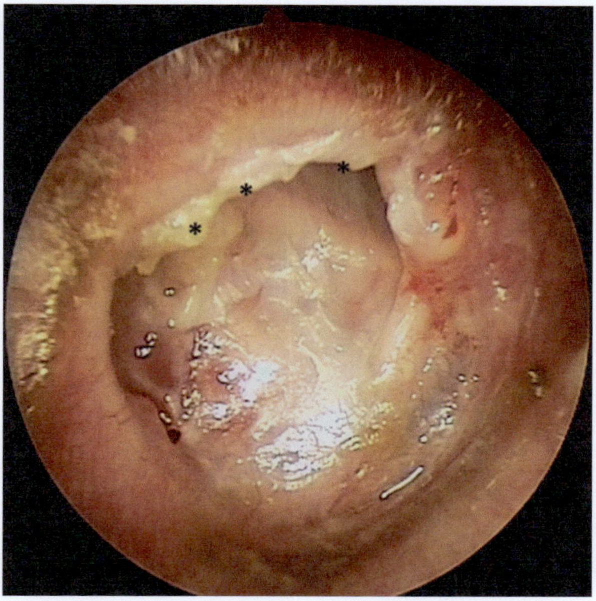

Fig. 4.12 Right ear showing adhesive otitis media associated with attical cholesteatoma (*), incus and stapes are eroded, skin lying directly on the facial nerve

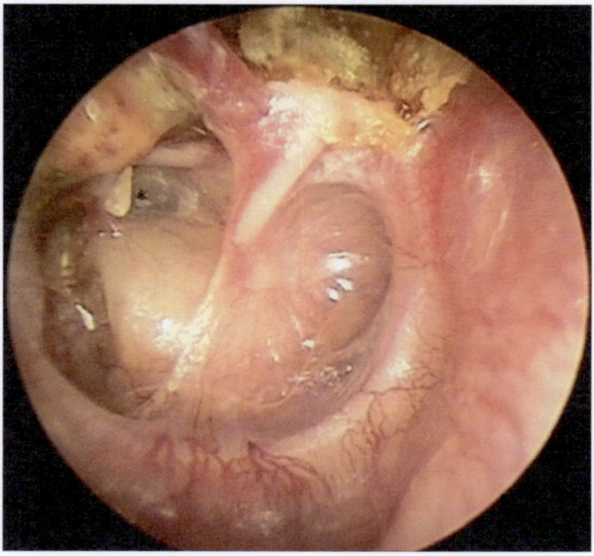

Fig. 4.13 Right ear adhesive otitis media with attical cholesteatoma, erosion of the incus and stapes superstructure; footplate (*)

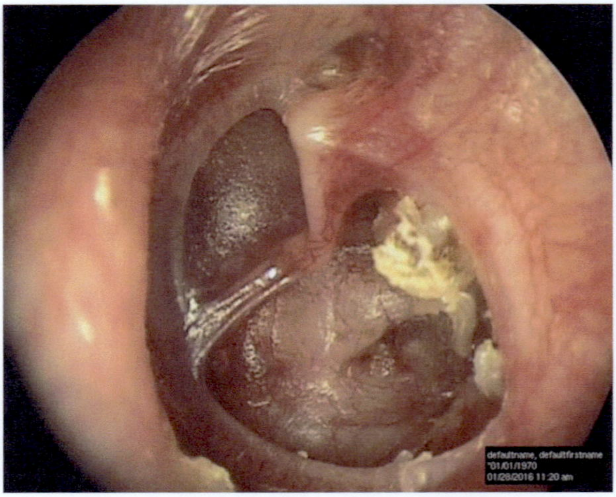

Fig. 4.14 Left ear adhesive otitis media with mesotympanic cholesteatoma

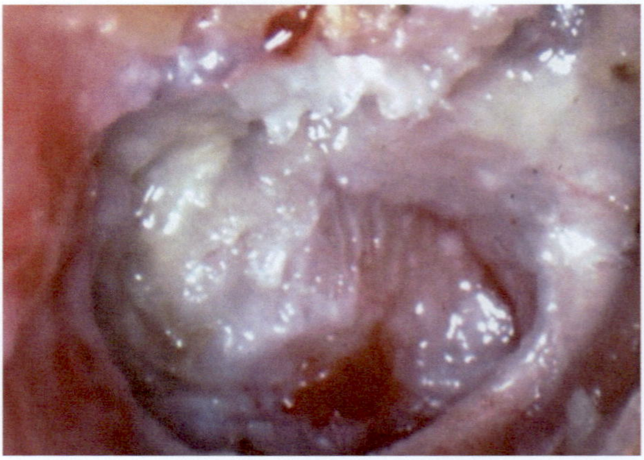

Fig. 4.15 Keratinized tympanic membrane: difficult differentiation between mesotympanic cholesteatoma and adhesive otitis media!

4.6 Imaging

Imaging of adhesive otitis media is not contributive, unless complicated by cholesteatoma or demonstrating associated attic pathology. In adhesive otitis media, the mastoid is almost constantly sclerotic (Fig. 4.16).

4.7 Management

Treatment should be primarily preventive in order to avoid atelectasis and progression to adhesive otitis media, encumbered with a bad functional prognosis.

Once adhesion has occurred between TM and middle ear mucosa and ossicles, treatment becomes quite difficult.

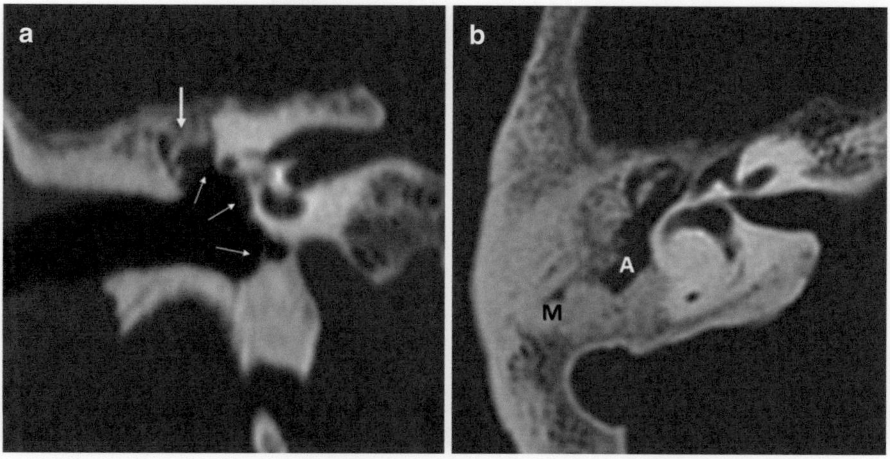

Fig. 4.16 CT of adhesive otitis media: (**a**) the adhesive stage of the whole pars tensa (*white arrows*) on the medial wall of the tympanic cavity, small attic with sclerosis (*thick arrow*), (**b**) sclerotic mastoid (M), condensated antrum (A)

4.7.1 Preventive Treatment of Adhesive Otitis Media

If we admit the sequence of: Eustachian tube dysfunction → effusion → recurrent infection → atelectasis → adhesive otitis media, all measures have to be taken as early as possible to arrest and reverse the process before reaching the end stage of severe adhesive otitis media.

4.7.1.1 Treatment of Eustachian Tube Dysfunction

Several therapeutic methods are proposed to correct Eustachian tube dysfunction: This topic is very wide and is a subject of controversy regarding its benefits, still it is out of the main scope of this chapter. It is understood that the multiplicity of the therapeutic attempts proves their doubtful results. Nevertheless adenoidectomy helps in many occasions to improve tubal function [27, 29].

Laser ablation of some pathological findings observed at the posterior half of the tube, in cases of tubal tonsil, could be beneficial [28].

Balloon dilatation of the tube was studied by Poe in 2011, for safety and efficacy in long standing cases of serous otitis media and proved significantly beneficial without major adverse effects [30].

Cleft palate repair has variable results on the tubal function [31–34].

The impact of septal deviations on the middle ear has been demonstrated, it would reflect a tubal dysfunction caused by turbulent inspiratory air at the nasopharynx. The beneficial effect of septoplasty on tubal fonction have been demonstrated by several studies [35, 36], however, it may come out without any major help.

4.7.1.2 Treatment of Atelectasis

Middle ear atelectasis may be reversible with ventilating tubes. Ventilation of the ME may reverse the atelectasis and bring back the TM to its normal position and

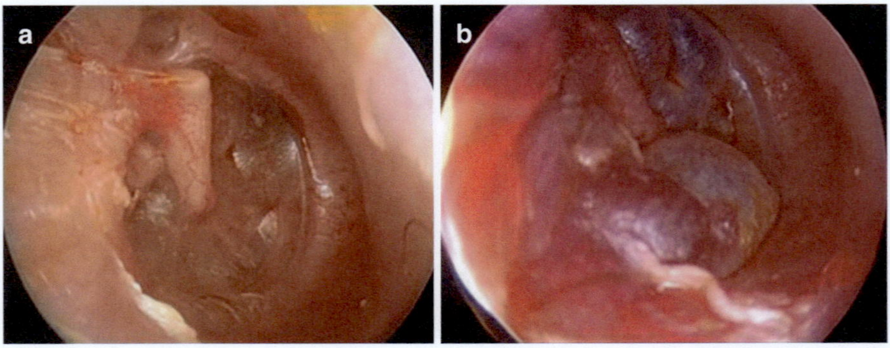

Fig. 4.17 (**a**) Right ear showing atelectasis, (**b**) the same ear after nitrous oxide inhalation during anesthesia which brings the major part of the tympanic membrane to its normal position. This maneuver makes grommet insertion possible and it is a good prognostic sign

restore its consistency thus preventing its progression to adhesive otitis media [17, 18, 37–39].

During insertion of the tube, atelectatic tympanic membranes can be restored to their normal position by administration of nitrous oxide during general anesthesia helping in the insertion of a ventilating tube (Fig. 4.17).

4.7.2 Definitive Treatment of Adhesive Otitis Media

Once adhesions between the TM and middle ear mucosa and ossicles have formed, the treatment of adhesive otitis media becomes challenging.

There is no consensus in the literature concerning the best treatment strategy of adhesive otitis media. Medical treatment has been proved to be ineffective.

Surgical treatment is controversial.

In our practice, *recurrent and refractory otorrhea in adhesive otitis media, is a sign of an unstable ear, and is an absolute indication for surgery.* Significant conductive hearing loss is another indication for surgery having counselled the patient about the alternative option of a hearing aid.

Hearing aid may impair ventilation and increase ear canal humidity, creating a favorable condition for infection of retained debris in the fundus with resultant otorrhea.

In practice a significant number of patients with hearing loss related to adhesive otitis media would select the surgical option after an unsatisfactory trial of hearing aid use.

Patients with a stable condition and without major hearing deficit do not need treatment; but a follow up of long duration is always indicated because a starting cholesteatoma is unpredictable.

Surgical treatment is justified only in cases with significant conductive hearing loss and/or recurrent infection with persistent otorrhea.

4.7.3 Surgery of Adhesive Otitis Media

Surgery consists of careful dissection of the adherent skin from the posterior and medial wall of middle ear followed by a perichondrium/cartilage reinforcement of the drum. A ventilation-tube is inserted through the cartilage graft. Ossicular reconstruction is performed when needed.

Otorrhea control is obtained by the resulting smooth and regular drum surface that facilitates the epithelial migration and the restoration of the self-cleaning function of the canal skin. Different results of otorrhea control have been reported by different authors: (94%) by Y.M. Shen et al. [40], (78%) by Ichimura et al. [41], and (55%) by Yu et al. [42].

Nevertheless this procedure carries the risks of inducing a sensorineural hearing loss and possible iatrogenic cholesteatoma [3, 4, 43–52].

In 2004, Yu et al. reported good results for the postoperative ABG closure, 58.5% showed a nearly normal tympanum. More recently, Ichimura et al. reported 78% of audiologically successful results [42]. Y.M. Shen et al. on 2010 reported after treatment with tragus cartilage tympanoplasty over 25 dB ABG closure at 1 year [40].

One of our authors [26] achieved in 58 patients a closure of ABG to within 20 dB in 83.6% of operated ears by using tragal cartilage graft with concomitant placement of a ventilation tube. Such good postoperative results could be partly due to the restoration of a permanent ventilation of the middle ear by the inserted ventilation tube. Long term success of surgery in ears with Eustachian tube dysfunction, including adhesive otitis media, is significantly dependent on maintaining an aerated middle ear (Fig. 4.18).

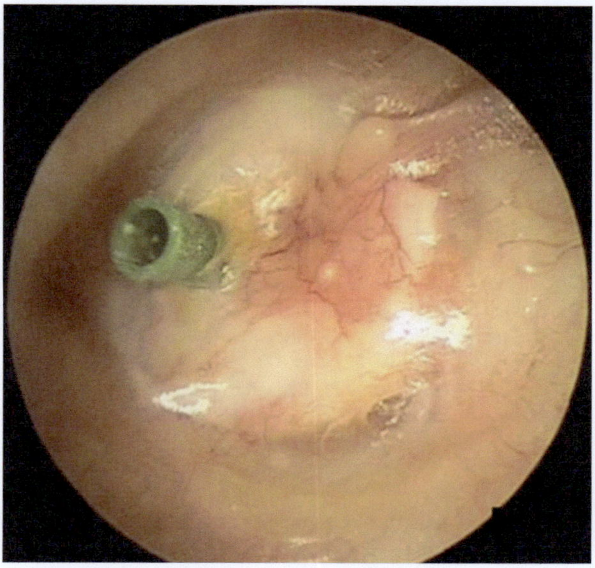

Fig. 4.18 Postoperative endoscopic examination of left ear, 18 months after the surgery, showing a healed tympanic membrane in a proper position together with an aerated middle ear. Note the T-tube and the integration of the malleus handle in the V-notch created in the cartilage graft

In cases of adhesive otitis media associated to cholesteatoma, surgical treatment with a canal wall down mastoidectomy (open technique) is the best option without raising the adhesive tympanic membrane. The objective is to favor leveling between the middle ear floor and the mastoid, to salvage sulci and corners from skin growth and keratin accumulation.

Conclusion

Middle ear aeration must be the major concern of every routine ear examination in the childhood or young adults. Every step must be undertaken to prevent global or selective dysventilation syndromes in order to avoid such destructive process in the middle ear.

Collaboration between family physicians, pediatricians and otologists is contributive in this regards.

References

1. Von Troeltsch A. Textbook of otolaryngology. Leipzig, Germany: FCW Vogel; 1873.
2. Politzer A. Traite desmaladies de l'oreille. Paris: Doin; 1884.
3. Palva T. Surgical treatment of adhesive tympanum. Acta Otolaryngol Suppl. 1964;188:70–4.
4. Siirala U. Pathogenesis and treatment of adhesive otitis. Acta Otolaryngol Suppl. 1964;188:9–18.
5. Bremond G, Magnan J, Bonnaud G. L'otite adhésive. Otorhinolaryngologie. Encycl Méd Chir, 20-182-G-30. Paris: Elsevier SAS; 1985. 8 p.
6. Dommerby H, Tos M. Sensorineural hearing loss in chronic adhesive otitis. Arch Otolaryngol Head Neck Surg. 1986;112:628–34.
7. Sadé J, Berco E. Atelectasis and secretory otitis media. Ann Otol Rhinol Laryngol. 1976;85(Suppl 25 pt 2):66–72.
8. Moller P, Dingsor G, Breck P, Thomassen R. Tympanic membrane changes and retraction pockets after secretory otitis media. In: Tos M, Thomsen J, Peitersen E, editors. Cholesteatoma and mastoid surgery. Amsterdam: Kugler and Ghedini Publications; 1989. p. 351–5.
9. Fujita A, Sato H, Nakamura H, Yagi N, Honjo I. The etiological role of the retraction pocket in cholesteatoma. In: Tos M, Thomsen J, Peitersen E, editors. Cholesteatoma and mastoid surgery. Amsterdam: Kugler and Ghedini Publications; 1989. p. 421–4.
10. Guerrier Y, Charachon R, Dejean Y, et al. Pathologie fonctionnelle du voile du palais et sa réhabilitation. Rapport Société Française d'ORL et pathologie cervicofaciale. Paris: Arnette; 1978. p. 154–65.
11. Deggouj N, Gersdorff M. Bilans otologique et orthophonique et fente labiopalatine. Rev Laryngol Otol Rhinol. 1994;115:257–9.
12. Bluestone CD. Role of Eustachian tube function in otitis media: current concepts and relation to management. Ann Otol Rhinol Laryngol Suppl. 1985;120:48–9.
13. Daly K. Risk factors for otitis media sequelae and chronicity. Ann Otol Rhinol Laryngol Suppl. 1994;163:39–42.
14. Paparella MM, Yoon TH, Schachern PA. Pathology and pathogenesis of retraction pockets and cholesteatoma. In: Tos M, Thomsen J, Peitersen E, editors. Cholesteatoma and mastoid surgery. Amsterdam: Kugler and Ghedini Publications; 1989. p. 401–11.
15. Sadé J. Atelectatic tympanic membrane: histologic study. Ann Otol Rhinol Laryngol. 1993;102:712–6.
16. Zechner G. Adhesive otitis media. J Laryngol Otol Suppl. 1983;8:59–62.
17. Tos M. Experimental tubal obstruction. Changes in middle ear mucosa elucidated by quantitative histology. Acta Otolaryngol. 1981;92:51–61.

18. Tos M, Stangerup SE, Larsen PL, Siim C, Hvid G, Andreassen UK. The relationship between secretory otitis and cholesteatoma. In: Tos M, Thomsen J, Peitersen E, editors. Cholesteatoma and mastoid surgery. Amsterdam: Kugler and Ghedini Publications; 1989. p. 325–30.
19. Tos M. Atelectasis, retraction pockets, and cholesteatoma. Ann Otol Rhinol Laryngol Suppl. 1985;120:49–51.
20. Maw AR, Bawden R. Tympanic membrane atrophy, scarring, atelectasis and attic retraction in persistent, untreated otitis media with effusion and following ventilation tube insertion. Int J Pediatr Otorhinolaryngol. 1994;30(3):189–204.
21. Tay HL, Mills RP. Tympanic membrane atelectasis in childhood otitis media with effusion. J Laryngol Otol. 1994;109:495–8.
22. Prades JM, Martin C, Dumollard JM, Dubreuil C. Histologie et histopathologie de la trompe auditive. In: Martin C, Magnan J, Bebear JP, editors. La trompe auditive (la trompe d'Eustache). Paris: Arnette-Blackwell SA; 1996. p. 43–65.
23. Bremond G. L'otite adhésive. J Fr ORL. 1987;36:301–3.
24. Martin C, Martin H, Prades JM, Desermeaux JC. Du traitement de l'otite fibro-adhésive et des séquelles adhésives d'otite. Cah ORL. 1984;19:797–810.
25. Sadé J, Ar A. Middle ear and auditory tube: middle ear clearance, gas exchange, and pressure regulation. Otolaryngol Head Neck Surg. 1997;116:499–524.
26. Haidar H, Alsaadi A, Larem A, et al. Tympanoplasty in adhesive otitis media: a descriptive study. Laryngoscope. 2016;126(12):2804–10.
27. Magnan J, Chays A, De Gasquet R, Bremond GA. Adhesive otitis: clinical and surgical sides. In: Sadé J, editor. The Eustachian tube, clinical aspects. Amsterdam: Kugler and Ghedini Publications; 1991. p. 323–6.
28. Sedlmaier B, et al. The improvement of middle ear ventilation by laser ablation of the epipharyngeal eustachian tube: a prospective study. Lasers Med Sci. 2009;24:793–800. Springer
29. Morgon A, Narcy P, Dejean Y, et al. L'otite séro-muqueusecet ses complications. Rapport Société Française d'ORL etcpathologie cervicofaciale. Paris: Arnette; 1985. p. 123–62.
30. Poe DS, et al. Balloon dilation of the cartilaginous Eustachian tube. Otolaryngol Head Neck Surg. 2011;144(4):563–9.
31. Sellari-Franceschini S, Bernardini M, Bruschini P, Berrettini S, Massei A, Massei P. Eustachian tube function in children with cleft palate: effect of palatoplasty, a preliminary report. In: Sadé J, editor. The Eustachian tube, clinical aspects. Amsterdam: Kugler and Ghedini Publications; 1991. p. 201–3.
32. Muntz HR. An overview of middle ear disease in cleft palate children. Facial Plast Surg. 1993;9:177–80.
33. Smith TL, Di Ruggiero DC, Jones KR. Recovery of Eustachian tube function and hearing outcome in patients with cleft palate. Otolaryngol Head Neck Surg. 1994;111:423–9.
34. Duroux S, Devars F, Patuano E, Bondonny JM, Traissac L. Division palatine et pathologie inflammatoire de l'oreille moyenne. Rev Laryngol Otol Rhinol. 1993;114:165–9.
35. Deron PB, Clement PA, Derde MP. The influence of septal deviation and septal surgery on tubal function. In: Sadé J, editor. The Eustachian tube, clinical aspects. Amsterdam: Kugler and Ghedini Publications; 1991. p. 217–20.
36. Low WK, Wilatt DJ. The relationship between middle ear pressure and deviated nasal septum. Clin Otolaryngol. 1993;18:308–10.
37. Hashimoto S. A guinea pig model of adhesive otitis media and the effect of tympanostomy. Auris Nasus Larynx. 2000;27:39–43.
38. Buckingham RA, Ferrer JL. Reversibility of chronic adhesive otitis media with polyethylene tube, middle ear air-vent, kodachrome time lapse study. Laryngoscope. 1966;76(6):993–1014.
39. Valtonen H, Qvarnberg Y, Nuutinen J. Tympanostomy in young children with recurrent otitis media. A long-term follow-up study. J Laryngol Otol. 1999;113:207–11.
40. Shen YM, Sun WQ, Shen H, Li YH. Tragus cartilage tympanoplasty for treatment of adhesive otitis media. Nan Fang Yi Ke Da Xue Xue Bao. 2010;30:1382–4.
41. Ichimura K, Ishikawa K, Nakamura K, Saito C. Cartilage palisade tympanoplasty for adhesive otitis media. Nihon Jibiinkoka Gakkai Kaiho. 2009;112:474–9.

42. Yu LS, Qi ZM. Operative therapy of the adhesive otitis media. Zhonghua Er Bi Yan Hou Ke Za Zhi. 2004;39:40–3.
43. Dogru H, Tuz M, Uygur K, Candir O, Yariktas M. Tympanostomy preceding tympanoplasty: could it be a new approach for the management of adhesive otitis media. J Otolaryngol. 2003;32:411–4.
44. Tos M. Tympanoplasty in chronic adhesive otitis media. Acta Otolaryngol. 1972;73:53–60.
45. Vartiainen E, Harma R, Karjalainen S. Surgery of chronic adhesive otitis media. Clin Otolaryngol Allied Sci. 1985;10:163–4.
46. Nielsen KO, Bak-Pedersen K. Otosurgery of incipient adhesive otitis media in children. J Laryngol Otol. 1984;98:341–5.
47. Yu LS, Qi ZM. Operative therapy of the adhesive otitis media. Chin J Otorhinolaryngol. 2004;39:40–3.
48. Politzer A. Traite des maladies de l'oreille. Paris: Doin; 1884.
49. Sade J, Avraham S, Brown M. Dynamics of atelectasis and retraction pockets. In: Sade J, editor. Cholesteatoma and mastoid surgery. Amsterdam: Kugler Publications; 1982.
50. Charachon R, Gratacap B, Vuarnet J. Classification and surgical treatment of fibroadhesive otitis. AJO. 1985;6:305–10.
51. Tos M. Obliterative otitis media. J Laryngol Otol. 1979;93:569–73.
52. Bremond G, Magnan J. L'otite adhesive. Ann Oto-Laryngol (Paris). 1977;94:73–82.

Tympanosclerosis

5

Contents

S. Mansour et al., *Middle Ear Diseases*,
https://doi.org/10.1007/978-3-319-72962-6_5

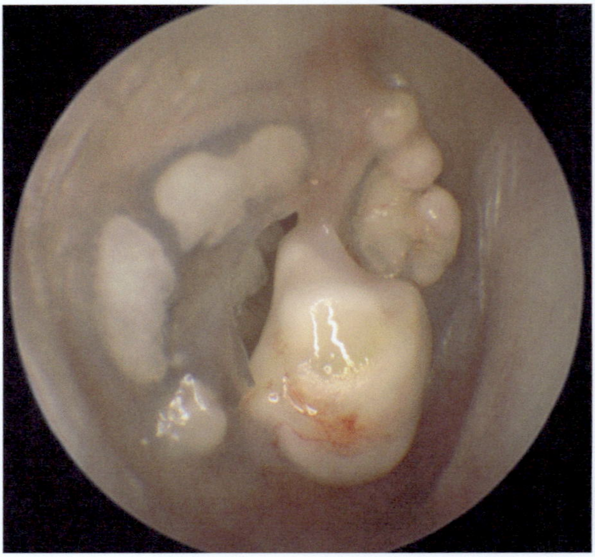

Fig. 5.1 Right ear showing tympanic membrane and middle ear cavity white nodules and plaques which are typical of tympanosclerosis

5.1 Introduction

Tympanosclerosis is a common clinicopathological entity of the middle ear cleft, typically presents as white plaque-like lesions, involving discrete regions of the tympanic membrane and/or middle ear (Fig. 5.1). Its pathogenesis and optimal management have eluded the otologists since its description by von Troeltsch in 1863 [1]. He described it as "a stiffness of the fibrous tissue of the middle ear mucosa." Then in 1955, Zollner and Beck addressed this pathology as a distinguished entity [2, 3]. It is now universally accepted that tympanosclerosis is a hyaline degeneration of the fibrous layer (lamina propria) of the tympanic membrane and the basement membrane of middle ear mucosa.

In this chapter, we will review the most recent advances concerning its etiopathogenesis, its clinical manifestations, the correlation between the sites of middle ear involvement and the degree of hearing loss. Clinico-radiological correlations in regard to the therapeutical strategies are emphasized. The main surgical approaches and rehabilitation of hearing are presented.

5.2 Definition

Tympanosclerosis is an abnormal condition of the middle ear cleft where hyaline calcareous deposits are found on the tympanic membrane, in the tympanic cavity, on the ossicular chain, the ligaments and occasionally in the mastoid (Fig. 5.2). Relative to the extent of calcification and its invasion of the ossicular chain, the resultant degree

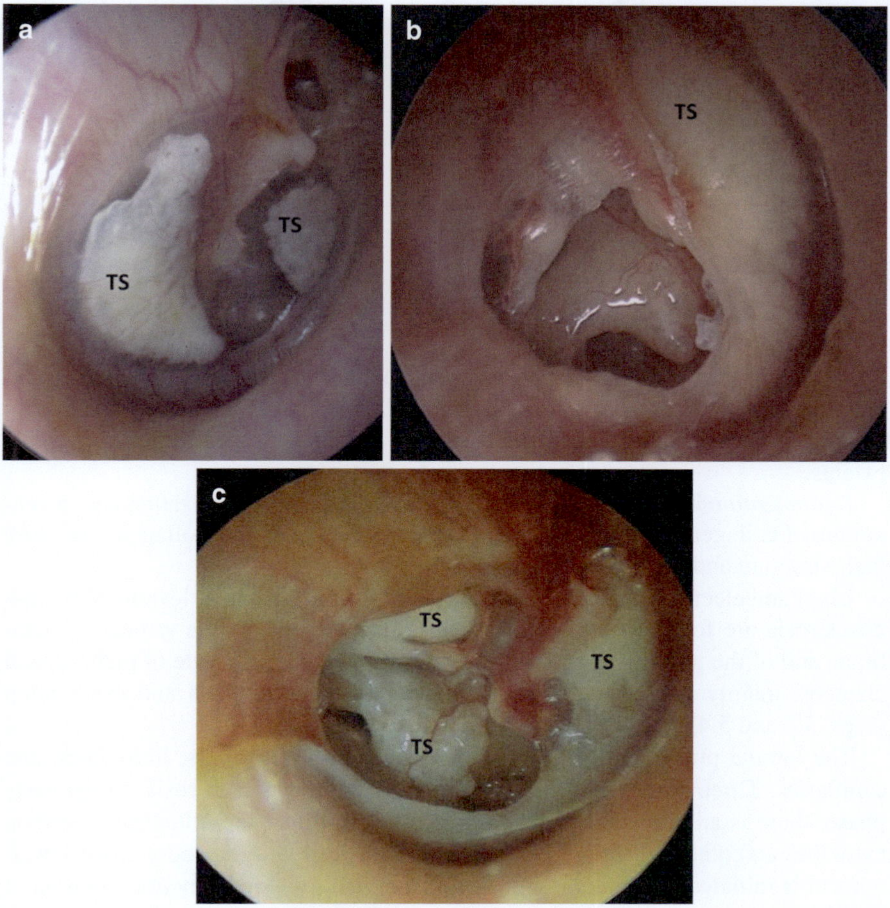

Fig. 5.2 Various forms of tympanosclerosis (TS). (**a**) right ear tympanosclerosis limited to an intact tympanic membrane (TS), this pathology is asymptomatic; (**b**) right ear more severe form of tympanosclerosis of the tympanic membrane with posterior perforation; (**c**) right ear extensive tympanosclerosis (TS) extended into the middle ear cavity, involving the stapes and the promontory

of conductive hearing loss varies. Tympanosclerosis is considered as long term irreversible sequelae of an ill resolved inflammatory process in ears where a long standing and silent chronic otitis media has generated pathologic insults.

Tympanosclerosis affects the tympanic membrane either alone, then it is called *myringosclerosis* or in association with other structures of the middle ear cleft. In the middle ear, tympanosclerosis has a predilection for certain cul-de-sac areas where mucosal cells have minimal glandular activity with diminished ciliary activity [4]. Stapes-Oval window area, upper promontory, epitympanum, incus-malleus joint, Fallopian canal and sub Fallopian groove are the common predilective sites of the disease. Hypotympanum and mastoid cavity are rarely involved (Table 5.1).

Table 5.1 Main features of tympanosclerosis

Main features of tympanosclerosis
• Irreversible end product of chronic middle ear inflammation
• Does not destroy the ossicles, but leaves fixation
• Commonly found along ligaments and in "cul de sac" areas
• mainly found in the attic and in the OW niche

5.3 Histology

Tympanosclerosis is a pathologic degenerative condition of the middle ear that is characterized by an excessive deposition of collagen fibers, the presence of hyalinization of connective tissue with calcifications and possible ossification in variable extents.

Hyalinization is a pathological process that consists of vacuolization and degeneration of collagen fibers with disorganization of fibrous tissue. Collagen fibers lose their structure and fuse into a homogeneous mass.

Light and electron microscopy have established that the basic lesions of tympanosclerosis are found in the lamina propria (submucosa) of the tympanic membrane and of the middle ear mucosa. The lamina propria is the site of pathological changes, mainly hyalinization, necrosis, fibrosis, calcifications and ossification (Figs. 5.3 and 5.4).

The lamina propria is normally composed of collagen fibers, fibroblasts, and capillaries. Three phases exist in the formation of tympanosclerosis. In the early phase, there is an alteration of the lamina propria: Under the influence of certain cytokines and other regulatory factors, the initial phase of tympanosclerosis development is initiated by an *increased fibroblast activity*, followed by degeneration of the fibrous skeleton and formation of abnormal fibrils (Fig. 5.4). This is followed by hyalinization of this layer, which characterizes the intermediate phase. The final phase is the stage of maturation of the plaque, with or without calcification or even ossification.

During otitis media, inflammatory macrophages are the first cells to invade middle ear mucosa followed by T-cells and B-cells; all these cells express *inducible nitric oxide synthase*. The inducible nitric oxide synthase and the inflammatory cells conjugate series of sequences leading to collagen degeneration; the fibers lose their structure and merge to become a homogeneous (hyaline) mass [5]. Then the activated *macrophages* initiate the process of calcification: they express osteopontin and differentiate into osteoclasts to produce calcium deposits and ossification [6, 7] (Fig. 5.5).

Macroscopically, two types of tympanosclerotic plaques are described according to their consistency and surgical detachment feature [8]:

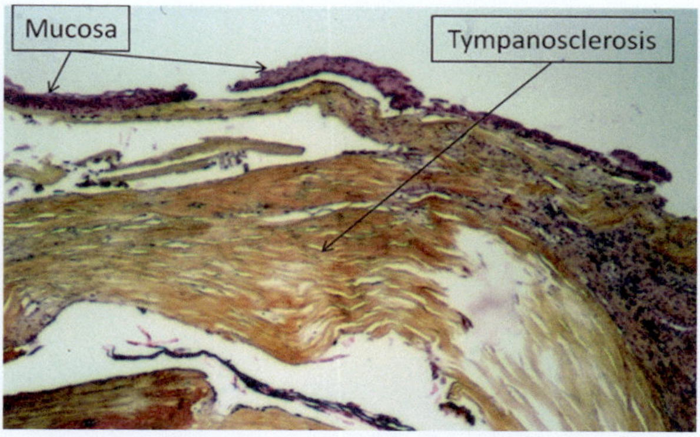

Fig. 5.3 Optic microscope: middle ear tympanosclerosis: Lying in the submucosa immediately under the thin atrophic cuboidal mucosa of the middle ear, a lamellated mass of hyalinized collagen is found (arrow) with few fibrocytes

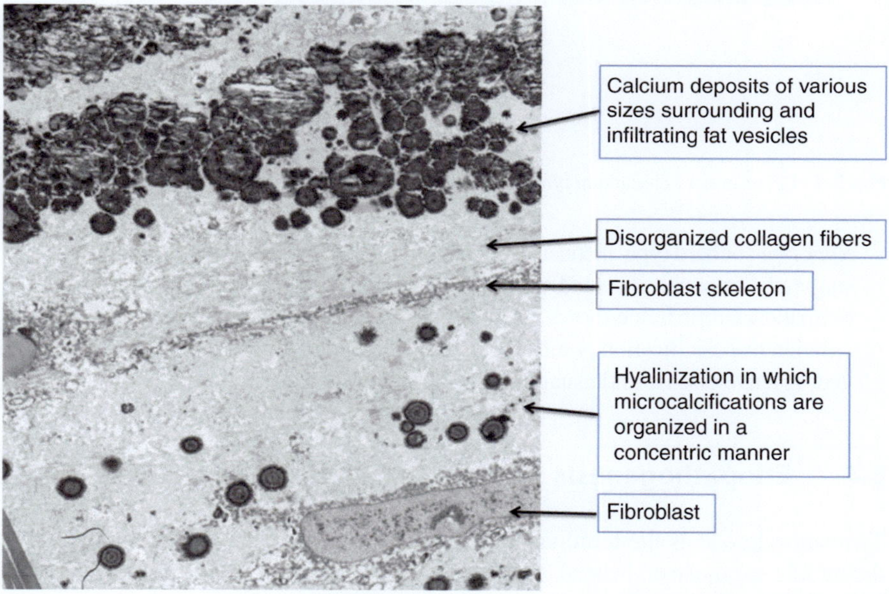

Fig. 5.4 Electronic microscopy of a tympanic membrane with myringosclerosis showing hyalinization of the lamina propria, disorganization of collagen fibers and calcifications of various sizes

– *Chalk type*: or soft type, it exhibits lamellar morphology and is soft on palpation and easily removable. Light microscopic evaluation of this type of tympanosclerotic tissue usually shows that fibroblasts and collagen fibers are equally abundant in typical loose connective tissue. A few small calcium crystals could be seen. In this type of tympanosclerotic disease, even if complete resection of sclerotic tissue is performed, the underlying process may go on and new sclerotic tissue formation can be expected.

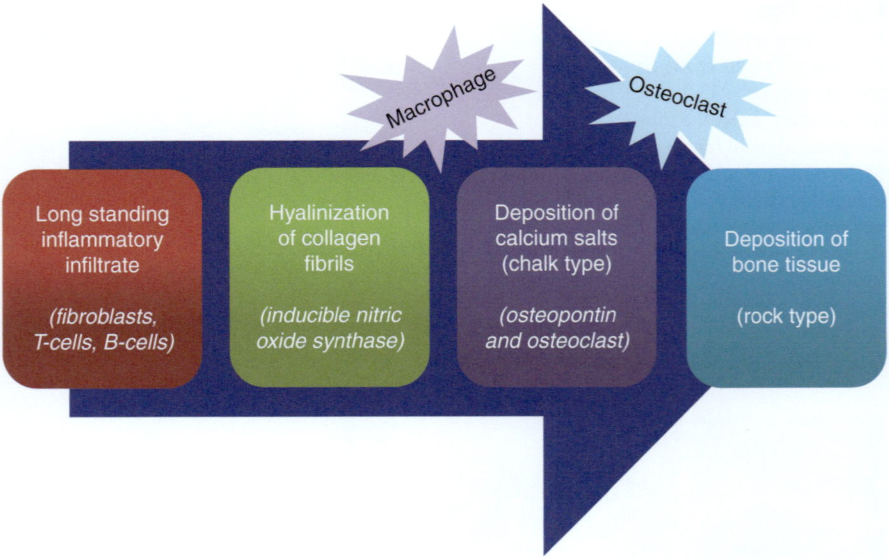

Fig. 5.5 Inflammatory cascade in tympanosclerosis

– *Rock type*: or hard type, it consists of hard white plaques which are difficult to remove surgically from the involved tissues. Light microscopic evaluation of this type of tympanosclerotic tissue shows round shaped condroblast-like cells located in lacunae with intense calcification points. Rock type tympanosclerosis is associated with limited, inactive disease and usually doesn't progress or recur after removal.

5.4 Etiopathogenesis

Tympanosclerosis is the terminal stage of an inflammatory process taking place in the middle ear mucosa; instead to regress, the inflammation heals through an abnormal scarring process with hyalinization, calcification and osteogenesis. It is an irreversible phenomenon. It may occur following surgery on the tympanic membrane such myringotomy and tube placement (insults to the lamina propria) or in response to a long standing chronic middle ear infection.

The etiology of tympanosclerosis is still not fully understood. Immunological reactions, genetic predisposition, infection, trauma and free oxygen radicals are possible underlying causes of tympanosclerosis [9].

Generally, middle ear inflammation may resolve properly or may resolve with abnormal scarring (TS) or may induce complications. The outcome of a middle ear inflammatory process is determined by the type of generated inflammatory mediators that depends on the individual immune and genetic profile [10]. In some individuals, a special profile of the inflammatory process (immune cells and inflammatory mediators) induces a cascade of events that causes differentiation of *macrophages to osteoclasts* and finally leads to tympanosclerosis development [6]. Middle ear inflammation with high levels of *TNF-alpha* ends up with abnormal scarring and tympanosclerosis [11].

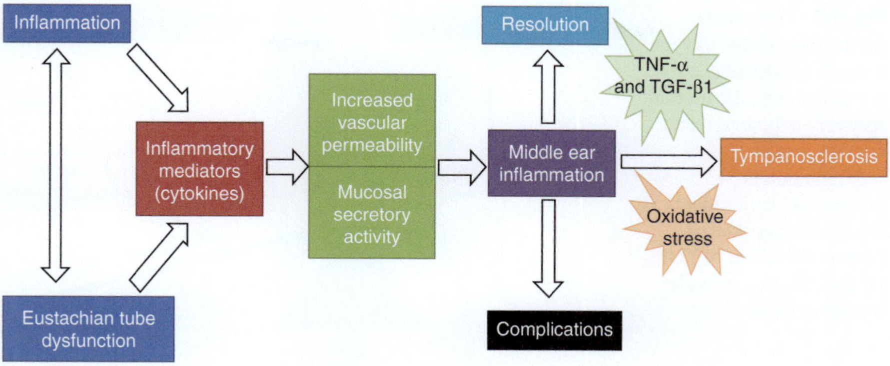

Fig. 5.6 Pathogenesis of middle ear tympanosclerosis

In addition, the expression of TGF-β1 is significantly increased in ears with tympanosclerosis which indicates that TGF-β1 plays an important role in the development and outcome of otitis media towards tympanosclerosis [12–14] (Fig. 5.6).

Free oxygen radicals **(FORs)** are an important etiological factor in the development of TS [15].

Middle ear inflammation and hyperoxia in a special inflammatory profile (special inflammatory cells and mediators) induce the production of ***FORs*** by the activated macrophages and other inflammatory cells. Excessive production of FORs causes tissue damage. Inducible nitric oxide synthase was seen more frequently in patients with tympanosclerosis [16–18] (Fig. 5.7).

FORs are normally battled by antioxidants (catalase, vit c,…). Oxidative stress is a status of antioxidants decrease or an increase of the production of oxidants (nitric oxide and FORs).

Tympanosclerosis develops in patients with chronic otitis media who have genetically determined ineffective anti-oxidant system to deal with free radicals generated by middle ear inflammation and by middle ear hyperoxia (from perforation or grommet) (Fig. 5.7). It is likely that *high inducible nitric oxide synthase* levels and low catalase levels play a role in the tympanosclerosis formation by increasing the production of nitric oxide and other free oxygen radicals (Fig. 5.7).

Moreover tympanosclerotic patients present larger mastoid air cell systems than patients with chronic otitis media without tympanosclerosis, possibly indicating that the more the mastoid is pneumatized, the more the production of free oxygen radicals is high, favoring the induction of the tympanosclerotic process [19].

Furthermore, the biological mechanism of calcification in tympanosclerosis is thought to be probably similar to that occurring elsewhere in other tissue calcifying processes such as in atherosclerosis. The rate of appearance of myringosclerosis in atherosclerotic patients has been found to be 66.6%. This is very high compared to the rate of 12% appearance of myringosclerosis in the normal population. Among atherosclerotic patients who suffer from middle ear infections, >80% have tympanosclerosis, while in non-atherosclerotic patients who suffer from middle ear infections; this rate is <20% [20, 21]. These findings indicate that there must be similar risk factors triggering pathogenesis in tympanosclerosis and atherosclerosis. Both

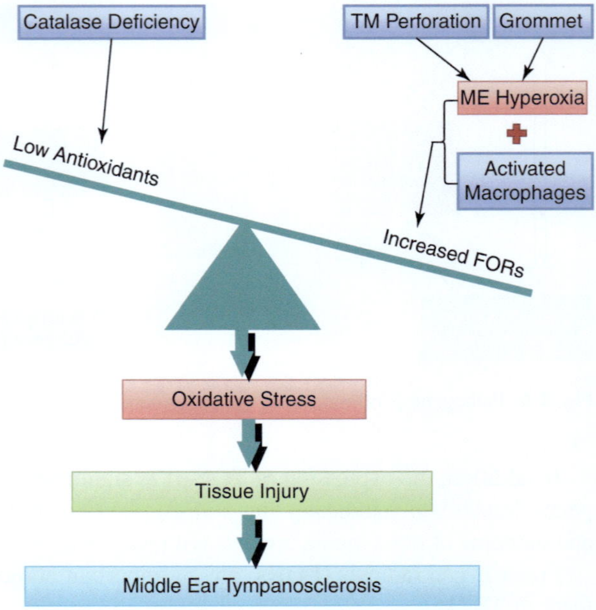

Fig. 5.7 The excess production of free oxygen radicals (FORs) causes tissue damage; the normal recovery is hindered and the duration of inflammation is prolonged. Antioxidants are substances that prevent the effect of FORs on the cells and provide oxidative balance

diseases are last reactions of inflammation in connective tissue and pathogenesis may follow the same route.

Some reports demonstrated that the up-regulation of TGF-β1 affects the prognosis of otitis media, and is thought to be the cause of tympanosclerosis. TGF-β1 promotes the development of fibrosis in various organs, such as the liver and the kidney, which appears to experience similar pathological alterations as in tympanosclerosis [22–25].

ACE inhibitor (ACEI) or angiotensin II receptor blocker (ARB), inhibit the progress of middle ear tympanosclerosis and organ fibrosis due to the reduction in the TGF-β1 expression [26–29].

Captopril and losartan exert preventive effects on tympanoscelrosis via down-regulation of the expression of TGF-β1, which may be one possible explanation for the histological amelioration of the middle ear mucosa and the partial recovery of hearing function [30].

In addition, topically applied calcium channel blockers showed to be able to reduce the progression of tympanosclerosis [31]. Thus the preventive therapy of calcium channel blockers in tympanosclerosis could be possible.

5.5 Prevalence of Tympanosclerosis

The clinical incidence of tympanosclerosis is 5–10% in patients who suffered from chronic otitis media [32–36]; but only 6% of these cases complained of hearing loss. Tympanosclerosis is bilateral in around 50% of cases [37].

Tympanosclerosis was seen most commonly in individuals over 40 years of age (86.7%). Tympanosclerosis prevalence is higher in the older age groups, showing an

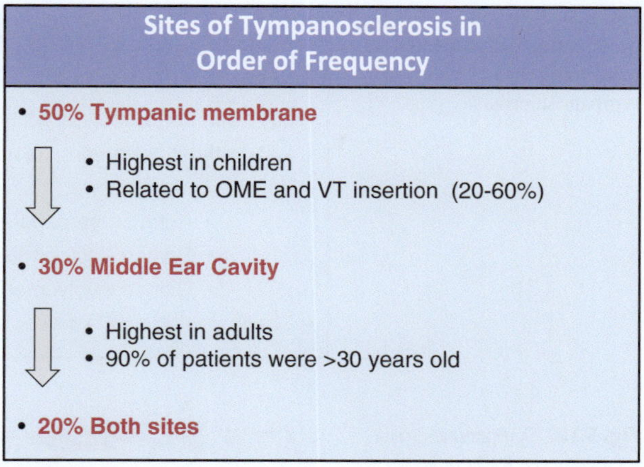

Fig. 5.8 Sites of tympanosclerosis in order of frequency

increased occurrence with age. It is more frequent in males 1.6:1 [38]. The incidence of myringosclerosis in children who had insertion of ventilation tubes, is between 28 and 61% [39].

5.6 Sites of Involvement in the Ear

Tympanosclerosis affects most frequently the tympanic membrane alone (50%). In 30%, middle ear structures are affected, as ossicular ligaments, interosseous joints, muscle tendons and submucosal areas, causing varying degrees of fixity of the ossicular chain [40]. In 20%, tympanosclerosis affects both, the tympanic membrane and the middle ear structures (Fig. 5.8). The difference in the anatomic architecture of the tympanic membrane and the middle ear mucosa explains the difference of incidence of tympanosclerosis at these sites. The pars tensa of the tympanic membrane has a well organized thick layer of fibrous tissue, however, the mucosa of the middle ear cavity has a loose subepithelial space, which accounts for the lower incidence of tympanosclerosis.

In the tympanic membrane, any part of the drum could be involved except the pars flaccida which is always spared. In the pars tensa, tympanosclerosis is found most commonly in the anterior and posterior inferior quadrants, and within these quadrants is seen most often in a central rather than a peripheral position [38]. The formation of tympanosclerosis requires a compact, well-formed, and well-differentiated middle fibrous layer. The middle fibrous layer in the inferior quadrants is compact and becomes looser as one approaches the annulus, umbo, and posterior superior quadrant. Anteroinferior involvement is common but usually not extensive [41]. By far the commonest otoscopic finding associated with tympanoscleoris is a central tympanic membrane perforation (80%); 20% of tympanosclerosis cases are associated with an intact tympanic membrane (Fig. 5.9).

In the middle ear cavity, tympanosclerotic plaques occur preferentially in dependent areas where the mucus glands population is lowest and the ciliary activity is low; so stagnation of inflammatory exudates is favored in such areas

Fig. 5.9 Sites of predilection of tympanic membrane tympanosclerosis

Tympanosclerosis of the Tympanic Membrane

- 80% with perforation (open tympanosclerosis)
- 20% without perforation (close tympanosclerosis)
- Zones of predeliction
    - Anterior tympano-malleolar ligament
    - Postero-*inferior* quadrant
    - Diffuse involvement
- **The Pars flaccida is never involved**

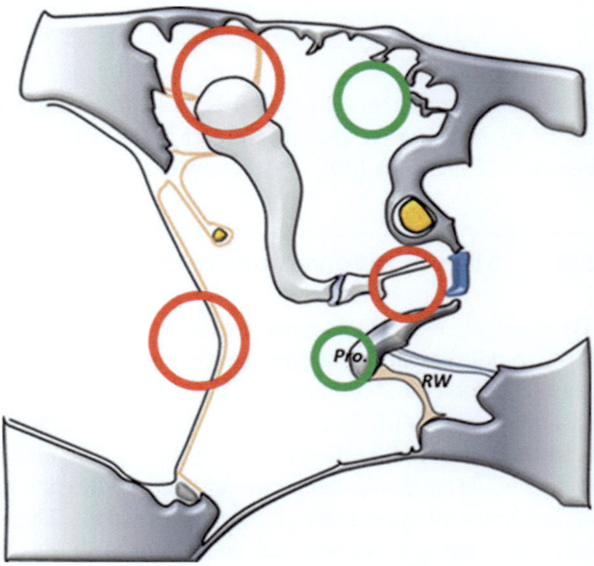

Fig. 5.10 Tympanosclerosis localizations: Red circles represent sites with possible hearing loss, and green circles sites of silent affection. Pro: promontory; RW: round window

Fig. 5.11 Localisations of intratympanic tympanosclerosis

Intratympanic Tympanosclerosis

- 80% around the malleus (most frequent)
- 45% around the incudomalleal joint
- 35% around the stapes
- 14% on the promontory

resembling "cul de sac" areas like the attic and the oval window niche [42]. The plaques typically occur in certain sites of predilection, most commonly the epitympanum and posterior mesotympanum. In the mesotympanum, the oval window, sinus tympani, facial recess, round window niche, promontory, malleus, and the incus are common sites of involvement. Tympanosclerosis of the Eustachian tube area, the hypotympanum and the mastoid are less encountered (Figs. 5.10 and 5.11).

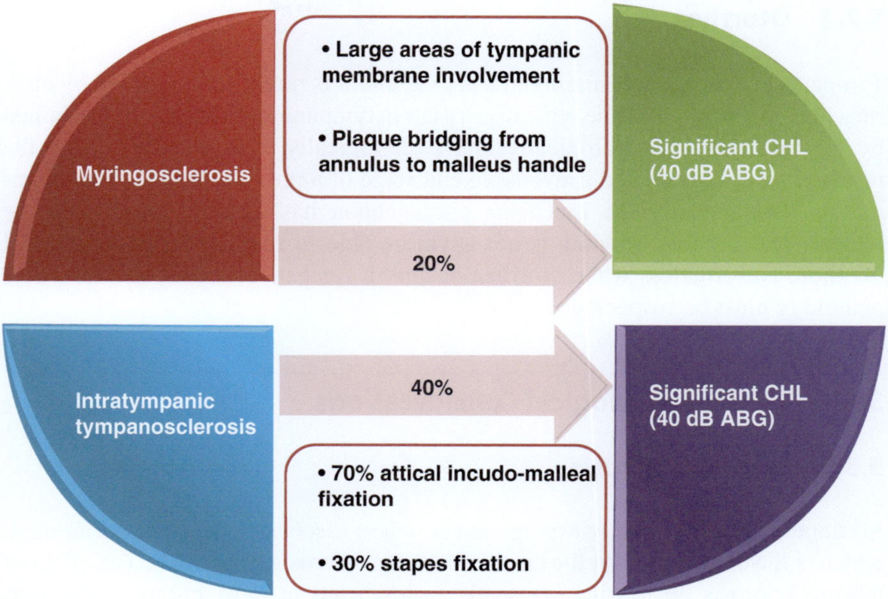

Fig. 5.12 Hearing loss depending on the different localizations of tympanosclerosis

The frequency of invasion of the ossicular chain by tympanosclerosis varies in the literature from 39 to 56% [32, 34–36]. More recently, Tsuzuki reported that the frequency of tympanosclerosis located in the epitympanum, above the tympanic diaphragm is 86%, and tympanosclerotic fixation of the stapes complex located below the tympanic diaphragm in the mesotympanum is less frequent (36.9%) [43] (Fig. 5.11).

Middle ear tympanosclerosis could be silent or could manifest with hearing loss depending on the site of involvement. The anatomical and physiological impairment is greater if the area of involvement is the epitympanum. If it involves the head of malleus and body of incus assembly, the fixation may induce 40 dB of conductive hearing loss. The stapes footplate may be fixed at the oval window by a tympanosclerotic plaque causing a "pseudo-otosclerosis" presentation (Fig. 5.12).

5.7 Clinical Manifestations

5.7.1 Hearing Loss

Tympanosclerosis remains often clinically silent until the hearing loss appears. The chief complaint for the majority of tympanosclerosis patients seeking medical advice is hearing loss. The hearing loss is usually of conductive type: the degree of hearing loss depends on the extent and location of the tympanosclerotic plaques. Mixed hearing loss can be observed and the sensorineural component could be due to the previous episodes of active middle ear inflammation or due to the involvement of the inner ear by tympanosclerosis toxins as suggested by Gibb et al. [37].

5.7.2 Otorrhea

Tympanosclerosis occurs mainly in a dry ear and it is rarely accompanied by otorrhea [32, 35, 36, 40, 44]. The typically dry ear in tympanosclerosis can be explained by the fact that, morphologically and pathologically, tympanosclerosis is the result of an exhausted and irreversible end stage of a previous middle ear inflammation. Dynamically the mucositis phenomenon has already ceased and the mucosa that became atrophic is not anymore able to react to further microbial invasion. Nevertheless when otorrhea occurs in tympanosclerosis, an associated pathology must be suspected.

5.8 Clinicopathological Considerations

5.8.1 Myringosclerosis

Myringosclerosis is usually asymptomatic unless associated with TM perforation, which is the case in 80% of the cases of myringosclerosis (Fig. 5.13). The effect of myringosclerosis on hearing is usually insignificant in most instances and it is asymptomatic in the absence of associated ear diseases. In some cases, extensive involvement of the drum results in significant conductive hearing loss (Figs. 5.12 and 5.13b).

When a simple myringosclerosis of an intact the eardrum is associated to a significant conductive hearing loss (Fig. 5.14), an intratympanic tympanosclerosis involvement should be suspected and CT Imaging becomes valuable.

The clinical diagnosis of extensive tympanosclerosis behind a closed tympanic membrane (pseudo-otosclerosis) in a patient with a significant conductive hearing loss is suspected according to the following clinical criteria:

1. Long history of recurrent otitis media
2. Negative family history of otosclerosis
3. Presence of tympanosclerotic plaques on the tympanic membrane (myringosclerosis)
4. CT-Imaging findings

5.8.2 Intratympanic Tympanosclerosis

Tympanosclerosis invading the tympanic cavity may have different degrees of extension. It is easily recognized when the middle ear is assessed during otomicroscopy or endoscopy examination looking through the perforation (Figs. 5.15 and 5.16). The eardrum perforation is mostly central. If the ossicular chain is involved by tympanosclerosis, the patient will have a hearing loss worse than the one expected from tympanic membrane perforation alone.

The following clinical criteria are contributive to suspect intratympanic tympanosclerosis with tympanic membrane perforation:

1. Hearing loss out of proportion to the size of perforation (over 30 dB)
2. Chalky patches seen on the promontory or oval window (Fig. 5.15).
3. An extensive myringosclerosis
4. A fixed manubrium found during gentle palpation under microscope

Ossicular involvement is usually seen in about 30–40% of cases of intratympanic tympanosclerosis [32, 34, 35]. Incudomalleal complex fixation by epitympanic tympanosclerosis is found in around 70% of all tympanosclerotic ossicular fixations

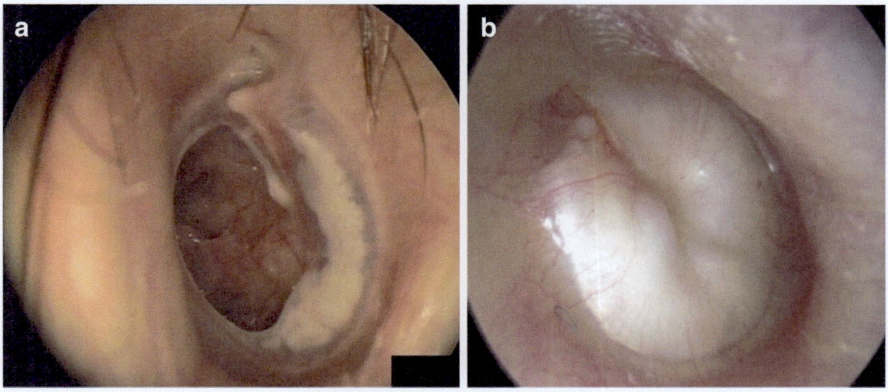

Fig. 5.13 (**a**) Right ear myringosclerosis with central TM perforation; (**b**) right ear massive and extensive myringosclerosis fixing the manubrium

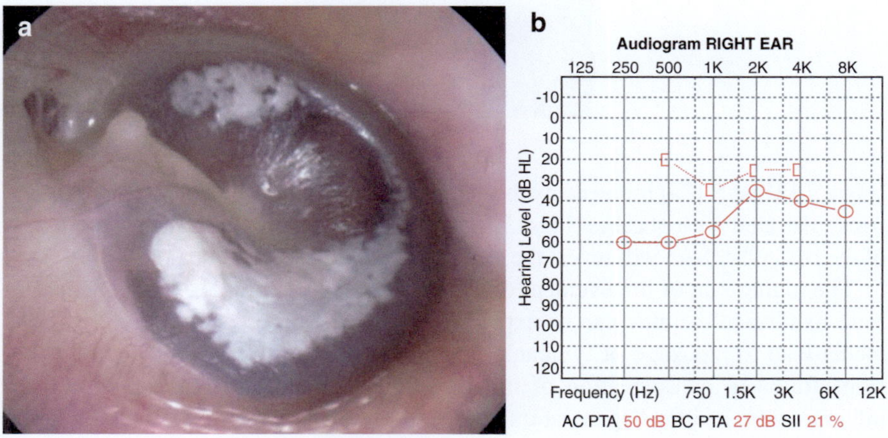

Fig. 5.14 (**a**) otoscopic image of a right ear with a large myringosclerosis (**b**) a moderate conductive hearing loss suggesting ossicular chain involvement

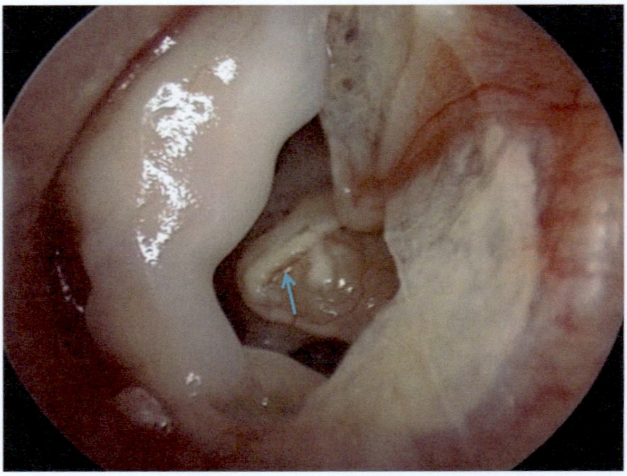

Fig. 5.15 Left ear tympanosclerosis on the promontory (blue arrow)

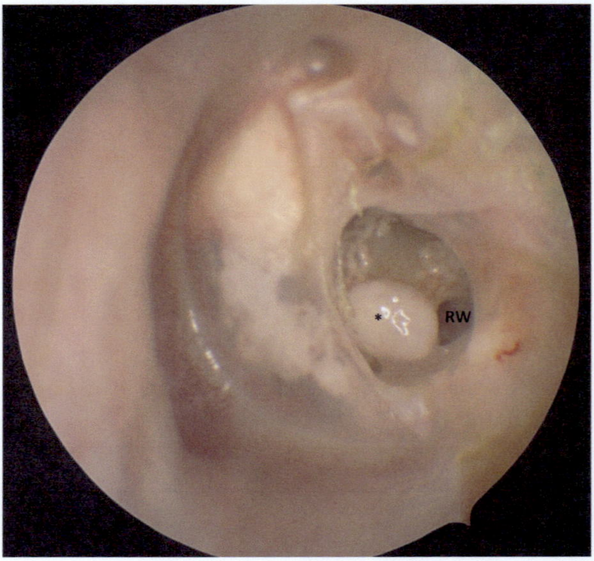

Fig. 5.16 Left ear showing myringosclerosis with intratympanic tympanosclerosis, visible through the perforation, and involving the promontory (*) and extending to the round window (RW)

(Figs. 5.12 and 5.17a) followed by the stapes fixation with oval window tympanosclerosis in around 30% of cases (Figs. 5.12 and 5.17b). Only intraoperative examination of the ossicular chain will reveal the exact status of the ossicular chain.

The higher rate of involvement of the incudo-malleal complex by tympanosclerotic fixation in the attic can be explained by the fact that recurrent bouts of otitis media lead to blockage of tympanic isthmi by secretions, granulations and adhesions followed by stagnation of inflammatory exudate with unresolved chronic inflammation, hyaline degeneration, tympanosclerosis leading to the fixation of the incudo-malleal complex.

Rarely tympanosclerosis may cause ossicular necrosis by ischemia due to a strangulation effect on the blood supply rather than by osteolytic necrotic destruction as in chronic infection. Erosion of the long process of the incus and stapes crura, found in tympanosclerotic ears could be also the result of the chronic active inflammatory process previous to the installation of the tympanosclerosis process (Fig. 5.18).

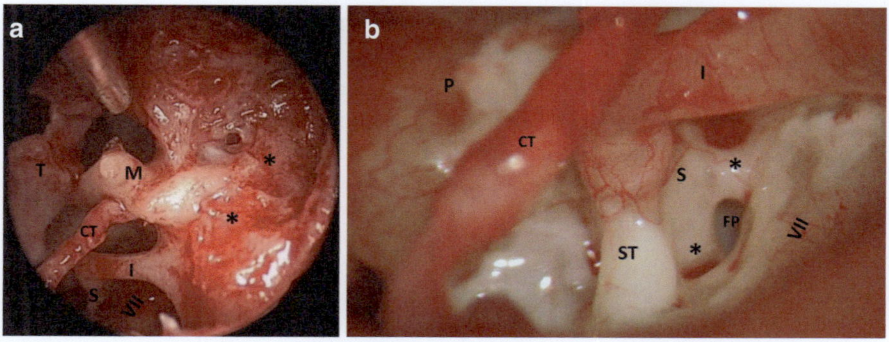

Fig. 5.17 (**a**) Left ear intraoperative endoscopy after raising the drum (T) and endaural atticotomy showing incudomalleal complex fixation by epitympanic tympanosclerosis (*) fixing the malleus (M) and the incus (I) the Stapes (S) is free. (**b**) left ear intraoperative microscopic exploration showing stapedial complex fixation by extensive tympanosclerosis (*) spreading from the facial nerve (VII) around the stapes (S) and stapedial tendon (ST) the promontory (P). *M* malleus, *FP* footplate, *I* incus, *CT* chorda tympani (*Courtesy Pr H Vijayendra)*

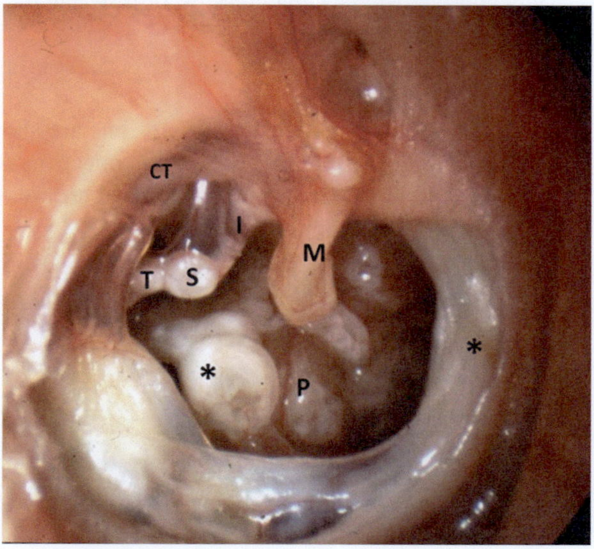

Fig. 5.18 Right ear endoscopy showing tympanosclerosis (*) involving the tympanic membrane, the promontory (P), the stapes (S) and stapedial tendon (T). Notice the necrosis of the long process of incus (I). *M* malleus, *CT* chorda tympani

5.9 CT-Imaging in Tympanosclerosis

Clinico-radiological correlations are of high interest to improve the positive and the differential diagnosis of tympanosclerosis: the degree of hearing loss, otomicroscopic evaluation and endoscopic findings correlated to CT imaging enlighten the strategy of its management.

5.9.1 Positive Diagnosis: Radiologic Signs of Tympanosclerosis

It is important to report to the radiologist the description of all tympanosclerotic plaques seen on otoscopy to orient the CT reading and facilitate the differential diagnosis of an associated conductive hearing loss. *The main imaging sign of tympanosclerosis on CT is the presence of calcified hyperdense plaques on the eardrum or inside the cavity.*

5.9.1.1 Myringosclerosis

Calcified plaques on the tympanic membrane may vary from very tiny spots of calcifications to large thickened calcified plaques (Fig. 5.19).

5.9.1.2 Calcified Material Inside the Tympanic Cavity

Tympanosclerosis inside the tympanic cavity may manifest as a calcification of the ligaments, folds and tendons (Fig. 5.20), in form of bandlike structures, that cross the cavity (Fig. 5.21a), calcifications of the capsule of the incudomallear joint (Fig. 5.21b).

Tympanosclerosis can manifest by diffuse calcifications throughout the tympanic cavity and its recesses (Fig. 5.22a) or even calcified block formations with narrowing of the lumen of the cavity (Fig. 5.22b), or extend to the Antrum and Mastoid (Fig. 5.23).

However, not all tympanosclerotic lesions are shown by CT as calcified formations, especially the chalk type, which appears as condensation images hardly differentiated from other soft tissue or chronic inflammatory pathologies (Fig. 5.24).

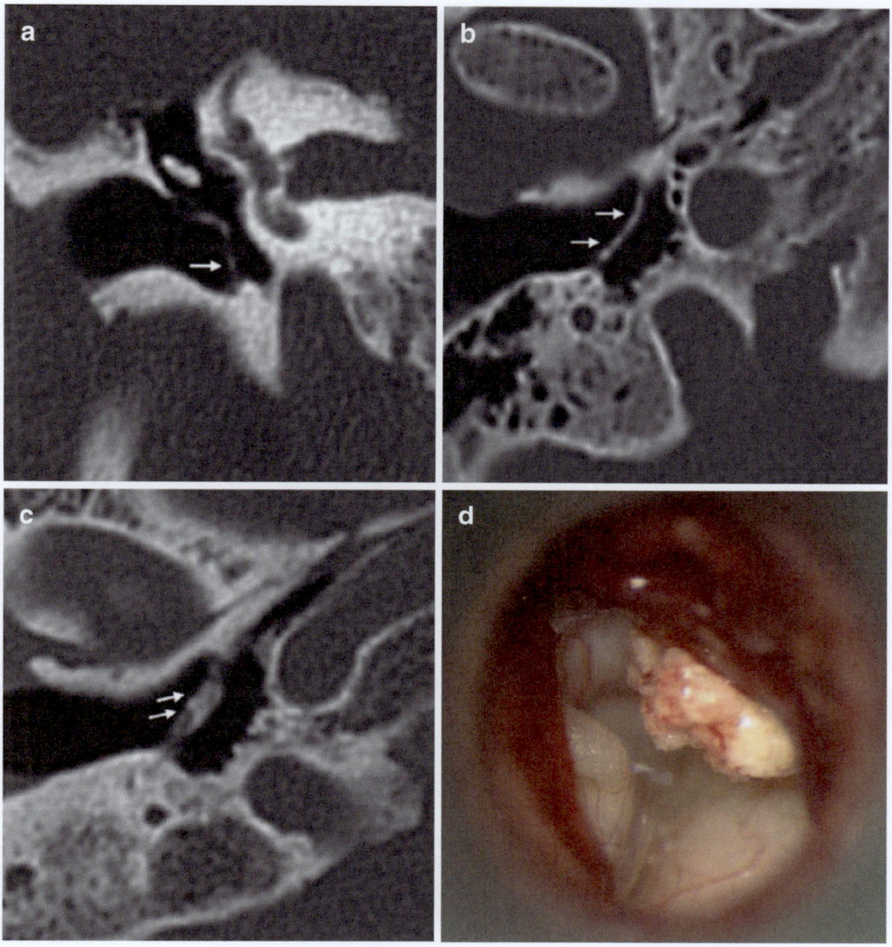

Fig. 5.19 (**a**)–(**c**) Different aspects of myringosclerosis on CT- images: (**a**) Coronal CT view of a thin tympanic membrane with a very tiny spot of calcification (arrow) (**b**) axial CT- image of a right ear: moderate thickening and calcification of the whole tympanic membrane (arrows) (**c**) axial CT image of a right ear: important heterogeneous thickening of the tympanic membrane with calcified plaques (arrows) (**d**) otoscopic view of the huge myringosclerotic plaque in (**c**)

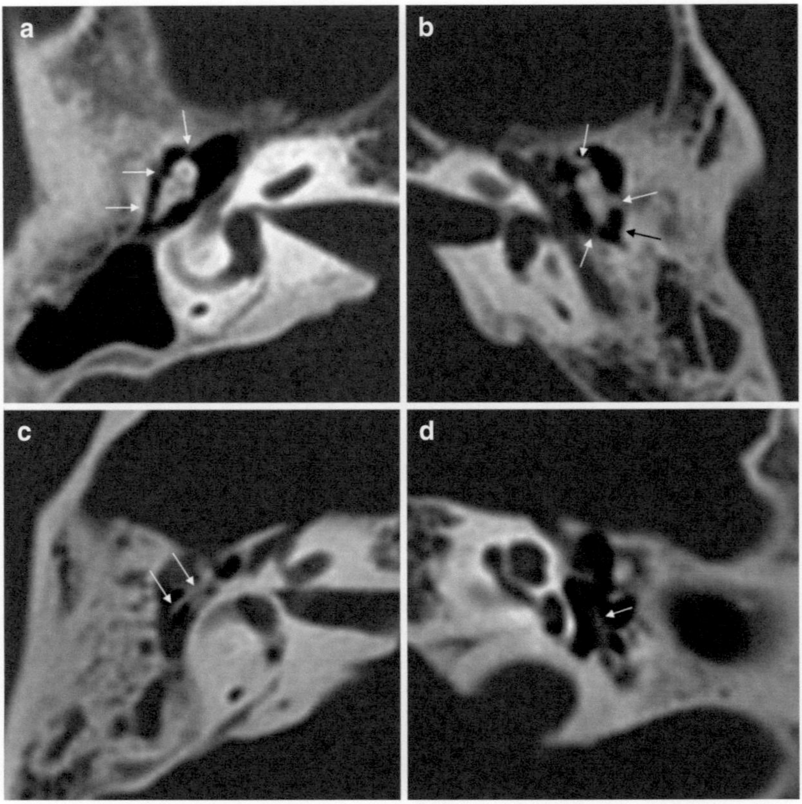

Fig. 5.20 Tympanosclerosis of the ossicular ligaments, seen on axial CT images (**a**) of the right ear as thickening of the ligaments (arrows), in (**b**) of a left ear as calcification of the ligaments (arrows). (**c**) right ear, calcification of the superior incudal fold, (**d**) left ear, thickening of the stapedial muscle tendon (arrow)

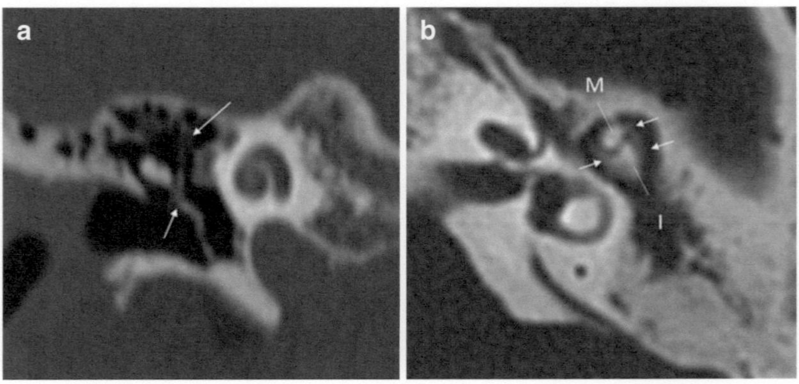

Fig. 5.21 (**a**) coronal CT-image showing a long calcified band extending from the calcified tympanic membrane (short arrow) to the attic wall (long arrow) (**b**) axial CT-Scan of a left ear: images of tympanosclerosis around the incudomalleal joint: *M* head of the malleus, *I* incus, arrows tympanosclerosis

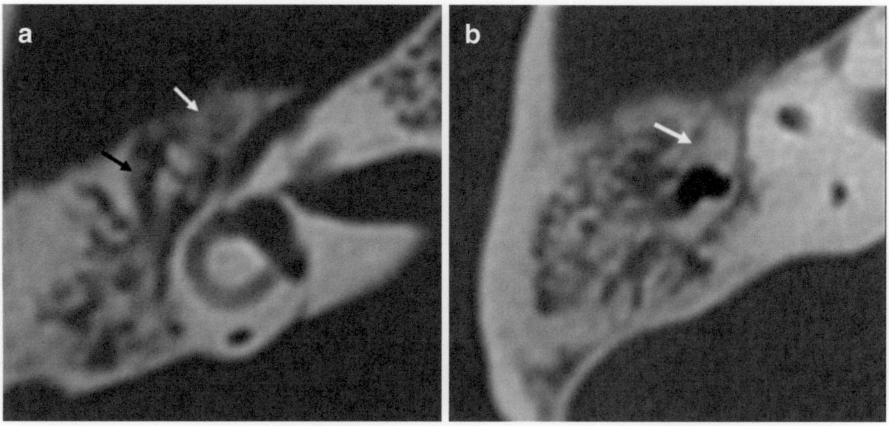

Fig. 5.22 (**a**, **b**) Axial and coronal view of a different right ears: (**a**) calcified tympanosclerotic material in the epitympanum: external attic (black arrow), anterior epitympanic recess (white arrow) (**b**) large attic calcification (arrow) filling the epitympanum

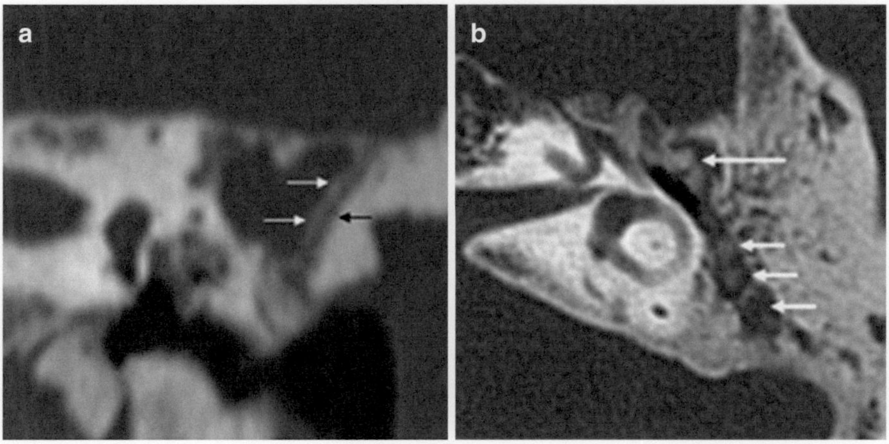

Fig. 5.23 (**a**) Coronal CT-image of a left ear: mucosal thickening of the antrum (black arrow) covered by a thin rim calcification (white arrows) (**b**) axial CT-image of a left ear: the antrum is filled with tympanosclerotic blocks (short arrows) occupying nearby all the antrum lumen. Incudo-malleal chain (long arrow)

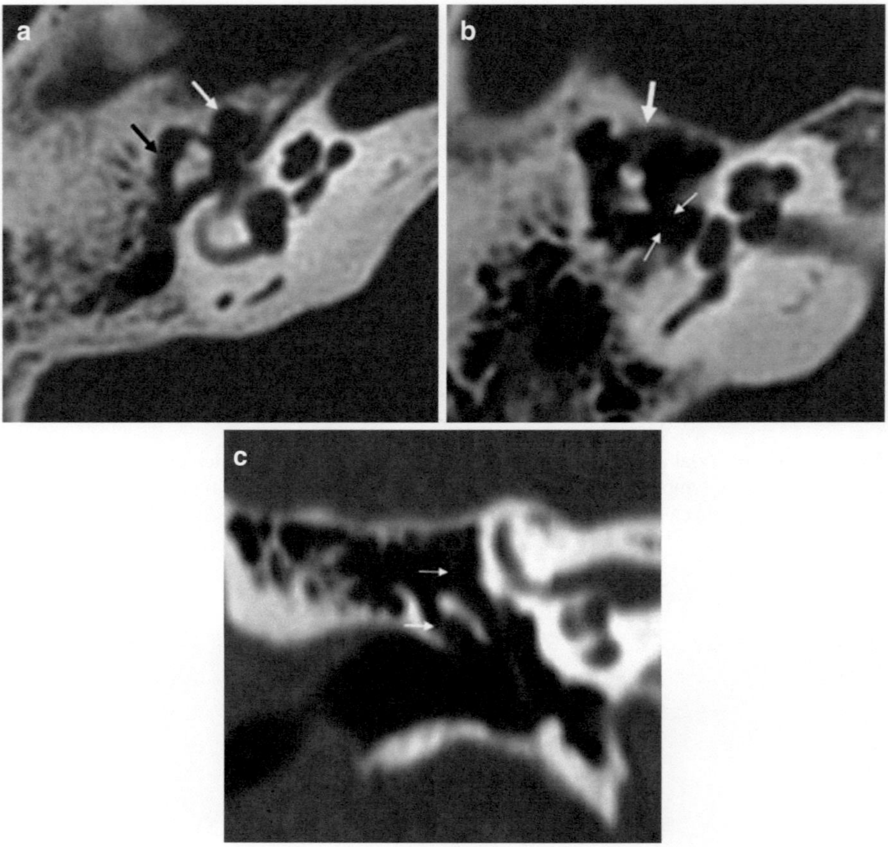

Fig. 5.24 (**a**) Axial CT-image of the right ear: Condensation images without visible calcifications in the lateral attic (black arrow) and the AER (white arrow). Tympanosclerosis was confirmed only during surgery. (**b**) axial and (**c**) coronal CT Scan of the right ear of another patient with conductive hearing loss, myringosclerosis and a tiny tympanic membrane perforation: small weblike condensations inside the cavity (small arrows), important thickening of the anterior malleal ligament (thick arrow): the per-operative finding was tympanosclerosis extended into the attic and calcifications around the malleus and incus

5.10 Surgical Treatment of Tympanosclerosis

Surgical treatment of tympanosclerosis is challenging, especially in invasive stages. It still suffers from a lack of consensus among otologists who have maintained unwavering faith in the value of surgery and its cost-benefit [32, 35, 40, 42, 45].

There is a big disagreement about surgical treatment and the choice of an optimal approach [46]. Some of the leading otologists, Austin, Sheehy, House, Tos advocate surgical treatment, while others, Schukhnecht, Morrison and Smyth, consider tympanosclerosis as the last disease of the middle ear to be surgically managed [47].

Our long-standing experience in middle ear surgery favored the attitude that tympanosclerosis needs to be surgically managed: first aiming the complete eradication of the pathological process and secondly the restitution of the transmission apparatus.

Surgery is based on the assumption that tympanosclerosis usually does not recur after its "total and complete" removal. Thus the favorable postoperative hearing results should be stable for a long duration. However surgery of tympanosclerosis is demanding and includes complex counseling: since the surgeon often does not know what procedure is likely to be performed until the exact extension of the lesions has been accurately evaluated through a meticulous surgical exploration. It is agreed that:

- *Surgery of the incudomalleal complex tympanosclerosis is generally simple and easy to manage;*
- *In contrary, its association to a stapedial complex involvement may require staging and various stapes surgeries;*
- *Stapes surgery may expose to possible failure, to more postoperative risks, and complications. Therefore more definite strategy and surgical expertise are required.*

5.10.1 Management of Tympanic Membrane Tympanosclerosis:

Tympanic membrane tympanosclerosis is usually asymptomatic and doesn't warrant treatment. Removal of the tympanosclerotic plaques from the tympanic membrane is required only if there are extensive plaques affecting the compliance of the tympanic membrane. Plaques on the tympanic membrane briding from the annulus to the malleus and disturbing its mobility should be also removed.

Plaques are removed either through the edges of perforation or after raising the tympanomeatal flap. A small tunnel is made with angled pick between the plaque and lateral epithelium and thereby gradually undermining the whole plaque which is then removed with a grasping forceps. Small plaques do not in any way affect graft uptake or hearing restoration.

5.10.2 Management of Isolated Incudo-Malleal Complex Tympanosclerotic Fixation

Two major procedures are in use:

5.10.2.1 Mobilization (Preserving the Integrity of the Ossicular Chain)

Complete and total removal of tympanosclerotic plaques around and over the ossicles could restore ossicular mobility and lead to surgical success in case of incudomalleolar complex fixation.

Mobilization is possible when the disease is of limited degree; but the surgical dissection of the plaques from the malleus, especially anteriorly and around the joint may cause sensorineural deficit secondary to a heavy manipulation. Smith [48] found Laser as a useful adjunct tool in performing accurate separation of TS layers surrounding the ossicles and avoiding heavy ossicular manipulation. Incudomalleal complex mobilization could be done preferably through a transcanal atticotomy approach (Figs. 5.17a, 5.25a) or through a transmastoid atticotomy approach (Fig. 5.25b).

When it is impossible to mobilize the ossicular chain to a satisfying extent or when the chain is disrupted, a bypass technique should be applied.

5.10.2.2 Bypass Technique

Often, the Bypass technique is preferred; then it is necessary to disarticulate the incudo stapedial and incudo malleolar joint, remove the incus and nip the malleus. This should be followed by making malleus to stapes horizontal assembly using an autologous freshened reshaped incus. A second option of vertical collumella using (PORP) could be applied. The bypass technique offers shorter operating time than the mobilization technique and it has a lower risk of postoperative sensorineural deterioration. Also Bypass may give a better and long-standing stable hearing improvement than mobilization of the ossicles.

In case of attic fixation and a concomitant erosion of the long process of the incus, the bypass procedure is the method of choice (Fig. 5.26).

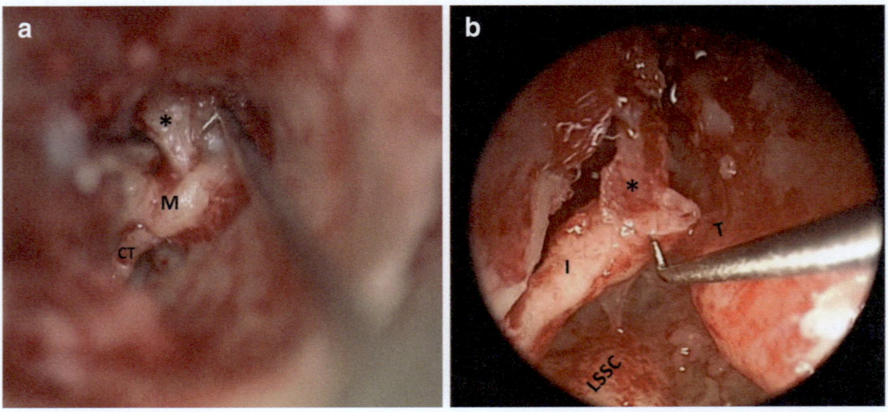

Fig. 5.25 Mobilization. (**a**) Left ear microscopic removal of tympanoscleoric plaques from anterior malleal ligament (*). (**b**) left ear endoscopic removal of tympanosclerotic patch (*) fixing the malleus head and incus body (I) to the tegmen (T). *M* malleus, *CT* chorda tympani, *LSCC* lateral semicircular canal

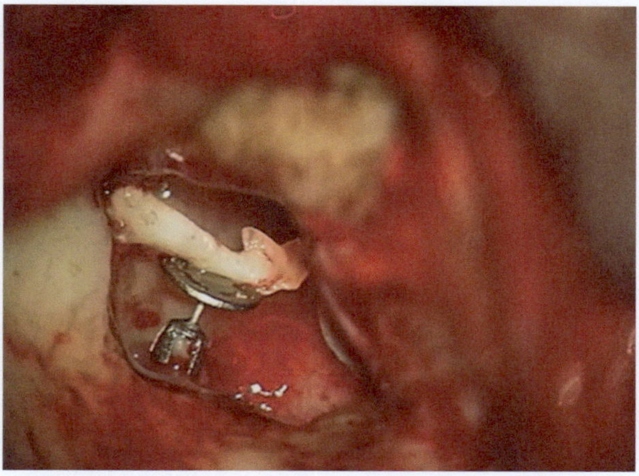

Fig. 5.26 Left ear ossiculoplasty (PORP) insertion between the drum and stapes to bypass incudo malleal fixation

5.10.3 Management of Stapes Complex Tympanosclerotic Fixation

Stapes fixation in tympanosclerosis is encountered in around 30% of the intratympanic disease ossicular involvement [44]. Although in some cases, the disease process is localized and confined to the stapes complex, more often it represents the center of a widespread tympanosclerosis involving the meso and epitympanic areas along with the tympanic membrane (see Fig. 5.40).

The prevailing belief is that tympanosclerotic fixation of the stapes footplate is due to the disease invasion of the annular ligament between the footplate and oval window margin which is followed by calcification, possibly ossification and fixation [48–52]. The degree of involvement of the stapes by tympanosclerosis can be categorized in three types (Fig. 5.27). This classification is purely descriptive; it does not describe grades of evolution.

5.10.3.1 Conservative Management of the Stapedial Complex

A conservative attitude is based on the decision not to take any risk to expose the vestibule to a non sterile pathology avoiding any manipulation or opening the oval window for reconstruction. After closure of tympanic membrane perforation, patient's hearing is managed by a conventional hearing aid or BAHA depending on the severity and type of hearing loss (Fig. 5.28).

5.10.3.2 Surgical Management of the Stapedial Complex

During surgical exploration, stapes involvement by tympanosclerosis does not show the same surgical aspect of fixation encountered in stapedial otosclerosis, but the footplate looks merely as splinted by a surface layer of tympanosclerosis. This splinting phenomenon is sufficient to impair sound conduction.

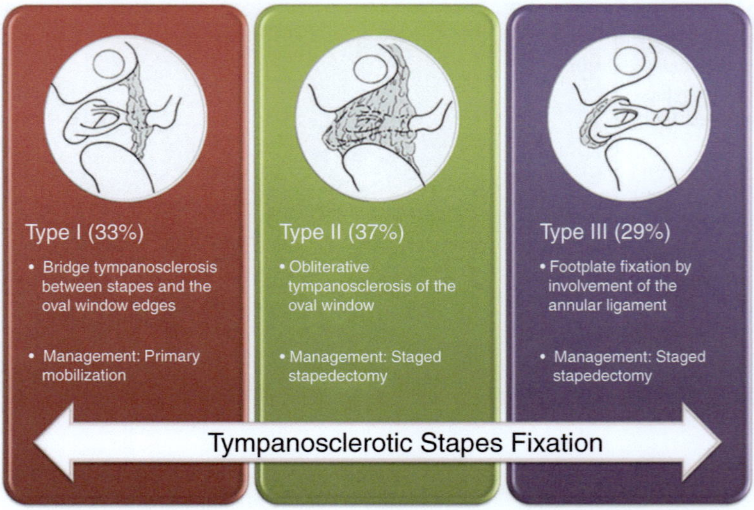

Fig. 5.27 The three types of involvement of the stapes by tympanosclerosis and their appropriate management

Fig. 5.28 Management of stapes fixation by tympanosclerosis

Management Options for Stapes Tympanosclerosis

- **Conservative management**
  No stapes surgery/post-tympanoplasty Hearing Aid
- **Surgical management**
  A Mobilization of the Stapes
  - With grafting of TM in one setting
  - Risk of SNHL

  B Stapedotomy
  - Relatively stable results
  - Staging in case of TM perforation
  - Risk of SNHL

Success in tympanosclerosis surgery depends largely on the degree of ossicular chain mobility and function restored.

According to the different disease status of the stapes, the following operative procedures are proposed (Fig. 5.28):

1. *Mobilization Procedure*: Peeling off the chalk soft plaques until the footplate recovers its complete mobility, taking care not to open the oval window or
2. *Stapes Surgery*: Creation of a small opening into the calcified plaques covering the oval window for a piston insertion [53] (Fig. 5.28).

Stapes involvement raises the most pronounced controversies regarding the surgical approach to tympanosclerosis, The question remains if mobilization of the fixed stapes plate is enough or if there is a need for stapedotomy.

Fig. 5.29 Hints and pitfalls in stapes mobilization

Hints and Pitfalls in Stapes Mobilization

- Preserve the incudostapedial joint till the end to avoid inadvertent cracking of the stapes
- Preserve the stapedial tendon till the end to avoid inadvertent dislocation of the footplate
- Peeling of TS from posterior to anterior direction
- Laser assistance is very helpful when available

Tos et al. and many other authors favor mobilization because of its advantage of being a one stage performance [54]. Smyth disagrees with that, thinking that the possibility of damaging the inner ear during mobilization either with hydrolic blast or perilymphatic fistula is very high, up to 36% [55]. Giddings and House have the same opinion giving the priority to stapedectomy [56]. Many authors accept both attitudes, documenting no difference between mobilization and stapes surgery [35].

According to our practice, the choice of mobilization or stapedotomy relies on the surgical skill and the extent of the disease.

Stapes Mobilization

Stapes mobilization was generally regarded as the first option for treatment of stapes fixation in the 1950s and early 1960s. Stapedectomy was retained for cases when mobilization failed to restore mobility. Stapes mobilization proceeds by piecemeal removal of hyalinized plaques. We recommend stapedial tendon resection in case of difficult approach to the posterio part of oval niche during removal of the plaques. Some hints and pitfalls in stapes mobilization are described in Fig. 5.29.

Some hard calcified plaques could be mixed with chalk plaques, rendering them friable, able to crack inadvertently. The footplate and the bone of the promontory may also crack to damage the inner ear structures resulting in sensorineural hearing loss.

The use of Laser is very helpful and avoids mechanical manipulation injuries to the ossicular chain and labyrinth and prevents inadvertent opening or fracture of the footplate. Improved long term hearing results, the technical ease and its safety were behind its popularity among otologist especially for tympanosclerosis surgery [46, 57] (Fig. 5.29).

Stapedotomy/Stapedectomy in Tympanosclerosis

Stapedotomy in tympanosclerosis is commonly planned as two staged surgery procedures since most tympanosclerosis cases are associated to tympanic membrane perforation. Care must be taken not to dislocate the incus in the first stage of the surgery in order to maintain the ability of stapedotomy in the later stage. Stapes surgery in tympanosclerosis requires a clear counseling especially in bilateral hearing loss because the results could be unsatisfactory.

Indications

The less favorable hearing improvement after stapedotomy in tympanosclerosis compared to otosclerosis makes the decision for this surgery somehow conflictual.

Therefore stapedotomy must be considered in tympanosclerosis only for patients with severe bilateral conductive hearing loss in the presence of an intact tympanic membrane.

Efficiency

The efficiency of stapes surgery in tympanosclerosis depends essentially on the preservation of mobile malleus and incus. A literature review reports a success rate (postoperative ABG < 20 dB) of only 70%, while success in otosclerosis stapedotomy is about 95% [52, 58], with a closure of ABG of 10 dB.

In 272 cases of tympanosclerosis operated by one of the authors [53] stapes fixation was demonstrated in 47% of the cases and required stapedotomy or stapedectomy in 36% of cases. Failure of stapes surgery was of 25% and was mostly due to the failure of ossiculoplasty between tympanic membrane and oval window.

- ***Large OW fenestra technique*** gives better closure of the ABG and long lasting improvement but carries higher risk of vestibular contamination and labyrinthitis from the inflammatory mediators of the unsterile plaques of tympanosclerosis.
- ***Small OW fenestra technique*** reduces labyrinthine insult but carries a greater risk of early ABG deterioration following initial postoperative success [59].

Safety

Some patients with tympanosclerosis may show high frequency bone conduction drop after stapedectomy, due to extensive drilling in the oval window region with 3% significant postoperative sensorineural hearing loss [52, 60, 61]. SNHL could be also due to the inflammatory reaction of the opened vestibule in contact with the disease itself. In one of the author's series only 2 out of 84 stapedotomies resulted in more than 20 dB loss of their bone conduction (2.3%) [53]. The author's surgical experience in such stage of the disease with stapedectomies demonstrated that the risk of bone conduction loss is by far lower than the one found after inadvertent dislocation of the footplate during mobilization.

Therefore mobilization is not recommended in obliterative tympanosclerosis.

Stability

Some hearing attrition may occur with time, after an early post-stapedotomy ABG improvement. Deterioration could be secondary to regrowth of the disease process around the prosthesis with recurrent fixation.

TS Footplate Fixation Associated to Incus Lysis

The association of stapes fixation and incus necrosis by tympanosclerosis could be encountered in about 50% of the cases of tympanosclerotic stapes fixation [56].

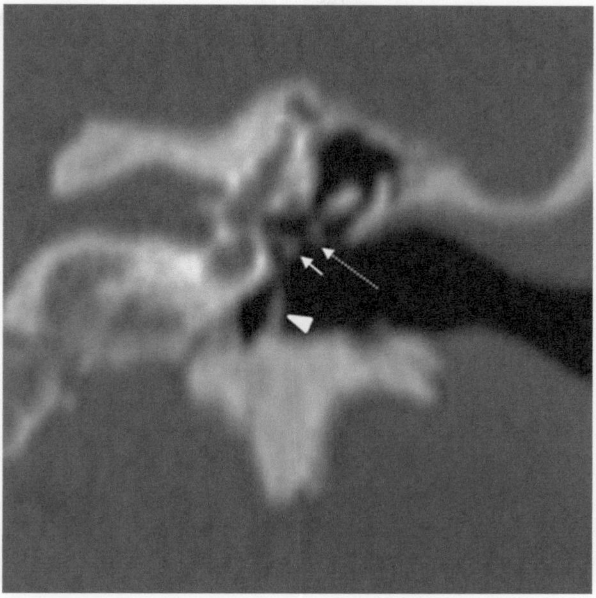

Fig. 5.30 Coronal CT-Image of a left ear: retraction of the partially calcified tympanic membrane (arrowhead) on the promontory, and on the incudostapedial chain, here with myringostapediopexy (short arrow) and lyses of the long process of the incus (long arrow)

Incus necrosis is rarely due to tympanosclerosis but usually a sequela of the previous chronic inflammatory otitis media before the tympanosclerotic process takes place (Fig. 5.30).

In such situation staged malleostapedotomy is the procedure of choice, however it remains challenging and may end up with a non-satisfactory closure of the ABG.

5.11 Clinico-Radiologic Inputs in Surgical Strategies

According to the clinical presentation, the microscopic and endoscopic examination, the audiometric evaluation and in coordination with the radiological findings, the management strategies facing variable TS aspects and localizations can be designed as follow:

5.11.1 Myringosclerosis Without TM Perforation and Almost Normal Hearing

Diagnosis: on otoscopy, the myringosclerosis can be limited or extended to a larger surface of the eardrum without a clinical consequences, imaging is not required.

Surgery: no indication for surgery.

5.11.2 Myringosclerosis with TM Perforation and CHL Below 25 dB

Diagnosis: Otoscopy and audiometry.

Surgery: Myringoplasty without removal of the eardrum plaques is to be considered.

The rationale behind the surgical indication is to close the tympanic membrane to eliminate middle ear hyperoxia status (persisting oxygen free oxygen radicals) aiming to control the progression of the disease.

During tympanic membrane grafting, removal of the tympanosclerotic plaques from the residual tympanic membrane is only indicated when they occupy a significant area of the tympanic membrane, impairing its mobility by a large plaque joining the tympanic annulus to the manubrium.

The graft "take" rate in tympanosclerosis is excellent; irrespective of whether plaques are excised or not, success rate is 90% [37]. Kinney [33], Tos et al. [40] and Gibb et al. [37] reported successful grafting in over 90% of cases and concluded that the presence of tympanosclerosis had no adverse influence on immediate grafting results.

5.11.3 Intratympanic Tympanosclerosis with Tympanic Membrane Perforation and CHL of 30 dB and Above

Diagnosis: Otoscopy, Audiometry + CT assessment as follows:

- Degrees of the extent of the tympanosclerosis on the incudo-malleal complex
  - Simple malleus head fixation
  - Incudo-malleal en bloc fixation
- Degree of extent of the tympanosclerosis on the stapedial complex
  - Global thickening of the suprastructure and the footplate
  - Calcifications on the footplate and/or condensation image on the oval window niche
  - Calcified stapedial tendon
- Combined tympanosclerosis of the incudomalleal complex and the stapedial complex
- Extensive tympanosclerosis to the round window niche
- Extensive tympanosclerosis into the epitympanum and mastoid

Despite the precious input of the CT scan in analyzing the extent of tympanosclerosis, it is only during the surgical exploration that the actual status of the functional structures and the different compartments involved could be accurately determined. In certain circumstances, the positive diagnosis of a mobile footplate could be only established after an excision of the ossified stapedial tendon or even after resection of the ossified crura.

***Surgery*:**

Middle ear reconstruction in Tympanosclerosis must be weighted according to a cost/benefit ratio, the risk of complications and the expected degree of hearing improvement from a planned surgical procedure.

Tympanoplasty, ossicular reconstruction and stapedoplasty are to be considered depending on the functional deficit, especially in bilateral tympanosclerosis (40–60% of cases); in these cases, surgery must start with the ear which offers better surgical conditions and higher chances of success for a hearing improvement.

The following paragraphs will explore the most accepted surgical treatment strategies:

5.11.3.1 Tympanosclerosis with Fixation of the Malleus Head

Audiometry: around 30 dB CHL.

CT Imaging: identifies the isolated calcification fixing the malleus head to the tegmen (Fig. 5.31).

Surgery: Through a large atticotomy, excision of the tympanosclerosis block fixing the malleus head to the tegmen could be achieved allowing adequate mobility of the malleus.

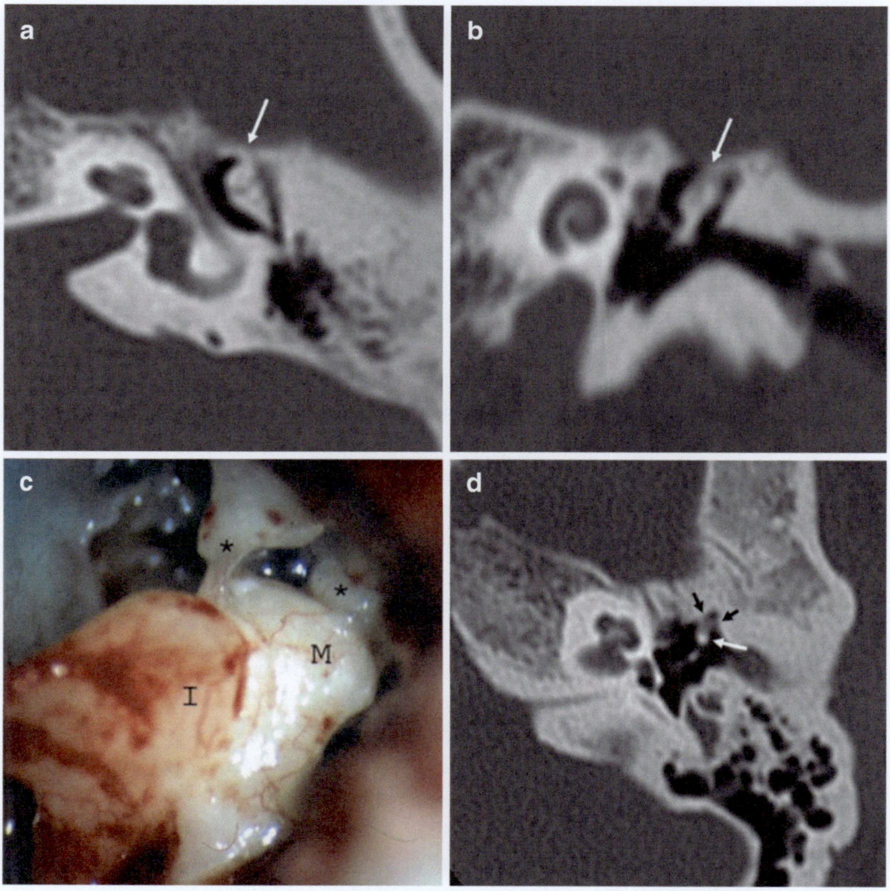

Fig. 5.31 (**a**) axial CT-image of a left ear: Isolated superior malleus head fixity (arrow) (**b**) coronal CT image of the fusion of the malleus head to the attic (**c**) surgical aspect of tympanosclerosis (*) fixing the malleus head (*M* malleus, *I* incus) (**d**) axial CT images passing by the neck of the malleus (white arrow) showing a thick and calcified anterior malleal ligament (small black arrows)

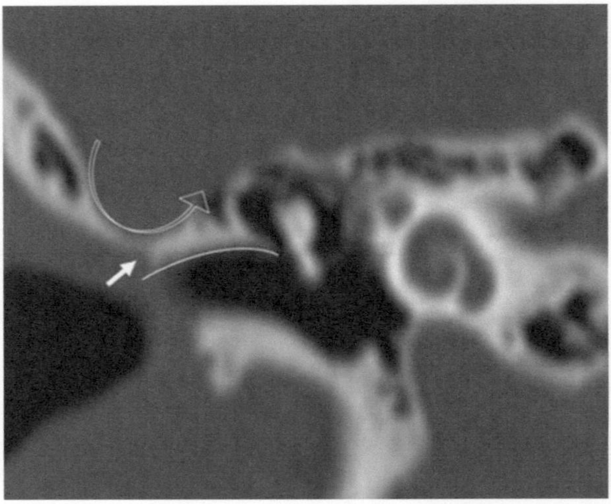

Fig. 5.32 Coronal CT-image of a right ear with an important tympanic slope from lateral to medial (curved arrow), the lateral tegmen is thin (short arrow), too tight to achieve an atticotomy without damaging the superior auditory canal wall (thin horizontal line)

Outcome: When adequately performed, good results are obtained for a long time.

Surgical Hint: In cases where the tegmen is very low and does not offer enough space for an adequate mobilization (CT- Fig. 5.32), a bypass technique is preferable with resection of the head of the malleus followed by an ossicular transposition/reconstruction of the ossicular chain.

5.11.3.2 Tympanosclerosis with Incudomalleal Complex Fixation

Audiometry: CHL about 30–40 dB.

CT-Imaging: variable signs of incudomalleal fixation, in the demonstrated case a large condensation encases the lateral side of the incudo malleal chain and fixing it to the lateral and anterior attic (Fig. 5.33a, b).

Surgery (Fig. 5.34): A masto-tympanoplasty after complete dissection and liberation of the ossicular chain through an adequate attico-epitympanotomy is able to close successfully the ABG with good longterm results (Fig. 5.33c).

5.11.3.3 Tympanosclerosis of the Stapedial Complex

***Audiometry*: CHL of 30–40 dB.

***CT-Imaging*:** The tympanosclerosis of the stapedial complex can be seen as a global thickening of the crura and the footplate (Fig. 5.35a), or with apposition of calcified material on the footplate (Fig. 5.35b) or by a diffuse obliteration of the oval niche with sclerotic material (Fig. 5.35c), or by calcified stapedial tendon (Fig. 5.35d), all are highly suggestive of tympanosclerosis.

CT may also show evidence of thickening of the stapes head associated to a calcification of the stapes muscle tendon (Fig. 5.35d).

Surgery: Different surgical steps are proceeded as follows:

1. Adequate debulking of the crura (advantages of Laser) or bilateral crurotomy
2. Excision of tympanosclerotic materiel from the oval window niche and the footplate

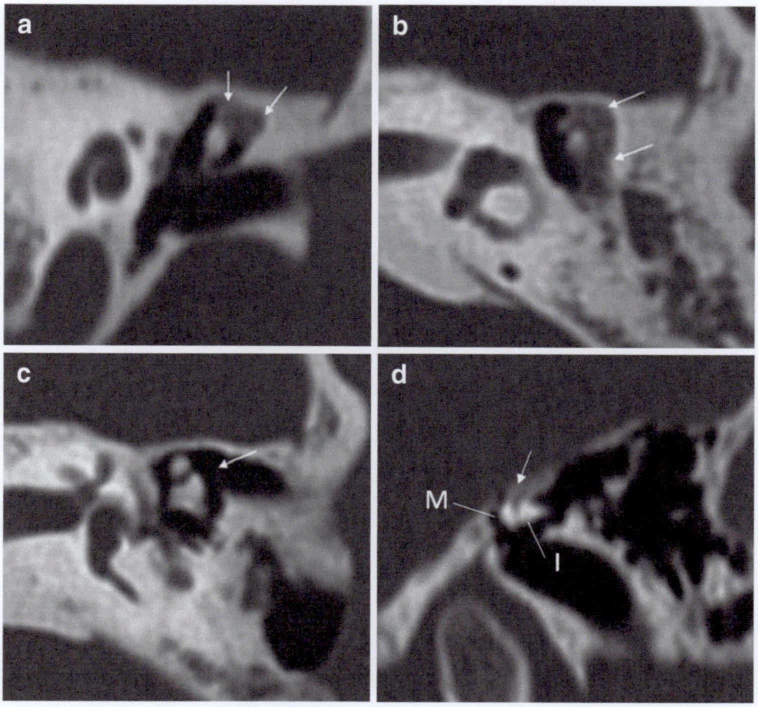

Fig. 5.33 CT images (**a**) coronal view of a tympanosclerotic plaque (arrows) in the outer and upper attic, fixing the incudomalleal chain. (**b**) axial view of the tympanosclerotic plaque (arrows) encasing the lateral side of the incudomalleal chain (**c**) postoperative follow up: the axial view does not show any tympanosclerotic recurrence several years after complete liberation of the lateral attic. (**d**) sagittal CT-reconstruction of another patient with a large attical tympanosclerotic plaque (arrow) encroaching the superior part of the malleus (M) and incus (I)

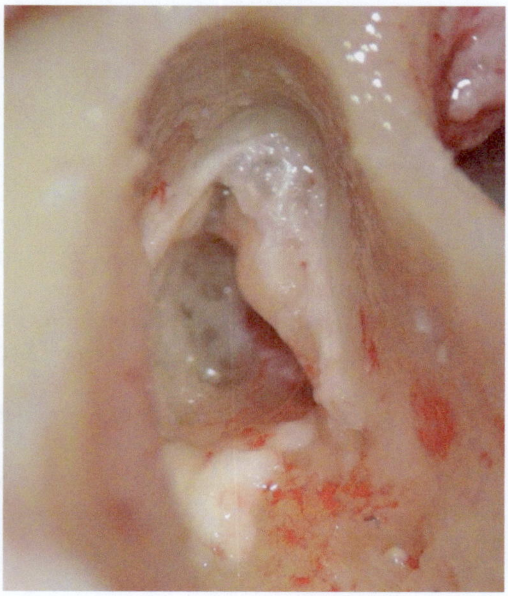

Fig. 5.34 Transmastoid atticotomy showing epitympanic tympanosclerosis fixing the incus body and head of the malleus (Courtesy Pr H Vijayendra)

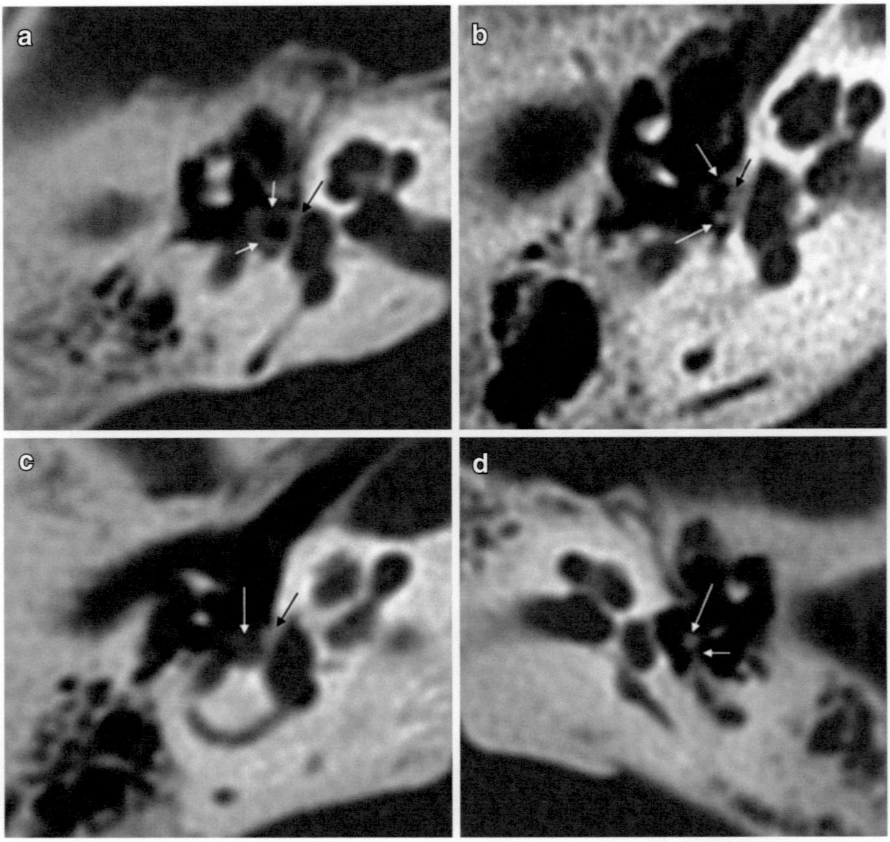

Fig. 5.35 Axial CT-images: (**a**) right ear: global thickening of the stapes crura (white arrows) and the footplate (black arrow). (**b**) apposition of tympanosclerotic material on the footplate (black arrow), the stapes crura are thickened and calcified (white arrows). (**c**) focal thickening of the footplate (black arrow) and obliteration of the oval window niche by dense condensations (white arrow). (**d**) very thick and dense head of the stapes (long arrow), calcified tendon of the stapes muscle (short arrow)

3. Resection of the ossified stapedial tendon
   (a) *Then, if the footplate becomes mobile*, the debridement procedure is completed, if stapes superstructure is absent, by a reconstruction with incus-footplate prosthesis on a perichondrium covering the free mobile footplate for protection.
   (b) *If the footplate remains fixed*, staging the surgery is a must: grafting the eardrum followed 6 months later on by a stapedotomy.

5.11.3.4 Tympanosclerosis of the Incudo-Malleal Complex and the Stapedial Complex

Tympanosclerosis of the stapedial complex is rarely isolated and most commonly associated to tympanosclerosis of the incudo-malleal complex (Figs. 5.36 and 5.37).

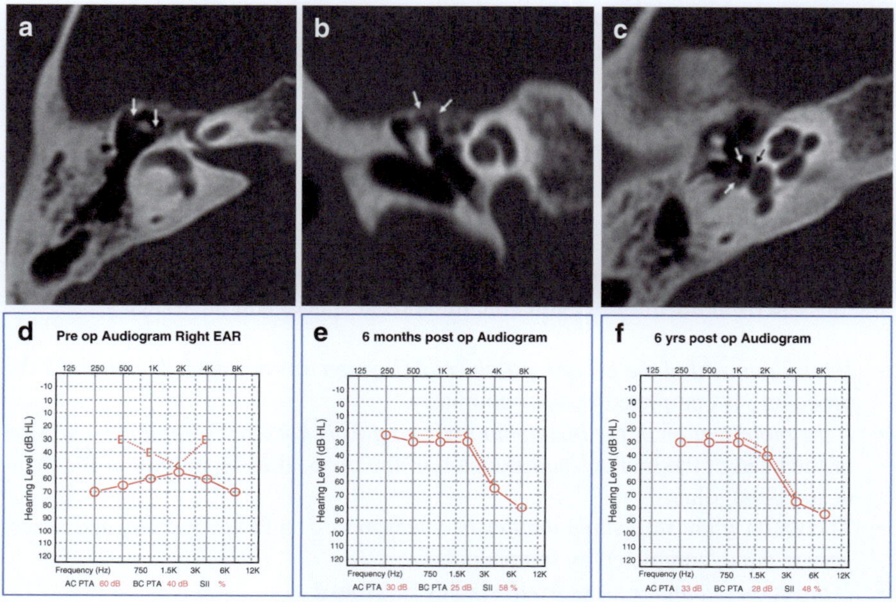

Fig. 5.36 A 55 years old patient with dry TM perforation and intratympanic TS who underwent attico-mastoidectomy with mobilization of the incudomalleal complex and stapes. The patient had complete and stable closure of the ABG with mild drop of high frequency BC due to manipulation. (**a**) axial CT-view: Fixed malleal head from both sides by large bands (arrows) of TS material to the cavity (**b**) coronal CT view: hypodense tissue between the head and the medial attic wall (arrows) (**c**) axial CT view of the stapes, showing slightly thickened crura (white arrows) and a dense footplate (black arrow) (**d**) Audiograms preop, (**e**) 6 months post-op and (**f**) 7 years postop

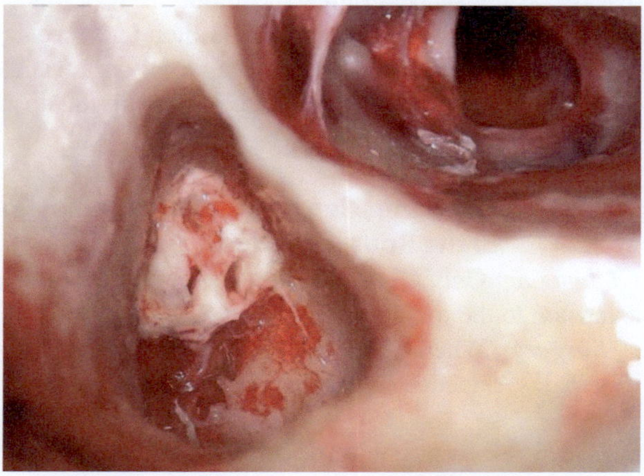

Fig. 5.37 Right ear operative view of atticomastoidectomy showing tympanosclerosis of the Incudo-Malleal Complex and the Stapedial complex (Courtesy Pr H Vijayendra)

Audiometry: the hearing loss is usually a pure conductive hearing loss of 50–60 dB, or a mixed type of hearing loss/with an important ABG still in favor of a beneficial surgery with postoperative hearing improvement.

CT-Imaging: CT is showing tympanosclerotic plaques in the attic fixing the incudomalleolar chain, associated to different signs of tympanosclerosis of the stapedial complex. In the demonstrated case (Fig. 5.36), the stapes suprastructure and the footplate showed a global thickening.

Surgery

1. *First stage surgery*:

Masto-atticotomy and malleus/incus mobilization to insure adequate removal of the disease from the mastoid, attic, the middle ear spaces and the ossicles.

- *If total removal of the lesions and the mobilization are successfully obtained*: the procedure is completed by tympanoplasty.
- *If the mobilization of the incudomalleal complex is not totally obtained*: excision of the head of the malleus and excision of the incus after separation of the incudostapedial joint.
- Then after *if the stapedial complex becomes mobile*: a PORP reconstructive surgery is done, completed by tympanoplasty.
- *If the stapes complex stays fixed*: staging is a must:

2. *Second stage surgery at least 6 months after the first stage*:

During second middle ear exploration, confirmation of the complete disease control without any remaining tympanosclerosis, then a stapedoplasty with large fenestration of the oval window and incus or malleus stapedoplasty could be engaged.

There is no consensus among otologists regarding surgery for such advanced disease, as the success of a stapedotomy is very low and the risk of postoperative neurosensorial deafness is high. The literature reveals conflictual opinions: some authors reject the indication of stapes surgery in advanced TS; others report satisfactory stable long term closure of the ABG with the opening of the footplate despite extensive forms of the disease.

5.11.3.5 Tympanosclerosis of the Stapedial Complex Extended to the Round Window

CT Imaging: Only CT is able to assess and preoperatively the real status of the TS extension to the round window (Fig. 5.38).

Surgery: When CT shows a complete obliteration of the round window (Fig. 5.38), stapedotomy is contraindicated.

5.11.3.6 Extensive Tympanosclerosis in the Epitympanum and Mastoid

CT-Imaging

The extension of the TS to the pneumatized attico-antral mastoid compartments is shown by CT, it can cover the LSSC, the facial nerve canal and/or fill in the anterior epitympanic recess (Fig. 5.39).

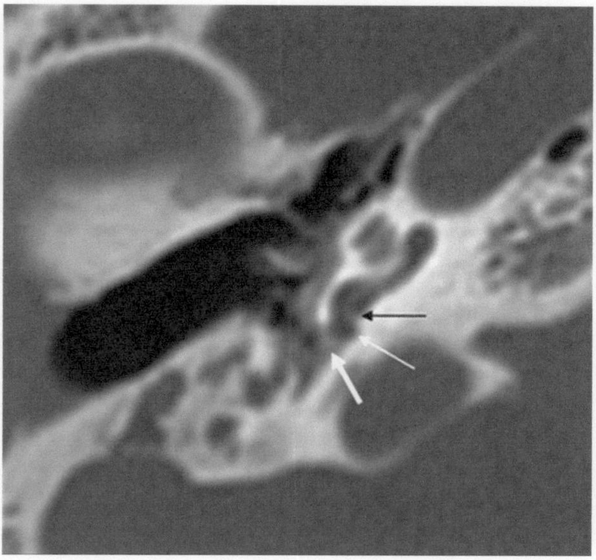

Fig. 5.38 Axial CT images of a right ear, calcified material covering the entry of the recess of the round window (thick white arrow), the round window recess itself (white long arrow), the round window membrane (black arrow)

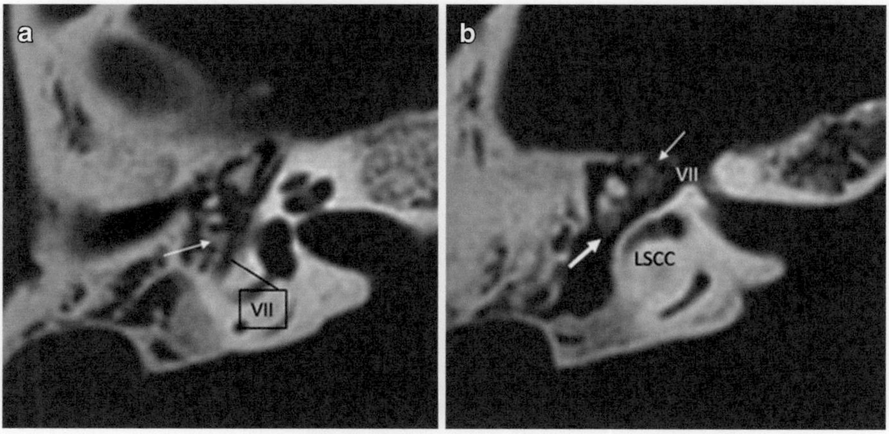

Fig. 5.39 CT images of a right ear: (**a**) massive calcified material (white arrow) covers the distal part of the second portion of the facial nerve (VII) (**b**) tympanosclerotic material covering the proximal part of the tympanic portion of the VII nerve (thin arrow) also covering the LSCC (thick arrow)

Surgery

Mastoidectomy, atticotomy and wide anterior epitympanotomy may insure complete excision of the extended disease. Reconstruction and/or stapes surgery (PORP/TORP/Staging) is selected as prescribed above.

With a clear counseling of the patient, a case by case decision is advised facing such extended pathology especially when and a hearing aid trial is not well tolerated.

5.11.4 Intratympanic Tympanosclerosis Behind a Closed Tympanic Membrane

Clinical presentation: Myringosclerosis and hearing loss above 30 dB.

CT-Imaging: behind an intact tympanic membrane, CT Scan is very appreciated to confirm the positive diagnosis of the TS inside the cavity as the cause of the hearing loss and to assess its different localisations and extensions as described above.

Counselling: Counselling remains complex depending of the actual status of the ossicular chain and the stapedial footplate invasion.

Surgery: the preserved tympanic membrane offers the advantage in such cases to enable **one stage surgery** whether a PORP, TORP, or a stapedotomy, to be performed without the need of staging [57] (Fig. 5.40).

Finally the surgical management of TS stages is summarized in Table 5.2.

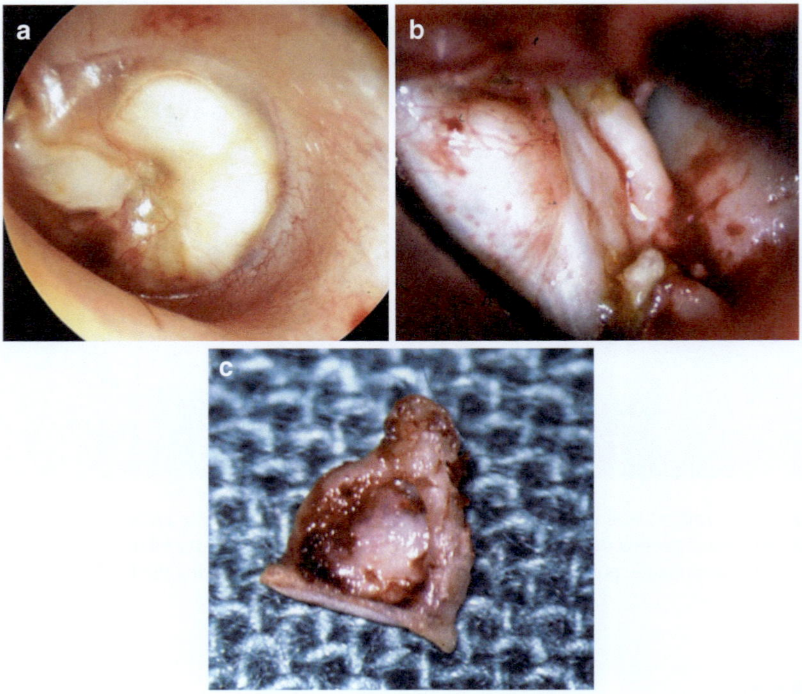

Fig. 5.40 Extensive tympanosclerosis of left ear behind a closed tympanic membrane (**a**) otoscopy showing the huge tympanosclerotic mass behind the intact tympanic membrane. (**b**) after elevation of the tympanomeatal flap, tympanosclerotic plaque filling the whole posterior mesotympanum. (**c**) stapes was removed and the obturator foramen was full with tympanosclerosis

Table 5.2 Algorithm of different clinical pictures and air bone gap levels in TS and their surgical management

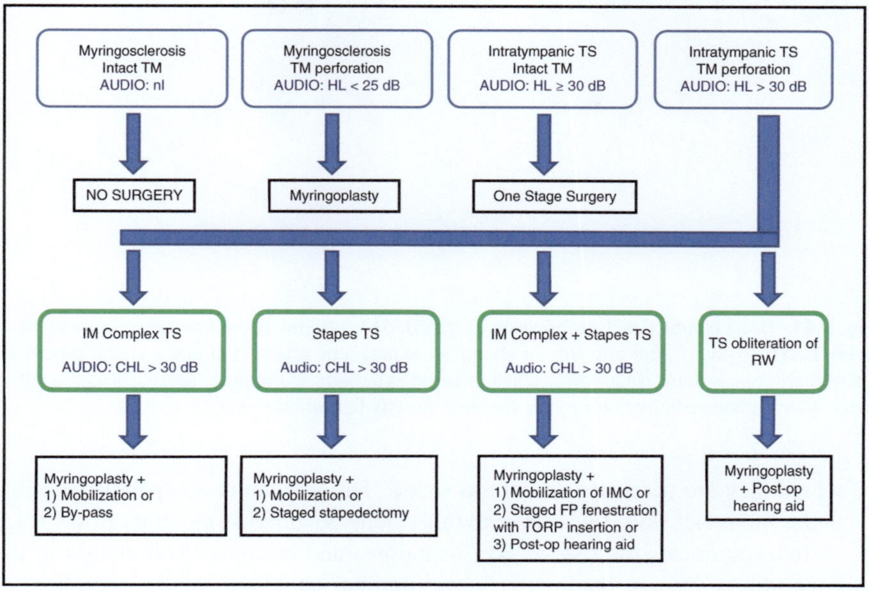

5.12 Non Surgical Rehabilitation of Hearing Loss in Advanced TS

Non surgical rehabilitation of a hearing loss due to tympanosclerosis by Hearing Aid must be considered every time the disease extension indicates a probable non satisfactory outcome from the surgical treatment and always when surgery carries a risk of sensorineural injury. When the conventional hearing aid is not helpful, the following rehabilitative measures could be helpful:

5.12.1 BAHA, or Bone Bridge in Tympanosclerosis

In cases of a conductive hearing loss or mixed hearing loss due to tympanosclerosis with eardrum perforation, a bone conduction hearing aid may be used to bypass the non-functional middle ear and amplify the sound that stimulates the cochlea directly through the bone (Fig. 5.41).

- **BAHA** offers amplification up to the cochlear reserve. It is regarded as a third option after surgery and hearing aids. However, patients with TS report only a moderate satisfaction with BAHA.
- **The BONEBRIDGE**, The Bonebridge is an innovative new bone conduction implant that transmits sound waves via the cranial bone directly to the inner ear,

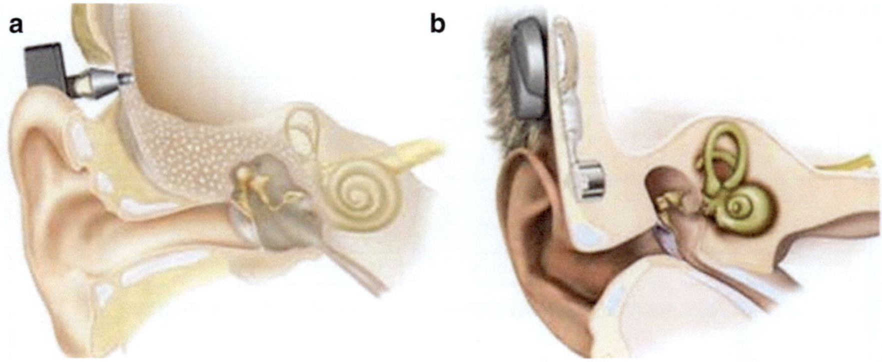

Fig. 5.41 Bone conduction hearing systems. (**a**) BAHA system: There are three components of every BAHA System. The implant, an abutment or magnetic attachment and a sound processor. (**b**) Bonebridge system. Bonebridge consists of an externally worn audio processor and a surgically-inserted bone conduction implant that lies directly beneath the skin

where they are perceived as natural sound. The implant is completely invisible under the intact skin. In contrast to other bone conduction systems, Bonebridge system minimizes the risk of skin irritations, and the direct stimulation of the bone (direct-drive technology) achieves optimal sound transmission results.

5.12.2 Middle Ear Active Implants in Tympanosclerosis

Vibrant soundbridge (VSB) is an active partly implantable hearing device that demonstrated good results in adults. The vibrating part of the vibrant Soundbridge (Floating mass transducer FMT) could be placed directly on the round window, or on the stapes or the incus, in order to amplify sound transmission to the cochlea. The advantage of the VSB over the BAHA is the avoidance of a percutaneous abutment and improved sensorineural gain especially in cases of mixed hearing loss. It seems that in some cases of tympanosclerosis VSB with application of FMT on the round window membrane could give better result than conventional hearing aid [62].

5.13 Other Pathologies Rarely Associated to TS

5.13.1 Tympanosclerosis and RP

Association of retraction pocket and tympanosclerosis was clinically reported as a possible reactive pathology into the pocket: the collagen fibers of the tympanic membrane in a retraction pocket, having disappeared, are replaced by a post inflammatory hyalinized process which is followed by calcium deposition and tympanosclerosis.

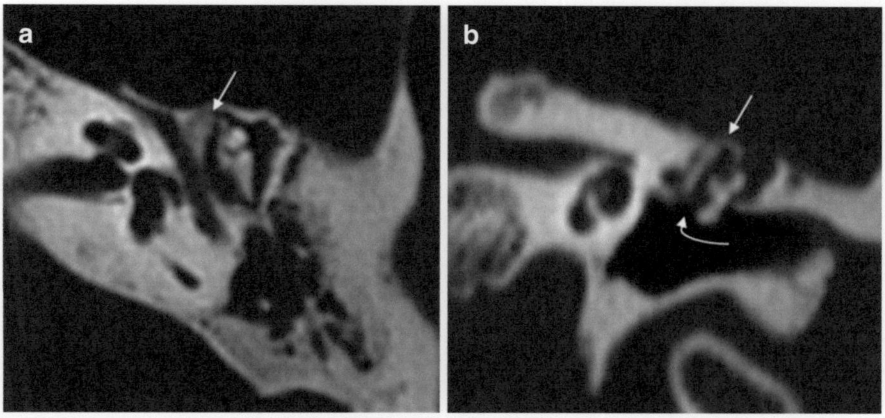

Fig. 5.42 CT images of a left ear: (**a**) axial image showing a calcified border of a pocket (arrow) in the inner attic, coming in close contact to the medial side of the incudomalleal chain (**b**) coronal image showing the origin of this retraction pocket (curved arrow), extending up to the tegmen (arrow)

TS in a RP may progress despite a stable status of the RP itself; TS associated to a stable RP may present different degrees of extension that are demonstrated by CT-Scan to help the surgical indication and planning (Fig. 5.42).

5.13.2 Tympanosclerosis and Cholesteatoma

The literature revue reports 2–4% of cases of cholesteatoma associated to TS [35–37, 63, 64].

Cholesteatoma and tympanosclerosis are two contradictory processes in the same ear with an underlying chronic inflammatory pathology [64, 65]: one, the cholesteatoma, is a destructive and lytic process, the other one is the end stage of a healing process following an inflammatory process in the submucosa (hyalinisation and calcification). The association of both pathologies must be considered when the clinical presentation of TS is associated to otorrhea. The expression of a tympanosclerotic reaction as a defense mechanism relies on a genetic and immunological individual background [66, 67].

The following case report is showing this association:

A 39 years-old female patient presented with left-sided hearing loss history of intermittent otorrhea. Otoscopic examination showed a dry ear with tiny tympanosclerotic calcifications occupying the postero superior quadrant; normal pars tensa and good aeration of the middle ear. Pure tone audiometry revealed a mixed hearing loss of 50 dB with a 35 dB air-bone gap (Fig. 5.43a).

CT-Imaging confirms the clinical diagnosis of TS with much extended attical manifestations of TS.

A rounded soft tissue mass was found in the antrum, without any lytic process associated, but the lobulated aspect of the mass was suggestive of cholesteatoma.

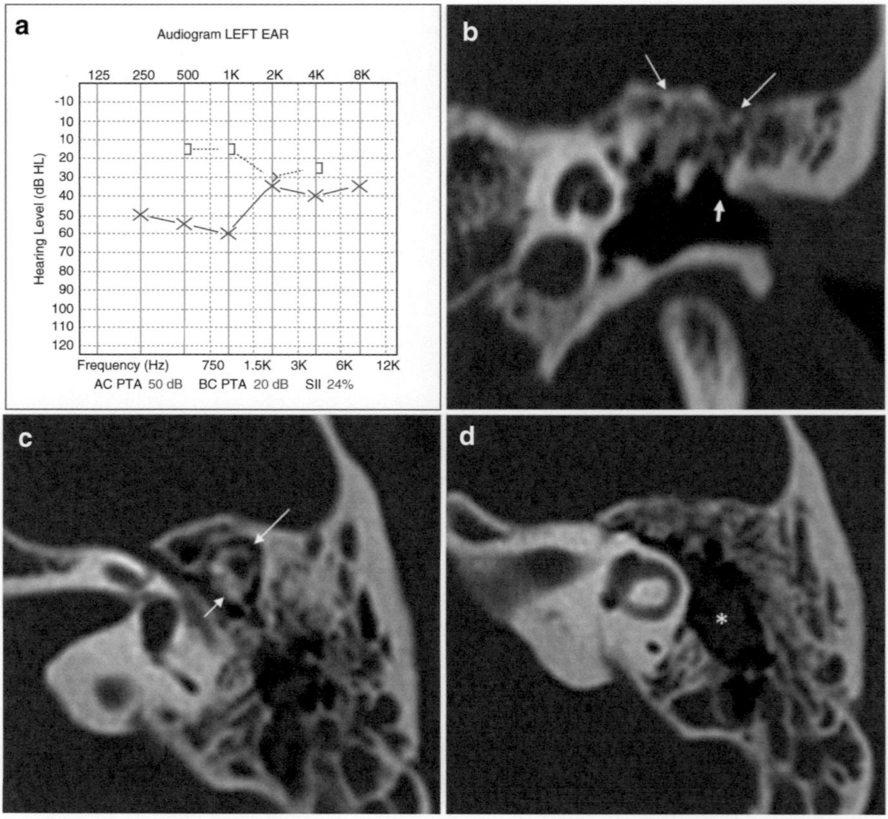

Fig. 5.43 CT of the left ear: (**a**) audiogram: 50 dB CHL (**b**) coronal CT-image: huge amount of tympanosclerosis in the superior attic (thin arrows), slight amputation of the scutum (small arrow) (**c**) axial CT-image at the level of the incudomalleolar chain: incus (short arrow), calcified wall of a retraction pocket in the lateral attic (long arrow) (**d**) a huge mass of tissue density, polylobulated, occupying the antrum, is suspicious of a cholesteatoma, that was confirmed at surgery. Non specific condensation of most of the mastoid cells (M) that were found to contain also cholesteatoma at surgery

5.13.2.1 Surgery

The intraoperative findings confirmed the cholesteatoma inside the antrum, that had even invaded the whole mastoid cells. A CWU with complete removal of the cholesteatoma and the tympanosclerosis was done. The lytic incus was removed and an ossicular reconstruction with PORP was done. The management of such associated pathologies must be primarily oriented by the specific strategy towards the cholesteatoma in order to insure a safe ear.

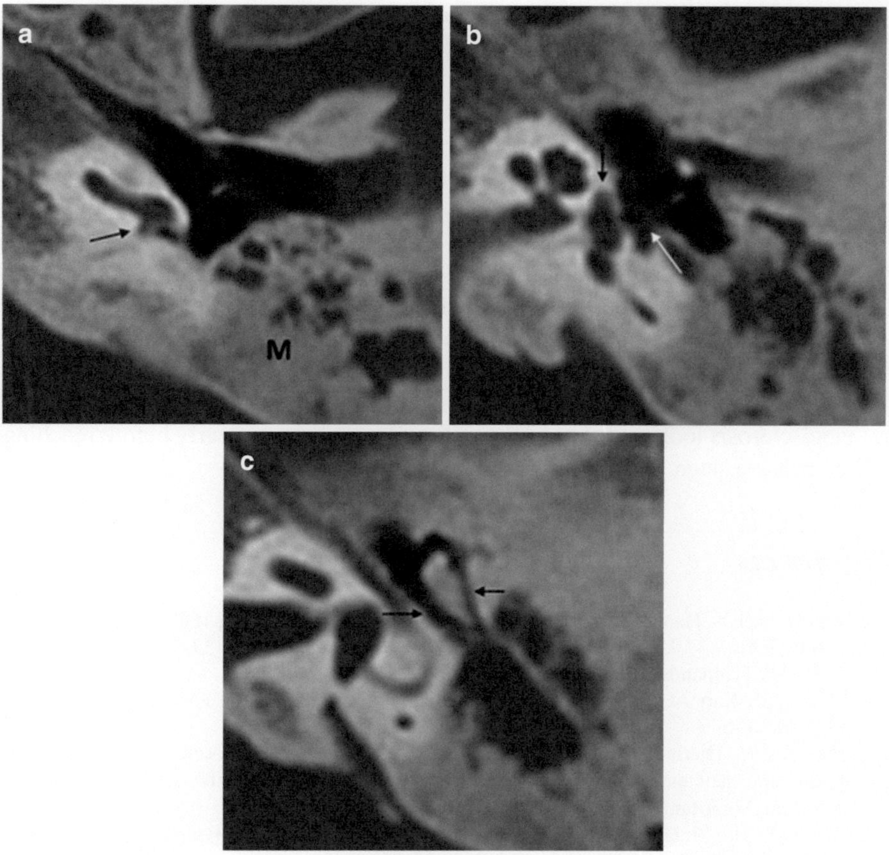

Fig. 5.44 Axial CT-image of the left ear, that showed myringosclerosis on otoscopy and 50 dB conductive hearing loss on audiogram (**a**) a typical otosclerotic focus at the abutment of the cochlear aqueduct to the basal cochlear turn (arrow), poorly developed mastoid (M) but fully condensed cells (**b**) typical otosclerotic ante fenestral focus (black arrow), associated to a global thickening of the footplate and the crura (long arrow) (**c**) attico antral condensation images (arrows) in favour of an attico antral extension of the tympanosclerosis. Surgery confirmed both pathologies in the same ear

5.13.3 Tympanosclerosis and Otosclerosis

A chronic ear can develop a tympanosclerosis as a superimposed post-inflammatory disease in an individual who is already affected by otosclerosis. Both are independent pathologies, but when suspected in the same ear, CT scan is helpful for their differential diagnosis in regard to the conductive hearing loss and management planning (Fig. 5.44).

Surgery: In such situation a clear counseling of the patient is mandatory. One stage surgery is possible because of the presence of a closed tympanic membrane.

Conclusion

Strategy for Tympanosclerosis in regard to the stapes involvement is conflictual and remains among the most difficult conditions that may face the otologist. A clear counseling for the patient is of a prime importance.

CT-Imaging in tympanosclerosis is very helpful to evaluate the middle ear pathology and its extent especially behind an intact tympanic membrane, however exploration surgery of the middle ear remains the most accurate diagnostic measure to orient the management.

Research studies are still awaited to find a reliable medical treatment of tympanosclerosis looking for an arrest of the disease progress early before reaching an invasive stage.

References

1. Von Troltsch A. Handbuch der Ohrenheilkunde. Leipzig: FCW Vogel; 1869.
2. Zollner F, Beck C. Die Paukensklerose. Z Laryng Rhin Otol. 1955;3:137–55.
3. Zollner F. Tympanosclerosis. J Laryngo. 1956;2:77–85.
4. Mckee GJ, Karr AG. Tympanosclerosis: a scanning electron microscopic study. Clin Otol. 1989;14:11–6.
5. Milojević M, Djerić D, Bijelić D. Prognostic significance of tympanosclerotic plaques localization and their morphological and histological characteristics for the outcome of surgical treatment. Vojnosanit Pregl. 2012;69(2):190–4.
6. Forséni Flodin M, Hultcrantz M. Possible inflammatory mediators in tympanosclerosis development. Int J Pediatr Otorhinolaryngol. 2002;63(2):149–54.
7. Makiishi-Shimobayashi C, Tsujimura T, Sugihara A, Iwasaki T, Yamada N, Terada N, Sakagami M. Expression of osteopontin by exudate macrophages in inflammatory tissues of the middle ear: a possible association with development of tympanosclerosis. Hear Res. 2001;153:100–7.
8. Harris I, Weiss L. Tympanosclerosis: superficial and embedded forms. Trans Amer Acad Opht Otolaryngo. 1962;6:683–714.
9. Tos M, Stangerup SE. Hearing loss in tympanosclerosis caused by grommets. Arch Otolaryngol Head Neck Surg. 1989;115:931–5.
10. Forséni M, Eriksson A, Bagger-Sjöbäck D, Nilsson J, Hultcrantz M. Development of tympanosclerosis: can predicting factors be identified? Am J Otol. 1997;18(3):298–303.
11. Mionskowski T, Kuczkowski J, Sakowicz-Burkiewicz M. Assessment of tumor necrosis factor alpha gene expression profile in selected structures of middle ear in patients with tympanosclerosis. Otolaryngol Pol. 2012;66(4 Suppl):20–4.
12. Guo W, Bai X, Han Y, Xu L, Liu W, et al. Expressions of TGF-beta1 and MMP-9 in a guinea pig model of tympanosclerosis: possible role in the pathogenesis of this disorder. Laryngoscope. 2012;122:2037–42.
13. Cooter MS, Eisma RJ, Burleson JA, Leonard G, Lafreniere D, et al. Transforming growth factor-β expression in otitis media with effusion. The Laryngoscope. 1998;108:1066–70.
14. Melhus A, Ryan AF. Expression of cytokine genes during pneumococcal and nontypeable Haemophilus influenzae acute otitis media in the rat. Infection and immunity. 2000;68:4024–31.
15. Forseni M, Hansson GK, Bagger-Sjöback D, Hultcrantz M. An immunhistochemical study of inducible nitric oxide synthase in the rat middle ear, with reference to tympanosclerosis. Acta Otolaryngol. 1999;119:577–82.
16. Forseni M, et al. Study of inflammatory mediators in the human Tympanosclerotic middle ear. Arch Otolaryngol Head Neck Surg. 2001;127(5):559–64.

17. Garça MF, Turan M, Avşar B, Kalkan F, Demir H, Kozan A, Bozan N. The evaluation of oxidative stress in the serum and tissue specimens of patients with chronic otitis media. Clin Exp Otorhinolaryngol. 2015;8(2):97–101.
18. Görür K, Vayisoglu Y, Ozcan C, Güner N, Yaroglu H, Tamer L. The glutathione-S-transferase and N-acetyltranferase gene polymorphism in tympanosclerosis. Int Adv Otol. 2012;8:38–44.
19. Koc A. The role of mastoid pneumatization in the pathogenesis of Tympanosclerosis. Int Adv Otol. 2012;8(3):426–33.
20. Ahmet Koç. · Cünyet Üneri Genetic predisposition for tympanosclerotic degeneration. Eur Arch Otorhinolaryngol, 2002, 259, 4, 180–183.
21. Pirodda A, Bruzzi C, Ferri GG, Modugno GC, Gaddi A. Otoscopic findings in hypercholesterolemic subjects. B-ENT. 2010;6(2):123–6.
22. Cordeiro MF. Beyond Mitomycin: TGF-beta and wound healing. Prog Retin Eye Res. 2002;21:75–89.
23. Paclik D, Lohse K, Wiedenmann B, Dignass AU, Sturm A. Erratum: Galectin-2 and -4, but not Galectin-1, promote intestinal epithelial wound healing in vitro through a TGF-beta-independent mechanism. Inflammatory Bowel Diseases. 2011;17:1449.
24. Gressner AM, Weiskirchen R, Breitkopf K, Dooley S. Roles of TGF-beta in hepatic fibrosis. Front Biosci. 2002;7:d793–807.
25. Xaubet A, Marin-Arguedas A, Lario S, Ancochea J, Morell F, et al. Transforming growth factor-β1 gene polymorphisms are associated with disease progression in idiopathic pulmonary fibrosis. American J Respir Crit Care Med. 2003;168:431–5.
26. Ruiz-Ortega M, Ruperez M, Esteban V, Egido J. Molecular mechanisms of angiotensin II-induced vascular injury. Curr Hypertens Rep. 2003;5:73–9.
27. Kim S, Ohta K, Hamaguchi A, Omura T, Yukimura T, et al. Angiotensin II type I receptor antagonist inhibits the gene expression of transforming growth factor-beta 1 and extracellular matrix in cardiac and vascular tissues of hypertensive rats. J Pharmacol Exp Therap. 1995;273:509–15.
28. Siegert A, Ritz E, Orth S, Wagner J. Differential regulation of transforming growth factor receptors by angiotensin II and transforming growth factor-β1 in vascular smooth muscle. J Mol Med. 1999;77:437–45.
29. Habashi JP, Doyle JJ, Holm TM, Aziz H, Schoenhoff F, et al. Angiotensin II type 2 receptor signaling attenuates aortic aneurysm in mice through ERK antagonism. Science. 2011;332:361–5.
30. Yan W, Li J, Chai R, Guo W, Xu L, Han Y, et al. Combining use of captopril and losartan attenuates the progress of *Streptococcus pneumoniae*-induced Tympanosclerosis through the suppression of TGF-β1 expression. PLoS One. 2014;9(10):e111620.
31. Selcuk A, Akdogan O, Ozcan I, Giray SG, Dere H, Ozogul C. Topical application of calcium channel blockers to reduce the progression of experimentally induced myringosclerosis and tympanosclerosis. Laryngoscope. 2008;118(4):697–705.
32. Sheehy JL, House WF. Tympanosclerosis. Arch Otolaryngol. 1962;76:151–7.
33. Kinney SE. Postinflammatory ossicular fixation in tympanoplasty. Laryngoscope. 1978;88:821–38.
34. Ho KY, Tsai SM, Chai CY, Wang HM. Clinical analysis of intratympanic tympanosclerosis: etiology, ossicular chain findings, and hearing results ofsurgery. Acta Otolaryngol. 2010;130(3):370–4.
35. Austin DF. Reconstructive techniques for tympanosclerosis. Ann Otol Rhinol Laryngol. 1988;97:670–4.
36. Asiri S, Hasham A, Anazy FA, et al. Tympanosclerosis: review of literature and incidence among patients with middle ear infection. JLO. 1999;113:1076–80.
37. Gibb AG, Pang YT. Current considerations in the etiology and diagnosis of tympanosclerosis. Arch Otorhinolaryngol. 1994;251:439–51.
38. Bhaya MH, Schachern PA, Morizono T, Paparella MM. Pathogenesis of tympanosclerosis. Otolaryngol Head Neck Surg. 1993;109(3 Pt 1):413–20. (ISSN: 0194-5998)
39. Wielinga EWJ, Kerr AG. Tympanosclerosis. Rev Clin Otolaryngol. 1993;18:341–9.
40. Pal I, Sengupta A. Clinicopathological and audiological study of tympanosclerrosis. Indian J Otolaryngol Head Neck Surg. 2005;57:235–9.
41. Jaisinghani VJ, Hunter LL, Li Y, Margolis RH. Quantitative analysis of tympanic membrane disease using video-otoscopy. Laryngoscope. 2000;110(10 Pt 1):1726–30.

42. Tos M, Bak-Pedersen K. Goblet cell population in the pathological middle ear and eustachian tube of children and adults. Ann Otol Rhinol Laryngol. 1977;86(2 pt. 1):209–18.
43. Tsuzuki K, Yanagihara N, Hinohira Y, Sakagami M. Tympanosclerosis involving the ossicular chain: mobility of the stapes in association with hearing results. Acta Otolaryngol. 2006;126(10):1046–52.
44. Zhang S, Ma F, Pan T, Ke J, Zhang K, Song Y, Jiang L. Clinical analysis of tympanosclerosis: characteristics and treatment. Lin Chung Er Bi Yan Hou Tou Jing Wai Ke Za Zhi. 2015;29(14):1238–42.
45. Yabe T, Moriyama H, Kamide Y, Honda Y. Tympanosclerosis—clinical and pathological investigation. Nihon Jibiinkoka Gakkai Kaiho. 1995;98(4):606–12.
46. Teufert KB, De La Cruz A. Tympanosclerosis: long-term hearing results after ossicular reconstruction. Otolaryngol Head Neck Surg. 2002;126:264–72.
47. Albu S, Babighian G, Trabalzini F. Surgical treatment of tympanosclerosis. Am J Otol. 2000;21(5):631–5.
48. Smith MFW. Tympanoplasty: ossicular reconstruction. In: Britton BH, editor. Common problems in otology. St. Louis: Mosby Year Book; 1991. p. 65–9.
49. Igarashi M, Konishi S, Alford BR, Guilford FR. The pathology of tympanosclerosis. Laryngoscope. 1970;80:233–43.
50. Morgan WC. Tympanosclerosis. Laryngoscope. 1977;87:1821–5.
51. Fraysse B, Rugiu MG, Vandeventer G, Deguine O. La tympanosclerose: argon laser et tympanosclerose. Rencontres Institut Georges Portmann (Bordeaux). 1992:35–38.
52. Vincent R, Oates J, Sperling NM. Stapedotomy for tympanosclerotic stapes fixation: is it safe and efficient? A review of 68 cases. Otol Neurotol. 2002;23(6):866–72.
53. Magnan J. Long term results and indications of tympanosclerosis. In: Charachon R, Garcia-Ibanez E, editors. Proceedings Politzer Society Conference. Amsterdam/Milano/New York: Kugler Publications; 1991.
54. Tos M, Lau T, Arndal H, Plate S. Tympanosc lerosis of the middle ear: late results of surgical treatment. J Laryngol Otol. 1990;104(9):685–9.
55. GDL S. Tympanomastoid disease. In: Gibb AG, MFW S, editors. Otology. London: Butterworths; 1982. p. 3–18.
56. Giddings NA, House JW. Tympanosclerosis of the stapes: hearing results for various surgical treatments. Otolaryngol Head Neck Surg. 1992;107:644–50.
57. Querat C, Richard C, Martin C. Labyrinthine fenestration for tympanosclerotic stapes fixation. Eur Ann Otorhinolaryngol Head Neck Dis. 2012;129(6):297–301.
58. Vincent R, Sperling NM, Oates J, Jindal M. Surgical findings and long-term hearing results in 3,050 stapedotomies for primary otosclerosis: a prospective study with the otology-neurotology database. Otol Neurotol. 2006;27(8 Suppl 2):S25–47.
59. Gormley PK. Stapedectomy in tympanosclerosis. A report of 67 cases. Am J Otol. 1987;8(2):123–30.
60. Celik H, Aslan Felek S, Islam A, et al. Analysis of long-term hearing after tympanosclerosis with total/partial stapedectomy and prosthesis used. Acta Otolaryngol. 2008;128(12):1308–13.
61. Stankovic MD. Hearing results of surgery for tympanosclerosis. Eur Arch Otorhinolaryngol. 2009;266(5):635–40.
62. Iwasaki S, Suzuki H, Moteki H, Miyagawa M, Takumi Y, Usami S. Experience with the Vibrant Soundbridge RW-Coupler for round window Vibroplasty with tympanosclerosis. Acta Otolaryngol. 2012;132:676–82.
63. Emmett JR, Shea JJ. Surgical treatment of tympanosclerosis. Laryngoscope. 1978;88:1642–8.
64. Plester D. Tympanosclerosis. Aust J Otolaryngol. 1972;3:325–6.
65. Gristwood RE, Venables WN. Cholesteatoma and tympanosclerosis. In: Sade J, editor. Cholesteatoma and mastoid surgery. Amsterdam: Kugler; 1982. p. 133–7.
66. Hara H, Hasegawa M, Matzuzawa S, Kodama K, Shinnabe A, Kanazawa H, Yoshida N. Clinical characteristics of middle ear cholesteatoma with sclerotic regions. Otol Jpn. 2011;21(3):222–6.
67. Hoshino T. Osteoplastic changes in attic cholesteatoma. J Laryngol Otol. 1995;109(8):703–6.

Chronic Suppurative Otitis Media (CSOM): A Middle Ear Mucosal Disease

6

Contents

S. Mansour et al., *Middle Ear Diseases*,
https://doi.org/10.1007/978-3-319-72962-6_6

6.1 Definitions and Terminology

Chronic suppurative otitis media (CSOM) is defined as a chronic inflammation of the middle ear and mastoid cavity, which presents with recurrent ear discharges or otorrhea through a tympanic membrane perforation. CSOM is also called chronic purulent otitis media, chronic otomastoiditis or chronic tympanomastoiditis. The mode of presentation is a chronic infection of the ear but the pathological process may be occasionally of acute form. The tympanic membrane perforation modifies the demarcation between middle ear and external ear canal and creates conditions of adverse interactions inducing different pathological processes.

The basic features of CSOM are (Fig. 6.1):

1. ***Otorrhea****: sign of an active ME chronic inflammatory/infectious process*
2. ***Perforated tympanic membrane: a sequela of the process***
3. ***Inflammatory middle ear mucosa***

Tympanic membrane perforations are named by their anatomic locations:

6.1.1 Central Perforation

A central perforation is located in the pars tensa surrounded by a residual eardrum or at least a preserved annulus (non marginal perforation). Relative to its position in relation to the handle of the malleus, a perforation can be anterior (Fig. 6.2), posterior (Fig. 6.3), inferior (Fig. 6.4) or subtotal (Fig. 6.5). Subtotal perforation indicates a large perforation with an intact annulus, the handle of the malleus is usually

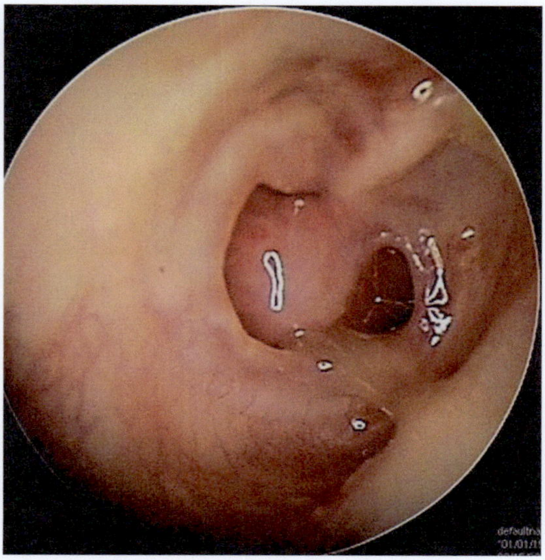

Fig. 6.1 Right ear with chronic suppurative otitis media showing: tympanic membrane perforation, inflammatory middle ear mucosa, and otorrhea

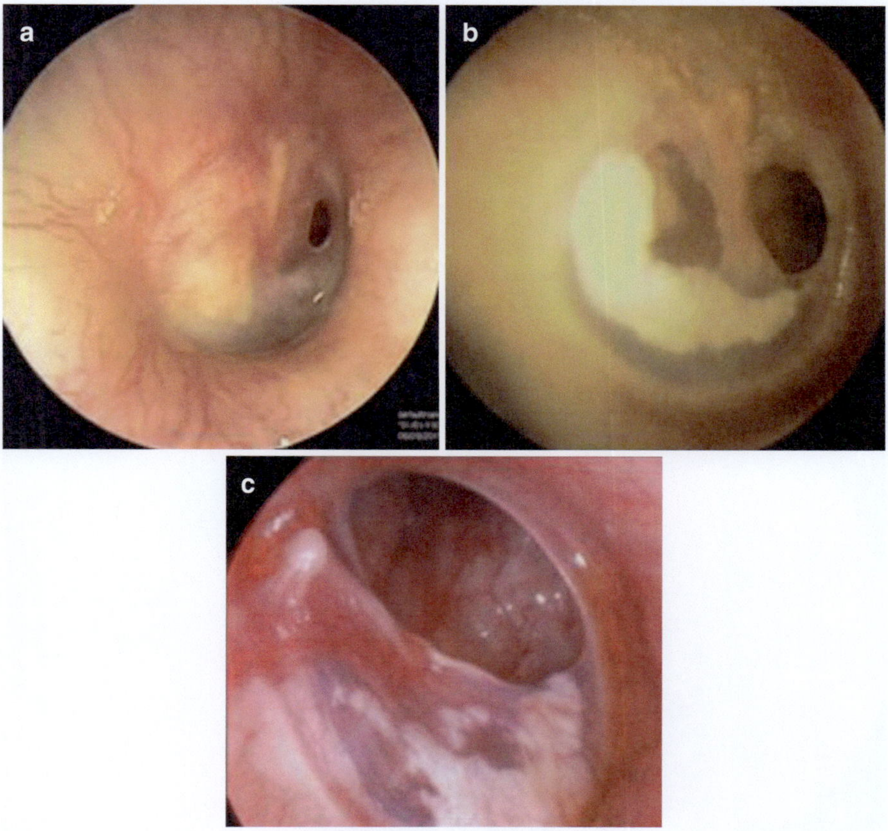

Fig. 6.2 Three left ears with a variable size of anterior perforations (**a**) small anterior perforation; (**b**) medium size anterior perforation; (**c**) large anterior perforation

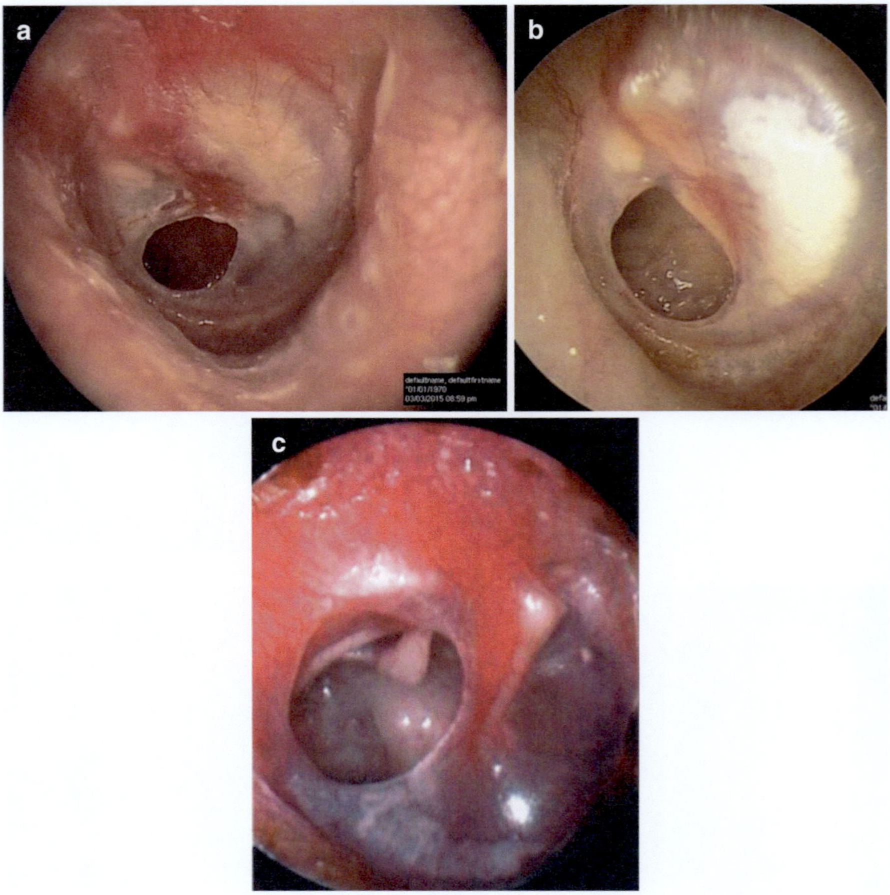

Fig. 6.3 Three left ears with posterior perforations. (**a**, **b**) Postero-inferior perforations and (**c**) posterosuperior perforation

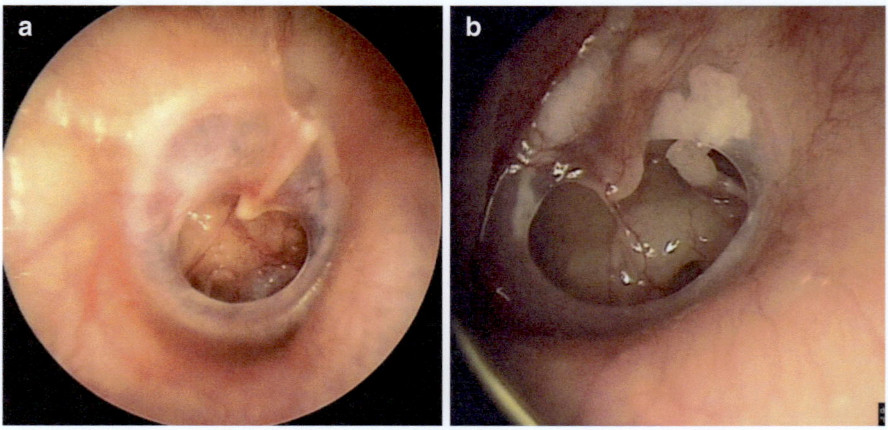

Fig. 6.4 (**a**) Inferior perforation of a right ear and (**b**) postero-inferior perforation of a right ear

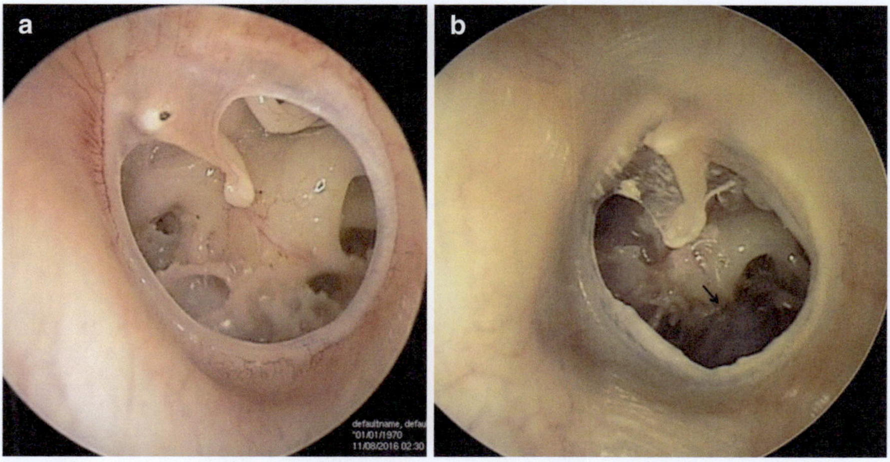

Fig. 6.5 (**a**) Subtotal perforation of a left ear, ossicular chain is visible and intact, malleus handle is medialized and (**b**) subtotal perforation of a left ear with high jugular bulb (black arrow)

medialized and all middle ear contents are visible even an occasional high jugular bulb (Fig. 6.5).

As central perforations expose the mucosa of the middle ear and Eustachian tube orifice, their presence was historically denoted by the term "*tubotympanic disease*" taking place below the tympanic diaphragm. Nowadays ears with a central perforation are called *"safe ears", which suffer from* ***a mucosal disorder*** [1], ***but without a cholesteatomatous pathology***.

6.1.2 Marginal Perforation

A marginal perforation is a posterior perforation with a contiguous pathological loss of the annulus allowing direct exposure of the bony canal wall (Fig. 6.6); or an attical perforation with a defect of the Pars Flaccida (Fig. 6.7).

Marginal and attical defects of the tympanic membrane expose the attic, the antrum and the mastoid cell system and are historically referred as "*attico-antral disease*", taking place above the tympanic diaphragm. Marginal and attical perforations are commonly associated with a cholesteatoma and for this reason they are presently termed as "*unsafe ears*", with risk of unfavorable prognosis and life threatening complications (Figs. 6.6 and 6.7) [1].

This chapter will review the advanced knowledge concerning CSOM mainly relative to safe ears and mucosal disorders. CSOM due to cholesteatoma (unsafe ears) is studied in the chapter of cholesteatoma (see Chap. 8).

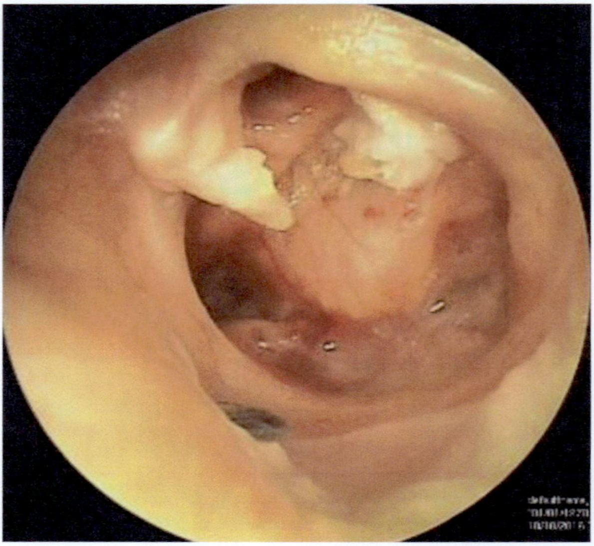

Fig. 6.6 Unsafe CSOM with subtotal and postero-superior marginal perforation of the left tympanic membrane with keratin debris migrating medially over the incudostapedial joint

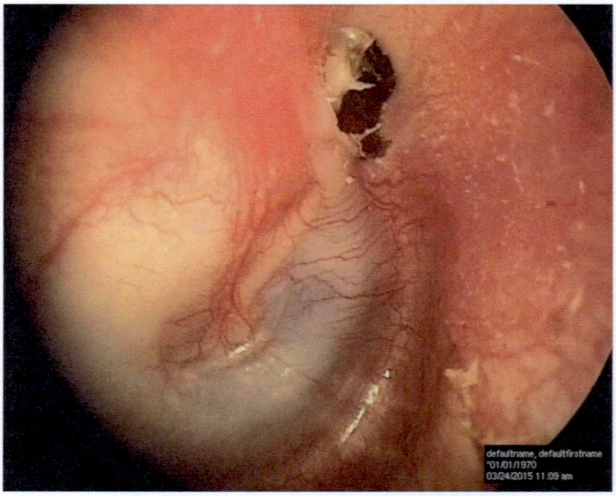

Fig. 6.7 Marginal anterior attical perforation of the right ear, visible after cleaning of the bottom of the ear canal, with a whitish mass behind the tympanic membrane highly suggestive of a cholesteatoma

6.2 Prevalence and Epidemiology

CSOM is thought to occur secondary to recurrent episodes of AOM in childhood: 70% of children in the USA have at least one AOM before the age of 3 years, which is a major risk factor for the development of CSOM [2]. Also, CSOM may occur as a sequela of otitis media with effusion (OME).

Estimates suggest that between 65 and 300 million cases of CSOM occur worldwide, 60% of these cases suffering of significant hearing impairment [3–5]. The prevalence of CSOM varies from one region to another. It is less prevalent in developed societies (USA and Europe) and when it occurs, it is often linked to tympanostomy tube (TT) insertion. In the UK, the prevalence of active chronic suppurative otitis media was reported by Browning as 0.6 % in the adult population [6].

It has been observed that males and females are equally affected [7]. Yearly a great number of deaths due to complications of CSOM are reported [8, 9]. In 1990, about 28,000 deaths all over the world and largely among developing countries were due to otitis media [10]; mortality and disabilities due to otitis media are primarily related to the complications of CSOM [11], particularly brain abscesses [12]. There is still an enormous financial burden, even in developed countries, associated with otitis media and its sequelae, including CSOM [13, 14].

Improved living conditions, along with the availability of specialized otological services in health care systems are behind a recent overall decrease of the prevalence of CSOM.

6.3 Etiology/Pathogenesis

CSOM is a multifactorial disease resulting from a complex series of interactions between environmental and host factors. CSOM is thought to occur secondary to recurrent episodes of AOM in childhood. The development of CSOM is mostly insidious, although the link between acute and chronic otitis media is frequently tenuous.

Risk factors for AOM, mostly implicated in the development of CSOM, include age, race, recurrent upper respiratory tract infections, poor access to otologic services, crowded living conditions, poor hygiene and nutrition, attendance at day care centers, bottle-feeding, exposure to passive smoking, and family history of otitis media. Risk factors especially for the developpement of chronic otitis media are represented in Fig. 6.8.

The middle ear is an organ that is highly prone to inflammation and human beings are considered highly susceptible to otitis media. Inflammation of the middle ear comprises a group of disorders that are highly prevalent in childhood and indeed are amongst the most common disorders of childhood.

The evolutionary forces that drive human susceptibility to middle ear inflammation cannot be considered in isolation, but rather exist in a complex interplay with the evolutionary forces affecting colonization, survival, and pathogenicity of bacteria living in the nasopharynx.

Bluestone has suggested that human susceptibility to otitis media is closely related to the evolution of craniofacial morphology, and in particular the angulation and caliber of the Eustachian tube. These ideas are premised on the notion that anatomy or function of the Eustachian tube is the major determinant of susceptibility to OM [15–18], but this premise is questionable and seems insensitive to the complexities of host and pathogen interaction. There is little evidence that the Eustachian tube is in some way abnormal in the OM susceptible population: in fact, most evidence suggests no difference [19, 20].

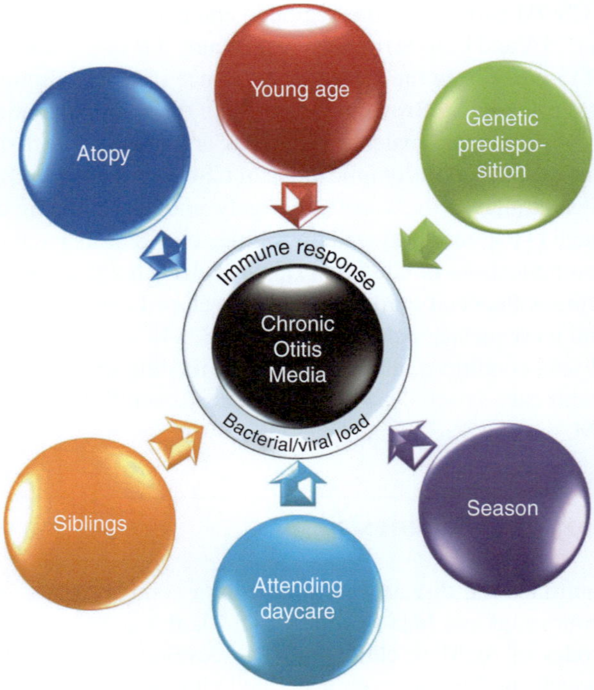

Fig. 6.8 Risk factors associated with chronic suppurative otitis media

Bluestone also suggests that otitis media is almost unique to humans [18], but actually OM is well documented by the veterinary community in small and large domestic animals, including dogs, cats, rabbits, ruminants, horses, pigs, and camelid, although it can be difficult to diagnose [21].

Otitis media remains prevalent because it is a complex infectious disease. Bacteria that normally reside silently in the human nasopharynx are the cause of AOM when they ascend up the Eustachian tube into the middle ear. The middle ear is an immunodeficient organ. The human middle ear is devoid of any immunocompetent cells in normal mucosa. The normal mucosa of the middle ear possesses neither immunocompetent lymphocytes nor associated lymphoid tissues [22, 23].

Antibodies detected in the middle ear during AOM derive predominantly from serum transudation and reflux of nasal secretions containing antibodies, with no evidence for independent, local antibody production [24].

Phylogenetically, the immune system is very ancient and appeared at very early stages during evolution. The adaptive immunity with specific immune cells and antibodies evolved with the vertebrate lineage [25] which is far earlier than the phylogenetic development of the middle ear which appeared at the Water–Land Transition when animals transitioned from an aquatic to a terrestrial existence.

The late phylogenetic appearance of the external and the middle ear rendered them immunodeficient organs. When the ME mucosa is exposed to injury or aggression, its mechanism of defense is very primitive and consists of increased mucociliary clearance which usually sweeps away most of the pathogens out of the ME. However, when the aggression is severe or persistent, ME mucosa reacts by metaplasia with a transition into mucus-secreting epithelium rich in secretory goblet cells with resultant decreased mucociliary clearance and mucus plug formation (see Fig. 6.15 below).

On the other hand, the bottom of the external ear canal, which is formed by a cavitation process of the same mesenchymal tissue associated to an invagination of the cutaneous epithelium and tympanic bone development, is the result of a delayed formation. Such delay is behind its fragile immune system and its vulnerability to inflammation.

In CSOM, the perforation of the tympanic membrane exposes both organs with a fragile immunity (tympanic membrane and middle ear mucosa) to a common battlefield, the same inflammatory process taking place at the same time. Where recurrences and chronicity depend of the individual immune competencies: "not anyone is subject to CSOM". These differences could be due to ethnic variations in socio-economic factors [26] or in illness-seeking behavior [27], as well as genetics.

6.3.1 Associated Features to Chronic Suppurative Otitis Media

(a) *ET dysfunction* in children: Cleft palate and Down's syndrome, also a patulous ET allowing nasopharyngeal reflux
(b) *Mucosal Immune System (MIS) deficiencies*, specific to URT mucosa immunity, atopy
(c) *Systemic immune deficiency*: Abnormalities of humoral immune system (e.g. hypogammaglobulinemia) and cell-mediated immunity (e.g. HIV infection).
(d) *Poor mastoid pneumatization*: A relationship between chronic middle ear disease and poor mastoid pneumatization was observed: Sade reported a rate of COM of 52.2% in low-pneumatized ears (<6 cm^2) and only 20% in well-pneumatized ears (>6 cm^2) in 72 adult patients who were followed up for 33 months [28]. Less pneumatized mastoids and ossicular diseases in elderly patients with chronic perforated otitis media suggest that they had longer lasting and more severe middle ear pathologies than did younger patients [29].

It is admitted that infection in infancy or early childhood prevents mastoid pneumatization, although infection within an already pneumatized cleft induces sclerosis, with obliteration of the cells and a secondary hypopneumatization.

In acute otitis media, a destruction process of the three layers of the tympanic membrane (epithelium, lamina propria, and mucosa) can take place and may lead further to a perforation. In most of the cases, the perforation heals spontaneously. The healing of a tympanic membrane perforation depends on the proliferation of the connective tissue and squamous epithelium at the margins of the defect.

The failure of healing of a tympanic membrane perforation leads to the development of CSOM. Multiple factors are implicated behind the healing failure:

(a) *Persistent infections* in the middle ear cavities with continuous purulent otorrhea (most of the pathogenic bacteria found in CSOM are those common to the external auditory canal) maintaining a "tympanic membrane-stoma" for drainage.
(b) *Eustachian tube obstruction* with the vicious circle of hypopressure in the tympanic cavity, local secondary hypoxia, and inflammation, creating conditions of a definitive breakdown of the epithelial lining.
(c) *Large size of perforations* causing failure of closure by spontaneous regeneration and epithelial migration which may impinge on the medial side of the tympanic membrane.
(d) *Formation of granulation tissue and polyps* within the middle ear space in response to the host attempt to resolve the infection or the inflammatory insult. A study by Wang et al suggested that in CSOM, T-cell-mediated cellular immunity plays a role in the formation of granulation tissue [30].

*Following the aggression on the mucosa of the ME (*ETD, infection, reflux, and genetic responses Fig. 6.9), *the chain of events presents the following sequences*

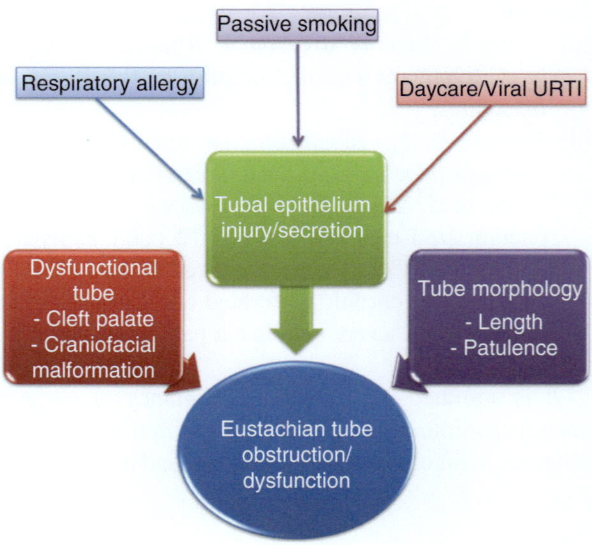

Fig. 6.9 Etiological factors responsible for Eustachian tube dysfunction in CSOM

Fig. 6.10 Chain of events that lead to the development of chronic inflammation of middle ear mucosa

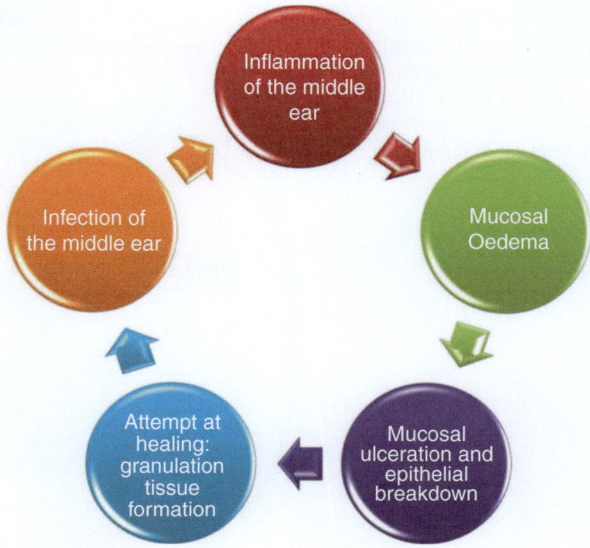

(Fig. 6.10): **Inflammation → hypoxia → oedema of the mucosa → ulcerations → reparative reaction → granulations → polyps → ossicular lysis.**

6.3.2 Inflammation in CSOM and Hypoxia

During otitis media, the large amount of inflammatory cells and the hyperplasia of the mucosa participate to the consumption of O2, leading to hypoxia. In addition, the ET is often blocked by oedema and secretions increasing the hypoxia.

Biomarkers of hypoxia are:

- The transcription factor hypoxia inducible factor 1α (**HIF-1α**) and
- The secreted protein vascular endothelial growth factor (**VEGF**) [31].

The stress response to hypoxia induces an overproduction of *oxygen radicals* called "*reactive oxygen species*" which react with several components of the cells (protein, lipids, DNA…) resulting in cell damage and perpetuating the vicious circle between hypoxia and inflammation in the middle ear epithelium (Fig. 6.11).

6.4 Molecular Biology of CSOM

- The immune system responds to injuries or hypoxia through an innate cascade mechanism known as inflammation which is mediated by multiple elements (mediators and cell responses). These elements are produced by epithelial cells, endothelial cells, and infiltrating inflammatory cells.

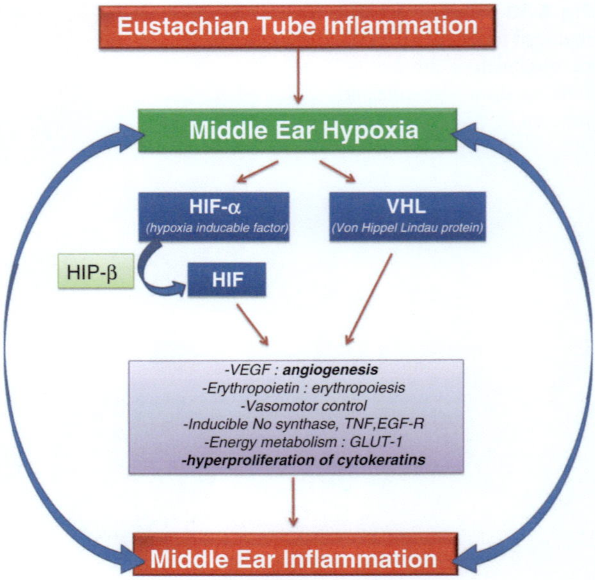

Fig. 6.11 The chain of events from Eustachian tube dysfunction and middle ear hypoxia that leads to the development of middle ear inflammation

- Bacterial endotoxins induce secretion of inflammatory mediators and stimulate *macrophages* to produce Tumor Necrosis Factors –alpha (**TNF-α**) and **Interleukines -1**.
- Infiltrating *immune cells* (neutrophils, monocytes and lymphocytes) and *local cells* (keratinocytes and mast cells) are capable of producing inflammatory mediators **such IL-1 and TNF-α**.
- Inflammatory mediators are a double-edged sword, having the potential to fight off infection, but also to damage the host. Such mediators are potential key factors responsible for the chronicity of otitis media.

6.4.1 Interleukine IL-1

- *IL-1 is an early-response cytokine, inducing the proliferation and differentiation of T-cells, B cells, monocytes, and macrophages.*
- *IL-1 is one of the most active substances* ***inducing bone resorption through osteoclast activation****.*
- *IL-1 stimulates the synthesis of TNF, IL-2, IL-6, and IL-8.*
- *IL-1 induces cell adhesion molecules (intercellular adhesion molecule -1 and vascular cell adhesion molecule -1) that in turn stimulate the migration of leukocytes.*
- *IL-lβ plays an important role in the pathogenesis of otitis media with effusion (OME).*

Hence a treatment that reduces the production of IL-1 may be an effective adjuvant in the early stage of OM in children.

6.4.2 Tumor Necrosis Factor (TNF)

- *TNF is a pair of cytokines originally called cachectin (TNF-α) and lymphotoxin (TNF-β) made by a wide variety of cells including fibroblasts, T cells and B cells.*
- *TNF-α was detected in human middle ear effusion: TNF-α is one of the most significant inflammatory mediators in otitis media.*
- Higher expression of TNF-α in human otitis media confers higher risks of recurrent episodes and longer courses of otitis media as well as the *chronicity of otitis media*

6.4.3 Other Cytokines

High levels of inflammatory cytokines such as IL-8 have been demonstrated in CSOM patients [32]. IL-8 plays a role in the development of chronicity of otitis media and has been related to bacterial growth. Increased levels of TNF-α, IL-6, and IFN-γ have been found in higher levels in the middle ear mucosa of CSOM patients compared with healthy individuals [33]. The secretion of these pro-inflammatory cytokines can cause tissue damage as well as transition from acute to chronic OM.

6.4.4 Immunoglobulines IgG and IgA

There is a need to characterize the role of immunity (both innate and adaptive) as it pertains to the transition from AOM to CSOM. IgG and IgA are the most important immunoglobulins in the defense mechanism against mucosal infections like in CSOM acting by their adherence to the bacterial wall, i.e. ***coating*** [34].

- Secretory IgA (sIgA) prevent bacteria from attaching to and colonizing the middle ear mucosa. Middle ear mucosa lacks the ability to secret local sIgA (See Sect. 6.3). Middle ear sIgA are synthesized by plasma cells in the mucosa of the nasopharynx (MALT) and are transported to the middle ear by nasopharyngeal reflux and transudate. *Children with atopy and CSOM may lack secretory IgA* [35].
- IgG-class immunoglobulins facilitate phagocytosis directly or via complement activation. IgG and IgG-subclass concentrations are age dependent [34]: children with recurrent upper respiratory tract infections may have low specific IgG-subclass (mostly IgG2) antibody levels (10–20% of cases) [36, 37].

In CSOM, intense sIgA and IgG coating of bacteria is common, but when P. aeruginosa is the causative agent of the infection, no bacterial coating is seen. This is because the immune adaptive response in the middle ear is initiated by bacterial-MALT encountered in the nasopharynx with resultant secretion and transportation of specific immunoglobulins to the middle ear. Bacteria reaching the middle ear through the nasopharynx, like Moraxella or Streptococcus, can have intense IgA and IgG coating in the middle ear. However, bacteria reaching the middle ear through a tympanic membrane perforation, like Pseudomonas aeruginosa, lack effective coating and can colonize middle ear mucosa chronically. This explains why infections caused by P. aeruginosa are difficult to eradicate from the middle ear [35, 38].

6.5 Genetics in CSOM

It is important to identify the genes that contribute to CSOM susceptibility. The identification of genetic and prognostic markers will help in predicting CSOM-susceptible individuals and possibly even novel therapeutic strategies.

Candidate gene studies have identified a handful of genes contributing to otitis media susceptibility, including several immune genes polymorphism, such as *IL10* and *TNF genes*, as well as *FBXO11*, which have been significantly associated with otitis media in several independent cohorts [39–41].

The first genome-wide association study looking at the otitis media phenotype has identified *CAPN14* and *GALNT14* on chromosome 2p23.1 and the *BPIFA* gene cluster on chromosome 20q11.21 as novel candidate genes which warrant further analysis [42].

6.6 Microbiology

Microorganisms found in otorrhea secretions gain access to the middle ear cavity from the EAC through the TM perforation. The commonest organisms isolated are gram neg. as *Pseudomonas aeruginosa, and Proteus* species (P. *mirabilis* and *P. vulgaris*). The *Staphylococcus aureus* is the most common gram positive organism. Other organisms found less commonly in chronically discharging ears include *Escherichia coli*, *Streptococcus pneumoniae*, *Diphteroids*, *Klebsiella* species and the anaerobic *Bacteroides* species (Fig. 6.12).

- **Pseudomonas aeruginosa** is the most prevalent germ present in CSOM. It uses pili to attach to the necrotic or diseased epithelium of the middle ear. Once attached, the organism produces proteases, lipopolysaccharides, and other enzymes to hinder normal immunologic defense mechanisms from fighting the infection. The ensuing damage from bacterial and inflammatory enzymes creates further damage, necrosis, and, eventually, bone erosions leading to the complications of CSOM. Pseudomonal infections are commonly resistant to macrolides, extended-spectrum penicillins, and first- and second-generation cephalosporins. This can complicate treatment plans, especially in children.

- **Staphylococcus aureus** is the second most common organism isolated from chronically diseased middle ears. Reported data estimate infection rates from 15 to 30% of culture-positive draining ears.

Klebsiella (10–21%) and *Proteus* (10–15%): they are gram-negative organisms.

Polymicrobial infections are seen in 5–10% of cases, often demonstrating a combination of gram-negative organisms and *S. aureus* (Fig. 6.12). The moist and humid environment and excessive usage of antibiotic ear drops favor superimposed fungal infections of the ear (Fig. 6.13).

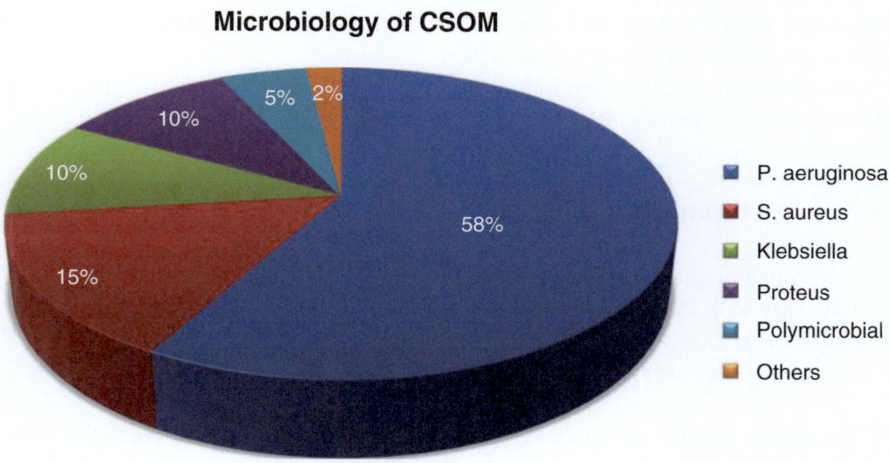

Fig. 6.12 Percentage of different pathogens in CSOM

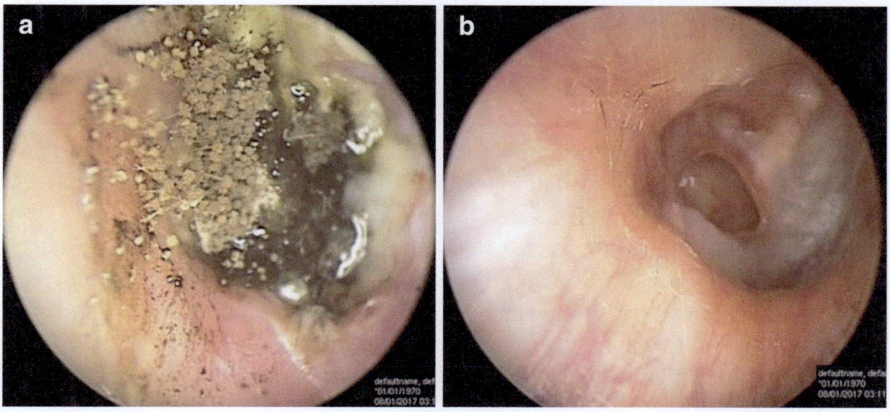

Fig. 6.13 (**a**) Fungal debris (aspergillus niger) and (**b**) after cleaning showing tympanic membrane perforation

6.6.1 Bacterial Biofilms

In the middle ear mucosa of patients with chronic otitis media, biofilm formation is common, especially when ear discharge history is present. Biofilms are a collective of one or more types of microorganisms in which cells stick to each other and adhere to a wet surface. These adherent cells are frequently embedded within a self-produced matrix of extracellular polymeric substance (EPS) acting as a protector. Bacteria, instead of being single, independent cells (planktonic), are organized into sessile aggregates called biofilms. The important hallmarks of chronic biofilm-based infections are their extreme resistance to antibiotics and the great capacity for evading the host defenses. Fungal biofilms can also cause infections by growing on otologic implanted devices or tympanostomy tubes.

Antibiotic treatment of biofilms may kill bacteria on the periphery, but deep organisms persist and act as a nidus for regrowth and periodic planktonic showers, that can result in a systemic infection [43].

Biofilm formation has been found in chronic, recalcitrant infection of the middle ear and mastoid mucosa, requiring surgical treatment.

6.7 Histopathology of CSOM

The histopathological changes observed in the mucosa of the middle ear with CSOM vary with the degree and the extent of the disease: the most intense inflammatory changes are seen in ears with lasting otorrhea.

The changes occurring in the middle ear cleft mucosa (Fig. 6.14) are as follows:

1. In normal middle ear mucosa, the distribution of the ciliated epithelial cells decreases from the Eustachian tube towards the mastoid antrum. The pseudostratified ciliary respiratory epithelium in the Eustachian tube changes progressively to an unicellular flat epithelium in the mastoid antrum. During infection, the mucosa shows rapid dynamic structure changes with an increasing number of ciliated cells and goblet-cells resulting in an increase in mucosal mucociliary clearance. These epithelial changes are associated with subepithelial lamina propria inflammatory changes which consist of an increased capillary permeability and infiltration of the lamina propria by lymphocytes, plasma cells, and histiocytes. The mucous secretion from secretory cells and newly formed glands is an important part of the discharge seen in chronic suppurative otitis media.
2. Inflammatory granulation tissue or aural polyps develop during the early stages of the healing process following tissue destruction. The polyp is usually covered by a ciliated columnar epithelium; occasionally polyps are covered with squamous epithelium, which may occur by metaplastic change. Although polyps are often a sentinel sign for an underlying cholesteatoma, aural polyps can occur in all types of CSOM.

Fig. 6.14 Different histopathological phases of CSOM

Different Histopathological Phases of CSOM

- Chronic inflammatory infiltrates associated with mucosal oedema
- ME epithelium ***metaplasia*** to ***respiratory*** type
- Increased number of goblet cells and mucus secretions
- Inflammatory granulation tissue develops during early stages of healing
- Fibrosis in late stages

TS is a special form of fibrosis often occurring in CSOM

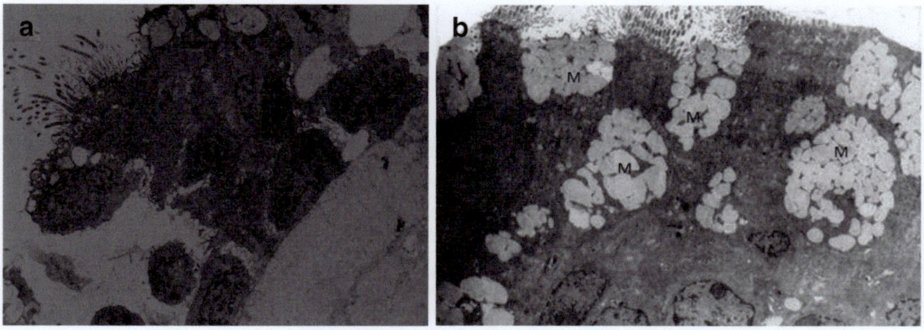

Fig 6.15 Electronic microscopic examination of middle ear protympanum mucosa in normal (**a**) and ears with CSOM (**b**). Notice the simple layer of pseudostratified ciliated epithelium in normal middle ears that transform by metaplasia to a thick mucosa with so many mucus secreting goblet cells (M) with resultant excessive mucus secretion that hinders the function of epithelial cilia and leads to formation of middle ear mucus plugs that can easily block the ET

3. The late stages of the disease are characterized by a decrease in vascularity and fibrosis. These changes are particularly well observed in the mastoid which is eburnated.
4. After a long duration process of quiescent CSOM, tympanosclerosis can occur.

In healthy subjects that did not have prior disease of the middle ear, very few mucus glands are usually observed, whereas in subjects that had a history of otitis media events, these glands are more numerous [44]. This suggests that mucus glands probably appear in the middle ear after several episodes of otitis media and then remain even after the disease resolution.

In patients with CSOM, the density of mucus glands is very high and appears as a sequela of CSOM [45] (Fig. 6.15).

6.8 Ossicular Chain Erosion in Chronic Suppurative Otitis Media

Different aspects of CSOM sequela on the ossicular chain are shown in Fig. 6.16. Ossicular erosion is much more common in unsafe CSOM than in safe CSOM. It was found in 14% in CSOM of safe ears. *An* excessive amount of inflammatory mediators in the tympanic cavity induces activation of osteoclasts and bone resorption resulting in ossicular lysis. The long duration of the inflammatory process appears to be the most harmful factor for the ossicles [46].

- *Incudal necrosis* is the most prevailing ossicular pathology in cases of CSOM and most frequently localized in the lenticular process (Fig. 6.17) followed by the long process (Fig. 6.18); necrosis typically spares the body of the incus. Tenuous blood supply and exposure to the external milieu especially in posterior perforations are factors behind the predilection of incus long process necrosis which is reported to be 8% in safe ears [46].
- *The stapes* lysis is uncommon in safe ears [46].
- *The malleus* is the most defiant and resilient middle ear ossicle. This can be attributed to the firm attachment of the handle to the tympanic membrane which acts as a mechanical barricade and allows adequate blood flow to the handle: such combined effect diminishes the risk of malleus handle necrosis. In case of subtotal perforations, the malleus handle is usually medialized due to the unopposed pull of the tensor tympani muscle (Fig. 6.19) [46]. Malleus handle necrosis may rarely occur in ears with a subtotal perforation and is reported to be of 2% in safe ears. Malleus handle necrosis in subtotal perforation is secondary to the decreased blood supply to the handle which is usually nourished by tympanic membrane vessels and due to the unprotected exposure of the malleus handle to the external environment (Fig. 6.20) [46].

6.9 Biomechanics of Chronic Ears

6.9.1 Hearing Loss Mechanisms in Tympanic Membrane Perforation

The sound pressure difference across the tympanic membrane is the driving force for middle ear sound transmission, a reduction of this sound pressure difference due to a perforation is the cause of hearing loss.

Voss et al. [47, 48] demonstrated that the major mechanism for hearing loss in most cases of tympanic membrane perforations is the loss of pressure difference across the tympanic membrane that occurs as the sound volume velocity travels through the perforation instead of the ossicular chain. Large perforations will reduce the efficiency of the tympanic membrane to a greater degree in reducing the sound pressure difference across the tympanic membrane (outside and inside the tympanic cavity). Hearing loss increases with the size of the perforation and not with its location [49].

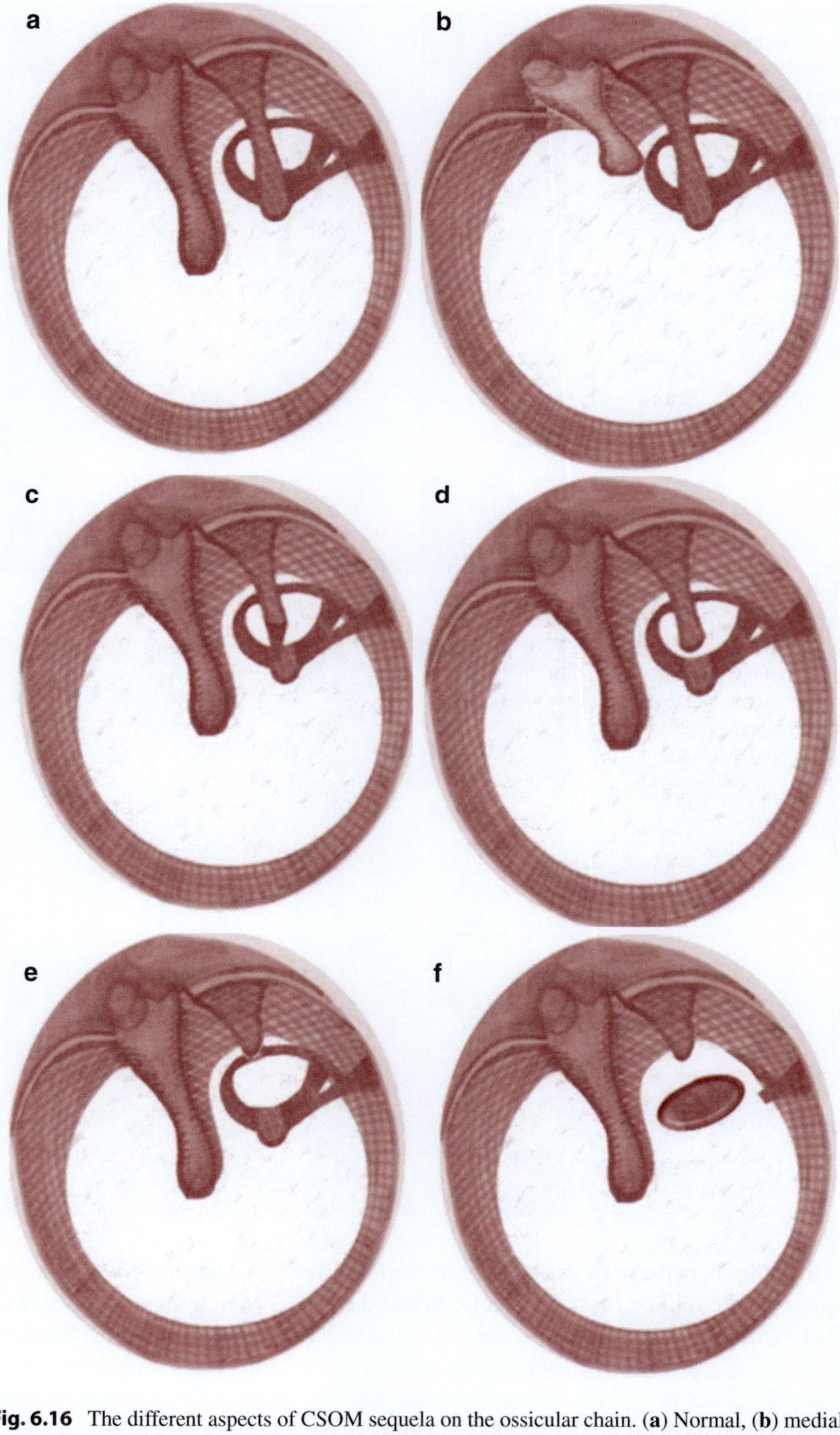

Fig. 6.16 The different aspects of CSOM sequela on the ossicular chain. (**a**) Normal, (**b**) medialized malleus, (**c**) fibrous band, (**d**) lenticular process resorption, (**e**) long process resorption and (**f**) stapes superstructure resorption

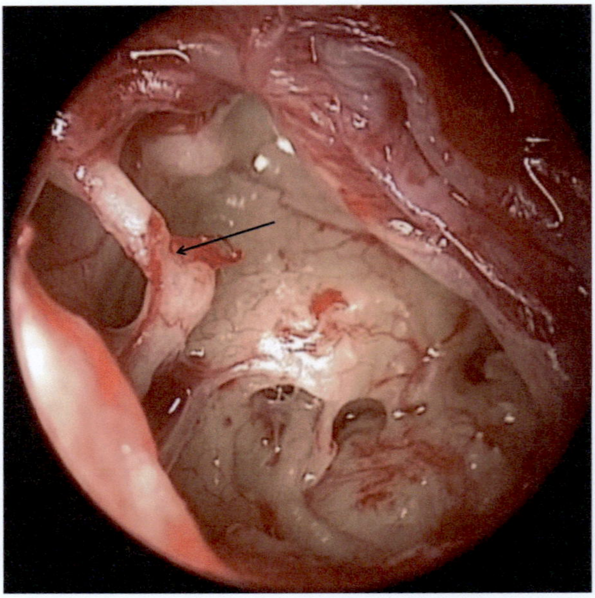

Fig. 6.17 Right chronic ear showing erosion of the lenticular process of the incus with residual fibrous band (black arrow) connecting incus and stapes

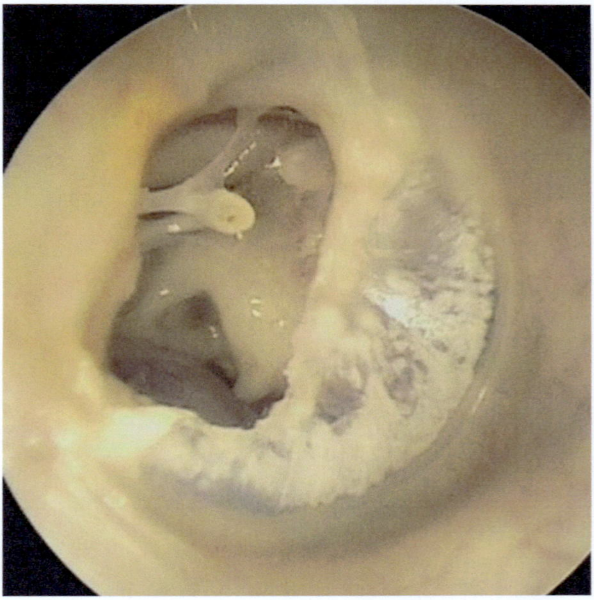

Fig. 6.18 Right CSOM ear with incus erosion (notice uncommon finding of a high jugular bulb seen during otoscopy through the perforation).

In addition, in the presence of a perforation, hearing loss varies inversely with the volume of the middle ear and mastoid. Mastoid and ME volume can vary from 1 to 20 cc with an average of 6 cc; in case of equal size and location of the perforation, the air-bone gap from a perforation can vary by up to 35 dB depending on that volume [49]. This can explain why similar tympanic membrane perforations in size and locations can have different degrees of hearing loss.

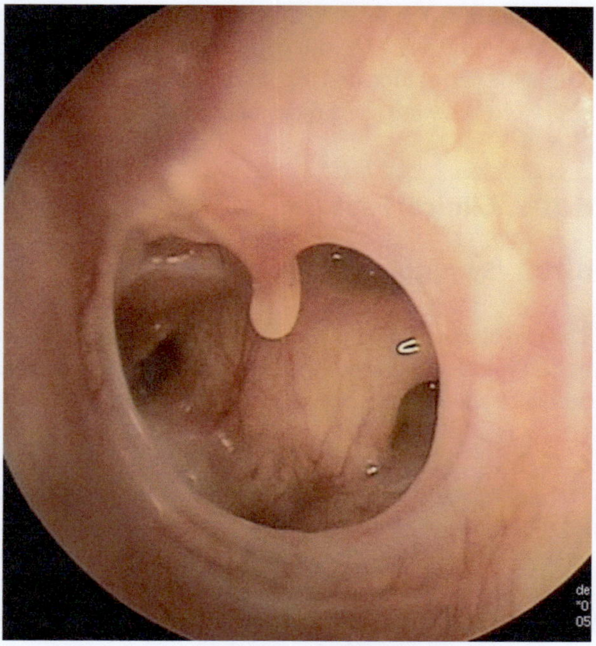

Fig. 6.19 Left ear with subtotal perforation and medialized malleus handle

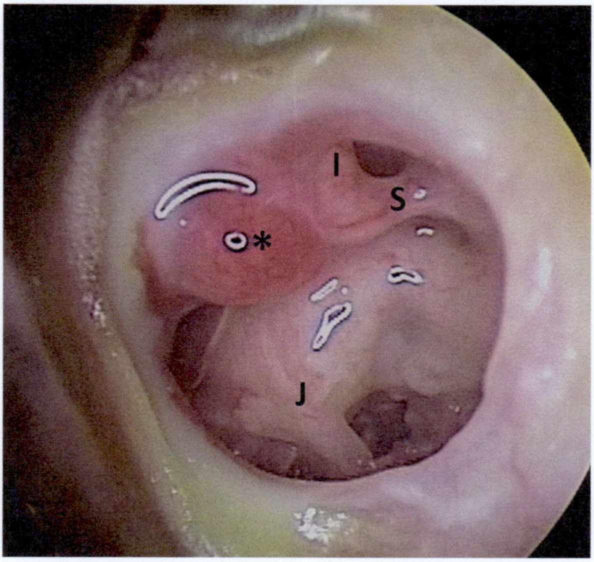

Fig. 6.20 Left ear otoscopy showing subtotal perforation with necrosis of the malleus handle which is replaced by a small granuloma (*). Both incus (I) and stapes (S) are still intact. J: Jacobson nerve

ME volumes smaller than 0.5 cc should lead to progressively larger gaps, whereas an increased volume above about 1.0 cc seems to provide little additional acoustic benefit.

At the lower frequencies, the hole in the tympanic membrane introduces a shunt path for volume velocity to flow directly into the middle ear cavity, and it is the compliant middle ear cavity that dominates the impedance. *When frequencies increase above about 0.5–1 kHz*, the perforation forms a resonance between the mass of air within the perforation and the air volume of the middle ear cavities and *at frequencies above this resonant frequency*, the ear's response approaches its normal value.

6.10 Clinical Features

6.10.1 Symptomatology

The two classic symptoms of chronic suppurative otitis media are otorrhoea and deafness. Typically, patients deny pain or discomfort. Reports of fever, vertigo, pain and headache should raise concern about intratemporal or intracranial complications.

6.10.1.1 Otorrhea

The ear discharge can be continuous or intermittent, serous or mucoid to frankly purulent, moderate or profuse draining through the external meatus. A viscous non-odorant, adherent and filiform discharge may render the ME toilet difficult. An increase in the amount of discharge can be precipitated by upper respiratory tract infections or swimming. Bloodstained discharge is associated to granulations over or around a ventilating tube, or to an aural polyp which is a predictor of underlying cholesteatoma.

6.10.1.2 Hearing Loss

CSOM can cause conductive hearing loss (CHL) as well as sensorineural hearing loss (SNHL). CSOM may contribute more than half to the global burden of hearing impairment, and eliminating it can potentially reduce the global burden by four-fifths.

CHL in CSOM

CHL in CSOM ranges from 20 to 60 dB. It is of the otologist's concern that all measures for an early cure of the disease, including surgery, should be considered promptly to prevent further hearing loss in these patients.

Factors that influence the degree of conductive deafness are the following:

1. HL and TM Perforations:
   (a) HL is largest at the lowest frequency and decreases with increasing frequency.
   (b) HL increases as perforation size increases.
   (c) HL does not depend on perforation location [49].

Mucosal oedema and granulation tissues can also influence the sound conduction, due to the aeration deficiency, which by itself could cause 40 dB CHL.

2. Ossicular Bone Necrosis
   (a) Mechanics of the middle ear differs in the presence of tympanic membrane perforation with partial or complete incus necrosis.
   (b) Complete ossicular disarticulation, in the presence of an intact tympanic membrane, leads to a reduction of middle ear transmission in the order of 40–60 dB depending on frequency [50, 51]. Peake et al. [52] showed that in

such a loss in ossicular coupling is consistent with a cochlea responding only to the pressure difference at its oval and round windows (i.e., acoustic coupling).

(c) Partial ossicular interruption, mostly replaced by connective fibrous tissue, associated to an intact tympanic membrane, results generally in higher ABG at high frequencies than at low frequencies (due to the decrease of stiffness) [51, 53].

SNHL in CSOM

Toxins and inflammatory mediators can penetrate the round window membrane causing damage to outer or inner hair cells, especially those at the cochlear base where the hair cells are sensitive to high-frequency sounds. A significant loss of outer and inner hair cells, as well as significant atrophy of the stria vascularis in the basal turn of the cochlea, have been observed in CSOM patients. The basal turn of the cochlea also demonstrated severe pathological changes that were consistent with the high-frequency SNHL in CSOM patients [54–56].

The majority of SNHL in CSOM patients is in the high-frequency range [57]. The percentage of CSOM patients with higher BC thresholds tended to increase with age [58]. The site and size of the tympanic membrane perforation have been correlated with the degree of SNHL, showing that posterior perforations have a greater decibel level loss, probably as a result of the direct exposure of the round window membrane to microbial agents [59].

6.10.2 Examination Findings

Microscopic otoscopy is always done with a minutious and cautious cleaning step which could be sometimes delicate and laborious, especially in children, avoiding any discomfort or painful maneuver. Otomicroscopic ear examinations should always start with the contralateral ear which is not the source of the patient's complaints. The clinical status of the contralateral ear likewise can provide insight into tubal maturity and function in the diseased ear. Cleaning the ear from otorrhea is an important step, abundant otorrhea must not delay an accurate otomicroscopy.

6.10.2.1 Different Caracteristics of Otorrhea (6.10.1.1)

The activity of the disease will be reflected by the degree of discharge:

- In active cases, the discharge can be mucoid or purulent.
- In severely infected cases, a pulsatile purulent discharge may occur (Fig. 6.21).
- In inactive cases, there is no discharge and the middle ear mucosa looks dry.

6.10.2.2 Different Aspects of Tympanic Membrane Perforation

The principal examination finding in CSOM is the tympanic membrane defect. A drawing of the tympanic membrane should be made in the case record; the description of the tympanic membrane must be the most objective possible (endoscopic pictures)

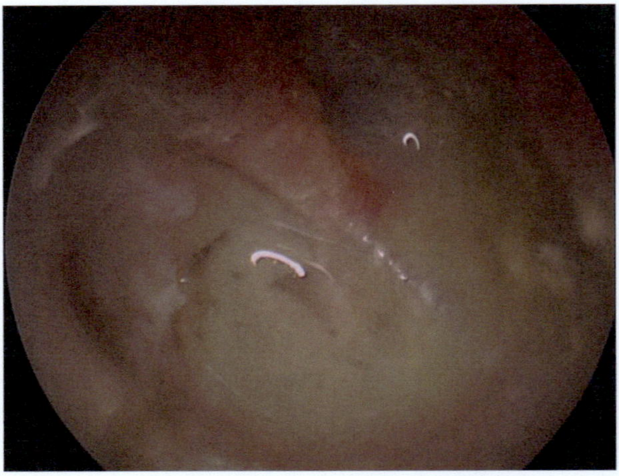

Fig. 6.21 Right CSOM with active mucopurulent discharge

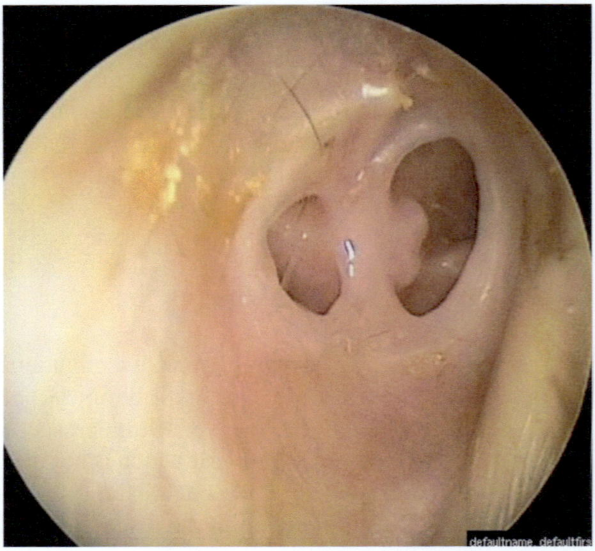

Fig. 6.22 Right ear with two tympanic membrane perforations and pale middle ear mucosa, suggestive of tuberculous otitis media

- Perforations can vary in size from a pin hole-type defect to a large subtotal defect.
- Perforation may be central or marginal (see Figs. 6.2, 6.3, 6.4, 6.5, and 6.7).
- Multiple tympanic membrane perforations in the same ear associated with a progressive and profound hearing loss and facial palsy suggest tuberculosis. Significant clinical features are the presence of abundant pale granulations, the presence of a normal mastoid cellular development on CT-Imaging and a past personal or family history of tuberculosis of any other organ localization (Fig. 6.22).

6.10.2.3 Status of the Middle Ear Cavity Mucosa

- Visualized through the perforation, the middle ear mucosa may be oedematous with different degrees of inflamed mucosa.

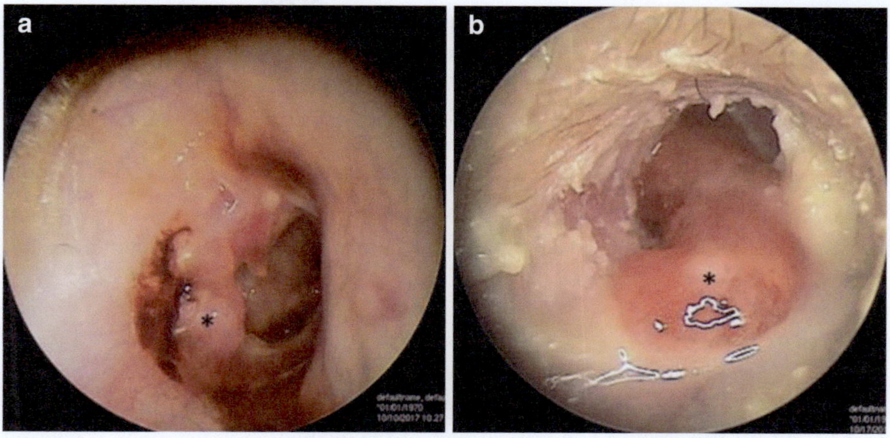

Fig. 6.23 (**a**) Right CSOM with small polyp (asterisk) arising through the posterior margin of the perforation and (**b**) large aural aural polyp (asterisk)

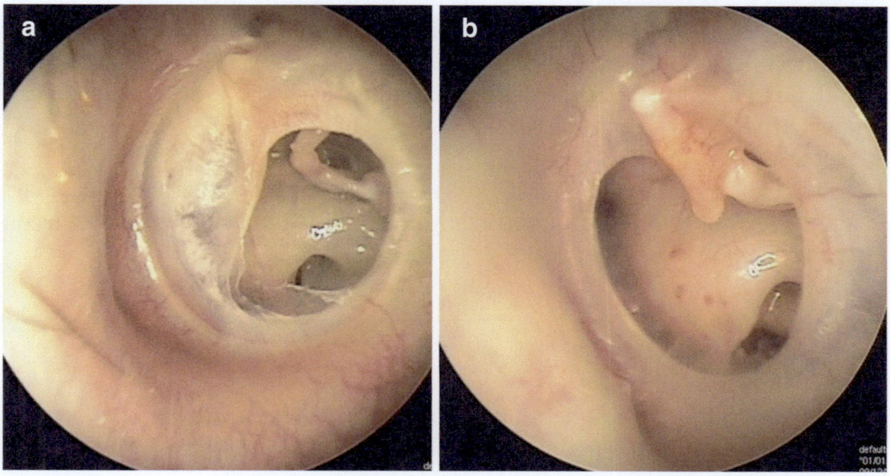

Fig. 6.24 (**a**) Left tympanic membrane posterior perforation with intact ossicular chain and (**b**) left subtotal perforation with incus erosion and medialized malleus

- Aural polyps may be present, arising from the middle ear mucosa or the margins of the perforation. In some cases the aural polyp may be as large as the external auditory canal and may manifest at the lateral meatus (Fig. 6.23).

6.10.2.4 Ossicular Chain Assessment

The integrity of the ossicular chain can often be observed through the perforation. The most commonly seen ossicular abnormalities are disruption of the incudostapedial joint, necrosis of the long incus long process; often a medialization and shortening of the malleus handle is observed, (Fig. 6.24).

6.10.2.5 Secondary Otitis Externa

Secondary otitis externa is reported in ears with earache and profuse discharge, rendering the otoscopy somehow uncomfortable. It should not be missed during ear examination. It must be treated adequately along with the ME infection.

6.10.2.6 Eustachian Tube Function Assessment

Eustachian tube plays a major role in the pathogenesis of CSOM. Its assessment remains clinical through a nasal examination looking for allergy, adenoiditis, and rhinosinusitis.

6.10.3 Hearing Assessment

- **512-Hz tuning fork**: it is a critical part of the evaluation to establish if hearing loss is present and whether it is conductive or sensorineural
- **Audiogram**: The expected conductive hearing loss with variable ABG is demonstrated. The variable AB -gap can be suggestive for the underlying pathology. Generally, a perforation will cause a conductive hearing loss between 5 and 40 dB depending on its characteristics [53]. The results of the audiogram should always be correlated with the physical exam, including Weber and Rinne tuning fork tests, especially when a masking dilemma is present. If the audiogram and tuning fork exam are not concordant, surgery should not be performed until correct testing.
- A mixed or sensorineural hearing loss may indicate more extensive disease and should alert the otologists of impending complications such inner ear extension of the disease (labyrinthitis).

6.11 Imaging Studies

For patients with CSOM, a high-resolution temporal bone CT scan may provide additional informations, especially when clinical findings are in favour of a safe ear but with complex clinical presentations as

- a long standing disease with recurrent episodes of active inflammation,
- being unresponsive to medical treatment
- with suspected complications

Along with the scanographic aspect of the middle ear cleft in patients with CSOM, the **preoperative clinico-radiological correlations** may also orient **the surgical strategy**.

The following situations may be met:

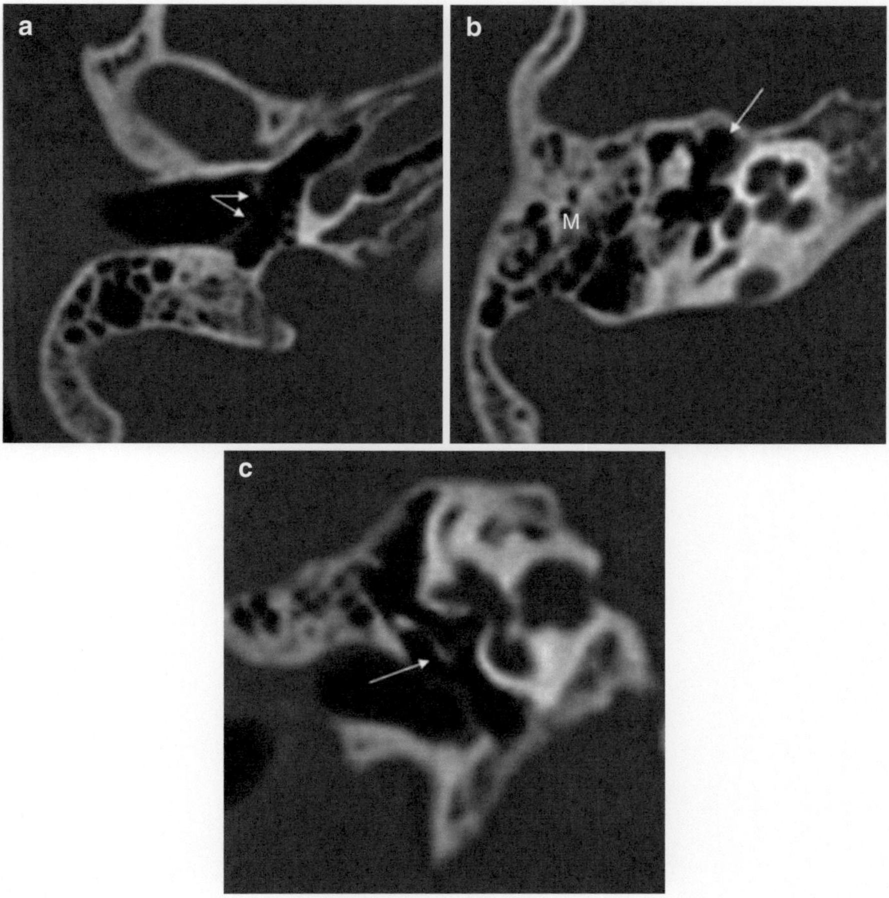

Fig. 6.25 CT images of a right ear of a 5 years old girl with CSOM: (**a**) axial view with a central inferior tympanic perforation (between the two arrows), (**b**) axial view passing by the incudomalleal chain: the AER is free (arrow), the mastoid is well aerated, without any condensation (M) and (**c**) coronal view with an intact ossicular chain, especially the incudostapedial joint

6.11.1 In Case of Anterior or Central Perforations, CT Confirms a "Safe Ear"

a) With an intact ossicular chain, or focal incudostapedial lysis and a good aeration of the supradiaphragmatic AAA spaces (Fig. 6.25)

→ ***Strategy*****: Sequelae repair only**

b) With an intact ossicular chain or incudostapedial lysis but *extended condensation images in the AAA spaces* (Fig. 6.26)

→ ***Strategy: in addition to sequelae repair, surgery should deal with the mucosal disease and free the ventilation pathways by mastoepitympantomy***

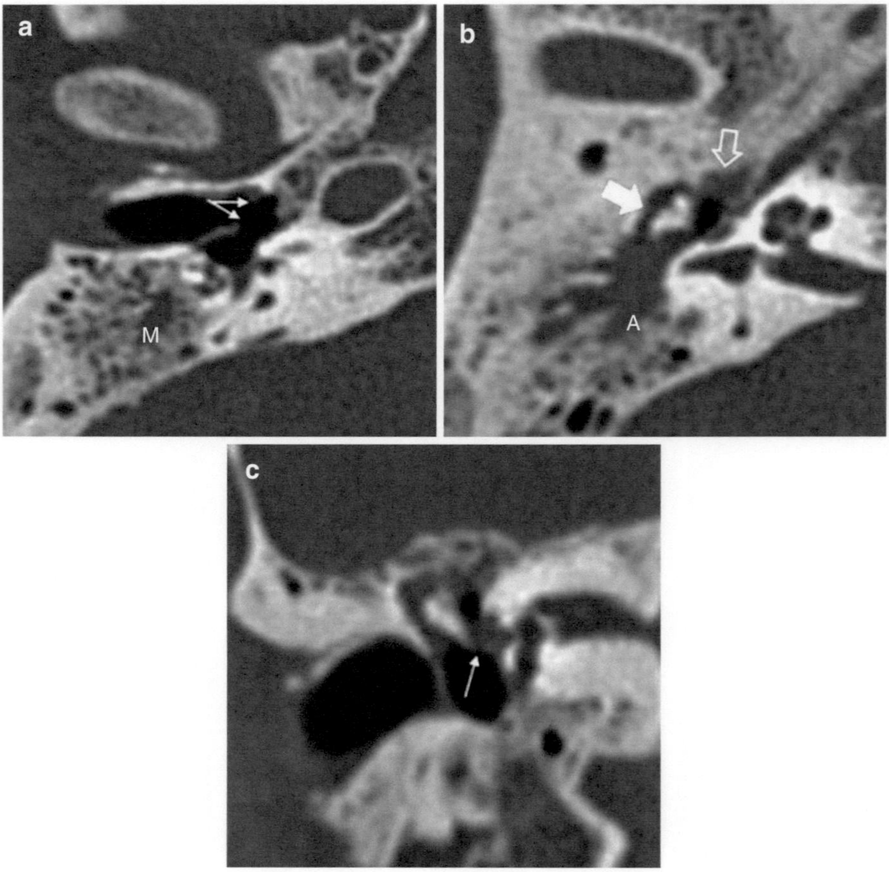

Fig. 6.26 CT-Imaging of the right ear of a 62 year-old patient with CSOM: (**a**) axial CT-image: anterior perforation of the thickened tympanic membrane with well visualized margins (between the two arrows); M = major mastoid cell condensation, (**b**) the axial CT-view passing by the incudomalleolar chain: the AER (empty arrow), the attic (plain arrow) the antrum (A) = the three AAA spaces are completely condensated and (**c**) coronal CT-reconstruction: interruption of the incudostapedial chain (long arrow)

6.11.2 In Case of Posterior or Any Marginal Perforations

a) CT is considered in favor of a "safe ear":

When the ossicular chain is intact, and the condensation images occupy most AAA spaces but do not demonstrate an appearance of round borders or a "mass effect" (Fig. 6.27).

→ ***Strategy*****: Surgery is oriented to a masto-epitympanotomy (aeration) and sequelae repair**

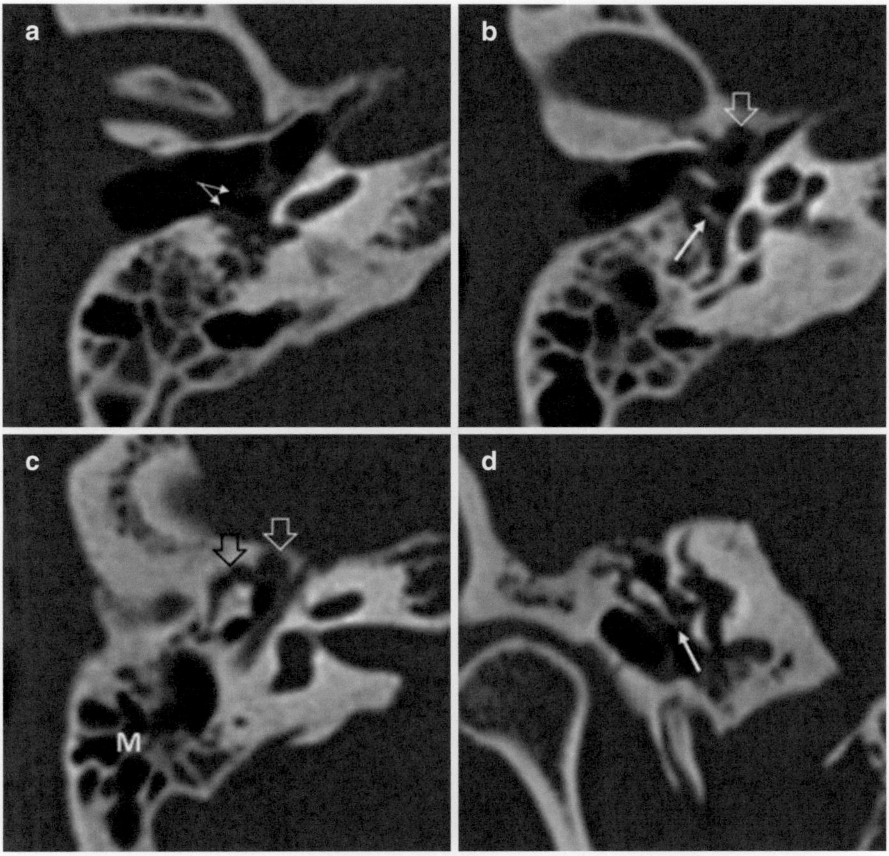

Fig. 6.27 CT-Imaging of the right ear of a 48 year-old patient with CSOM: (**a**) axial CT-image: posterior perforation (between two short arrows), (**b**) axial CT-image: continuity of the incudostapedial joint (arrow), condensation images around the ossicular chain and mucosal thickening of the supratubal recess (empty arrow), (**c**) axial CT-image: complete opacification of the AER (empty white arrow), condensations of the lateral attic (empty black arrow), partial condensations of the mastoid (M) and (**d**) coronal CT-reconstruction: intact incudo stapedial joint (long arrow)

b) CT becomes suspicious of an "unsafe" ear:

With advanced ossicular chain lysis and/or condensation images showing an aspect of "mass effect" (Fig. 6.28).

→ ***Strategy:*** **Surgery must be oriented to deal with a possible unsafe ear**.

c) CT becomes diagnostic for Cholesteatoma, if bony borders of the cavity became lytic, or the mastoid trabeculations disappear (Fig. 6.29)

→ **Strategy → see cholesteatoma treatment (see Sect. 8.10)**.

A summary of the clinico-radiologic assessment of ears with CSOM is given in Table 6.1.

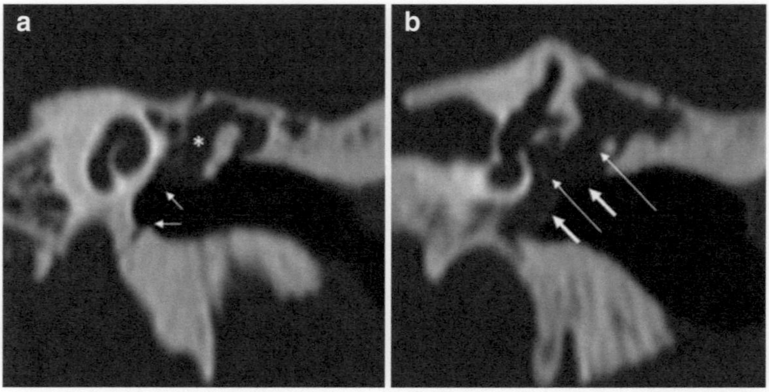

Fig. 6.28 CT with coronal reconstructions of a left ear of a 24-year-old patient with CSOM and a large antero-inferior perforation: (**a**) large antero-inferior perforation, likely marginal (between the two arrows), condensation of the whole attic (asterisk), (**b**) condensations of the cavity with rounded borders, “mass effect” (short thick arrows) and extended lysis of the long process of the incus (between the long arrows)

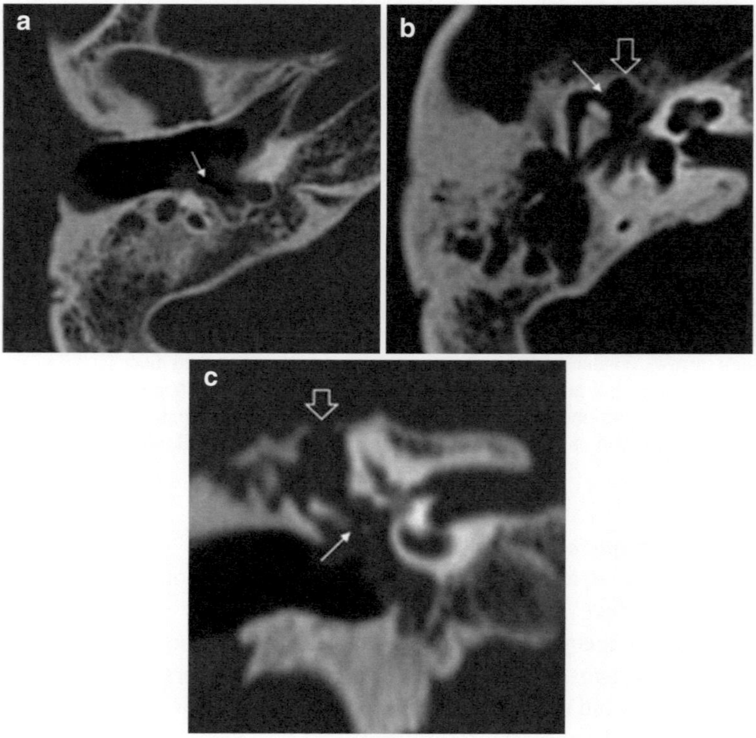

Fig. 6.29 Right ear of a 54 year old man, cholesteatoma developed on a posterior perforation. (**a**) Axial CT-image: posterior perforation (arrow), (**b**) axial CT-image: lytic cog (arrow), AER condensation (empty arrow) and (**c**) coronal CT: lyses of the incudostapedial chain (arrow), bony erosion of the tegmen (empty arrow)

Table 6.1 Clinico-radiologic assessment of TM-perforations

Site of TM perforation	CT: ossicular lysis	CT: condensations	Diagnostic features
Central perforation	No ossicular lysis	No condensations	Safe ear
Anterior perforation	Incudo stapedial lysis	AAA condensations, major condensations	Safe ear
Antero-inferior or posterior perforation	No ossicular lysis	AAA condensations (no rounded borders)	Safe ear
Marginal perforation	Any suspected ossicular lysis	Any condensation image with rounded borders	Suspicious of an unsafe ear
Marginal or posterior perforation	Ossicular lysis, bony lysis: mastoid septa, scutum, cog, tegmen	Condensations with rounded borders, mass effect, sometimes slightly hyper-dense, associated to TS	Unsafe ear (cholesteatoma)

6.12 Treatment of CSOM

6.12.1 Medical Treatment

The aim of the medical treatment is to obtain a dry ear as early as possible before the decision making of surgery aiming to repair the sequelae with tympanoplasty. The systemic medical treatment is of 10–15 days duration and topical medical treatment should be of 6 weeks duration in order to obtain complete resolution of the inflammatory process. If all modalities of the medical treatment fail to obtain a dry ear during the expected delay, this type of treatment must be ceased.

The primary treatment modality for CSOM is a combination of aural toilet and topical antimicrobial drops. Systemic oral or parenteral antibiotics, although an option, are less commonly used at the start of the disease due to the fact that topical antibiotics in combination with aural toilet are able to achieve significantly higher tissue concentrations (about 100–1000 times greater) than systemic antibiotics

Actually, CSOM is difficult to control only with a topical treatment, especially in recurrent disease; in most cases it requires at the first or second episode a combined systemic antibiotherapy and systemic corticotherapy of limited time period to get a dry ear; however, this combination does not prevent from recurrence of the inflammatory/infectious process.

Successful topical therapy consists of three important components:

1. Regular adequate aural toilet,
2. Selection of appropriate antibiotic/steroid drops,
3. Control of granulation tissues.

Excluding complications, CSOM is treated effectively in the outpatient setting

6.12.1.1 Aural Toilet

In children with CSOM, aural toilet and topical treatment are sometimes difficult to perform in proper conditions.

Nevertheless aural toilet must be always done when possible:

- In-office suctioning to remove discharge and debris,
- Placing an ear wick to keep open an oedematous canal.
- Ototopical drops instillation to be insured

6.12.1.2 Ototopical Antibiotics-Steroid combination

6.12.1.3 The fluoroquinolones and aminoglycosides are the topical antibiotics for gram-negative (Pseudomonas etc.) and gram-positive (Staph aureus etc.).

Quinolones

Topical quinolones carry a low side-effect of cochlear toxicity and vestibulotoxicity, which are attributed to aminoglycosides. Dexamethasone is often used in combination with ciprofloxacin to reduce inflammation. The efficacy and low side-effect of topical quinolone explain their popularity.

Aminoglycosides: Gentamicin/Dexamethasone, and Tobramycin

All aminoglycosides have a significant potential cochlear and vestibular toxicity. Recent informations suggest that the potential for vestibular toxicity may be much higher, especially if preparations containing gentamicin are used. Despite the conclusion of several studies that the incidence of aminoglycoside-related hearing loss is at worst low, preferably local aminoglycosides must be avoided.

Neomycin and Polymyxin B

Dohar's studies indicate that fewer than 20% of gram-negative organisms remain sensitive to neomycin; however, polymyxin B continued to be effective for gram-negative bacteria.

pH Level of Drops

While low pH is an advantage when treating infections in the external auditory canal, the advantage is lost in the middle ear because the normal pH of the middle ear is neutral. These drops can be extremely painful if they penetrate into the middle ear. Ciprofloxacin and hydrocortisone combinations have a pH of 4.5–5.0, as do tobramycin and dexamethasone combinations.

Viscosity of Drops

Preparations containing a steroid are often of considerably higher viscosity. Polyviscous solutions may effectively coat and remain in contact with the infected tissues for longer periods.

Steroid-Containing Drops

A combination of topical antibiotic/anti-inflammatory is always advised. Topical anti-inflammatory action offers an important advantage in every topical treatment of CSOM, especially when significant amounts of granulation tissue are present.

6.12.1.4 Granulation Tissue Control

Granulation tissues can prevent topically applied antimicrobial agents from reaching the site of infection. Topical steroids are important and hasten the resolution of middle ear granulation. Surgery could be indicated for adequate removal of extended and important granulation tissue formations filling the ME compartments, the antrum and epitympanum.

6.12.1.5 Failure of Topical Treatment

In CSOM the failure of topical treatment alone is common. Associated systemic treatment should be the first line treatment.

Failures of topical combined antimicrobial/steroid therapy are almost always failures of delivery and not because of antimicrobial resistance; infectious debris, granulation tissue, cholesteatoma, cerumen, … Culture and sensitivity are of little benefit.

6.12.1.6 Systemic Antibiotherapy and Corticotherapy

Systemic Antibiotherapy

In most cases of active CSOM, a systemic antibiotherapy should be associated to topical treatment in order to obtain rapid and good control of the disease. Generally cultures reflect the dominating flora of the external canal not the ME or mastoid: in practice the pseudomonas in CSOM is the activated saprophytic pseudomonas of the ear canal, a consequence of otorrhea and necrotic inflammation tissue.

Quinolones, mainly Ciprofloxacin, are the drugs of choice for treatment of CSOM, however, they should not be used in children below 12 years because of the potential side effect on growth problems related to tendons and joints.

Amoxil-Clavulanate could be prescribed but is not always efficient. **Erythromycin or Bactrim** are antibiotics that are recommended for children. **Macrolides** have a very good intra tissular penetration and concentration in inflammatory mucosa.

All systemic aminoglycosides should be avoided.

Systemic Corticotherapy

Systemic corticotherapy for few days followed by tapering doses for another few days enhances the therapeutic control of the active inflammatory process and reduces exudates and transudates secretion by middle ear mucosa. In medical practice, steroids proved to shorten the duration of otorrhea reaching rapidly a dry ear.

6.12.1.7 Eustachian Tube Management in CSOM

Different aspects of therapeutical procedures have been tried to deal with the ET inflammation process in order to obtain rapidly a dry ear either with ET cannulation through the nasopharyngeal orifice [60] or through catheterism from the tympanic ostium with antibiotic/steroid solutions. In adults, the placement of a transtubal catheter of 1mm of diameter, installed through the ET ostium passing by the tympanic membrane perforation under general anesthesia, has been done in the past by one of the authors. Repetitive Eustachian tube lavage with a combined solution of antibiotics and steroids (1 cc) during one week has been reported to be very helpful to control active forms of CSOM [61]. It remains that this form of treatment is not yet common in today's practice.

6.12.1.8 Bacteriophages Treatment

Bacteriophages are viruses that specifically and uniquely destroy bacteria. Bacteriophages can be a viable option for the treatment of bacterial infections due to the emergence of multidrug-resistant strains [62–64]. Bacteriophages are considered safe, economical, self-replicating and effective bactericidal agents [65, 66]. In a small controlled clinical trial with 24 patients, bacteriophages provided efficient protection and demonstrated efficacy against chronic otitis media caused by chemo resistant *P. aeruginosa* [67].

6.12.1.9 Summary of Medical Treatments (Fig. 6.30)

In summary, medical treatment of CSOM must be based, at the first episode of the disease, preferably on a combined topical and systemic antibiotic-steroid combinations to be maintained long enough (topical during 6 weeks and systemic not more

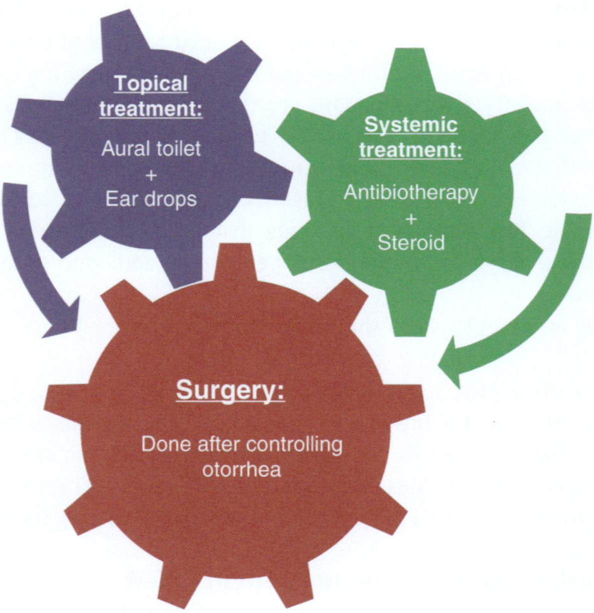

Fig. 6.30 Management strategy of CSOM

than 2 weeks) until achieving a dry ear. It is of utmost importance to face such disease efficiently at its initial phase in order to shorten the likelihood of a long duration of the inflammatory episode and at the same time avoid extensive structural and functional ME sequelae.

If CSOM fails to respond to a combination of topical and systemic therapy, surgery should be considered: tympanomastoidectomy with removal of granulations blocking the tympanic diaphragm can decrease the inflammatory process, eliminate infection and stop otorrhea in the majority of patients.

6.13 Surgery for Chronic Suppurative Middle Ear Without Cholesteatoma (Safe Ears)

Surgery of CSOM (Tympanoplasty) consists of treating the middle ear mucosal disease in addition to repair of CSOM sequelae, mainly eardrum and ossicles reconstruction.

6.13.1 Functional Considerations of Tympanoplasty

In order to insure the best possible hearing results when engaging the reconstruction of the middle ear, surgical procedures must be done according to the basic principles of ME mechanics and the mechanisms of acoustic sound gain.

Restoration of the "middle ear transformer mechanism" requires a secure connection between an intact tympanic membrane and inner ear fluids. The tympanic membrane should close an air-filled, mucosa-lined middle ear cavity. Traditional teaching attributes most of the middle ear gain to the hydraulic effect, which is the ratio of the effective vibrating area of the tympanic membrane to the area of the mobile stapes footplate. Round window protection to avoid phase cancellation (i.e., when sound impacts the oval and round windows at the same time) was also thought to be an important contributor to effective sound transmission to the inner ear. More recent investigations of human middle ear mechanisms modified these classic teachings.

Sound can be transmitted from the ear canal to the cochlea by two mechanisms: the ossicular and the acoustic coupling. Ossicular coupling is the sound pressure gain that occurs through the tympanic membrane and the ossicular chain. Acoustic coupling is the difference in the sound pressure that is acting directly on the oval and round windows. In normal ears (Fig. 6.31), acoustic coupling is negligible, but it may play a significant role in diseased and reconstructed ears (Figs. 6.32 and 6.33).

6.13.1.1 Ossicular Coupling

Ossicular coupling involves the transmission of sound pressure through the tympanic membrane and ossicular chain via the oval window. In such a state, sound pressure is deflected during passage through the air-fluid interface, resulting in a

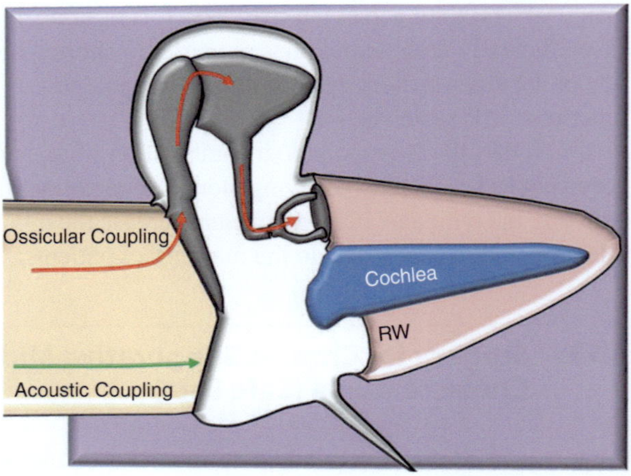

Fig. 6.31 Middle ear mechanics in normal ear

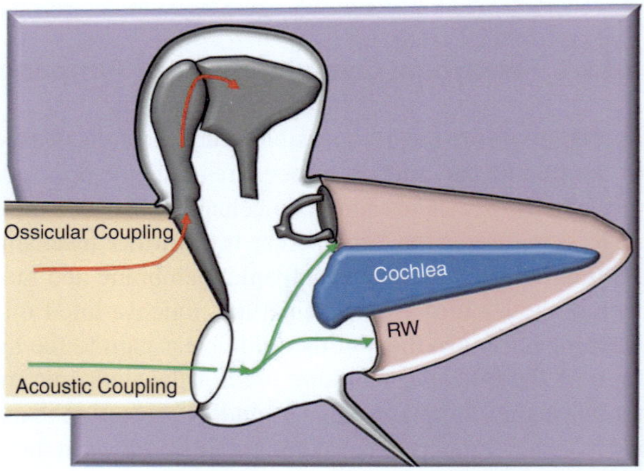

Fig. 6.32 Middle ear mechanics in ear with tympanic membrane perforation and ossicular chain discontinuity. Acoustic coupling with sound pressure difference on oval window and round window is the main mechanism for transmitting sound energy into the cochlea. Sound energy through ossicular coupling will not reach the cochlea

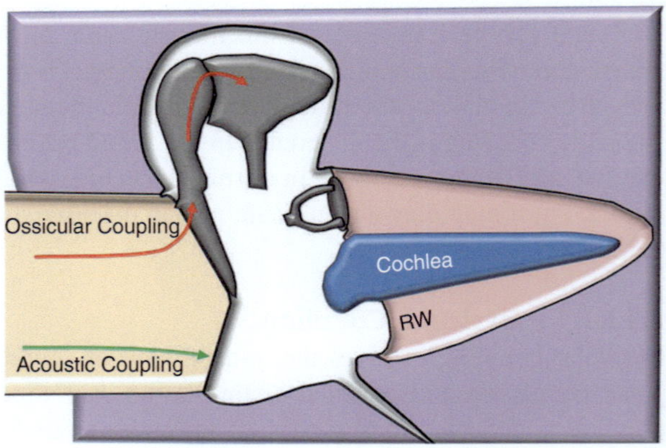

Fig. 6.33 Middle ear mechanics in ear with intact tympanic membrane and ossicular chain discontinuity. Sound energy will not reach the cochlea neither through ossicular coupling nor through acoustic coupling which will result in a maximal conductive hearing loss

loss of gain in the realm of 30 dB. The coupling effect of the tympanic membrane and ossicles overcomes almost this loss (Fig. 6.31).

Ossicular coupling has been attributed to the collective effect of three characteristics of the tympano-ossicular mechanism traditionally known as the *acoustic transformer theory*.

- The first and most significant of these characteristics is the *hydraulic lever effect* that results from the difference between the surface area of the tympanic membrane relative to that of the oval window (usually a ratio of nearly 21:1). This effect results in a compression of the sound energy and an increase in force at the oval window, equating to a theoretic approximate increase in gain of 26 dB.
- The second characteristic is the *malleoincudal lever effect* that results from the difference in length between the malleus manubrium relative to that of the long process of the incus along the axis of ossicular rotation (a ratio of 1.3:1). However, this effect only accounts for an additional 2 dB theoretical increase in gain.
- The final factor is the so-called *catenary lever effect* that is generated by the elastic stretching of the tympanic membrane from the annulus to the malleus manubrium (somewhat akin to the stretched strings across a tennis racquet). The specific degree of acoustic benefit derived from the catenary effect is not well understood but probably lies within a range similar to that of the malleoincudal lever).

The pressure gain that results from ossicular coupling in normal ears is frequency-dependent, and its magnitude is less than traditionally believed. The mean middle ear gain is about 20 dB between 250 and 500 Hz, reaches a maximum of about 25 dB around 1 kHz, and then decreases at about 6 dB at frequencies greater than 1 kHz.

A perforation of the tympanic membrane causes hearing loss by reducing the difference in sound pressure across the two sides of the tympanic membrane, causing decreased ossicular coupling. Hearing loss is proportional to the size of perforation and is frequency dependent, with the largest losses occurring at the lowest sound frequencies. It also varies inversely with the volume of the middle ear airspace (including the mastoid); this may explain why seemingly identical perforations in size and location produce different degrees of hearing loss, and why hearing loss may fluctuate in a given perforation with the presence or absence of otorrhea, which would decrease middle ear and mastoid airspace, thus increasing the hearing loss. More recent investigations also suggest that hearing loss does not vary appreciably with the location of perforation, in contrast to the long-held belief that posteroinferior perforations result in greater hearing loss than perforations at other locations owing to increased phase cancellation at the round window.

6.13.1.2 Acoustic Coupling

The sound stimulation of the inner ear involves direct passage of sound pressure via the oval and round windows without involvement of the tympanic membrane or ossicular chain. This is known as *acoustic coupling*. *Given an intact tympanic membrane and functional ossicular chain, this pathway is of only minor importance* (Fig. 6.31). However, in the various conditions of a diseased middle ear, acoustic coupling can be important (Fig. 6.32). This is why, for example, a conductive hearing loss will be greater in the case of ossicular discontinuity and an intact tympanic membrane (60 dB) compared with ossicular discontinuity and an absent tympanic membrane (40–50 dB). With the former, the intact tympanic membrane restricts the acoustic coupling pathway by blocking direct access of sound pressure to the oval and round window membranes (Fig. 6.33).

6.13.1.3 Phase Difference

A final relevant consideration in middle ear acoustic mechanics is that of *phase difference*. A sound stimulus to the inner ear is detected as the net difference in sound pressures applied to the round and oval windows that results in movement of intracochlear fluids. If these sound pressures are simultaneously applied to the round and oval windows with equal amplitude and phase, they will counteract each other and no resultant intracochlear fluid displacement will occur. In the normal situation, this does not occur due to the unbalanced selective effect of ossicular coupling upon the oval window, the acoustic shielding effect of the tympanic membrane upon the round window, and the uneven anatomical positioning of the round window versus the oval window relative to an incoming sound. However, when the tympano-ossicular mechanism is absent and acoustic coupling is primarily relied upon (as in the case of a type IV, or V tympanoplasty), an unshielded round window can yield significant negative acoustic consequences due to phase cancellation.

6.13.1.4 Middle Ear Aeration

Aeration of the middle ear plays an important role in sound transmission. In addition to contributing to normal stapes-cochlear impedance, aeration is crucial for normal ossicular coupling. The compressible air within the middle ear allows the tympanic membrane and the ossicles to move. In the normal human middle ear, sound pressure in the ear canal is higher than sound pressure within the middle ear; tympanic membrane motion is driven by this pressure difference.

Impaired middle ear aeration can adversely affect ossicular coupling by altering a pressure difference that is important to middle ear function. Reductions in middle ear air volume that result from disease or surgery lead to elevated middle ear airspace impedance and an increase in middle ear sound pressure. This leads to a reduction in the pressure difference across the tympanic membrane, with a subsequent reduction in tympanic membrane and ossicular motion. The minimum amount of air required to maintain ossicular coupling within 10 dB of normal hearing has been estimated to be 0.5 mL.

6.13.2 Tympanoplasty Types

Tympanoplasty is a surgical procedure performed to eradicate infection and restore the function of the middle ear.

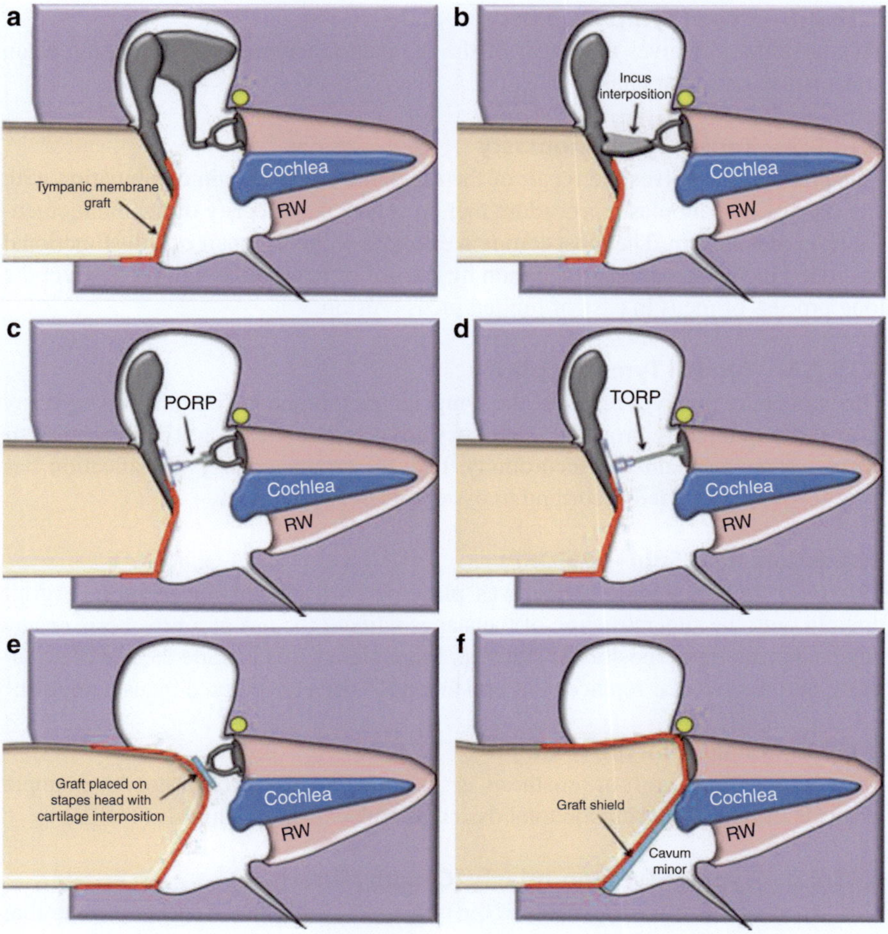

Fig. 6.34 Different types of tympanoplasty

Wullstein introduced a classification for tympanoplasty that is based on two factors:

1. The remaining structures of the middle ear after all pathology has been eradicated, and
2. How sound is transferred to the oval window while the round window is being protected.

Subsequent modifications of Wullstein's classification have been based on the underlying properties of acoustic mechanics associated with each tympanoplasty type (Fig. 6.34).

The presence of different tympanoplasty techniques is an indication that the otologic surgeon should be flexible when tailoring the procedure to fit the disease, rather than having a "one-size-fits-all" approach to surgery for chronic ear disease.

6.13.2.1 Type I Tympanoplasty

This procedure involves the repair of the tympanic membrane in the setting of an intact native ossicular chain.

6.13.2.2 Type II Tympanoplasty

This procedure involves the repair of the tympanic membrane in combination with any type of ossiculoplasty procedure that preserves the integrity of the malleoincudal lever mechanism. The most common example of this is repair of a dysfunctional or eroded incudostapedial articulation by the use of bone cement to reconstruct the long process of incus in case of limited incus erosion.

6.13.2.3 Type III Tympanoplasty

This procedure involves repair of the tympanic membrane in combination with any type of ossiculoplasty procedure that does not preserve the integrity of the malleo-incudal lever mechanism. Accordingly, type III tympanoplasty classification has been further subdivided according to ossiculoplasty technique.

Stapes Columella Subtype (PORP)

This type III tympanoplasty involves placement of a tympanic membrane graft directly onto the superstructure of the stapes *without* the use of a prosthesis or any other substantial interpositional material. Examples of this include the use of a synthetic partial ossicular replacement prosthesis (PORP) or sculpted incus autograft.

Major Columella Subtype (TORP)

The interpositional graft or prosthesis is set upon the stapes footplate. An example of this is the use of a synthetic total ossicular replacement prosthesis (TORP).

6.13.2.4 Type IV Tympanoplasty (Cavum Minor)

This procedure involves the repair of the tympanic membrane in such a manner that the boundary between the mucosal lining of the middle ear space and the epithelialized lateral compartment (external auditory canal, open mastoid cavity, epitympanum) is shifted in a way that renders the stapes footplate externalized as part of the latter. As a result, the tympanic cavity is divided into a smaller-than-normal aerated space in continuity with the Eustachian tube, termed the cavum minor, in which the round window is acoustically shielded, and an external component in which the mobile stapes footplate is covered by a thin epithelial layer and is directly exposed to incoming sound energy. It remains that this type of surgery is not fruitful as expected.

6.13.3 Selection of Cases for Tympanoplasty (Fig. 6.35)

Tympanoplasty should be considered when there is a conductive hearing loss of 30 dB or greater in an ear with COM that has a good cochlear function. Tympanoplasty is contraindicated in a dead ear or in an ear with poor cochlear function. Similarly,

Tympanoplasty

Indications	Contraindications	Relative Contraindications
• Marginal perforation • Recurrent otorrhea • Persistent otorrhea despite medical treatment • Conductive hearing loss • Disturbed quality of life (swimming, shower,...) • Imaging evidence of chronic otomastoiditis	• Only hearing ear or significantly better hearing ear • No cochlear function • Serious systemic illness	• Eustachian tube dysfunction • Very young age • Inactive disease with poor cochlear function • Diabetes

Fig. 6.35 Selection of cases for tympanoplasty

tympanic adhesive fibrosclerosis or tympanic epidermization is a contraindication because of the risks of non-aeration, prosthesis extrusion, and iatrogenic cholesteatoma.

Tympanoplasty carries a small risk of inducing a sensorineural hearing loss. Therefore it is important that the cochlear function in the contralateral ear is at an adequate level, and an only hearing ear or much better hearing ear is a contraindication for tympanoplasty.

Children younger than 5 years are poor candidates for tympanoplasty because of risk of subsequent failure from otitis media and poor Eustachian tube function. For the elderly, and for adults with serious medical problems, one has to determine whether the benefits of surgery outweigh the risks of anesthesia.

It is important to determine whether the CSOM in the considered ear is active or inactive.

Active CSOM should be treated medically to control infection and eliminate otorrhea, thus converting the process to inactive COM. Expectant observation for 6 months is recommended, and if the ear remains dry, then elective tympanoplasty may be performed. For patients who succeed to get a dry ear with the medical treatment and they are at their first episode of CSOM, the timing of surgery could be selected according to seasonal factors or patient preferences hoping that the ear remains dry while waiting for the surgery.

Failure of medical management in active CSOM generally indicates the need for combining mastoidectomy with tympanoplasty. When patients fail to get a dry ear despite a correctly applied medical treatment, surgery must be proposed without delay in order to avoid progress of sequelae.

Ears that drain intermittently need attention to obvious inciting events such as water exposure to control otorrhea. If there are no obvious predisposing events, then mastoidectomy is recommended in conjunction with tympanoplasty to eliminate infection and granulation in the mastoid tracts, antrum, and epitympanum. When patients report recurrent episodes of active otorrhea shortly after getting a dry ear and following repetitive medical treatment, surgery must be proposed without delay (within 8 weeks of a dry ear period) in order to avoid further episodes of suppuration.

In patients with bilateral COM, determining which ear to operate on first, depends on the severity of CSOM and the severity of conductive hearing loss. In general, the ear with more active disease should be chosen first. With bilateral inactive disease, the poorer hearing ear should be operated on first.

The hearing benefit perceived after tympanoplasty depends not only on the magnitude of improvement in air-bone gap but also on the level of cochlear function in the operated ear, the hearing level in the contralateral ear, and the symmetry of hearing levels between the two ears.

Patients may express disappointment that their hearing has not improved as much as they had expected. The following initial conditions seem most likely to result in dissatisfied patients with their hearing improvement:

1. Excellent hearing in one ear and a moderate-to-severe mixed type hearing loss in the surgical ear,
2. longstanding unilateral loss,
3. a postoperative hearing level that still requires a hearing aid despite of successful surgery, and
4. a conductive hearing loss as shown by audiometry but with a positive Rinne test at 256 and 512 Hz. In patients with these conditions, the degree of expected improvement must be fully discussed with them preoperatively to ensure that they have a realistic expectation of what can be achieved.

6.13.3.1 Special Considerations in Pediatric Patients

1. There is a need to free the nasopharyngeal area of the child: Adenoidectomy and possibly tonsillectomy must be evoked before engaging the ME ear surgery.
2. Eustachian tube catheterism could be of help to reduce oedema of the tube and recover aeration function; however mucosal ulceration and traumatic tubing of the ET must be prevented to avoid post cannulation stenosis or fibrosis
3. The authors' approach to pediatric patients is to avoid repairing the tympanic membrane during the otitis-prone years (≤5 years). ME reconstruction is preferably done at the age of 6–9 years old when the ET structure has reached its mature position and functions. Children have shorter, more horizontal tubes, immature floppy elastic cartilage, and larger adenoids compared with adults, which place them at a higher risk for obstruction and reflux of nasopharyngeal secretions and pathogens. The Eustachian tube in children usually reaches adult length by the age of 6 [68, 69]
4. In pediatric cases adjustment with school activities and swimming is important.

6.14 Surgical Techniques in Tympanoplasty (Middle Ear Reconstruction)

Modern tympanoplasty techniques have common ground in that they endeavor to

1. ***Reconstruct the tympanic membrane***
2. ***Perform proper reconstruction of ossicular chain (mechanics)***
3. ***Restore an adequate ME spaces aeration***

6.14.1 Tympanic Membrane Repair (Myringoplasty)

The common goals of tympanic membrane repair are to:

- Create a barrier between the dry lateral epithelialized compartment (eardrum, external auditory canal) and the moist medial mucosal compartment (middle ear, Eustachian tube)
- Provide reinforcement to correct tympanic membrane weaknesses in order to resist future disease processes (atelectasis, perforation)
- Create an optimized sound-conducting platform for ossicular coupling or a round window shield for acoustic coupling depending on tympanoplasty type
- Create a contour favorable for outward keratin debris migration

6.14.1.1 Surgical Approaches

Three main approaches are used in tympanoplasty: transcanal, endaural, and postauricular. The choice of the approach depends on the perforation size, the anatomy of the external auditory canal, and the surgeon's preference. The selection of any approach must be decided case by case and relative to the best comfortable experience of the surgeon. Most importantly, the selected approach should provide complete visualization of the perforation.

- The transcanal approach: it is the least invasive approach with the most rapid recovery. It is used for small posterior perforations or for medium-sized perforations, when the ear canal anatomy is favorable, and the entire perforation and an anterior tympanic membrane rim can be seen. The transcanal approach should be avoided in cases in which the anterior margin of the perforation is not well visualized, particularly in the hands of surgeons with less experience.
- The endaural approach can be used with all perforations and is more commonly used in Europe; it is most useful if a limited atticotomy is anticipated in conjunction with tympanoplasty.
- The postauricular approach: it can be used with all perforation sizes, and offers a better angle of visualization of the anterior tympanic membrane, even without canalplasty (Fig. 6.36).

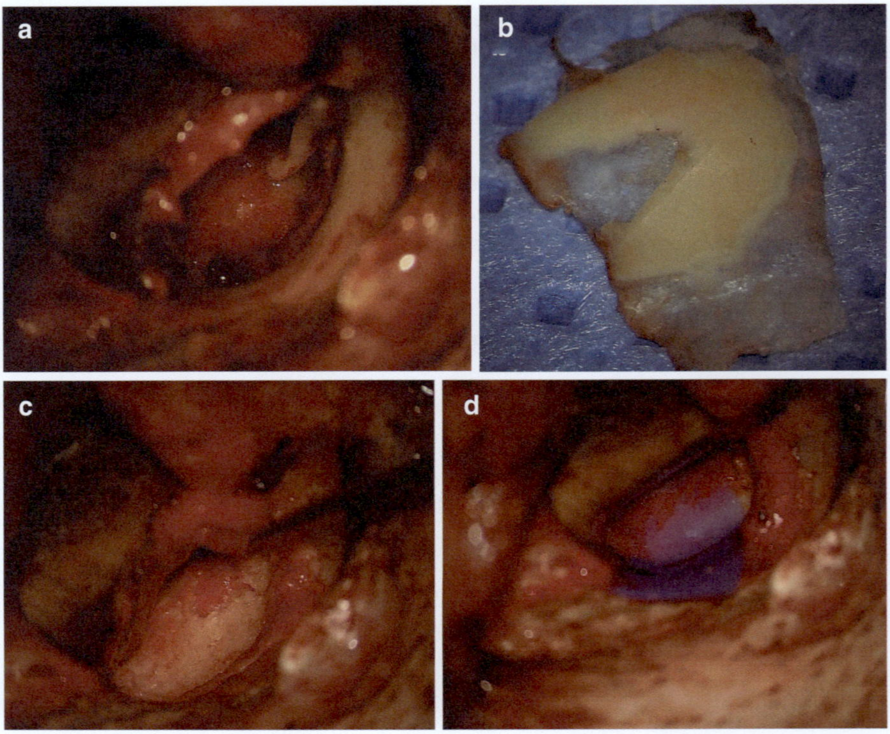

Fig. 6.36 Basic principles of tympanoplasty are shown on this left ear with subtotal perforation. (**a**) through a post-auricular approach, the edges of the perforation are refreshed and then the tympanomeatal flap is raised until we reach the anterior margin of the perforation. (**b**) a tragal cartilage is harvested with perichondrium on one side. a V-shaped notch is created to adapt the handle of malleus. (**c**) the cartilage is placed under the tympanomeatl flap and above the malleus. (**d**) the flap is returned back on the graft and a silastic sheet is placed above the flap

In case of anterior perforation, narrow ear canal, bulging of the anterior wall of the EAC, a bony drilling of the canal wall (canalplasty) enables the good exposure.

6.14.1.2 Graft Selection

Many different tissue grafts have been described for repair of the TM including temporalis fascia, perichondrium, cartilage, periosteum, and fat graft.

Temporalis fascia is the most commonly used material for the repair of tympanic membrane perforations. Temporalis fascia can be harvested at the time of tympanoplasty through a small incision posterosuperior to the helix in the hair-bearing scalp when using a transcanal approach. Tragal perichondrium is frequently used in tympanoplasty, particularly if there is no temporalis fascia available (e.g., in cases of multiple revisions) or if a composite cartilage/perichondrium graft is needed to prevent retraction of the reconstructed membrane when there is suspected persistent Eustachian tube dysfunction.

The fascia temporalis is the most commonly used graft, desired for its pliability with success rates between 93 and 97% in primary tympanoplasty, especially in well-aerated middle ears. One of the redraw of fascia is that it carries a risk of later re-perforation because of graft atrophy or infection.

Recently, the use of cartilage has been increasingly described for the reconstruction of large portions of the pars tensa of the tympanic membrane in cases of subtotal perforation or recurrent perforation. Although one might anticipate a significant conductive hearing loss with cartilage because of its thickness and rigidity, our clinical observations suggest no difference in hearing results with cartilage or fascia. Cartilage is well tolerated by the middle ear, and long-term survival is the norm. Cartilage graft seems to be nourished largely by diffusion and becomes well incorporated in the tympanic membrane. One major advantage of the cartilage graft is that it retains its rigid quality and resists resorption and retraction, even in the milieu of continuous Eustachian tube dysfunction (Figs. 6.37 and 6.38).

Different Graft Materials in Tympanoplasty	
Fascia	Good results, easiness
Perichondrium	Same properties, easy to manipulate for beginners
Cartilage	Stronger but needs to be thinned
	Revision procedure or primary when at risk
Fat	Small perforations, inlay, outpatient procedure

Fig. 6.37 Different graft materials used in tympanoplasty

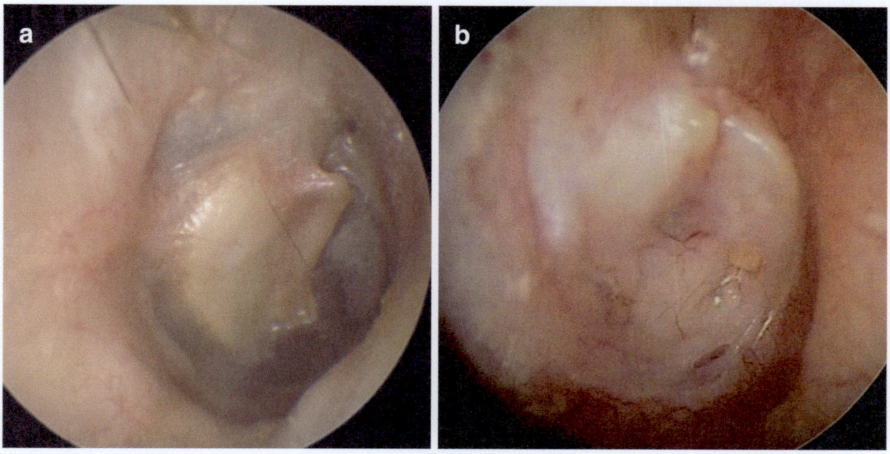

Fig. 6.38 (**a**) Two years after right ear cartilage tympanoplasty for posterior perforation. (**b**) One year after right ear cartilage tympanoplasty for subtotal perforation showing the good vascularization of the graft. The major advantage of cartilage graft is that it retains its rigid quality and resists to reperforation or retraction

Fat contains high population of multipotent cells referred as adipose-derived stem cells which are similar in activity to those of the bone marrow derived mesenchymal stem cells in the ability to differentiate into mesenchymal tissues such as endothelial and fibrous types promoting the healing process of the tympanic membrane [70]. Fat graft myringoplasty is an easy technique that is done under local anesthesia and has a good graft uptake rate. This justifies its use in the closure of small dry central TM perforations. Failure rate is higher in children and adult large perforations.

Two distinct techniques are commonly employed for cartilage reconstruction of the tympanic membrane: the perichondrium/cartilage island flap, which uses tragal cartilage, and the palisade technique, which uses cartilage from the tragus or cymba.

The palisade technique is preferred when ossicular reconstruction is needed with a malleus in place. In the remaining scenarios, the perichondrium/cartilage island flap is favored.

6.14.1.3 Graft Placement

Underlay and overlay techniques refer to the placement of the graft either medial or lateral to the tympanic membrane remnant. Although some surgeons advocate certain techniques for graft placement in a particular situation, the success of any technique depends on how well this technique is performed by the surgeon, rather than on the technique itself. Consequently, there should not be an absolute indication for a particular technique in a certain perforation. Underlay technique can be used to repair total perforations or in revision cases if done properly by an experienced surgeon.

The Underlay Technique (Fig. 6.39)

The underlay technique involves placing the graft material underneath (or medial to) the residual eardrum. The underlay technique requires:

- Refreshment of the edges of the perforation.
- Elevation of a tympanomeatal flap.

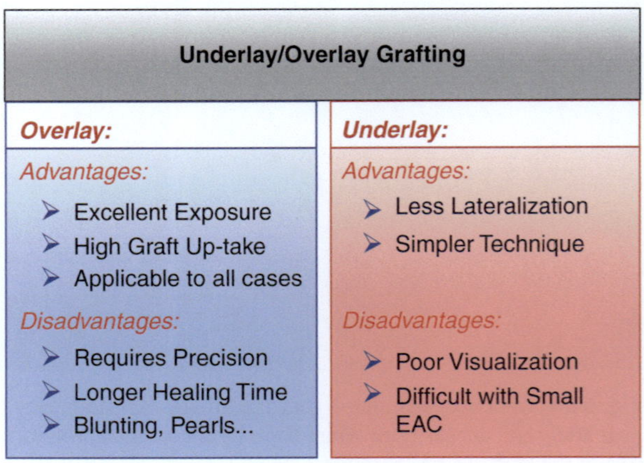

Fig. 6.39 Different graft placement techniques: advantages and disadvantages

- The graft material is tucked underneath the eardrum, supported with Gelfoam.
- The eardrum is flipped back to its normal resting position.
- The ear canal is filled with packing material.

The Overlay Technique (Fig. 6.39)

In the overlay technique, the graft is placed lateral to the fibrous layer of the tympanic membrane remnant, but medial to the malleus handle. This technique requires complete removal of the squamous epithelium from the lateral surface of the tympanic membrane remnant to avoid iatrogenic cholesteatoma formation. During elevation of the tympanomeatal flap, the annulus is left in the tympanic sulcus, and the dissection is transitioned from the bony external canal onto the lateral surface of the tympanic membrane, separating the superficial squamous layer from the middle fibrous layer. If the perforation is of medium size, the dissected epithelium can be left attached anteriorly and can be replaced on top of the graft. In total perforations, it is usually necessary to remove the skin of the external canal completely to ensure complete removal of squamous epithelium.

Although the graft is placed lateral to the annulus, it should be placed medial to the malleus handle to prevent lateralization. This is usually accomplished by cutting a vertical slit in the anterosuperior corner of the graft to accommodate the malleus handle. The trimmed anterior canal skin is repositioned with its thin medial part overlying approximately 1 mm of the graft. The anterior tympanomeatal angle should be maintained at an acute angle ($\leq 90°$) by placing pressed, rolled, and dry Gelfoam in the sulcus during healing. If the graft is placed on the anterior canal wall, or the acute anterior tympanomeatal angle is not preserved, a dead space is created that gets filled with fibrous tissue, resulting in blunting.

The vascular strip skin is placed back, with care taken to unfurl the skin edges to avoid burying epithelium.

6.14.1.4 Tympanic Membrane Repair Outcome

Success Rate

The success rate for tympanoplasty is considered quite high; it is usually reported as upwards of 90% in myringoplasty. It is instructive to note that, the few studies in the literature having assessed postoperative long-term hearing results and its changes, show a progressive and systematic decline in the initial hearing gain as a function of time [70–73].

There may be a higher failure rate in children, although this is not universally agreed upon. Tympanoplasty failure can be due to the following conditions:

1. Reperforation,
2. Graft lateralization,
3. Atelectasis,
4. Postop myringitis.

Any or all of the above can occur together.

Reperforation

The causes of **reperforation** may occur early or late. Early causes of reperforation are most often due to a faulty technique; late causes of failure are usually due to infection or ET dysfunction.

There are many reasons that could be attributed to a **faulty technique**. Inappropriate approach selection may have resulted in inadequate exposure of the tympanic membrane and surrounding structures, thus limiting visibility during the procedure. The graft may have been made too small. The graft may also have been placed improperly, allowing an edge to pull away from the supporting tympanic membrane remnant or to fall into the middle ear space.

Late causes of reperforation often relate to infection or graft atrophy. Persistent middle ear disease is undeniably the most common factor underlying a late graft reperforation. Persistent mucosal disease and disease in the mastoid cell system are major contributing factors. The common denominator for all middle ear disease is ultimately Eustachian tube dysfunction.

Graft Lateralization

Failure may also occur with **graft lateralization**. This most often occurs with the overlay technique of tympanic membrane grafting and is an inherent complication of the technique itself. Graft lateralization creates insufficient conduction of sound through the middle ear and can be quite difficult to reconstruct satisfactorily at a subsequent operation.

Atelectasis

The third way in which a tympanoplasty can fail is by postoperative atelectasis. This may be technical, caused by using a too thin graft, not reinforcing the graft with other materials, such as cartilage, or not ventilating the ear at the primary surgery. Although technical factors may play a role, the most common cause of postoperative atelectasis is the disease process, specifically, the Eustachian tube dysfunction.

Postoperative Myringitis

Postoperative myringitis is another condition that should be considered to be a graft failure. Hearing may be satisfactory and the middle ear protected; however, the patient may complain of pain, fullness, or otorrhea; this is a granular reaction of the lateral surface of the tympanic membrane graft. It can have a red or a velvety pink appearance. The etiology is uncertain, although an autoimmune response, reaction to topical agents used intraoperatively (including packing material), or a postoperative infection may be factors. If topical antibiotics, débridement, or silver nitrate cautery is not successful, revision tympanoplasty with excision of the diseased area may be necessary.

6.14.2 Ossicular Chain Reconstruction (Ossiculoplasty)

Best tympanoplasty results are obtained when the ossicular chain is intact; when the ossicles are disconnected; ossiculoplasty should be done in order to restore a stable sound transfer mechanism in the middle ear space. Ossicular chain reconstruction can be achieved by an allograft (bone or cartilage) or by a synthetic prosthesis. Most synthetic prostheses are divided into partial ossicular replacement prostheses (PORPs), to be used with an absent incus but a present stapes superstructure, and total ossicular replacement prostheses (TORPs), which are used when both the incus and stapes superstructure are absent or in poor anatomical position. A PORP usually consists of a head to make contact to the tympanic membrane and/or malleus and a shaft or cradle to fit the stapes capitulum and superstructure. A TORP is similar in design but with a shaft or wire that runs directly to the footplate.

6.14.2.1 Biomechanics of Ossiculoplasty

Several factors influence the results in ossiculoplasty, including the middle ear environment, the surgical technique, and the qualities of the prosthesis. The first factor is the most important determinant of long-term hearing outcomes with ossiculoplasty in the chronic ear. The next most important factor influencing results is surgical technique. By combining a fundamental understanding of middle ear mechanics and the consistent anatomical relationships that exist in even the diseased middle ear, the surgeon has a direct impact on results.

A-Biological Factors

There are a number of factors to be considered in reconstructing the middle ear. Biologic factors include the biocompatibility of the prosthesis, environment of the postoperative middle ear, and healing process.

1. Biocompatibility of the Prosthesis

Otology has been in search of the ideal ossicular replacement prosthesis via a variety of biologic or biocompatible materials. Biocompatibility depends on a prosthetic device remaining inert and stable in a biologic environment. If a material used in ossiculoplasty is perceived as foreign material by the human body, the prosthesis could become a nidus for chronic inflammation resulting in a failure of its objectives.

Polyethylene used in reconstruction in the late 1950s to early 1960s had some good initial results; however, this material was noted to induce an inflammatory reaction [74, 75].

Additionally, plastipore implants were criticized by studies that show frequent histologic evidence of multinucleated giant cells on plastipore implants [76, 77].

Titanium and hydroxylapatite prostheses are the most widely used and successful implants available at this time and have good mechanical properties, low extrusion rates, and good hearing results. More prospective trials will help delineate the differences between implants. Titanium prostheses are somewhat more “user friendly” and have therefore become more popular in recent years.

An interface of cartilage should be placed between all of the currently available prostheses and the tympanic membrane to minimize extrusion. Also it has been hypothesized that the cartilage acts to increase the “effective” area of the graft that is coupled to the stapes, which leads to an increase in the middle ear gain of the reconstructed ear [78]. Patients who underwent ossicular reconstruction with PORPs had slightly better postoperative hearing than did patients with TORPs. Postoperative hearing was essentially unchanged in approximately 55% of both groups.

2. Middle Ear Environment

The environment of the reconstructed middle ear must be conducive to optimal sound transfer. This includes repairing perforations and reconstructing a tympanic membrane that is capable of vibrating freely in response to acoustic energy. Middle ear negative pressure, effusion or granulation tissue in the middle ear, and fibrosis with tethering of the tympanic membrane or prosthesis, all can be detrimental to prosthetic extrusions and reconstruction failure.

(a) Status of Middle Ear Mucosa

Fibrotic middle ear mucosa and denuded mucosa during surgery are detrimental to hearing results compared with that of normal middle ear mucosa.

(b) Condition of the Ossicles

The presence of a malleus or stapes can also have different impact on the hearing outcome of ossiculoplasty.

The presence of stapes superstructure is very important for favorable hearing results. Clipping of PORP on the head of stapes offers a more stable connection, better coupling and less slippage compared with only a direct insertion on the footplate.

The presence of malleus is theoretically important for a favorable hearing outcome. The malleus is thought to provide better hearing results if incorporated in the reconstruction by preservation of the catenary lever.

Our clinical observation as well as that of other authors, however, did not report a substantial difference in the outcomes of ossiculoplasty relative to the presence or absence of the malleus [79].

B-Mechanical Factors

There are a number of mechanical factors to be considered in reconstructing the middle ear.

The primary goal of ossicular reconstruction is to reach a maximum of coupling the stapes footplate to the tympanic membrane to re-establish the hydraulic lever effect, which is the most significant mechanism of acoustic gain of the middle ear mechanism. This gain results from the difference between the surface area of the tympanic membrane relative to that of the oval window (usually a ratio of nearly 21:1).

1. Prosthesis Axis

The positioning of prosthesis appears to be important to its function [80]. Measurements in human temporal bone preparations suggest that the angle between the stapes and a prosthesis should be less than 45° for optimal sound transmission [81, 82], and that the neck of the malleus is a good contact point for TORPs [83] (Fig. 6.40).

While it is ideal to attach a prosthesis to the manubrium, experimental data show that acceptable results can occur with a prosthesis placed against the postero-superior quadrant of the tympanic membrane as long as approximately 3–4 mm of the prosthesis' diameter contacts the TM [84–86].

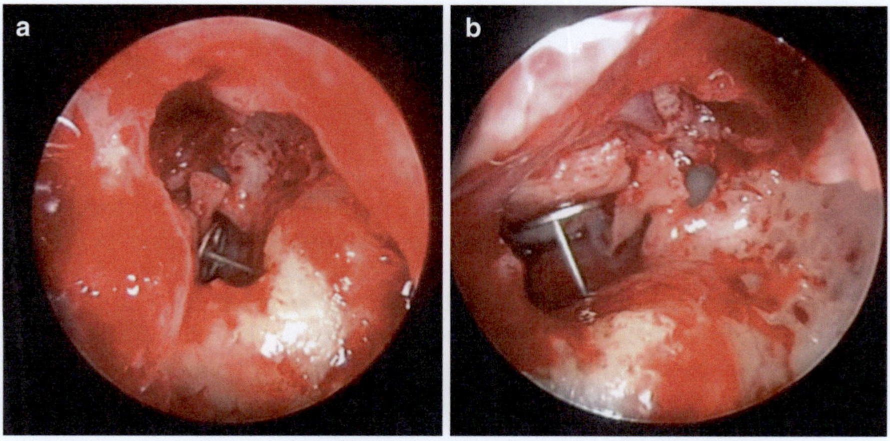

Fig. 6.40 Left ear TORP ossiculoplasty. (**a**) After middle ear reconstruction ended and ear pack is placed, a 30° scope was placed in the attic to visualize the prosthesis axis and was found to be inappropriate and (**b**) then the prosthesis was readjusted and checked again from the attic using angled scope to assess its appropriate axis

2. Tension

   The tension the prosthesis creates in the middle ear, which is generally a function of prosthesis length, appears critical in determining the hearing result [86].

   A prosthesis that is too long would stiffen the ME tympano-ossicular system resulting in a reduction of motion and of the closure of the air–bone gap.

3. Coupling

   Coupling refers to how well prosthesis adheres to the footplate or TM, and the degree of coupling will determine whether or not there is slippage at the end of the prosthesis. Thus, prosthesis transmits sound effectively only if there is good coupling at both ends. Clinical observations indicate that it is rare to obtain a firm union between a prosthesis and the stapes footplate. Hence, inadequate coupling at the prosthesis–footplate joint may be an important cause of a persistent postoperative air–bone gap. In order to achieve proper coupling, a Vario Kurz titanium prostheses is used where a pin on the head of the prosthesis is kept. Partial Ossicular Replacement Prosthesis (PORP) is crimped on the head of stapes and Total Ossicular Replacement Prosthesis (TORP) is coupled to the footplate by a cartilage shoe. Both prostheses are coupled to the drum by embedding a pin on the head plate of prosthesis in a full thickness broad cartilage palisades graft.

   Stable and reliable coupling between prostheses and the remaining ossicular rudiments is essential in order to achieve satisfactory hearing results following ossiculoplasty. Tilting and/or dislocation of the prosthesis, which prevents direct prosthesis–bone contact, are the major causes of poor postoperative audiometric results.

   Apart from biological reasons, prosthesis displacement is the most common cause of unsatisfactory hearing after such surgery.

In order to manage more successfully cases of type III tympanoplasty with a preserved stapedial arch, the use of the residual incus with good and adequate remodeling remains highly valuable regarding long term viability and hearing recovery. In addition a self-retaining, lightweight titanium prosthesis, fastened onto the stapes head with a clip mechanism is selected. In PORP, the cup is tighten to be clipped on the head of stapes for further stability. If the stapes suprastructure is missing, stable coupling of the prosthesis to the footplate is more complicated. Total ossicular replacement prostheses (TORPs) is performed with adequate coupling. A cartilage "shoe" of adequate dimensions, which fits into the oval window niche with a central perforation, guides the prosthesis onto the footplate centre and prevents dislocation. The cartilage shoe stabilises the TORP on the centre of the footplate surface, which is the optimal site for energy transfer.

6.14.2.2 Ossiculoplasty Strategies and Techniques (Fig. 6.41)

Basic Situation in Practice: *Medialized Malleus

In cases where the malleus handle is much medialized, the excision of the umbo is not recommended in order to avoid manubrium lysis and losing the good support of the graft (mechanics). In such situation, section of the tensor tympani ligament is accomplished to free and lateralize adequately the manubrium for better reconstruction. In every case of ossicular reconstruction, the malleus must be preserved for better success and stability.

Basic Situation in Practice: *Partial Erosion of Incudostapedial Joint

Distal erosion of the incus with an intact stapes superstructure is a common finding in CSOM ears. Our preferred technique involves the use of bone cement (Fig. 6.42).

The use of bone cement ossiculoplasty is very attractive because it preserves the configuration of native ossicles.

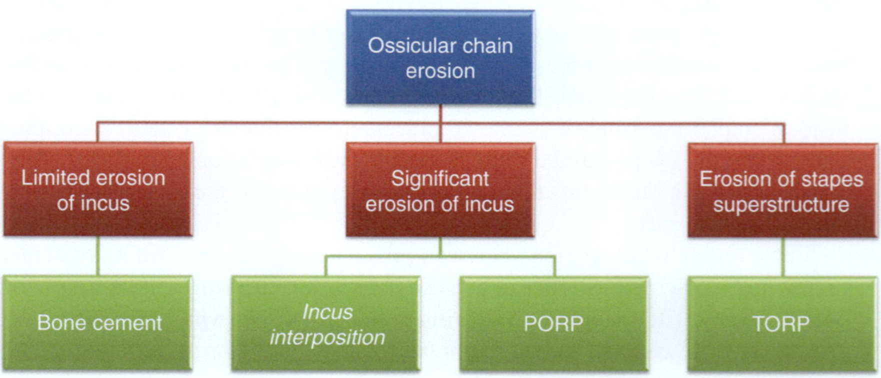

Fig. 6.41 Ossiculoplasty strategies

Good hearing results have been published using bone cement with more than 90% of the reconstructions showing an ABG closure of 20 dB or better [87–90].

No extrusions have been reported, probably because of the absence of contact between the cement and the tympanic membrane.

Basic Situation in Practice: *Eroded malleus

In case of selective erosion of handle of malleus, bone cement is to reconstruct the handle (Fig. 6.43).

Basic Situation in Practice: *Malleus and Stapes Present, Incus Missing

- ***Incus Interposition***

Incus interposition is the preferred type of reconstruction in this situation. An autologous incus is used whenever possible (Fig. 6.44). The incus interposition can

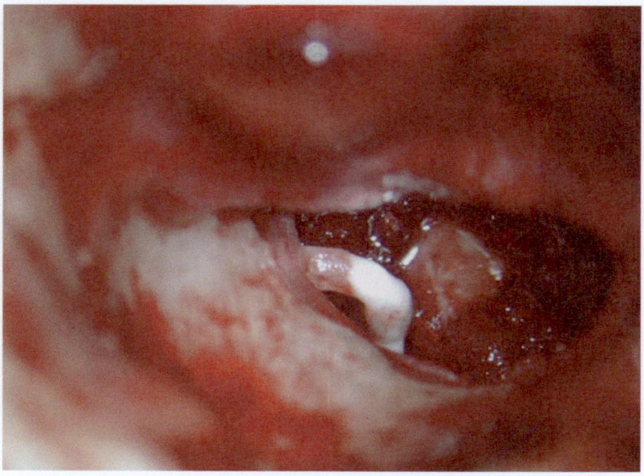

Fig. 6.42 Right ear intraoperative view showing reconstruction of the incudostapedial joint with bone cement

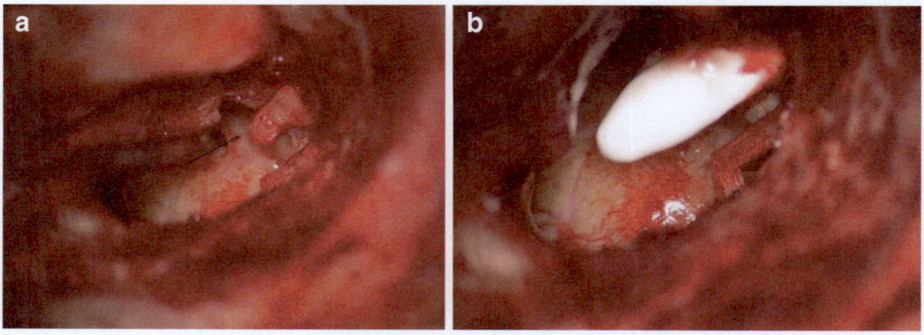

Fig. 6.43 (**a**) Left ear intraoperative view showing necrosis of the malleus handle (black arrow) and (**b**) after reconstruction of the handle with bone cement

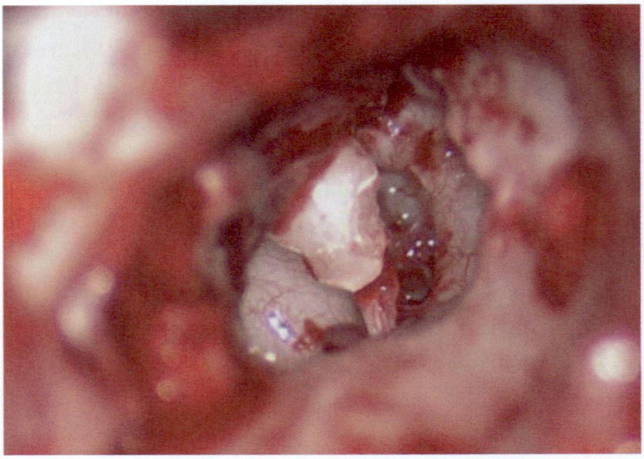

Fig. 6.44 Ossiculoplasty in left ear using incus interposition

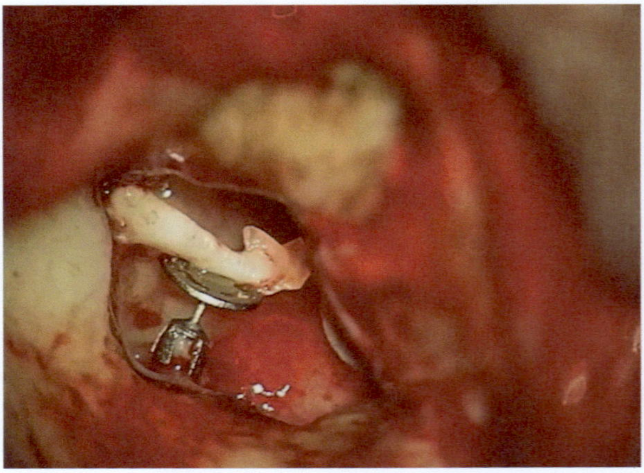

Fig. 6.45 Ossiculoplasty in right ear using PORP of titanium in case of unavailable incus

be done easily, except when the anterior half of the tympanic membrane is absent. A large anterior perforation destabilizes the malleus handle and eliminates the tension necessary to secure the reconstructed ossicular chain.

- ***Alternative Technique with Titanium Prosthesis***

Titanium prosthesis is used when the autologous incus is not available (Fig. 6.45).

Basic Situation in Practice: *Missing Stapes or An Inappropriately Oriented Stapes Superstructure

When the stapes superstructure is inappropriately oriented or damaged, TORP must be used. In order to achieve successful hearing outcomes after ossiculoplasty, the prosthesis must be attached in a firm and stable manner. Establishing a stable TORP-footplate coupling is mandatory for successful reconstruction and we use a cartilage shoe graft for this reason (Fig. 6.46). After placement of the TORP, the graft and the

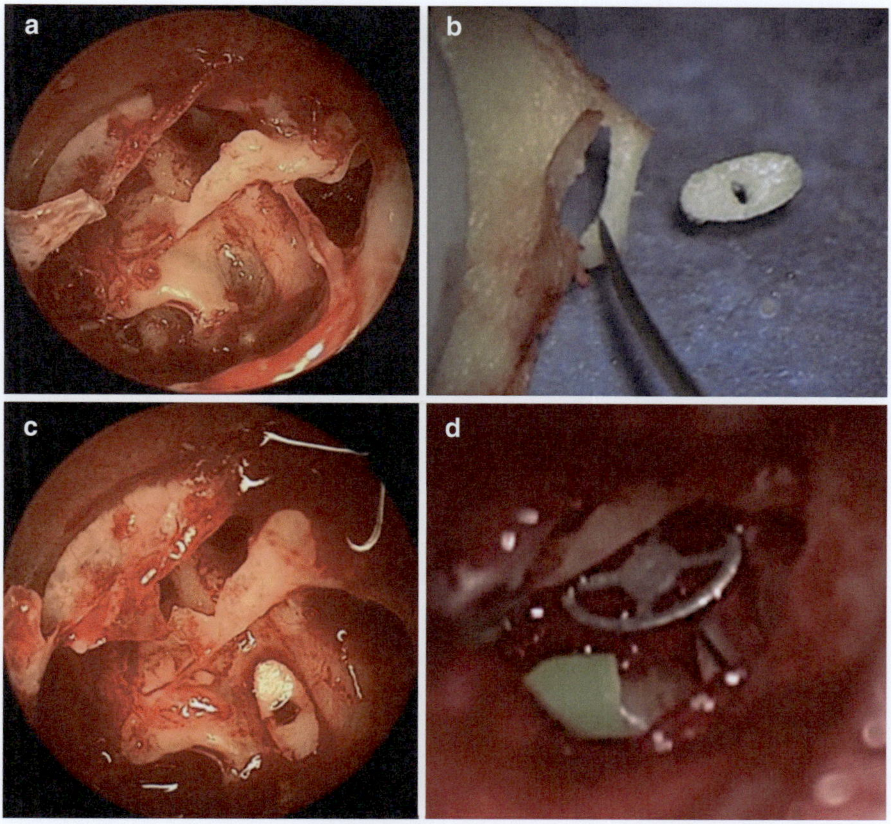

Fig. 6.46 Left ear ossiculoplasty using TORP and cartilage shoe. (**a**) footplate is exposed. (**b**) a cartilage shoe is harvested. (**c**) cartilage shoe is placed on the footplate. (**d**) TORP is placed in the cartilage shoe and under the handle of malleus

tympanometal flap, and after packing of the ear canal, the position and stability of the TORP should be checked through the mastoidectomy, if done, using a 30° scope before closure (Fig. 6.47).

Basic Situation in Practice: *Missing Malleus, Incus, and Stapes with Fixed Footplate

In such situation, ossiculoplasty should be staged. After 6 months, a revision surgery is planned, the footplate should be fenestrated and then covered with fascia. A TORP is then placed between the TM and the footplate fenestration (Fig. 6.48).

6.14.2.3 Outcomes of Ossiculoplasty

Ossiculoplasty Success

Postoperative hearing outcomes are considered successful, if the postoperative air-bone gap is within 20 dB.

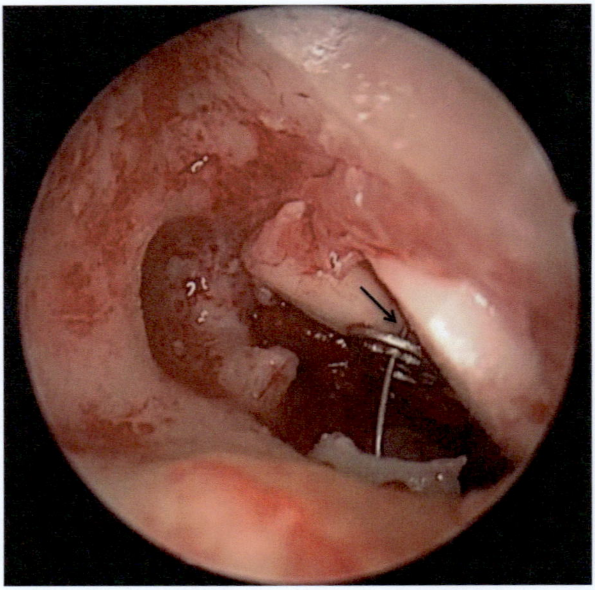

Fig. 6.47 Right ear ossiculoplasty using TORP and cartilage shoe. After finishing middle ear reconstruction and packing the ear canal, a 30° scope is placed in the mastoid attic to look into the middle ear cavity; the TORP is in proper position and is stable. Notice the pin (black arrow) on the headplate of the TORP which is kept intentionally so the TORP will incorporate in the TM cartilage

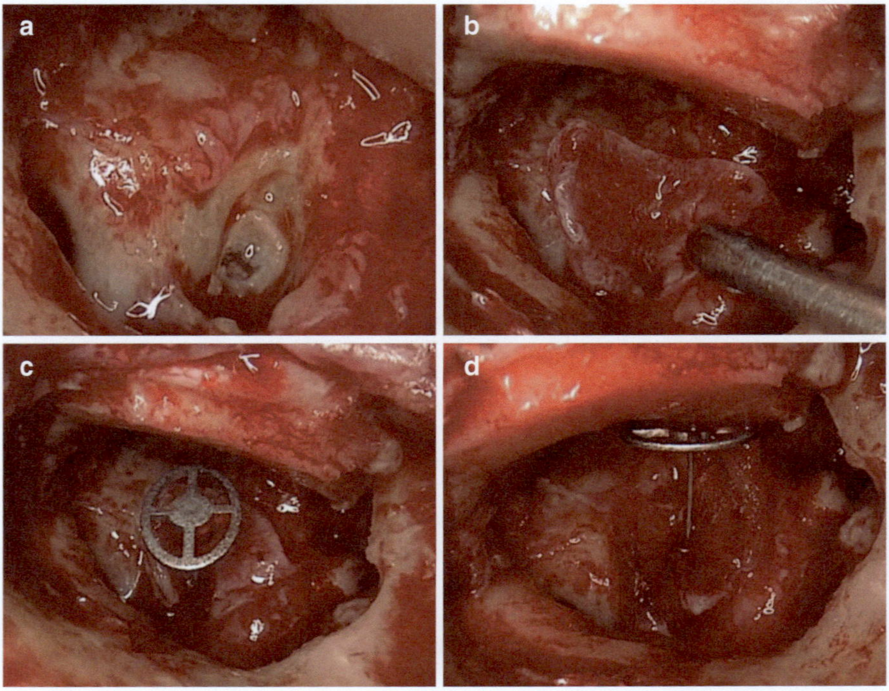

Fig. 6.48 Ossicular reconstruction in a left ear with *missing malleus, incus, and stapes and with fixed footplate.* (**a**) *Fenestration,* (**b**) *fenestration is covered by a fascia,* (**c**) *TORP is placed on the fascia,* and (**d**) *TM cartilage is reflected back on the TORP*

Our data showed that, a postoperative air-bone gap (ABG) ≤20 dB is achieved in more than 75% of the cases. Success rate is higher in PORP ears (80%) as compared to TORP ears (68.8%) [91].

Ossiculoplasty Failure

Ossiculoplasty may fail for one of three basic reasons: a problem with the prosthesis, postoperative adhesions, and recurrent disease.

Ossiculoplasty may fail essentially by a displacement of the prosthesis, due to numerous factors:

The first cause of failure, a problem with the prosthesis, may be immediate or delayed. Immediate failure is most likely due to technical pitfalls. The prosthesis may have been measured inappropriately; a too long prosthesis may lead to slippage or dislocation into the vestibule, and a too short prosthesis may lead to inadequate sound conduction. There may be an unrecognized fixation of the stapes footplate.

Lateron, the ossicular remnant (malleus or stapes superstructure) to which the prosthesis is attached, may become eroded and the prosthesis falling inside the ME cavity.

Delayed failure can also be due to slippage of the prosthesis within the middle ear space. This can be from inadequate contact with supporting ossicles.

Unrelated to the prosthesis itself, non-otologic events can cause prosthesis displacement after proper insertion. These include postoperative head trauma, simple sneeze or other Valsalva episodes, which are sometimes unavoidable.

It is also possible to have a malfunction of the prosthesis by reabsorption. This is rather uncommon with most biomaterials, except when cartilage is used to reconstruct the ossicular chain.

Extrusion of the prosthesis can occur with any implant and can result from a foreign body reaction to the prosthesis. The incidence of extrusion of a synthetic prosthesis may be reduced by using a cartilage interface between the prosthesis and the tympanic membrane graft (Fig. 6.49).

In addition, Prosthesis extrusion can result from the disease process recurrence around the prosthesis. The persistence of cholesteatoma, granulation tissue, reperforation of the tympanic membrane, or persistent otorrhea can cause a failure in ossiculoplasty. Scar tissue, adhesions, or tympanosclerosis can fix the prosthesis secondarily.

Atelectasis and non-aeration of the middle ear affect the transformer mechanism of the middle ear, although the ossiculoplasty itself may be intact. A major cause of failure in ossiculoplasty is from postoperative adhesions in the middle ear (Fig. 6.50).

6.14.3 Aerating Surgery of the Middle Ear

Critical to the success of CSOM surgery is the ability of the middle ear to maintain normal aeration, which prevents restriction of movement of both the tympanic membrane and the round window.

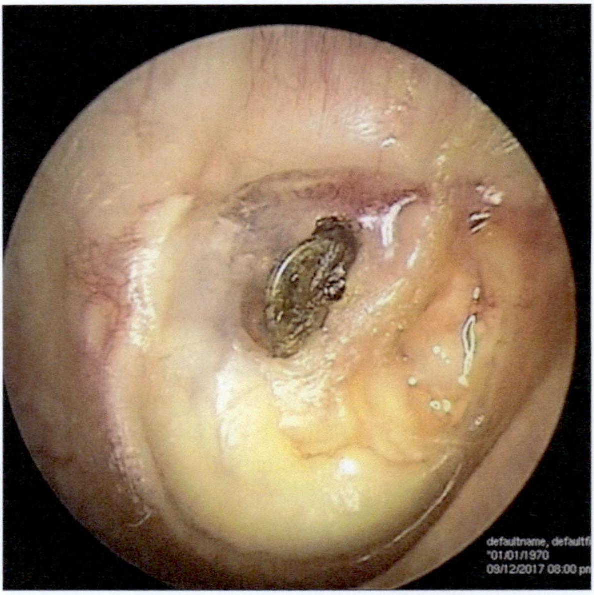

Fig. 6.49 Right ear, 1 year post-op showing partial extrusion of the prosthesis

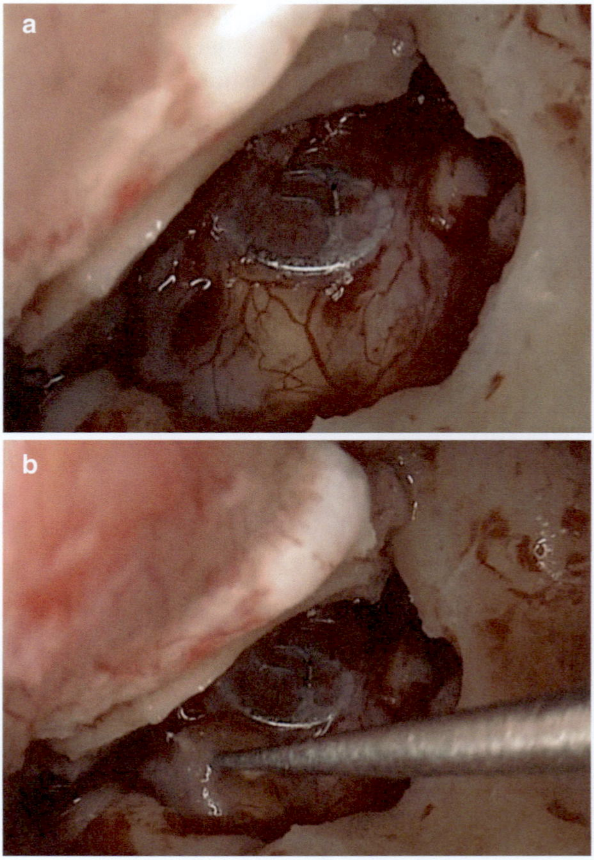

Fig. 6.50 A failing TORP ossiculoplasty. (**a**) Although that the prosthesis is not displaced, however (**b**) it is surrounded by intense fibrotic adhesions that freeze the prosthesis (seen in front of the pick instrument)

In a clinical study of middle ear mechanics in tympanoplasties, Merchant reported a 35- to 55-dB conductive hearing loss in those with non-aerated middle ear spaces [92]. *The aeration of the ME and the Mastoid has a positive predictive value in long-term surgical outcome after tympanoplasty* [93].

Global dysventilation of ME from ETD and poor ventilation of the different air spaces within the temporal bone is believed to be at the center of active CSOM etiopathogenic process.

Combined tympanomastoidectomy with exenteration of air cells and restoration of microventilation pathways is considered as the cornerstone for successful chronic ear surgery.

Beyond any Eustachian tube dysfunction, there are multiple opportunities for obstruction within the narrow ventilation pathways of the tympanic cavity, which result in selective poor ventilation of the areas proximal to these sites. Preoperative CT scan can show the location of dysventilated compartments and can orient the surgeon for the selection of the appropriate treatment and approach.

In cases where the CSOM has produced extensive mucosal disease into the mastoid antrum and the attical spaces, obstruction of the aeration pathways (anterior and posterior) is manifest and becomes the main cause of graft retraction, adhesion and failure of the middle ear reconstruction (epitympanum gas diffusion). At this level mastoidectomy is done not only to remove organized unhealthy mucosa but also it must be oriented to open the tympanic diaphragm, remove all folds and cog enabeling complete excision of the tensor tympani fold to get a full aeration function (AER surgery).

TB CT can assess the aeration status of three important zones: Anterior epitympanum, Posterior epitympanum, and Mastoid antrum.

CT images showing condensations of the mastoid cells, the antrum, the attic and/or the AER (called all together the “AAA spaces”) orient the surgeon to perform mastoid clearance and AER surgery (see Sect. 7.13.2.2.e).

The reestablishment of a complete aeration of the ME compartments, the mastoid cells and especially the anterior epitympanum is the basic solution to guarantee the regeneration of a functioning mastoid cell mucosa capable of an adequate gas diffusion exchange (buffer). Fibrosis in the attic and mastoid after mastoidectomies, reported by some authors, is the result of an inadequate mastoid surgical procedure with an insufficient clearance technique and not because the mastoidectomy is not helpful or not relevant: not all mastoidectomies are the same, mastoidectomy differs from surgeon to surgeon [94].

The influence of the mastoidectomy on the physiologic functions of the ME has been investigated. Yetixser and Karapinar [95] found that a significantly higher number of patients achieved normal ME ventilation in the first 3 months postmastoidectomy when compared with a group of patients without mastoidectomy.

In most cases, especially when surgery is done on active inflammation after failure of medical treatment that had not succeed to obtain a dry ear, the excessive swelling of the ME mucosa (mostly the promontory) is a major issue to deal with. Freeing the tympanic diaphragm to insure good aeration and the use of thin silastic sheets is considered to avoid adhesions; also underlay technique with a graft lying on the malleus handle and under the tympanic annulus is selected to avoid blunting and insure better hearing recovery. Ventilation tube installed in the remaining

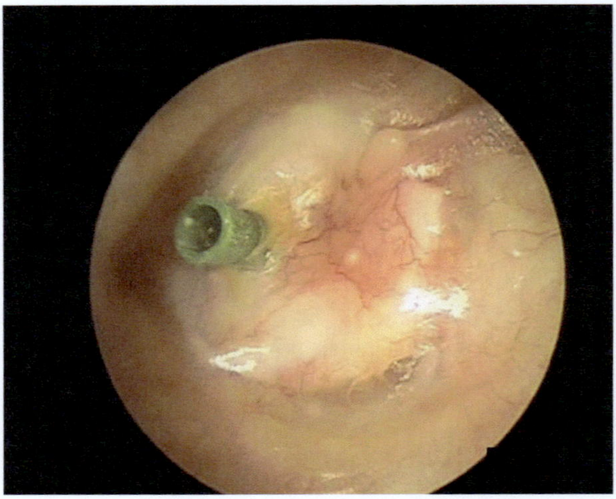

Fig. 6.51 Ventilation tube through the cartilage graft

eardrum or in the cartilage graft could be done at the same time of grafting (Fig. 6.51). Nevertheless mucosal disease is best managed by aeration pathway recovery.

6.14.4 Biologic and Pathologic Considerations in Tympanoplasty

The biology and pathology of Chronic Otitis Media can have significant effects on hearing results after tympanosplasty.

- **Aeration of the middle ear spaces** remains a major issue in the group of patients with disturbed mucosal immune system deficit: over the long term, a negative pressure leads to retraction and atelectasis of the reconstructed TM and functional compromise, as well as a predisposition to displacement or extrusion of ossicular prostheses.
- **Different materials placed in the middle ear**: In response to materials placed in the middle ear (Gelfoam, hyaluronic acid, Silastic, and Teflon GelfoamTM), a host inflammatory response, leading to its resorption, results in adhesions, especially when the middle ear mucosa is deficient with residual edema. Further, GelfoamTM is resorbed within 2 weeks, which is probably an insufficient time for mucosal regeneration to occur. Silastic and Teflon sheeting are relatively inert but they are not resorbed and can sometimes extrude. *There is a serious need for an auxiliary material that will remain in place for several weeks to allow sufficient time for mucosal regeneration, thereafter undergo degradation and resorption, so that the ear can become aerated without fibrosis.*
- **Histopathologic responses** of the ear to various ossicular grafts and prostheses play an important role in determining the outcome of tympanoplasty; these include a foreign body giant cell response to synthetic materials that may lead to a breakdown and resorption of parts of the implant [96].

6.14.5 Overall Results After Middle Ear Surgery

Tympanoplasty and mastoidectomy surgery for CSOM are quite successful in controlling infection and preventing recurrent disease, with success rates in excess of 80–90%. However postoperative hearing results vary widely, depending on the extent of TM and ossicular lesions, mucosal disease, and Eustachian tube function. Also smoking is a cause for lower rate of success in overall results of tympanoplasty [97] due to the effect on the mucociliary apparatus, such as altered viscosity or quantity of the mucus, destruction of auditory tube and middle ear hair cells, and altered ciliary function.

When only TM reconstruction is needed, 80–90% of patients will have an air–bone gap of 20 dB or less. When ossicular reconstruction is necessary, long-term closure of the air–bone gap to less than 20 dB is achieved in 80% of cases when the stapes is intact, and only in about 65% in which the stapes superstructure is missing [91].

The widespread pathological tissue changes in ears with CSOM have important implications for tympanoplasty. For example, postoperative mucosal fibrosis, formation of new bone, and development of negative static pressure in the middle ear, which can occur over the course of months or years, can have a detrimental effect on the outcome of tympanoplasty. These factors are responsible for the overall modest nature of tympanoplasty results, especially in comparison to outcomes after stapedectomy for otosclerosis.

It is a consensus that tympanoplasty remains an effective surgical modality of management in patients with CSOM sequelae; however persistent mucosal disease and bilateral affected ears continue to present a guarded prognosis still facing the otologists [98].

6.14.6 Complications of Tympanoplasty

Graft failure rates range from 10 to 20% depending on the surgical care attributed during surgery to establish the anatomical aeration pathways of ME and the skill of the surgeon. Complications of tympanoplasty may include the following:

- Infection.
- Hematomas can develop with postauricular incision.
- Taste disturbance occurs secondary to damage to the chorda tympani nerve.
- Ear numbness of the pinna and lobule.
- Conductive hearing loss can occur secondary to lateralization of the graft and failure of middle ear spaces aeration (40 dB loss secondary to loss of ME aeration and granulations).
- Sensorineural hearing loss, a serious complication, due to excessive manipulation of the ossicular chain).
- Vertigo can occur, if it is severe or persistent, further workup may be necessary.

6.14.7 Complications of Mastoidectomy or Tympanomastoidectomy

Complications of the mastoidectomy or tympanomastoidectomy include, in addition to the above, the following:

- CSF leak may occur if the dura is violated during the dissection; this can often be repaired if recognized during surgery.
- Meningo encephaloceles secondary to a large tegmen injury.

Iatrogenic meningoencephalocele results from a bony defect in the tegmen tympani or tegmen mastoideum due to a trauma from the drill at the time of the original surgery and could stay clinically silent for a long period of time. A brain hernia could present at a revision surgery for CSOM as a meningoencephalocele or an encephalocele. This condition must be carefully recognized, inspected and repaired at the time of surgery.

Imaging: When suspected, it can be well assessed with a CT and/or MRI. CT evaluates the size of the tegmen bony lysis and the MRI demonstrates the soft tissue content of the hernia and the site of the CSF leak (Fig. 6.52).

Surgical repair of such complications are mostly done through the epitympanum within the mastoid surgery without the need of an intracranial approach. Resection of the encephalocele is terminated with a perichondrium/ cartilage and autogenous bone graft when the hernia is large. Mastoid obliteration could be indicated.

6.15 The Future in CSOM

Present research addresses mainly the prevention of CSOM in high-risk populations.

1. ***Targeting biofilms***: an attempt to reduce the burden of disease caused by CSOM. One study in Western Australia is looking at using **dornase alfa** (a drug used in cystic fibrosis to reduce viscosity of secretions and shown to improve lung function) at the time of TT insertion to breakdown neutrophil extracellular traps (NETS), which harbor live bacteria and biofilm [62]. Directly degrading the DNA, **dornase alfa** may improve bacterial clearance from the ME by reducing biofilm stability and causing bacteria to return to their planktonic form which becomes more susceptible to locally (or systemically) administered antimicrobials and host immune mechanisms.
2. ***Mucosal vaccination*** using Mucosal immune system (*M cells as career*) as a medium against the primary pathogens of OM. The heptavalent PCV vaccine against *Streptococcus pneumoniae* has been shown to provide some protection against OM while significantly reducing frequency of otitis, ME effusion and the need for TT placement in affluent populations [63]. However there is little evi-

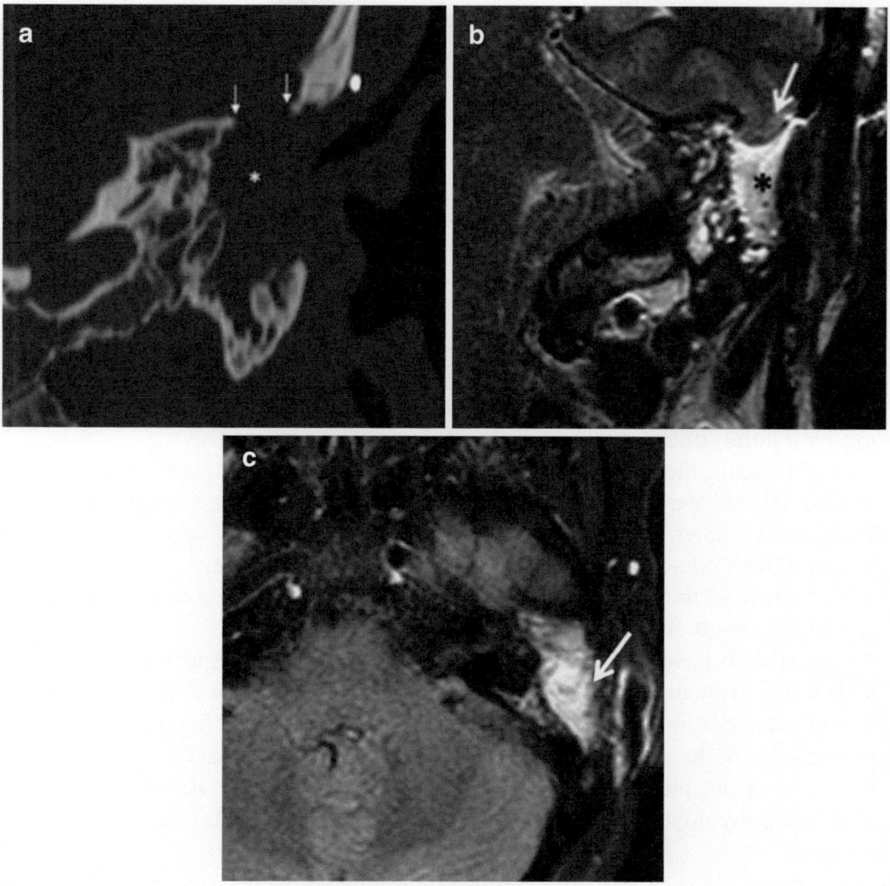

Fig. 6.52 55 year old lady that has underwent left mastoidectomy for CSOM. (**a**) Coronal CT image showing the tegmen defect (between the two arrows) and non specific condensation images inside the cavity, (**b**) T2 weighted coronal T2 image: herniation of cerebral tissue (white arrow) into the attic through the tegmen defect, the whole underlying mastoid cavity is filled with hyper-intense material and (**c**) axial MR image on FLAIR showing the same hyperintense signal in the mastoid cavity, in favour of liquid/granulations, and not an encephalocele with CSF fluid that should be hypointense on FLAIR!

dence to suggest a reduction of CSOM and this is especially the case in high-risk groups. This may be partially due to replacement of OM disease by non-vaccine serotypes and *H. influenzae*. The outcome of the use of a 10-valent pneumococcal Haemophilus protein mD conjugate vaccine and a 13-valent PCV that target these two groups of pathogens is much anticipated [64].

3. ***New surgical techniques***, such as the use of b-FGF (***fibroblast growth factor***) on **gelatin sponge** held in position by fibrin glue, which can be highly successful at treating even large perforations, are promising [65].

6.16 Chronic Suppurative Otitis Media: Some Unusual Presentations

6.16.1 Tuberculous Otitis Media

The true incidence of tuberculous otitis media is unknown in view of the highly selected material in various reports. Tuberculosis of the middle ear and mastoid is very rare nowadays. It would appear from the literature that the clinical presentation of tuberculosis of the middle ear has altered over the last three to four decades and multiple perforations of the drum which were thought to be the characteristic feature (Fig. 6.22) are no longer seen. The typical feature of the disease at presentation is profuse otorrhoea, most commonly painless which fails to respond to both topical and systemic antimicrobial therapy in combination with aural toilet.

In all patients, there was a disproportionate hearing loss compared with the clinical findings and the majority had pale exuberant granulations. Complications are significantly higher (facial palsy, sensorineural hearing loss, labyrinthitis) when compared with non-cholesteatomatous suppurative otitis media.

The spread of the disease into the middle ear is thought to be either through the Eustachian tube or haematogenous.

Diagnosis is based upon a high index of suspicion and, in particular, a history of previous exposure to the disease or a past history of active disease. The presence of a discharging ear in a patient from the Asian ethnic minority should alert the clinician to the possibility of tuberculosis. Bacteriological culture is usually time consuming and Ziehl-Neelsen staining is unreliable. Final diagnosis is established by histology of the granulation tissue, which may need to be repeated.

The treatment is by modern antituberculous chemotherapy and usually involves a course of multiple chemotherapeutic agents to prevent development of resistance to the organisms. However, surgery may also be required, not only to remove sequestra but also to allow adequate drainage and reconstruct hearing.

6.16.2 Immune Deficiency

Immune deficiency may be idiopathic or secondary to various immune depressant drugs.

The idiopathic hypogammaglobulinemia is characterized by a deficiency in the IgG fraction of serum globulin which often presents with recurrent upper respiratory tract infections and otitis media at an early age. In some of these patients, a chronic discharging ear could well be the presenting symptom, a clinical dilemma also observed in IgA deficiency. If the condition is not recognized, all attempts of combined medical and surgical treatment will result in repeated failure. Recognition of such immune deficiencies is of paramount importance.

The management of chronic discharging ears in such patients should include:

1. CWU approach to minimize wound contamination.
2. If CWD procedure is preferred, stabilization of the cavity is achieved by skin grafting.
3. Appropriate correction of IgG and IgA fractions by pre- and postoperative replacement therapy guided by repeated plasma estimations of the above fractions.
4. Bactericidal antimicrobial therapy pre-, per- and postoperatively.

In the drug-induced immune deficient patient associated with chronic suppurative otitis media, where the patients are quite ill, myringoplasty with an onlay technique under a local anaesthetic could be successful. Pre- and postoperative antibiotic cover is essential.

Chronic ear disease is sometimes observed in Job's syndrome (also referred to as lazy leucocyte syndrome) and is associated with recurrent "cold" staphylococcal abscesses, purulent nasal discharge and sinusitis, pulmonary infection and elevated IgE in peripheral blood.

6.16.3 Wegener's Granulomatosis

Wegener's granulomatosis is characterized by the presence of granulomatous deposits in the upper and lower respiratory tracts together with multi-system involvement, particularly the kidneys. Histologically, it presents as a vasculitis with granulomatous changes and is thought to be a hypersensitivity disorder.

Middle ear infection, either as a primary or secondary involvement of the disease, has been described. Secondary involvement is much more common and results from infection in the nasal fossa or the sinuses and commonly presents as middle ear effusion.

Almost half of patients with Wegner granulomatosis had either active or resolved otitis media and a few have chronic suppurative otitis media.

Diagnosis is established by being aware of the possibility of Wegener's granulomatosis in patients with recurrent middle ear infection/discharge associated with persistent mucopurulent rhinorrhoea and an elevated erythrocyte sedimentation rate (ESR) and positive C-ANCA. Final diagnosis is established by histology on suspected lesions within the nose.

Treatment consists in a combination therapy with cyclophosphamide and prednisolone. Middle ear infection improves parallel with the response to systemic treatment.

6.16.4 Histiocytosis X (Langerhans Cell Histiocytosis)

Histiocytosis X involvement of the middle ear is rare and manifest as recurrent otitis with aural polyps. An elevated ESR is of particular significance in suspecting the disease; however, the diagnosis is confirmed by biopsy. Treatment is by a combination of steroids and chemotherapy (vinblastine sulphate).

References

1. Mawson S, Ludman H. Disease of the ear. a textbook of otology. 4th ed. London: Edward Arnold Publication; 1979.
2. Kraemer MJ, Marshall SG, Richardson MA. Etiologic factors in the development of chronic middle ear effusions. Clin Rev Allergy. 1984;2:319–28.
3. Acuin J. Chronic suppurative otitis media. BMJ Clin Evid. 2007;2007. pii 0507
4. Monasta L, Ronfani L, Marchetti F, Montico M, Vecchi Brumatti L, Bavcar A, Grasso D, Barbiero C, Tamburlini G. Burden of disease caused by otitis media: systematic review and global estimates. PLoS One. 2012;7:e36226. https://doi.org/10.1371/journal.pone.0036226.
5. Morris P. Chronic suppurative otitis media. BMJ Clin. 2012;2012:0507.
6. Browning GG, Picozzi GL, Calder IT, Sweeney G. Controlled trial of medical treatment of active chronic otitis media. Br Med J. 1983;287(6398):1024.
7. Matanda RN, Muyunga KC, Sabue MJ, Creten W, Van de Heyning P. Chronic suppurative otitis media and related complications at the University Clinic of Kinshasa. B-ENT. 2005;1:57–62.
8. Acuin J, World Health Organization Department of Child and Health Adolescent Health and Development and the Team for Prevention of Blindness and Deafness of the World Health Organization Blindness. Chronic suppurative otitis media: burden of illness and management options. Geneva: World Health Organization; 2004.
9. WHO. Investing in health research and development. Report of the Ad Hoc Committee on health research funding relating to future intervention options. Geneva: World Health Organization; 1996.
10. Murray CJL, Lopez AD. Deaths by age, sex and cause (thousands), 1990. In: Murray CJL, Lopez AD, editors. Global burden of disease. Geneva: World Health Organization; 1996. p. 433–68.
11. Berman S. Otitis media in children. N Engl J Med. 1995;332(23):1560–5.
12. Chotmongkol V, Sangsaard S. Intracranial complications of chronic suppurative otitis media. Southeast Asian J Trop Med Public Health. 1992;23(3):510–3.
13. Coticchia JM, Chen M, Sachdeva L, Mutchnick S. New paradigms in the pathogenesis of otitis media in children. Front Pediatr. 2013;1:52.
14. Taylor PS, Faeth I, Marks MK, Del Mar CB, Skull SA, Pezzullo ML, Havyatt SM, Coates HL. Cost of treating otitis media in Australia. Expert Rev Pharmacoecon Outcomes Res. 2009;9:133–41.
15. Bluestone CD. Impact of evolution on the eustachian tube. Laryngoscope. 2008;118:522–7.
16. Bluestone CD, Bluestone MB, Coulter J. The eustachian tube: structure, function, role in otitis media. Hamilton: B C Decker; 2005.
17. Bluestone CD, Klein JO. Otitis media in infants and children. Hamilton: B C Decker; 2007.
18. Bluestone CD, Swarts JD. Human evolutionary history: consequences for the pathogenesis of otitis media. Otolanryng Head Neck. 2010;143:739–44.
19. de Ru JA, Grote JJ. Otitis media with effusion: disease or defense? A review of the literature. Int J Pediatr Otorhinolaryngol. 2004;68:331–9.
20. Sade J, Ar A. Middle ear and auditory tube: middle ear clearance, gas exchange, and pressure regulation. Otolanryng Head Neck. 1997;116:499–524.
21. Kahn CM, Line S. The merck veterinary manual. New Jersey: Merck; 2010.
22. Ichimiya I, Kawauchi H, Mogi G. Analysis of immunocompetent cells in the middle ear mucosa. Arch Otolaryngol Head Neck Surg. 1990;116:324–30.
23. Lim DJ, Chun YM, Lee HY, et al. Cell biology of tubotympanum in relation to pathogenesis of otitis media—a review. Vaccine. 2000;19(Suppl 1):S17–25.
24. Kaur R, Kim T, Casey JR, Pichichero ME. Antibody in middle ear fluid of children originates predominantly from sera and nasopharyngeal secretions. Clin Vaccine Immunol. 2012;19(10):1593–6.
25. Buchmann K. Evolution of innate immunity: clues from invertebrates via fish to mammals. Front Immunol. 2014;5:459. https://doi.org/10.3389/fimmu.2014.00459.

26. Vernacchio L, Lesko SM, Vezina RM, et al. Racial/ethnic disparities in the diagnosis of otitis media in infancy. Int J Pediatr Otorhinolaryngol. 2004;68:795–804.
27. Park CH, Kogan MD, Overpeck MD, et al. Black-white differences in health care utilization among US children with frequent ear infections. Pediatrics. 2002;109:E84.
28. Sade J, Fuchs C. Secretory otitis media in adults: II the role of mastoid pneumatization as a prognostic factor. Ann Otol Rhinol Laryngol. 1997;106(1):37–40.
29. Hasegawa MI, Shinnabe A, Kanazawa H, Iino Y, Yoshida N. Clinical characteristics of chronic perforated otitis media in different age groups. J Int Adv Otol. 2017. https://doi.org/10.5152/iao.2017.3513. [Epub ahead of print]
30. Wang DN, Li J, Zhao SQ, Wang Y, Yang L. Role of FOXP3 CD4 CD25 T cells in otitis media with effusion. Chin Arch Otolaryngol Head Neck Surg. 2013;20:126–8.
31. Sekiyama K, et al. The role of vascular endothelial growth factor in pediatric otitis media with effusion. Auris Nasus Larynx. 2011;38(3):319–24.
32. Elmorsy S, Shabana YK, Raouf AA, Naggar ME, Bedir T, Taher S, Fath-Aallah M. The role of IL-8 in different types of otitis media and bacteriological correlation. J Int Adv Otol. 2010;6:269–73.
33. Si Y, Zhang ZG, Chen SJ, Zheng YQ, Chen YB, Liu Y, Jiang H, Feng LQ, Huang X. Attenuated TLRs in middle ear mucosa contributes to susceptibility of chronic suppurative otitis media. Hum Immunol. 2014;75:771–6. https://doi.org/10.1016/j.humimm.2014.05.009.
34. Stenfors LE, Raisanen S. Opsonization of middle ear bacteria during chronic suppurative and secretory otitis media. Acta Otolaryngol. 1992;112(1):96–101.
35. Stenfors LE, Raisanen S. Immunoglobulin-coated bacteria in effusions from secretory and chronic suppurative otitis media. Am J Otolaryngol. 1991;12(3):161–4.
36. Veenhoven R, Rijkers G, Schilder A, Adelmeijer J, Uiterwaal C, Kuis W, et al. Immunoglobulins in otitis-prone children. Pediatr Res. 2004;55(1):159–62.
37. Gross S, Blaiss MS, Herrod HG. Role of immunoglobulin subclasses and specific antibody determinations in the evaluation of recurrent infection in children. J Pediatr. 1992;121(4):516–22.
38. Stenfors LE, Raisanen S. Secretory IgA- and IgG-coated bacteria in chronically discharging ears. J Laryngol Otol. 1991;105(7):515–7.
39. Segade F, Daly KA, Allred D, Hicks PJ, Cox M, Brown M, Hardisty-Hughes RE, Brown SD, Rich SS, Bowden DW. Association of the FBXO11 gene with COME/ROM in the Minnesota COME/ROM family study. Arch Otolaryngol Head Neck Surg. 2006;132(7):729–33.
40. Rye MS, Wiertsema SP, Scaman ES, Oommen J, Sun W, Francis RW, Ang W, Pennell CE, Burgner D, Richmond P, Vijayasekaran S, Coates HL, Brown SD, Blackwell JM, Jamieson SE. FBXO11, a regulator of the TGFb pathway, is associated with severe otitis media in Western Australian children. Genes Immun. 2011;12:352–9.
41. Rye MS, Blackwell JM, Jamieson SE. Genetic susceptibility to otitis media in childhood. Laryngoscope. 2012;122(3):665–75.
42. Rye MS, Warrington NM, Scaman ES, Vijayasekaran S, Coates HL, Anderson D, Pennell CE, Blackwell JM, Jamieson SE. Genome-wide association study to identify the genetic determinants of otitis media susceptibility in childhood. PLoS One. 2012;7(10):e48215.
43. Ehrlich GD, Veeh R, Wang X, Costerton JW, Hayes JD, FZ H, Daigle BJ, Ehrlich MD, Post JC. Mucosal biofilm formation on middle-ear mucosa in the chinchilla model of otitis media. JAMA. 2002;287(13):1–5.
44. Tos M, Caye-Thomasen P. Mucous glands in the middle ear—what is known and what is not. ORL J Otorhinolaryngol Relat Spec. 2002;64(2):86–94.
45. Tos M, Bak-Pedersen K. Density of mucous glands in a biopsy material of chronic secretory otitis media. Acta Otolaryngol. 1973;75(1):55–60.
46. Haidar H, Sheikh R, Larem A, Elsaadi A, Abdulkarim H, et al. Ossicular chain erosion in chronic suppurative otitis media. Otolaryngol (Sunnyvale). 2015;5:203. https://doi.org/10.4172/2161-119X.1000203.
47. Voss SE, Rosowski JJ, Merchant SN, Peake WT. Middle-ear function with tympanic-membrane perforations: I—measurements and mechanisms. J Acoust Soc Am. 2001;110:1432–44.

48. Voss SE, Rosowski JJ, Merchant SN, Peake WT. How do tympanic-membrane perforations affect human middle-ear sound transmission? Acta Otolaryngol. 2001;121:169–73.
49. Mehta RP, Rosowski JJ, Voss SE, O'Neil E, Merchant SN. Determinants of hearing loss in perforations of the tympanic membrane. Otol Neurotol. 2006;27(2):136–43.
50. Merchant SN, Ravicz ME, Puria S, Voss SE, Whittemore KR Jr, Peake WT, Rosowski JJ. Analysis of middle-ear mechanics and application to diseased and reconstructed ears. Am J Otolaryngol. 1997;18:139–54.
51. Nakajima HH, Pisano DV, Roosli C, Hamade MA, Merchant GR, Mafoud L, Halpin CF, Rosowski JJ, Merchant SN. Comparison of ear-canal reflectance and umbo velocity in patients with conductive hearing loss: a preliminary study. Ear Hear. 2012;33:35–43.
52. Peake W, Rosowski JJ, Lynch TJ. Middle-ear transmission: acoustic versus ossicular coupling in cat and human. Hear Res. 1992;57:245–68.
53. Sheikh R, Haidar H, Abdulkarim H, Aslam W, Larem A, Alsaadi A, Alqahtani A. Preoperative predictors in chronic suppurative otitis media for ossicular chain discontinuity: a cross-sectional study. Audiol Neurootol. 2016;21(4):231–6.
54. Huang M, Dulon D, Schacht J. Outer hair cells as potential targets of inflammatory mediators. Ann Otol Rhinol Laryngol. 1990;(Suppl 148):35–8.
55. Cureoglu S, Schachern PA, Paparella MM, Lindgren BR. Cochlear changes in chronic otitis media. Laryngoscope. 2004;114:622–6. https://doi.org/10.1097/00005537-200404000-00006.
56. Joglekar S, Morita N, Cureoglu S, Schachern PA, Deroee AF, Tsuprun V, Paparella MM, Juhn SK. Cochlear pathology in human temporal bones with otitis media. Acta Otolaryngol. 2010;130:472–6. https://doi.org/10.3109/00016480903311252.
57. Jensen RG, Koch A, Homøe P. The risk of hearing loss in a population with a high prevalence of chronic suppurative otitis media. Int J Pediatr Otorhinolaryngol. 2013;77:1530–5. https://doi.org/10.1016/j.ijporl.2013.06.025.
58. Yoshida H, Miyamoto I, Takahashi H. Is sensorineural hearing loss with chronic otitis media due to infection or aging in older patients? Auris Nasus Larynx. 2009;36:269–73. https://doi.org/10.1016/j.anl.2008.07.004.
59. Vaidya S, Sharma JK, Singh G. Study of outcome of tympanoplasties in relation to size and site of tympanic membrane perforation. Indian J Otolaryngol Head Neck Surg. 2014;66:341–6. https://doi.org/10.1007/s120-014-0733-3.
60. Gluth MB, McDonald DR, Weaver AL, Bauch CD, Beatty CW, Orvidas LJ. Management of eustachian tube dysfunction with nasal steroid spray: a prospective, randomized, placebo-controlled trial. Arch Otolaryngol Head Neck Surg. 2011;137:449–55.
61. Bremond G, Wayoff M, Jost G. Les étapes du traitement de l'otite chronique chez l'adulte Librairie Arnette, Paris; 1966. 256 pages, p. 192–3.
62. Samson JE, Magadán AH, Sabri M, Moineau S. Revenge of the phages: defeating bacterial defences. Nat Rev Microbiol. 2013;11:675–87. https://doi.org/10.1038/nrmicro3096.
63. Viertel TM, Ritter K, Horz HP. Viruses versus bacteria—novel approaches to phage therapy as a tool against multidrug-resistant pathogens. J Antimicrob Chemother. 2014;69:2326–36. https://doi.org/10.1093/jac/dku173.
64. Qadir MI. Review: phage therapy: a modern tool to control bacterial infections. Pak J Pharm Sci. 2015;28:265–70.
65. Golkar Z, Bagasra O, Pace DG. Bacteriophage therapy: a potential solution for the antibiotic resistance crisis. J Infect Dev Ctries. 2014;8:129–36. https://doi.org/10.3855/jidc.3573.
66. Jassim SA, Limoges RG. Natural solution to antibiotic resistance: bacteriophages 'The Living Drugs'. World J Microbiol Biotechnol. 2014;30:2153–70. https://doi.org/10.1007/s11274-014-1655-7.
67. Wright A, Hawkins CH, Anggård EE, Harper DR. A controlled clinical trial of a therapeutic bacteriophage preparation in chronic otitis due to antibiotic-resistant *Pseudomonas aeruginosa*; a preliminary report of efficacy. Clin Otolaryngol. 2009;34:349–57. https://doi.org/10.1111/j.1749-4486.2009.01973.x.
68. Bluestone CD. Studies in otitis media: Children's Hospital of Pittsburgh-University of Pittsburgh progress report—2004. Laryngoscope. 2004;114:1.

69. Healy GB, Rosbe KW. Otitis media and middle ear effusions. In: Snow Jr JB, Ballenger JJ, editors. Ballenger's otorhinolaryngology head and neck surgery. 16th ed. Hamilton, ON: BC Decker Inc; 2003. p. 249.
70. Zuk PA, Zhu M, Ashjian PV, et al. Human adipose tissue is a source of multipotent stem cells. Mol Biol Cell. 2002;13:4279–95.
71. Colletti V, Fiorino FG, Sittoni V. Minisculptured ossicle grafts versus implants: long-term results. Am J Otolaryngol. 1987;8:553–9.
72. Blanchard J, et al. A longterm view of myringoplasty in children. J Laryngol Otol. 1990;104:758–62.
73. Vartiainen E, Nuutinen J. Long-term hearing results of one-stage tympanoplasty for chronic otitis media. Eur Arch Otorhinolaryngol. 1992;249(6):329–31.
74. Goldman DJ, Nalebuff J, Druss JG. Experimental observations on prosthetic materials in stapedial surgery with special reference to the use of Teflon. Laryngoscope. 1962;72:169–81.
75. Withers BT, Hatsfield SE, Richmond RW. Drum and middle ear grafts in cats. Laryngoscope. 1963;73:1022–43.
76. Yung MW. Literature review of alloplastic materials in ossiculoplasty. J Laryngol Otol. 2003;117:431–6.
77. House JW, Teufert KB. Extrusion rates and hearing results in ossicular reconstruction. Otolaryngol Head Neck Surg. 2001;125:135–41.
78. Mehta RP, Ravicz ME, Rosowski JJ, Merchant SN. Middle-ear mechanics of Type III tympanoplasty (stapes columella): I. Experimental studies. Otol Neurotol. 2003;24(2):176–85.
79. Brackmann DE, Sheehy JL, Luxford WM. TORPs and PORPs in tympanoplasty: a review of 1042 operations. Otolaryngol Head Neck Surg. 1984;92:32–7.
80. Murugasu E, Puria S, Roberson JB Jr. Malleus-to-footplate versus malleus-to-stapes-head ossicular reconstruction prostheses: temporal bone pressure gain measurements and clinical audiological data. Otol Neurotol. 2005;26(4):572–82.
81. Vlaming MS, Feenstra L. Studies on the mechanics of the reconstructed human middle ear. Clin Otolaryngol Allied Sci. 1986;11(6):411–22.
82. Nishihara S, Goode RL. Experimental study of the acoustic properties of incus replacement prostheses in a human temporal bone model. Am J Otolaryngol. 1994;15(4):485–94.
83. Puria S, Kunda LD, Roberson JB Jr, Perkins RC. Malleus-to-footplate ossicular reconstruction prosthesis positioning: cochleovestibular pressure optimization. Otol Neurotol 2005;26(3):368–79.
84. Goode RL, Nishihara S. Experimental models of ossiculoplasty. Otolaryngol Clin N Am. 1994;27(4):663–75.
85. Bance M, Campos A, Wong L, Morris DP, van Wijhe R. How does prosthesis head size affect vibration transmission in ossiculoplasty? Otolaryngol Head Neck Surg. 2007;137(1):70–3.
86. Morris DP, Bance M, Van Wijhe RG. How do cartilage and other material overlay over a prosthesis affect its vibration transmission properties in ossiculoplasty? Otolaryngol Head Neck Surg. 2004;131(4):423–8.
87. Babu S, Seidman M. Ossicular reconstruction using bone cement. Otol Neurotol. 2004;25: 98–101. 1188
88. Elsheikh MN, Elsherief H, Elsherief S. Physiologic reestablishment of ossicular continuity during excision of retraction pockets. Arch Otolaryngol Head Neck Surg. 2006;132:196–9.
89. Goebel JA, Jacob A. Use of Mimix hydroxyapatite bone cement for difficult ossicular reconstruction. Otolaryngol Head Neck Surg. 2005;132:727–34.
90. Ozer E, Bayazit YA, Kanlikama M, et al. Incudostapedial rebridging ossiculoplasty with bone cement. Otol Neurotol. 2002;23:643–6.
91. Altamimi Z, Haidar H, Larem A, et al. Innovation in otology: stability of ossicular reconstruction. J Bioeng Biomed Sci. 2016;6(5 (Suppl))
92. Merchant SN, McKenna MJ, Mehta RP, et al. Middle ear mechanics of type III tympanoplasty (stapes columella): II. Clinical studies. Otol Neurotol. 2003;24:186–94.
93. Kanazawa Y, Naito Y, Tona R, et al. Predictive value of middle ear aeration before second-stage operation in staged tympanoplasty with soft-wall reconstruction. Acta Otolaryngol. 2014;134:135–9.

94. Mansour S, Nicolas K, Naim A, Yamine F, Moukarzel N, Nehme A. Inflammatory chronic otitis media and the anterior epitympanic recess. J Otolaryngol. 2005;34(3):149–59.
95. Yetixser S, Karapinar U. Middle ear ventilation function in patients with myringoplasty alone and myringoplasty plus mastoidectomy. Kulak Burun Bogaz Ihtis Derg. 2011;21:179–83.
96. Bahmad F Jr, Merchant SN. Histopathology of ossicular grafts and implants in chronic otitis media. Ann Otol Rhinol Laryngol. 2007;116(3):181–91.
97. Onal K, Uguz MZ, Kazikdas KC, Gursoy ST, Gokce H. A multivariate analysis of otological, surgical and patient-related factors in determining success in myringoplasty. Clin Otolaryngol. 2005;30(2):115–20.
98. Nambiar SS. Tympanoplasty type I evaluation of the surgical results and its impact as the treatment modality in chronic otitis media. J Evid Based Med Health. 2017;4(58):3507–11. https://doi.org/10.18410/jebmh/2017/699.

Retraction Pocket

7

Contents

S. Mansour et al., *Middle Ear Diseases*,
https://doi.org/10.1007/978-3-319-72962-6_7

7.1 Introduction

Tympanic Membrane Retraction Pockets (TMRPs) refer to an otoscopic descriptive pathology of a retracted weak part of the tympanic membrane having lost its lamina propria and collapsed into the middle ear cavity [1, 2].

The most common sites are the posterosuperior part of the pars tensa (PT) and the pars flaccida (PF) [3]. RPs are often bilateral and symmetrical. Association of RPs in both tympanic parts of the same ear can occur.

The collapse of the total surface of the tympanic membrane is called atelectasis [3]. When the entire atelectatic membrane becomes adherent to the middle ear floor, it is called adhesive otitis media.

A chronic inflammatory process with hypoxia in the middle ear is the underlying promoter of the pathologic condition. TMRPs are potential precursors in the pathophysiology of cholesteatoma formation. Therefore, a correct evaluation of the TMRPs and its related management are essential in the prevention of middle ear cholesteatoma.

Despite numerous staging classifications, there is still a confusing methodology between otologists for the physical assessment of a retraction pocket. Consequently these classifications failed to predict its evolution. Retraction pockets can resolve spontaneously, they can stay stable and safe for a long period of time or become unstable to go on and invade the middle ear structures and even the mastoid.

Until now literature lacks objective criteria, not only for the positive diagnosis of RP and its assessment, its variable evolution or its management decisions, but also for its post-operative behavior and follow-up.

In this chapter, a comprehensive review of the recent literature regarding its prevalence, its etiopathogenesis, and advanced findings concerning its molecular biology will be presented. Advances in CT-Imaging assessment regarding its diagnosis and prognosis permitted to establish clinico-radiologic correlations serving, not only as a new methodology to differentiate between safe and unsafe pockets. In addition, these correlations could be used as a guideline to orient the surgical indication (timing and approach) to better deal with tympanic membrane retraction pockets.

7.2 Related Anatomy and Physiology of the Middle Ear Cleft

7.2.1 Middle Ear Ventilation Anatomy

The following review of the functional anatomy of the middle ear is essential to understand the pathophysiology and pathogenesis of retraction pocket pathology. For more details please refer to "The Comprehensive and Clinical Anatomy of the Middle Ear" (Springer, 2013).

From a ventilatory point of view, the ***tympanic diaphragm*** divides the middle ear physically into two compartments, the antero-inferior compartment and the postero-superior one.

7.2.1.1 The Antero-Inferior Compartment

It consists of the protympanum, mesotympanum, hypotympanum, the inferior part of the retrotympanum, and the lower unit of the attic (Prussak's space). The antero-inferior compartment is widely open to the Eustachian Tube which ensures direct aeration to the mesotympanic and hypotympanic spaces. In the antero-inferior compartment of the middle ear cleft, the mucosa is an extension of the mucosa of the rhinopharynx; the epithelial layer is pseudostratified; there are mucous and ciliated cells decreasing in number from anterior to posterior. The connective tissue is relatively dense. The role of the antero-inferior compartment in transmucosal gaze exchange is minimal and is devoted primarily to mucociliary clearance [4].

7.2.1.2 The Postero-Superior Compartment

It consists of the upper unit of the attic and the mastoid air cell system. It is situated away from the direct air stream of the ET and it is aerated only through a constant opening in the tympanic diaphragm called the tympanic isthmus. In 40% of cases there is accessory route of aeration through a defect in the tensor tympani fold (TTF) (Figs. 7.1 and 7.2) [5].

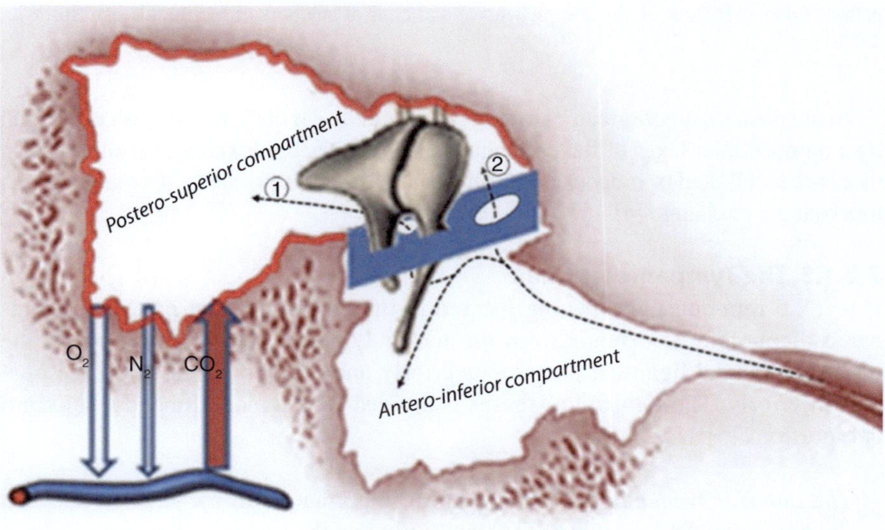

Fig. 7.1 The tympanic diaphragm divides the middle ear physically into two compartments, the antero-inferior compartment and the postero-superior one. The anterior inferior compartment is ventilated directly from the Eustachian tube. The posterosuperior compartment is ventilated from the antero-inferior compartment through an opening in the tympanic diaphragm known as the tympanic isthmus (1). In 40% of cases there is accessory route of aeration through a defect in the tensor tympani fold (2). The mucosa of the postero-superior compartment is specialized for gas diffusion from the middle ear

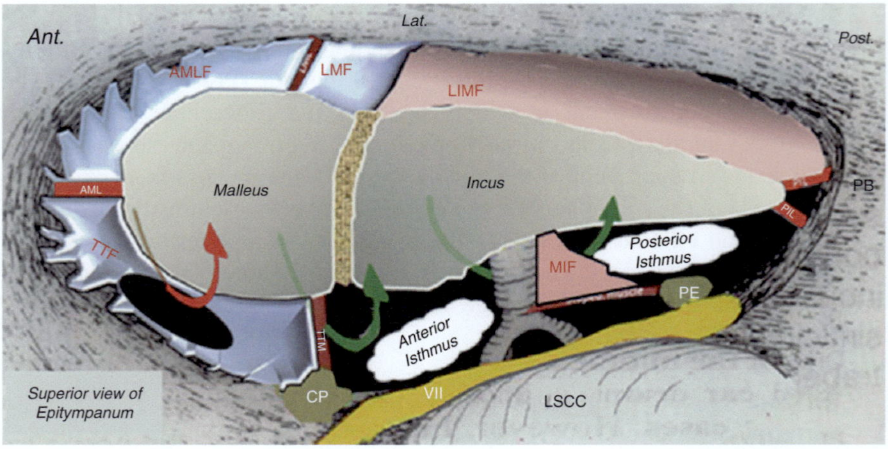

Fig. 7.2 Superior view of a right middle ear tympanic diaphragm showing a common variation of this structure. The tensor tympani fold (TTF) is incomplete and represents an accessory route of attic aeration (red arrow) from the protympanum. The green arrows represent the constant attic aeration through the tympanic isthmus. AMLF anterior malleal ligamental fold, MIF medial incudal fold, LMF lateral malleal fold, LIMF lateral incudomalleal fold, AML anterior malleal ligament, LML lateral malleal ligament, PIL posterior incudal ligament, TTM tensor tympani muscle tendon, CP cochleariform process, PE pyramidal eminence, LSCC lateral semicircular canal, PB petrous bone. (Mansour et al.: Comprehensive and clinical anatomy of the middle ear, Springer, 2013.)

In the postero-superior compartment of the middle ear cleft, the mucosa is covered by a monocellular layer of flat epithelial cells with a richly vascularized submucosa; there are no ciliated or mucous cells. This compartment is primarily devoted to transmucosal gas exchange [4].

7.2.1.3 The Tympanic Isthmus

It is a 2.5 mm constant opening located in the postero-medial part of the tympanic diaphragm, it extends from the tensor tympani muscle anteriorly to the posterior incudal ligament postero-superiorly and the pyramidal eminence postero-inferiorly. The tympanic isthmus is divided by the medial incudal fold into two portions [5]:

- *The anterior tympanic isthmus*, the most important pathway, situated between the tensor tympani muscle (TTM) anteriorly and the stapes postero-inferiorly.
- *The posterior tympanic isthmus,* less important, situated between the short process of the incus and the stapedial muscle. It is a communication between the mesotympanum and the *upper part of the retrotympanum, which is situated above the diaphragm.*

7.2.2 Middle Ear Ventilation and Pressure Regulation

Nowadays, the most commonly accepted theory of ME pressure regulation in healthy ears is the bi-directional gas diffusion over the ME mucosa, aided by intermittent pressure equilibration via the ET [6–8].

The net result of mucosal gas exchange is gas absorption from the ME to the mucosa of the postero-superior compartment of the ME. Continuous absorption of gas in the ME cleft through the mucosa leads to a physiologic gas deficit. In normal conditions, the intermittent ET ventilation serves to equilibrate the continuous loss of gas from the ME. A small imbalance between ventilation and diffusion could be buffered by a big mastoid volume (Fig. 7.3).

Air coming from the ET to the anteroinferior segment, can only pass to the postero-superior compartment through *the tympanic isthmi* (anterior and posterior isthmus). This route of ventilation of the postero superior compartment of the middle ear is called the *posterior microventilation pathway.*

Another possible opening is a congenital defect in the tensor tympani fold (**TTF**), situated anterior to the cog, in the anterior epitympanic recess. The TTF defect, present in 60% of ears, ventilates also the postero-superior compartment. In 40% of normal ears, this auxiliary *anterior microventilation pathway* is absent because their TTF is anatomically complete (Fig. 7.4).

- *The upper unit of the attic* and the mastoid air cells are ventilated through the anterior tympanic isthmus and through a defect in the TTF, when present. The upper retro-tympanum, also part of the upper unit of the attic, is ventilated through the posterior tympanic isthmus. Air passes from the mesotympanum through the posterior tympanic isthmus and around the ossicular chain

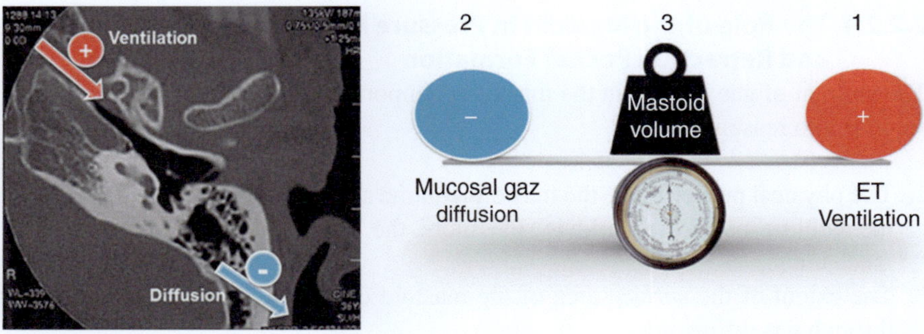

Fig. 7.3 Continuous absorption of gas in the ME cleft through the mucosa (diffusion) leads to a physiologic gas deficit. In normal conditions, the intermittent ET ventilation serves to equilibrate the continuous loss of gas from the ME. A small imbalance between ventilation and diffusion could be buffered by a big mastoid volume

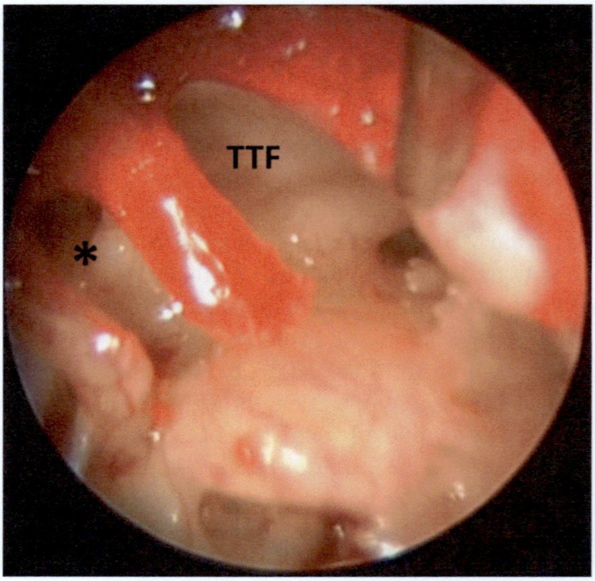

Fig. 7.4 Endoscopic view of a right middle ear showing the isthmus (*) and the tensor tympani fold (TTF) which is complete in this case

complex to reach the upper retrotympanum compartment. Prominent promontory and tilted stapes may constrict this micro ventilation pathway; the promontory becomes closer to the incus and malleus, facilitating its blockage, generating effusion, stagnation granulation tissues and adhesions.

– *The lower unit of the attic*, the Prussak's space, is ventilated from the mesotympanum through the posterior *pouch of von Troeltsch.* Hence any blockage of the later deprives the Prussak's pouch from ventilation.

7.2.2.1 The Role of the Mastoid in Pressure Regulation and Retraction Pocket Formation

The amount of gas present in the mastoid is important in regulating ME cleft pressure for two reasons:

1. The physical properties of the mastoid volume affect the compliance: the greater the volume of the mastoid is, the more the ME system is compliant (ME mechanics).
2. The extent of the surface area of the mastoid cavity affects mucosal exchange through gas diffusion.

Both factors are concerned in the development of TM retraction.

The mastoid air system constitutes the major part of the volume of the ME cleft and thus also represents the major part of the mucosal area available for transmucosal gas exchange [9].

In addition, the mastoid, as a gas reservoir, acts passively to compensate the pressure variations of the ME cavity together with the opening of the Eustachian tube [9–13].

Thus the mastoid cell system would be like a container or an extra volume serving to buffer ME pressure changes. According to the ideal gas law (PV = nRT), a drop in the amount of gas present in a big container (well pneumatized mastoid) has a little impact on pressure change; in contrary when the mastoid is small (diploic mastoid) the same change in amount of gas will lead to a higher drop in pressure. If in cases of sclerotic mastoids, the ET fails to open for a long duration of time, this will decrease the ME pressure (negative pressure) this is why the volume of mastoid in an ear plays a role in the genesis of RP: the gas exchange fails to be compensated by a functioning ET.

7.3 Middle Ear Dysventilation

The ME could be a victim of the two types of ventilation disorders: the global and/or the selective dysventilation syndromes. Two elements play the major role in the middle ear dysventilation.

7.3.1 Eustachian Tube Dysfunction: Global Middle Ear Dysventilation Syndromes

Eustachian tube dysfunction could be the result of:

- *Intrinsic pathologies*: due to a mucosal edema in case of reflux, atopy or allergy, infections, ciliary disease or mechanical palatal deformity or muscular dysfunctions.
- *Extrinsic pathologies*: adenoid hypertrophy or nasopharyngeal tumors.

However the most common cause of tubal dysfunction is the mucosal inflammation in relation to an "inadequate mucosal immune system" (MIS) syndrome with inflammation involving the upper respiratory tract (URT) mucosa with clinical signs of atopy. Due to a tubal dysfunction, the resultant negative pressure in the whole ME may manifest by *secretory otitis media, atelectasis or adhesive otitis media.*

→ This is called the **Global ME Dysventilation Syndrome** (Figs. 7.5 and 7.6b).

7.3.2 Mucosal Dysfunction

7.3.2.1 Impact on the Gas Exchange

Mucosal inflammation is the most common underlying cause of middle ear mucosal dysfunction. It is frequently encountered in patients suffering from an inadequate

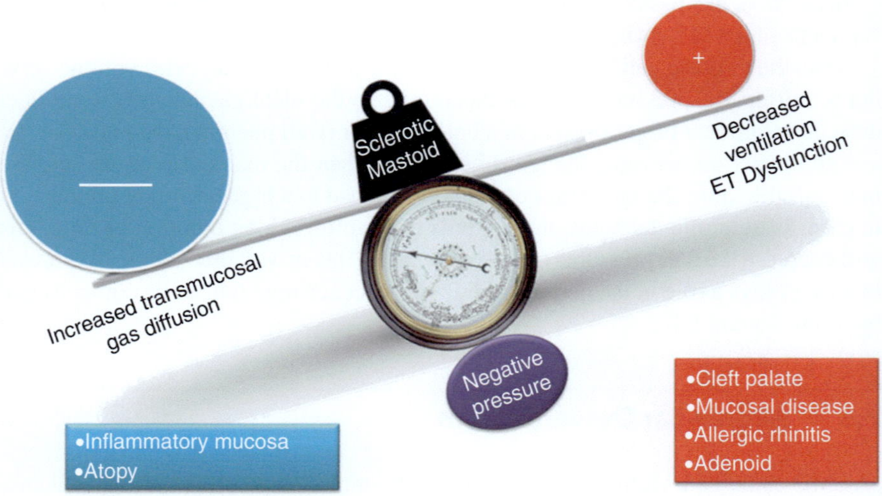

Fig. 7.5 Middle ear dysventilation is due to imbalance between ventilation and diffusion in an ear with sclerotic mastoid (small volume) that can't buffer this imbalance

mucosal immune system (MIS) syndrome of the upper respiratory tract especially in **atopy**. Hypoxia and Inflammation of the posterosuperior compartment produce an increase of both number and diameter of the blood vessels in its corresponding mucosa [14–16], causing a greater gas exchange with a decreased gas pressure inside the restricted compartment: The higher the degree of impairment of the trans-mucosal gas exchange is, the greater is the decrease in the total pressure of the middle ear cleft [16, 17].

Gas diffusing out from the ME into mucosal blood vessels could be insufficiently counterbalanced by ET ventilation either due to an excessive increase of the gas diffusion (mucosal inflammation) or insufficient ME ventilation by the oedematous ET or both of them (Fig. 7.5) [18–20].

7.3.2.2 Impact on the Middle Ear Gas Circulation

In addition, during inflammation the mucosa of the antero-inferior compartment becomes edematous, thick and even polypoid with a metaplastic transformation that increases the production of mucus and simultaneously reduces the fluidity of the sol layer. This leads to the formation of mucous plugs able to close any of the micro ventilatory pathways through the tympanic diaphragm (posterior or anterior pathway or both), causing a decreased pressure in the corresponding compartment above the tympanic diaphragm. The aeration deprivation of such restricted area of the ME ear space, may progress to cause a focal retraction of the correspondent part of the tympanic membrane despite an

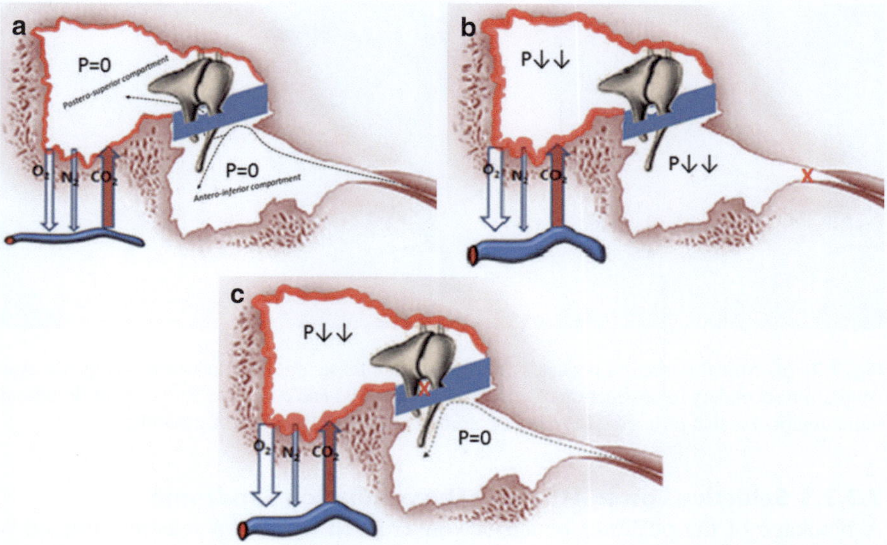

Fig. 7.6 (**a**) Normal middle ear ventilation; (**b**) global middle ear dysventilation due to ET dysfunction (X) and inflammatory mucosa; (**c**) selective epitympanic dysventilation, anteroinferior compartment is well aerated through the ET; however the epitympanic compartment is not properly ventilated due to obstruction of tympanic diaphragm with inflammatory mucosa

adequate re-aeration of the rest of the middle ear cavity by a well functioning ET or a ventilation tube.

Thus Retraction pocket is actually a disease of the folds of the tympanic diaphragm and less of the Eustachian Tube.

→ This is called the **Selective ME Dysventilation Syndrome** (Fig. 7.6c).

7.3.3 Middle Ear Dysventilation Syndromes

The pressure deficit in a given condition could manifest as the following:

7.3.3.1 Selective Dysventilation of the Retrotympanum

A blockage of the posterior tympanic isthmus may lead to a selective upper retrotympanum dysventilation with a resultant postero-superior PT RP.

7.3.3.2 Selective Upper Attic Dysventilation Syndrome

A blockage of the anterior tympanic isthmus in ears having a complete TTF (absence of anterior route) may result in an attic dysventilation with a resultant PF RP, or association of PF RP and PT RP.

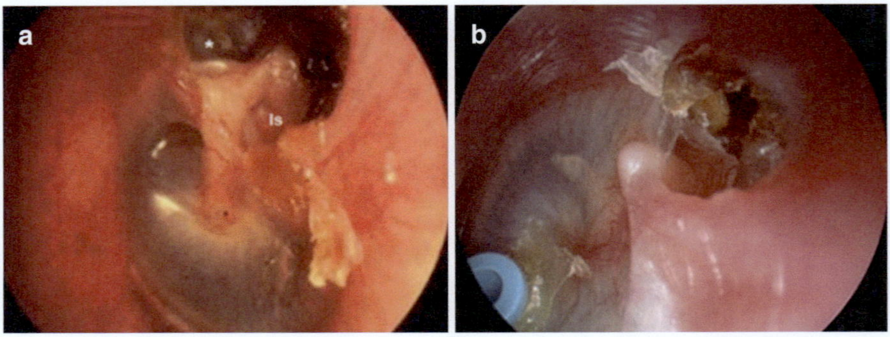

Fig. 7.7 (**a**) Attical retraction pocket, with normal pars tensa, due to selective epitympanic dysventilation secondary to obstruction of tympanic isthmus (Is) and complete TTF (*) and (**b**) attical retraction pocket that progressed to cholesteatoma even after placement of grommet

7.3.3.3 Selective Lower Attic Unit Dysventilation Syndrome

A blockage of the posterior pouch of von Tröltsch leads to a selective Prussak's space dysventilation (Fig. 7.7a) with the result of a limited PF RP that may progress to cholesteatoma despite grommet placement (Fig. 7.7b).

7.4 Epidemiology of Tympanic Membrane Retraction Pockets

Numerous studies, concerning mostly the pediatric population, agreed on the fact that frequent acute otitis media increases the frequency of tympanic membrane pathologies:

Tos and Poulsen (1980), while re-examining children who had secretory otitis media 3–8 years before, noticed that 34% of their ears have developed different degrees of attic retractions [21] in 1994 Max and Bowden [22] found, in a follow up of children for a period of 12 years, 40% of pars flaccida and 17% of pars tensa retractions.

Also Stangerup (1994) reported in a study of 294 healthy children from 5 to 16 years old, the prevalence of tympanic membrane retractions to be rising from 14 to 26% in the pars flaccida and only from 0.3 to 3.7% in the pars tensa [23].

The most important longitudinal cohort study actually available has been done on almost 7000 children from birth to ten years old by Maw et al. They found retraction of the pars flaccida in 9.6% and retraction of the pars tensa in 7.9%. Most of these retractions have been staged as mild, with only *few severe cases* [24]. On the other hand, de Beer, exploring children from 8 to 18 years, realized that many tympanic membrane abnormalities present at the initial screening, disappeared substantially after 10 years follow up [25].

Further studies showed that a PF RP present in one ear was frequently associated to a PT RP in the same ear; a pars flaccida retraction pocket is rarely found *without* any pars tensa retraction [24]. Also bilateral RP in the same patient are frequently found.

7.5 Etiology of Retraction Pockets

Three factors are implicated:

1. A weak anatomic structure of certain areas of the tympanic membrane. Collagenase and elastase secreted by inflammatory cells during AOM or OME can destroy the lamina propria of the tympanic membrane rendering it atrophic and prone to retraction [26, 27].
2. A *micro dysventilation syndrome* [28, 29] as explained above.

7.5.1 Formation of Pars Tensa Retraction Pocket

During OME, the chronic inflammatory process taking place in the area of the ossicular chain is more severe than in other areas of the ME due to the difficult drainage of the effusion, stagnation and granulation tissue formation [30]. This granulation tissue may obstruct the posterior tympanic isthmus pathway with the result of a dysventilation of the retrotympanum despite restoration of a normal ET function.

Moreover some anatomical predispositions in ME Structures facilitate the PTRP formation such:

- **The Retrotympanum**: The constricted frontiers and the variations of the depth of the retrotympanum (dependent of the degree of mastoid pneumatization) are the predisposing factors for a long term entrapment of effusion in this space and persistent inflammatory adverse reactions on the PT [31].
- **The Promontory**: The promontory inclines gently forward anteriorly toward the anterior wall of the tympanic cavity, but it is more steeply stopped posteriorly. In some ears, the promontory could figure at the same height of the long process of the incus and reach almost the level of the malleus handle or even the level of the stapes head. Consequently cases with a high promontory and deep retrotympanum favor the entrapment of the effusion for a long duration. Then a retracted PT comes easily in touch at the same time with the incus and the promontory favoring hereby a rapid adhesion to the incus or the incudostapedial joint with restrictive spoliation of the space aeration.

7.5.2 Formation of a Pars Flaccida Retraction Pocket

A selective epitympanic dysventilation syndrome occurs when a blockage of the anterior tympanic isthmus associated to a complete Tensor Tympani Fold causing a complete isolation of the epitympanum from the mesotympanum. This event induces a gas deficit, a selective decrease of the gas pressure in the attic, a subsequent Pars Flaccida retraction toward the attic and a retraction pocket formation independently of the well functioning ET.

Marchioni confirmed that an isthmus blockage is present in more than 96% of patients with attic disease compared to 6% in the control group (patients without attic disease). In addition, the TTF was found complete in more than 96% of patients with attic disease compared to 19% in the control group [32].

Aimi considered that occlusion of the anterior route of aeration is a predisposing factor for the development of acquired cholesteatoma when most patients with attic cholesteatoma demonstrate a near normal Eustachian tube function [33, 34].

Palva et al. investigated the aeration pathways of the anterior epitympanic recess and demonstrated that an incomplete TTF prevented the development of an extensive pathology around the malleus and incus body (attic) even in the presence of chronic otitis media [35].

A prospective study done by the authors demonstrated the implication of the AER in the recurrence of mucoid middle ear effusion that persists or recurs despite repetitive myringotomies with tube insertion; in addition they observed that the complete control of a retraction pocket is not obtained even with a cartilage tympanoplasty procedure or a reconstruction of the lateral attic wall if an adequate aeration surgery of the AER with excision of the cog and the TTF was not completed [36].

Ars reported that the solid tympanic diaphragm (complete TTF) with the absence of the anterior aeration pathway function is thought to be a predisposition for a retraction pocket and acquired cholesteatoma. He even suggested that the tympanic diaphragm predetermines the topography and localization of the tympanic membrane retraction pocket [13].

Morimutsu et al. advocated that removal of the cog and excision of the tensor tympani fold through an anterior tympanotomy to open the anterior route of ventilation, reduce the recurrence of retraction pocket and cholesteatoma from 17% to 5%. He supposed that the pathogenesis of cholesteatoma secondary to a retraction pocket is not related to an Eustachian tube dysfunction but rather to the tympanic diaphragm, the cog and the tensor tympani fold [37].

In conclusion: most of the studies demonstrated that in response to a blockage of the aeration pathways through the tympanic diaphragm, the weak part of the corresponding tympanic membrane starts invagination, with a possible progress to a retraction pocket formation.

7.6 Histopathology of the Retraction Pocket

The dominant histological feature in retraction pockets is the loss of the double collagen fibrous layer in the lamina propria due to a continuous inflammatory process (Fig. 7.4) [2, 24, 25, 38].

The following changes are observed [39]:

(a) **In the lamina propria**: A loss of the double collagen fibrous layer (Fig. 7.8).
(b) **In the mucosa**: when the membrane of the RP becomes adherent, the mucosal layer of the retracted part disappears.
(c) **In the epidermal layer**:
    - A sub-epithelial chronic inflammation, although the inflammatory process is ubiquitous in all stages of RP, it is more severe in advanced stages.

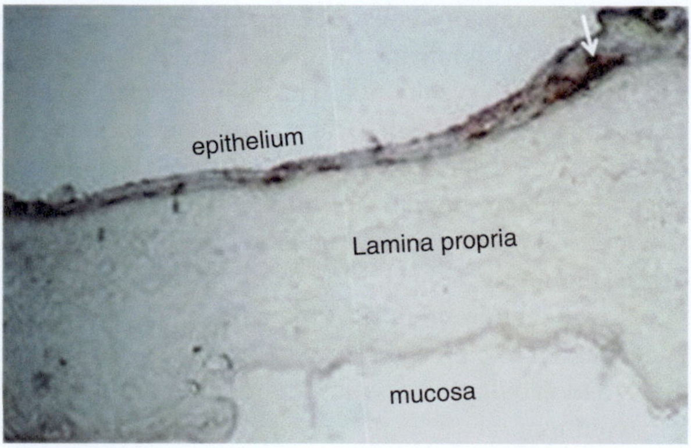

Fig. 7.8 Histology of a retraction pocket using optic microscope with specific coloration for macrophage of the skin showing infiltration of the epithelium by macrophages (*white arrow*) and focal reduction of the lamina propria thickness

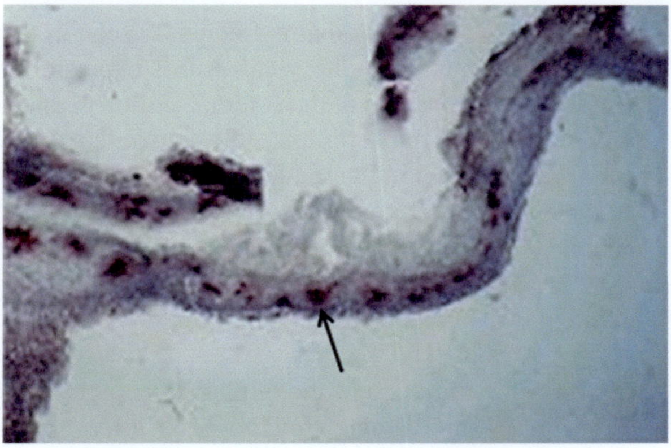

Fig. 7.9 Histology of a RP which became a precholesteatoma with specific staining of Langerhans cells showing infiltration of the epidermis with Langerhans cells (*black arrow*) and hyperplasia of the keratinizing squamous epithelium

- An infiltration of the epidermis by inflammatory cells, especially Langerhans' cells (Fig. 7.8). The more the Langerhans cells are increased in number, the more the RP is active and advanced (Fig. 7.9) [40].
- Hyperplasia and hyperkeratosis of the outer epithelial layer of the RP with the formation of epithelial cones in the deeper sections of the epithelium in advanced stages of RP (Fig. 7.9).
- A reduced self-cleaning potential of the squamous epithelium in the basal epithelial layer of epidermis in advanced stages of RP.

7.7 Pathogenesis and Molecular Biology of the Retraction Pocket

1. *Inflammation with negative pressure and gas exchange deficit in the middle ear spaces.*
2. *Localized disorganisation of the collagenic frame followed by invagination of the tympanic membrane.*
3. *Implication of two main molecular factors:* ***Keratin 10 and Id1****.*

The inflammatory cells as Langerhans' cells, T-Cells, Macrophages and others, migrate into the tympanic membrane, invade the nearby area of the ME, generating gas deficit and dysventilation. The tympanic membrane becomes retracted and suffers of disturbance of the self-cleaning mechanism. Peeled epidermal debris starts to be collected inside the fundus of the pocket with secondary bacterial superimposed infections which stimulate the infiltration of the epithelium by immune cells closing a vicious circle of inflammation, epithelial cell proliferation, retraction, collection of debris and infection [41]. Moreover, the process of chronic inflammation stimulates the growth and proliferation of keratinocytes in the eardrum, active promoter of the RP evolution into precholesteatoma and later on to cholesteatoma.

Two molecular factors play an important role in the development process and the RP evolution:

Keratin 10 and Id1

- ***Keratin 10***: is a protein that is frequently seen in the stratified squamous epithelium of the external auditory canal. It is expressed in RP. This suggests that the origin of RP is the skin of the external auditory canal invading the ME cavity [42].
- ***Id1 Protein***: is a transcription proliferative factor as a "keratinocytes growth factor" [42]. Chronic inflammation stimulates the growth and proliferation of keratinocytes in the external auditory skin canal and activates their migration into the retracted eardrum, since biologically proliferating cells are migratory.

These two molecular factors act in the process of retraction pocket as follows:

1. Chronic inflammation of the tympanic membrane activates Id1 protein.
2. Id1 triggers the cellular growth and proliferation process of basal cells of the retraction pocket membrane.
3. Loss of the self cleaning mechanism with deposition of debris in the fundus enhances the infection and inflammatory process in the fundus of the RP.
4. Under the above molecular stimulation, increased epithelial cell proliferation might take place with formation of basal epithelial cones, cone fusion and formation of lakes of keratin.

7.8 Clinical Features of a Retraction Pocket

7.8.1 Symptoms of a Retraction Pocket

A retraction pocket can be clinically silent for a long period of time and found during a systematic ear examination. However, the reported symptoms of a RP depend on its extent and severity. Hearing loss and otorrhea are the most common symptoms in history taking of the patient. Earache and dizziness are very rare symptoms. **Otorrhea** is mostly intermittent and can be spontaneous or following an exposition to water during swimming or bathing. **Hearing loss** is mostly of conductive type and can reach up to 45–55 dB in some cases. It is agreed that there is no correlation between hearing threshold and retraction stages [43]. Some authors suspect that cases with adhesion of the RP to the promontory increase the hearing threshold more than the adhesion to the incus [44].

7.8.2 Examination of the Pocket

On otomicroscopy, a complete and meticulous description of the RP is the baseline for its documentation in order to maintain a good evaluation of the pocket and to follow correctly its evolution over time. The same methodology of description must be strictly adopted by the disciplined examiner in every case of RP.

The otoendoscopy is a valuable and precious tool for this clinical description, because it permits better identification of the **limits, extensions, depth and relationship of the pocket with the hidden structures**. It assesses better the bottom of the retraction pocket and finally offers better quality of pictures for the chart documentation (Figs. 7.10 and 7.11).

The examination of the RP must give a precise description of the following:

7.8.2.1 Localization: PF or PT

- marginal (the bony boundary is the margin of the retracted membrane),
- non marginal (the annular ligament is the margin of the retraction),
- PF and PT in the same ear
- bilateral pathology

7.8.2.2 Adherences of the Pocket

Pocket membrane mobility can be tested by Valsalva maneuver with a Siegle speculum, or with a delicate suctioning taking care not to disrupt the pocket membrane.

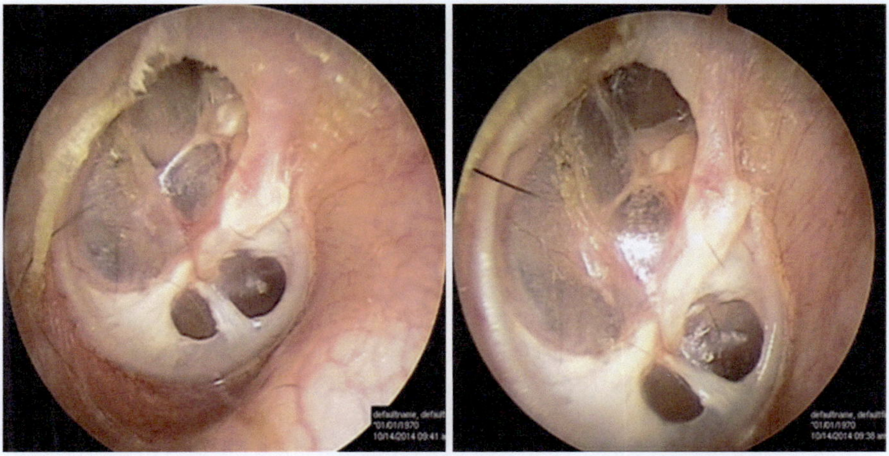

Fig. 7.10 Zero scope: fundus non visible vs. 30°: fundus visible, clean without debris or signs of inflammation

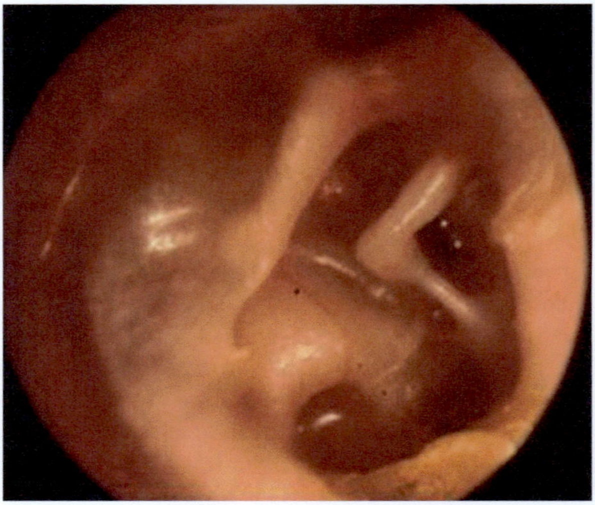

Fig. 7.11 Otoendoscopy examination of right ear showing PT RP collapsed and adherent to the intact ossicles and the promontory and extending into the sinus tympani. The sulcus tympani is eroded and enlarged at the posterosuperior quadrant. Notice that with the endoscope the whole retrotympanum is fully visualized and the fundus of the RP is visible and clean. *This can be hardly obtained with the microscope only*

- PT RP: Adhesion to the long process of the incus, to the incudostapedial joint, to the stapes, to the stapedial tendon, into the facial recess, to the sinus tympani, adhesion to the promontory, deep into the retrotympanum especially with high or very lateralized promontory (Fig. 7.11).
- PF RP: adhesion to the malleus neck, to the malleus head, deep in the attic (Fig. 7.13).

7.8.2.3 External Auditory Canal Status

- Skin status: presence of keratin accumulation at the margin of the RP, presence of skin redness or granulations proximal to the annulus: skin **suffering** (Fig. 7.12).
- Evident or suspected bone erosion of the scutum in the postero-superior quadrant (Figs. 7.12 and 7.13).
- Otorrhea: present or not during the examination.

7.8.2.4 Bottom of the RP

It is assessed by endoscopy, bottom fully visible or not, self-cleaning or not, crusting, presence of debris accumulation (Figs. 7.10, 7.11, and 7.12).

7.8.2.5 Neck of the RP

- *Large and wide open neck*: empty pocket, no debris accumulation despite a deep bottom. When the neck of the PF RP stays very large and wide enough, capable of self-cleaning, the RP may enlarge and extend into the epitympanum; the pocket membrane may get slowly thicker and thicker without becoming a real cholesteatoma matrix.
- *Constricted neck*: a constricted neck of a retraction pocket results in debris accumulation under tension inside the pocket, becoming highly suspicious of cholesteatoma formation. A constricted neck of the pocket may obscure the endoscopic input.

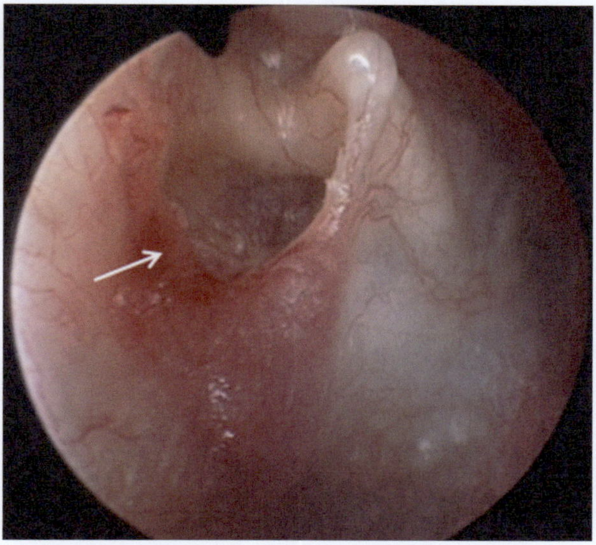

Fig. 7.12 Otoendoscopy of the right ear showing attic retraction pocket with large open neck of the pocket. Absence of keratin debris in the fundus of the pocket (hardly confirmed with microscope) but sign of skin suffering (*arrow*)

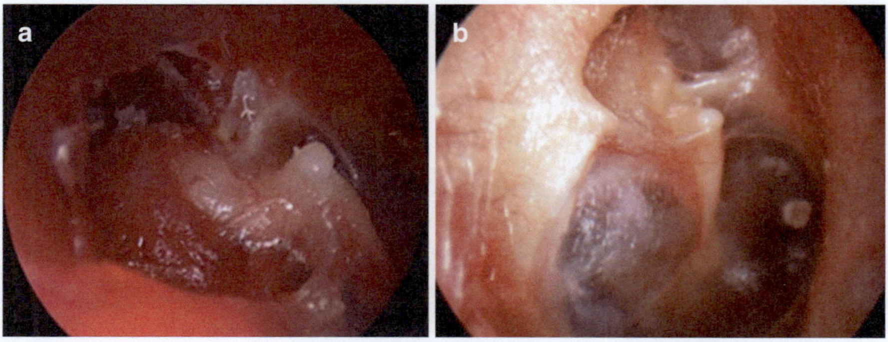

Fig. 7.13 (**a**) Otoendoscopy of a right ear showing an attic retraction pocket with a spontaneous atticotomy (bone erosion of the scutum). Notice the inflammatory skin canal (skin suffering) of the ear and retraction pocket, an evident sign of an aggressive behavior of the RP (precholesteatoma). (**b**) Otoendoscopy of a right ear showing almost the same degree of attical retraction as (**a**) with spontaneous atticotomy but without skin suffering

7.8.2.6 Ossicular Status (Figs. 7.14 and 7.15)

Otomicroscopy and endoscopy must analyze the correct status of the ossicular chain.

(a) Focal lysis of the incus
(b) Interruption of the incudo-stapedial joint
(c) Myringostapedopexy
(d) Lysis of the stapes

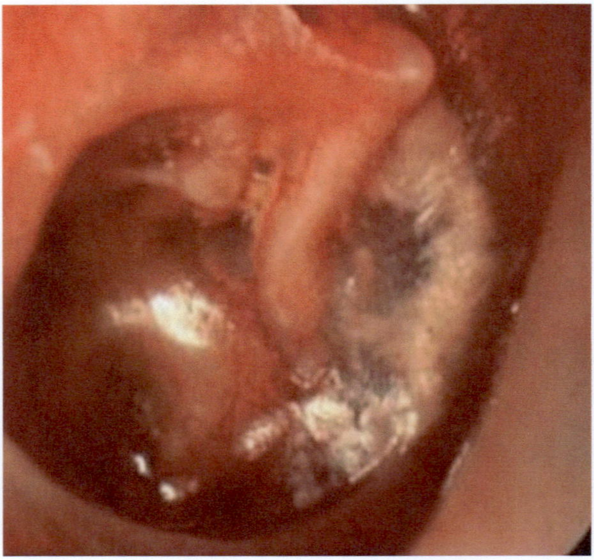

Fig. 7.14 Right ear, PT RP with intact ossicular chain and myringo-incudopexy

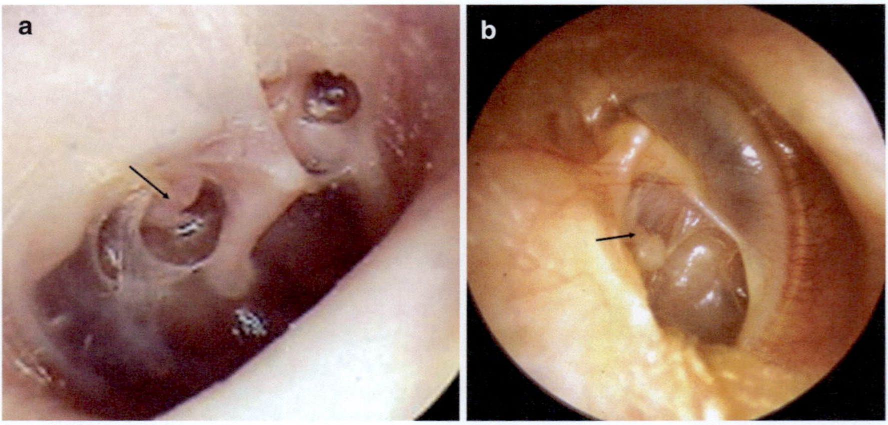

Fig. 7.15 (**a**) Otoendoscopy of left ear showing marginal erosion of the long process of the incus (*arrow*). (**b**) Otoendoscopy of left ear with incus erosion and myringostapedopexy and adhesion of the pocket on the promontory

7.9 Ossicular Erosion in Retraction Pockets

Ossicular erosion is a frequent finding in advanced RP; but it has been reported in the past only in a rate of 30% of cases [45, 46]. More recently, Jesic et al. stated that *destruction at the level of the long incus process in PT RP without cholesteatoma is present in more than 60% of cases*. The incidence of destruction of the two ossicles, the long process of the incus and the stapes superstructure, is found in a higher proportion in cases having combined PT RP and PF RP in the same ear [47].

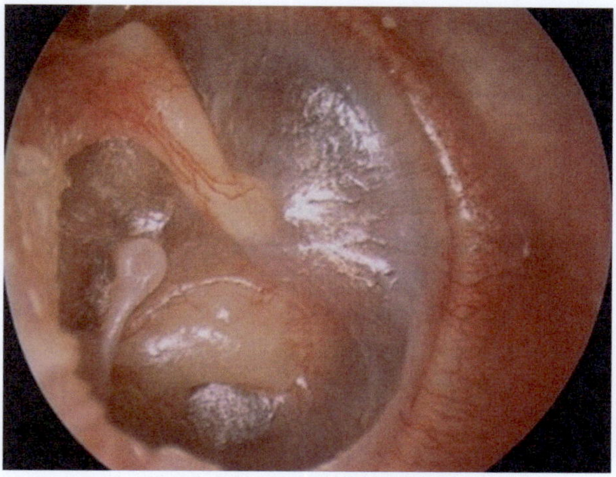

Fig. 7.16 Right ear PT RP with incus erosion and myringostapedopexy; some marginal keratin debris is indicating an advanced RP or precholesteatoma

2- The ossicular necrosis is most probably due to the:

(a) Continuous mechanical pressure effect of the RP layer on the ossicles,
(b) Osteoclastic enzymes released from the adherent epithelial layer of the RP
(c) Bacterial activity in case of associated infections.

Primarily the ossicular necrosis involves the long process of the incus and less frequently the stapes superstructure (Fig. 7.16). A functional hearing deficit is not constant and seldom important: necrosis of the long process of the incus may not induce a hearing loss due to the resultant myringostapedopexy (Fig. 7.16).

Most cases of RP with ossicular necrosis show moderate conductive hearing loss with a mean air–bone gap (ABG) of around 12 dB ± 10 dB [48]. Nevertheless a possible postoperative hearing loss greater than the preoperative deficit must be suspected and mentioned to the patient during counseling for surgery, especially in bilateral pathologies.

7.10 Classification of Retraction Pockets

Staging of retraction pockets was thought to be helpful for comparative assessment over time when the RP progresses. It was considered that grading a RP is a good protocol for the evaluation of the risk factors to progress to a cholesteatoma. However, there was no universally accepted nor adopted staging system for retraction pockets. The widely known classifications for the PF RP are of four stages according to Tos and Paulsen (1980), also of four stages according to Sade (1979) for the PT RP. Several other classifications enlarged the first ones, but did not either enjoy consensus (Charachon, Gerssdorf, *Dornhoeffer, Kakehata).* [49, 50].

All currently proposed classifications suffer from a high degree of interobserver variability [49, 50] and do not include the functional deficit.

All staging classifications describe the size, the extension and the depth visibility of the RP; but these descriptive characteristics - even informative—are not determinant to predict its fate because they are unable to disclose correctly and objectively the underlying inflammatory aspects which are the actual promoters of the RP evolution.

7.11 Fate of the Retraction Pocket

In the majority of cases, a retraction pocket is a stable otoscopic finding; but it can move to a dynamic pathology with variable outcome. An untreated retraction pocket may behave as follows:

1. it may stay unchanged in the majority of cases.
2. it may show spontaneous resolution, observed in about 40% of mild retraction cases [46, 48]. However, spontaneous resolution of the retraction pocket is very unlikely when adhesion of the epithelium is already present.
3. it may continue to progress towards a pre-cholesteatomatous stage in (15–20%) [21, 51, 52] and further to a cholesteatoma stage (see chapter 8).

As explained above, the determinant factor involved in the fate of a given RP is the dynamic, active and persistent inflammatory process inside the concerned ME spaces and its action on the neighboring segment of the tympanic membrane. The resolution of the inflammatory process implies stabilization or even regression of the RP whereas the exacerbation of the inflammatory process leads to a progression of the RP to more advanced stages. Therefore the duty of the otologist in front of an RP is to identify the presence and extension of an underlying inflammatory process both clinically and by imaging.

The following otoscopic and endoscopic descriptive signs during the evaluation of a RP are to be considered as **clinically adverse features**, that must be looked for as signs of an unfavorable future of the RP:

1. Otorrhea and Hypoacusia
2. Canal skin suffering, retention of keratin debris.
3. Fixity of the RP membrane to the eroded bony sulcus or bony scutum

It is of an utmost importance to identify the site of the causative underlying inflammatory process early enough before the advanced clinical bony destruction or other clinical features would take place. Clinical criteria remain dependant on the subjective observations skills and subject to the inter-observer findings. This is why objective criteria are needed to determine correctly the fate of a retraction pocket early enough to complete the subjective findings.

In a recent study done by the authors [36], TB CT has been found to contribute essentially to such aim, showing that:

(a) A poor pneumatization status of the mastoid favors the formation and progress of the RP.
(b) The presence on the CT of condensation images in selected ME spaces represent radiological signs of an ongoing inflammatory process, indicating an unfavorable evolution of the RP.

7.12 Imaging in Retraction Pockets

Recent literature lacks appreciable and specific studies relative to clinico-radiologic correlations in cases of RP. Nowadays CT-Imaging of ears with RP may enrich the clinical examination findings by additional imaging features. Facing the inability to predict clinically which retraction pocket will develop into an advanced stage or to even a cholesteatoma, CT scan may elucidate the disease dynamic status prior to its clinical morphologic manifestations and allow more sensitive pathological findings.

CT Imaging of a RP includes the following major inputs:

(a) *The morphologic assessment of the RP*
(b) *The pneumatization status of the temporal bone*
(c) *The aeration status of the middle ear cleft*
(d) *The topographic localisation of condensation images* found in the different middle ear spaces.

The above radiologic contributions, when analyzed in close clinico-radiological correlations will be the baseline to determine ***new objective criteria*** and establish a new strategy for the diagnosis, the prognosis and the management of retraction pockets.

7.12.1 Morphologic Assessment of the Retraction Pocket by CT

7.12.1.1 CT of the Pars Tensa Retraction

The pars tensa is easily identified on CT images, best in the transverse or coronal plane, dependent of the site of adhesions:

- A retraction of the central part of the pars tensa, adherent on the promontory is best seen on coronal reconstructions (Fig. 7.17a).
- A retraction of the pars tensa on the posterior wall of the retrotympanum and the condensation images of the underlying retrotympanic spaces are best assessed on the transversal plane (Fig. 7.17b).

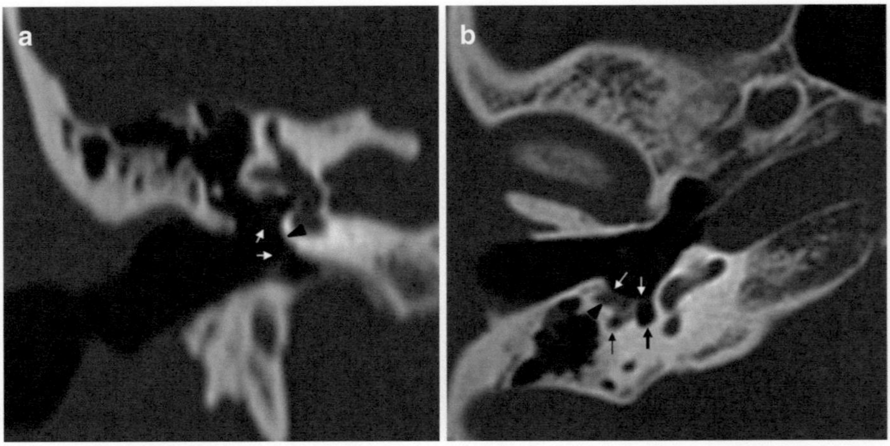

Fig. 7.17 (**a**) Coronal CT reconstruction: the tympanic membrane (*arrows*) is retracted on the promontory (*arrowhead*) and (**b**) transversal CT view: the retracted tympanic membrane (*white arrows*) is covering the facial recess which is fully condensated (*arrowhead*). The sinus tympani is still aerated (*thick black arrow*). VII nerve (*thin black arrow*)

- A retraction of the pars tensa on the incudostapedial ossicular chain is best analyzed on coronal images: the tympanic membrane may come into close contact to the incudostapedial ossicular chain (Fig. 7.18a), without any lysis, or may cause several degrees of lysis (Fig. 7.18b, c).

7.12.1.2 CT of the Pars Flaccida Retraction

The pars flaccida, when retracted, will be delimited by the bony borders: laterally by the lateral attic wall and medially by the lateral side of the incudomalleolar chain. As there is no air space left between the invaginated pocket and the bony borders, identification of the limits of this pocket is scanographically impossible (Fig. 7.19b); however there is one infallible stigmate of the retraction pocket: the amputation of the scutum! This sign must always be searched for on the coronal view. The RP can be seen if the pocket fundus has not yet reached the tegmen - as a thin dense band in the lateral attic separating the air in the pocket fundus and the air around the top of the pocket (Fig. 7.19a). When the membrane becomes thickened, or the fundus starts to collect the epidermal debris, it becomes more easily recognized on CT-Scan (Fig. 7.19c).

7.12.2 Pneumatization Status of the Mastoid

As explained above mastoid pneumatization status is involved in the formation and evolution of a retraction pocket due to the implication of the total air volume available in the middle ear cleft and the buffer role of the mastoid in the gas exchange conflicts;

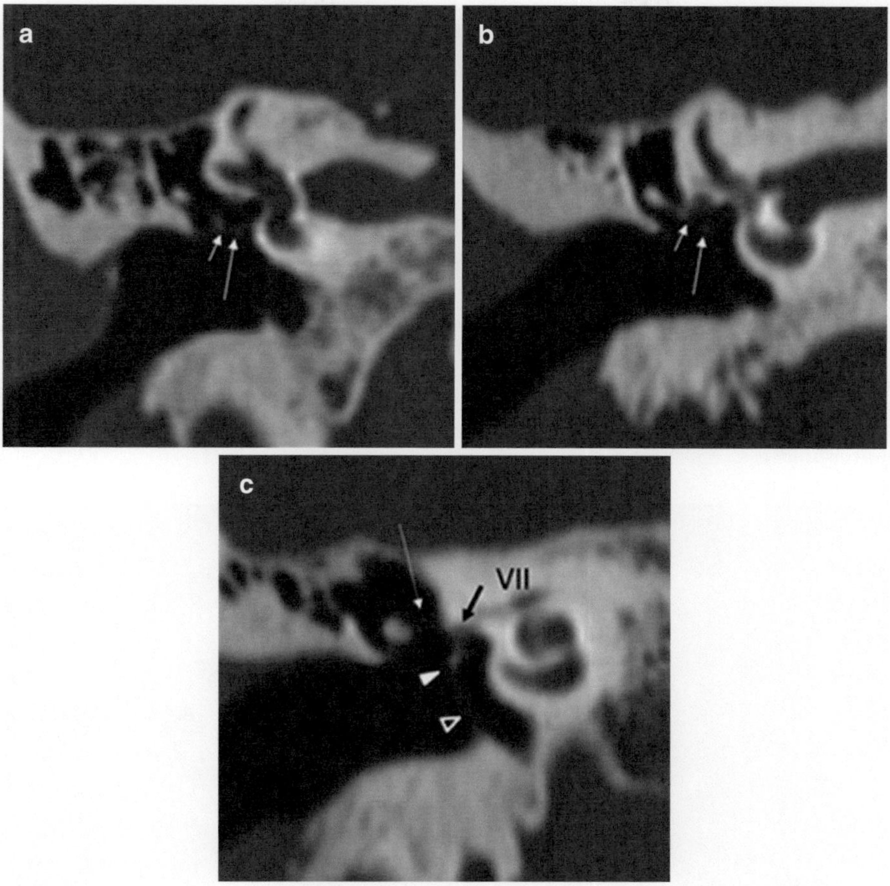

Fig. 7.18 Coronal CT reconstructions of different right ears with retraction of the tympanic membrane. (**a**) On the incudo-stapedial joint with lysis of the long process of the incus (*short arrow*) and the head of the stapes (*long arrow*). The space between the interrupted ossicular chain is filled by the thickened retracted membrane (between the two *arrows*), (**b**) on the incudostapedial joint with evident lyses of the long process of the incus (*short arrow*). Tympanostapedopexy (*long arrow*), but the tympanic membrane is very thin, difficult to visualize between the two arrows and (**c**) more advanced lyses of the long process of the incus, that is absent, the retracted tympanic membrane is herniated behind the incus (*long dashed arrow*), then retracted on the facial nerve canal (*black arrow*). Tympanostapedopexy (*full arrowhead*), the inferior pars tensa is in place (*empty arrowhead*)

1. The pneumatization status of the mastoid is commonly divided into three different aspects: sclerotic, diploic and well pneumatized mastoids. The antrum is the first developed mastoid space with its definite size at birth and does not grow significantly with age. Comparison of different ears at the antrum level evaluates the number and extension of pneumatized periantral cells. The transversal CT-images passing by the antrum and the incudomalleal chain are easily found and reproducible along with the different attic compartments (Fig. 7.20)

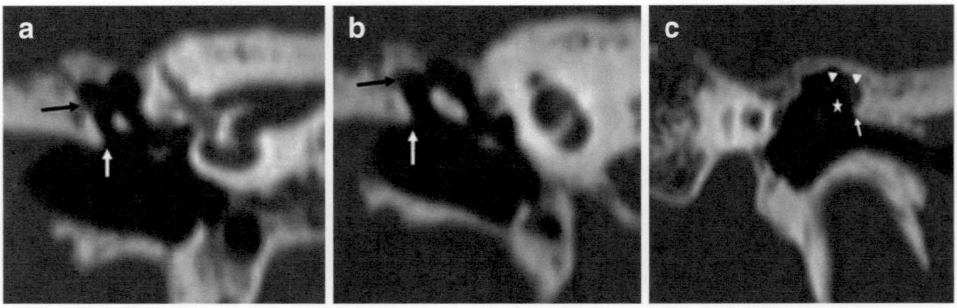

Fig. 7.19 Coronal CT reconstruction of pars flaccida retraction pockets: one common sign of all PF retraction pockets: the amputation of the scutum (*white arrows*). (**a**) Right ear PF RP: air space is left above and beneath the fundus of the pocket (black arrow), allowing its delineation, (**b**) right ear PFRP ear when extended to the tegmen, the fundus of the pocket (*black arrow*) is not any more individualized and (**c**) left ear PFRP (*) surrounded by condensation images at the pocket fundus (*arrowheads*)

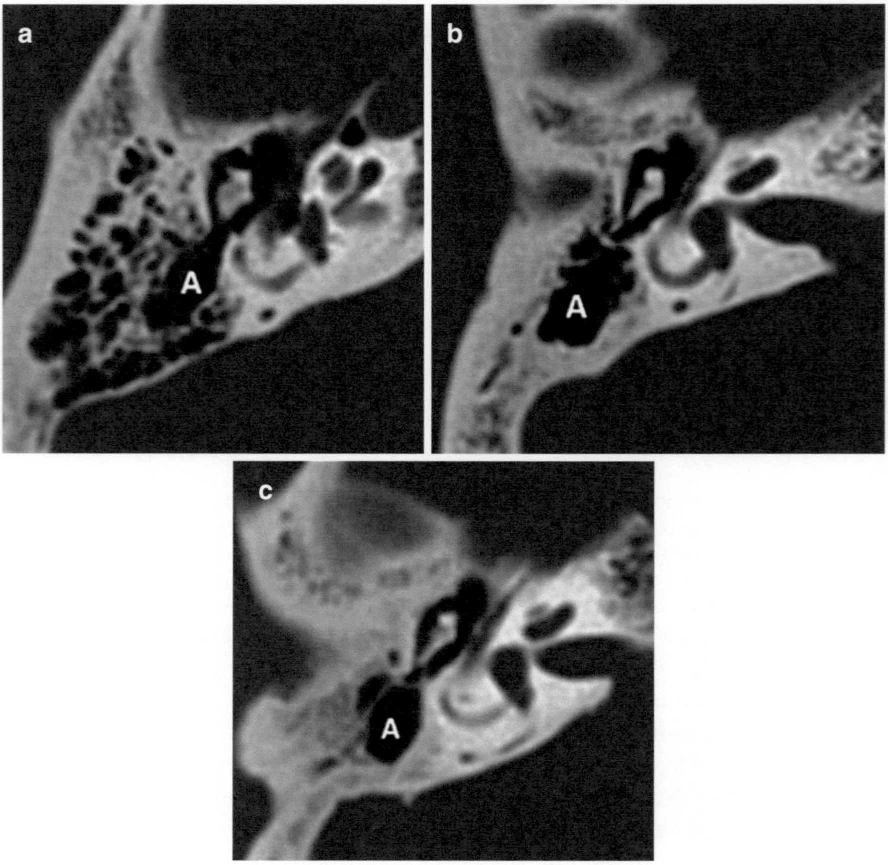

Fig. 7.20 Different pneumatization status of the mastoid compared on a transversal view passing by the antrum (A) of three different ears: (**a**) well pneumatized, (**b**) diploic = poorly pneumatized, (**c**) sclerotic = only the antrum is developed

7.12.3 Aeration Status of the Air Cell System of the ME Cleft

1. As the microdysventilation syndromes with blockage of one or both aeration pathways through the tympanic diaphragm cause retraction and invagination of the corresponding parts of the tympanic membrane into the **Attic**, this space is the essential part of the tympanic cavity to be evaluated.
2. As the obstruction of the anterior and posterior route of aeration engages the AER in the inflammatory process behind the RP, and takes place when the TTF in the Anterior epitympanic recess is complete, assessment of the **AER** is also crucial.
3. Condensation of the **Antrum** and the periantral cells indicates the obstruction of the tympanic isthmus, and an inflammatory condition of the mastoid cell system.

A transversal view passing by the upper part of the middle ear cavity, precisely by the **A**nterior epitympanic recess, the **A**ttic and the **A**ntrum, represents the crucial supradiaphragmatic spaces and the central portion of the mastoid cell system on one **"key image"**, representing at the same time the global pneumatization and the aeration status of the ear on one solely view, that we named the **"AAA" view** (Fig. 7.21a, b).

Isolated Pars tensa retraction pockets have been much more frequently found on CT-Scan imaging than Pars flaccida retraction pockets; in addition most of the Pars flaccida pockets showed an association to a Pars tensa retraction in the same ear. The study data are resumed in the following (Fig. 7.22):

- ***RP pathology is frequently associated with sclerotic or poorly pneumatized mastoids***
  93% of PFRP and 62% of PTRP were associated to sclerotic or diploic mastoid
  →*Thus sclerotic or poorly pneumatized mastoids are predisposing conditions for RP-formation and evolution*
- ***The AER pneumatization was found to be self- independent***:
  Even when the mastoid was poorly pneumatized, the AER was almost always well pneumatized and of normal dimensions.
- ***Condensation images of the AAA spaces were found in 80% of PFRP and 50% of PTRP***
- ***The AER (space A1) was condensed in 80% of PFRP and in 50% of PTRP***

The condensation status of the AAA spaces on the CT-Imaging represents an objective reliable imaging criteria to assess an underlying inflammatory process in the middle ear cleft. Normal aeration of the AER and/or the AAA spaces is almost always indicative of an arrest of the inflammatory process.

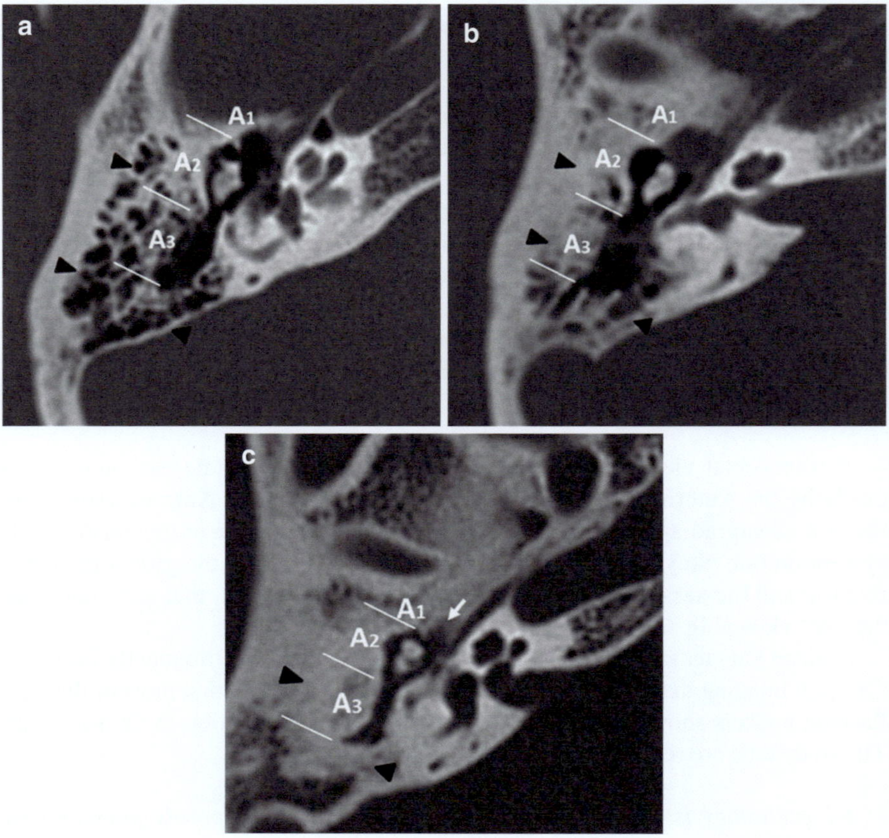

Fig. 7.21 The "AAA" view. (**a**) Normal pattern of the temporal bone pneumatization and aeration on the "AAA" view: A1 = AER, A2: Attic, A3: Antrum. Periantral mastoid air cells are well aerated (*arrowheads*), (**b**) A1: AER completely condensated, A2: lateral attic aerated, A3: antrum partially condensated. Moderately developed periantral mastoid air cells are partially condensated (*arrowheads*) and (**c**) totally sclerotic mastoid (*arrowhead*) and all three AAA spaces are completely obliterated, note the reduced size of this REA (*arrow*) along with the advanced sclerosis of the mastoid

Pneumatisation Status and Condensations in the Tympanic Cavity and the Mastoid

- RP pathology is frequently associated with sclerotic or poorly pneumatized mastoids
- AER pneumatization was found to be self-independent.
- Condensation images of the AAA spaces: 80% of PFRP and 50% of PTRP
- The AER was condensed in 80% of PFRP and in 50% of PTRP

Fig. 7.22 Pneumatisation status and space condensations in RP

7.13 Management of Retraction Pockets

Historically and because of the lack of objective criteria for a better diagnostic and prognostic methodology of RPs, there was no consensus among otologists concerning the indications, timing and surgical strategies for an adequate management of tympanic membrane retraction pockets. A recent systematic review stated that there is no high level of evidence to support any surgical intervention over watchful waiting in the management of tympanic membrane retraction pocket. In addition there is no good evidence to favor one particular treatment over the others.

In fact, the main problem is not the surgical decision taking, its timing or the proposed procedure, but is to know the actual clinical diagnosis of a given RP by itself: for the same otoscopic aspect of RPs, different otologists give different appellations such as retraction pocket, atelectasia, pre cholesteatoma … Often with relatively acceptable arguments by everyone, using one name or the other: "a confused diagnosis for a given RP results in a confused surgical strategy".

After reviewing the already proposed treatment modalities of RPs described in the past, and in order to offer a consensual therapeutical approach, a new strategy is proposed mainly based on the clinico-radiologic correlation through an evaluation of the status of the AAA spaces. Such evaluation offers the so called "objective criteria" aiming to avoid subjective inter observers differences and conflicts.

7.13.1 Watchful Observation

A conservative 'wait and see' or "wait and scope" policy is commonly adopted as a first-line strategy based on the presumption that retractions may resolve spontaneously in a large number of cases.

This attitude of "wait and see" should be applied, when the following conditions are found:

- No active inflammatory skin suffering in the external auditory canal, no otorrhea
- No functional deficit (CHL less than 30 dB)
- Aerated AAA spaces on the CT.

In this situation, the RP is almost asymptomatic. The absence of any inflammatory stigmata on the CT indicates that the RP has ceased its progress and there is no significant risk of degradation; consequently this ear can be considered as safe.

This policy is often coupled with medical therapies and environment control aiming to improve the specific mucosal immune system (MIS) of the upper respiratory tract and enhance the Eustachian tube function (i.e. nasal decongestant, oral antihistamines and steroids) [53, 54], or inflation devices (i.e. the Otovent® balloon) [55].

7.13.2 Surgical Management

7.13.2.1 Indications for Surgery

The indications for a surgical treatment decision of a given RP rely on *the presence of one or more* of the following adverse features:

1. Clinical description of the RP: debris collection, otorrhea, skin suffering, granulations.
2. Audiological Evaluation: Conductive hearing loss of more than 30 dB with an AB of 30 dB or more
3. CT-findings: Bony erosion of the scutum, condensation images of the AER alone or condensation in the **AAA spaces**.

A functional deficit of more than 20 dB could be an indication for surgery in order to improve hearing and repair the lytic sequelae of the retraction. However the surgical indication for a functional repair is relative and must be formally studied and counseled.

7.13.2.2 Surgical Procedures

Classical and minor surgical procedures have been practiced in the past to assist the ventilation function of the ET. Options included the insertion of a ventilation tube such as a grommet or T-tube which may be done alone or in combination with tympanic membrane reconstruction [56]. The affected segment of tympanic membrane can also be excised and replaced with a fascia graft or with a stronger graft such as cartilage harvested from the pinna or tragus. [57–59]. In children adenoidectomy may improve the Eustachian tube function, however there are conflicting reports regarding this assumption [60–62].

(a) ***Myringotomy with tubes***

Myringotomy with tube insertion is indicated for early stages of RP associated to a middle ear effusion during a watchful observation protocol.

Tubing can be associated with excision of the RP. This technique has been described first by Marquet in 1996—after insertion of the ventilation tube, he advised progressive suction of the atelectatic tympanic membrane to convert the retraction pocket into a lateral epithelial sac, and then cutting of the everted RP. According to his description, in less than 8 days the tympanic membrane regains normal appearance [63]. Excision should be done if retraction is limited to one quadrant. Care is to be taken not to excise too large areas of TM because a too large defect may persist. Pars flaccida RP are not excised since there is a risk of ingrowth of squamous epithelium and cholesteatoma formation at that area.

Patients must be followed long enough after extrusion of the tube to search for RP recurrence. Recurrence after tubing and even after simple removal of the RP and tympanoplasty is frequently encountered.

(b) ***Sub-annular ventilation tubes***

The technique consists of drilling in the posterior bony canal wall, after dissection of the skin flap together with the annulus, a bony depression to lodge a permanent fixed aerating tube communicating with the ME cavity without opening the tympanic membrane [64]. This procedure ensures a long term ventilation of the middle ear without the risk of a residual tympanic membrane perforation as compared to traditional T-tube insertion. Although this procedure has been reported to have a good and lasting control of retraction pockets; nevertheless it remains that this procedure is not without complications such as chorda tympani injury, otorrhea, occlusion of the tube with debris or granulations [65–67]**. Therefore** this procedure is indicated after repeated transtympanic tube extrusions and recurrence of the retraction pocket.

However, we consider that tubing does not respond adequately to the underlying causes *responsible of the* RP formation (microdysventilation).

(c) Tympanoplasty

In case of RP with adverse features, most authors advocate cartilage tympanoplasty. The RP should be separated, elevated and supported with cartilage graft [68–70]. In his 10-years follow-up of 63 RP reconstructed with perichondrium or temporalis fascia, **Buckingham** [71] **reported *recurrence in 80%* of the ears repaired with fascia and in 40% of those grafted with perichondrium**.

Utech H, first introduced cartilage in middle ear surgery in 1959 [72]. In 1982, Glasscock and al, first described the successful use of cartilage/perichondrial autograft for the surgical treatment of severe atelectasis and retraction pocket. Cartilage contributes much less to inflammatory tissue reaction; it is rigid and resists to resorption and it is largely nourished by diffusion with a very low metabolic rate. Cartilage resists firmly to middle ear pressure variations, even in the case of severe Eustachian tube dysfunction. Cartilage helps greatly in building back the lateral wall of the ME and the scutum.

Different techniques of cartilage tympanoplasty were described, from cartilage/perichondrium island graft, to cartilage shields or palisade techniques with cartilage thickness of less than 1 mm [73]. Nevertheless the reported recurrence rate of retraction with this procedure varies from *5% to 45% of cases* [58, 59, 74]. Also cartilage has some disadvantages such stiffness which gives some impairment of the high tone transmission; it is less compliant and has negative impact during higher sudden pressure variations. The most important criticism about this procedure is that the opaque cartilage graft may hide a possible cholesteatoma formation and does not relieve the ME from its causal pathology; cartilage tympanoplasty does not treat the underlying disease behind RP as explained above, especially in relation to the impact of normal aeration on ME mechanics (which may still lacking behind a non compliant eardrum graft.)

(d) Resection of the RP and Mastoid Obliteration

Mostly proposed for an advanced RP or even a precholesteatoma stage, the concept of this surgery is to reduce the degree of mucosal gas-exchange of the ME: the more the mucosa is extended the more the gas exchange is important [75]. The aim of the total mastoid obliteration is to create a small aerated tympanic cavity and to maintain an intact external ear canal wall to prevent recurrence of cholesteatoma secondary to the retraction pocket. The indication of this procedure relies on the grade of aeration of the tympanum shown by the CT of the temporal bone.

(e) Masto-Atticotomy with Anterior Epitympanotomy (AER Surgery)

As explained above, RP is not only a pathology of the tympanic membrane per se, but it is a consequence of a selective dysventilation syndrome taking place in one or more spaces or compartments in relation with the tympanic diaphragm obstruction. All means must be oriented to recover permanent aeration routes.

AER surgery provides an opportunity for the operator to divide folds, to free the physiologic ventilation pathways and to ensure the adequate gas exchange of the ME cleft particularly for the spaces situated above the tympanic diaphragm such the epitympanum and the retrotympanum in order to avoid recurrence of the PT RP and PF RP.

This is a functional surgery for the RP pathology in relation to the adverse clinico- radiologic aspects described above.

Anterior epitympanotomy procedure (AER) is indicated when the TTF is anatomically complete which is the case in 40% of ears [5]. The TTF can hardly be seen on the CT, unless it is pathologique [36], but it should be considered as complete in cases when the CT shows condensation images of the AER. *Taking in account the objective criteria of AAA condensation images even of an isolated AER condensation on the CT-evaluation, illustrating an ongoing inflammatory process, and along with the clinical findings as described above, the decision making of an AER surgery is favorable for so called* "high risk pockets".

The ***concept of AER surgery*** aims primarily to open the routes of aeration: first the posterior route of aeration (opening of the tympanic isthmus with reestablishment of the communication between the upper lateral attic and the lower lateral attic/atticotomy) and secondly the anterior route of aeration (anterior epitympanotomy with removal of the cog and the TTF) always with conservation of the ossicular chain (*this approach is called the direct approach*).

Anterior attico-tympanotomy is done through atticotomy following the tegmen until the zygoma anteriorly. *After resection of the cog, the TTF is excised* along with the inflammatory tissue filling the AER. During the progress of this surgery, attention must be paid to the tympanic segment of the facial nerve and the geniculate ganglion medially and at the same time a full respect of the ossicular chain is to be maintained to avoid iatrogenic trauma. Surgery is considered completed when a water aspiration test demonstrates a free water irrigation passage between all spaces of the attico-mastoid, the medial and lateral attic, the AER, the STR, the protympanum and the ME mesotympanum [36] (Fig. 7.23).

In cases where the long process of the incus is eroded, and a stapes – incus discontinuity is identified, incudo-malleal dislocation is done to render the anterior tympanotomy easier: a resection of the head of the malleus, resection of the cog and resection of the TTF are performed (*this approach is called the indirect approach*). During this indirect approach, after the AER surgery has been correctly performed, an incus/stapes transposition or a PORP procedure is done. Tympanic membrane grafting with perichondrium reinforced by thin and very small cartilage strips left

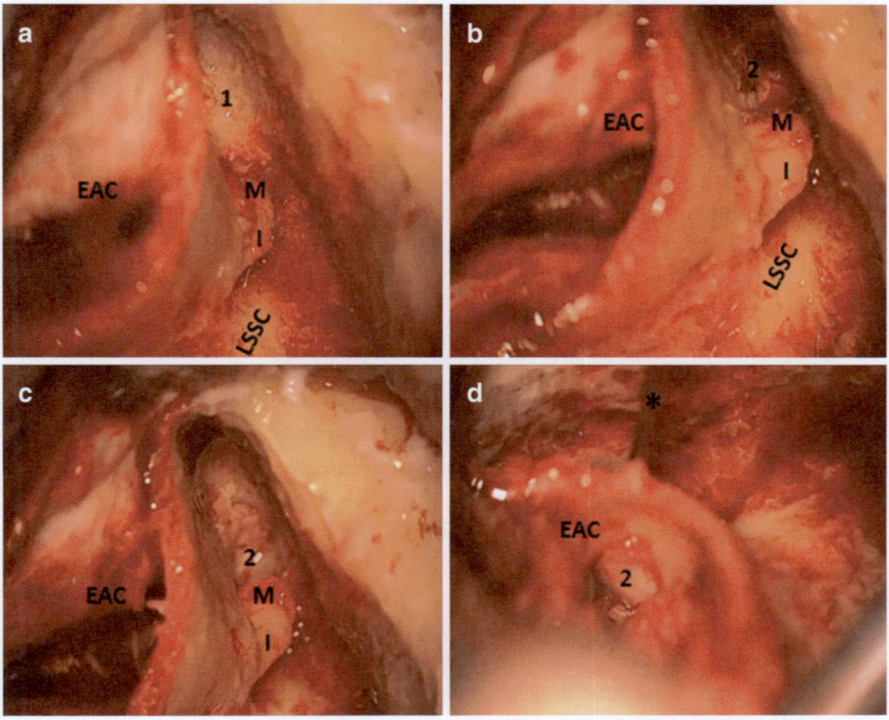

Fig. 7.23 Left ear surgical steps of AER approach and TTF removal. (**a**) Transmastoid anterior atticotomy till the cog (1) anterior to the head of malleus (M), (**b**) after drilling the cog, the TTF (2) is exposed, (**c**) closer view of the TTF (2) which appear thick and complete and (**d**) removal of the TTF (*) I: incus; LSSC: lateral semicircular canal; EAC: reconstructed external auditory canal

attached to the perichondrium. A probable lateral attic wall reconstruction is done using a strong piece of cartilage.

Some authors suggested that transcanal endoscopic technique could reach the anterior epitympanic recess and accomplish a resection or an opening of the TTF without the need to do posterior atticotomy (direct or indirect approach) [76]. This endoscopic approach could be feasible in cases where an evolving or advanced chronic inflammatory ME disease with granulations filling the AER is not in place. The anatomic topography of the AER when filled with granulation tissues and especially having a TTF of variable inclinations and thickness render the TTF hardly accessible and reachable from anteromedially (STR or protympanum), whatever the surgical tool used to perform correctly its complete resection. In addition the TTF needs to be resected, and not only transgressed, along with the excision of thick bony Cog, granulations and inflammatory mucosa in order to obtain a large and permanent opening for the anterior route of aeration and avoid the recurrence of the RP.

This is why we consider that the direct or indirect surgical AER approach is the key of success in dealing with RP.

Conclusion

Tympanic Membrane Retraction Pocket suffered of a lack of consensus among otologists. The concept of RP started in 1974 with Sade thanks to the microscopic examination and later by better documentation with the endoscope.

Advanced knowledge of the morpho-functional partition and the complex compartmentalization of the ME with its ventilation disorders followed by active inflammation and destruction, helped to understand the main causes behind the RP formation and its etiopathogenesis.

Most otologists elaborated various classifications which remained more theoretical than practical. Actually the tympanic membrane retraction pocket requires mostly a very careful and detailed physical otoscopic description.

A comprehensive assessment of the RP includes actually the input of TB CT, that can tell the otologist on one "key image" all about the pneumatization and relevant condensations above the tympanic diaphragm. When the so defined "AAA spaces" (**A**ER, **A**ttic and **A**ntrum) are entirely free of condensations, CT is then in favor of the absence of any evolutive inflammatory process: clinico-radiologic correlations permit to describe these pockets as stable and to elect for a conservative treatment.

In contrary, when the TB CT shows condensations in the AAA spaces, or even isolated condensations in the AER, coupled with clinically features of instability, the pocket has to be considered as unstable and probably evolutive. In these cases, a surgical treatment is proposed in order to prevent further evolution towards a cholesteatomatous process.

Better and more stable surgical results are obtained by an AER surgery. This functional surgery permits to all compartments of the middle ear to recover their aeration by the opening of the posterior and anterior routes. This is a determinant condition to eliminate RP recurrence.

A long term follow up of more than 5 years of the operated patients for RP must be the rule.

References

1. Tran Ba Huy P. Otites moyennes chroniques. Histoire e'le'mentaire et formes cliniques. EMC-Oto-rhino-laryngologie. 2005;2(1):26–61.
2. Yoon TH, Schachern PA, Paparella MM, Aeppli DM. Pathology and pathogenesis of tympanic membrane retraction. Am J Otolaryngol. 1990;11(1):10–7.
3. Sadé J, Avraham S, Brown M. Atelectasis, retraction pockets and cholesteatoma. Acta Otolaryngol. 1981;92(5–6):501–12.
4. Prades JM, Dumollard JM, Calloc'h F, Merzougui N, Veyret C, Martin C. Descriptive anatomy of the human auditory tube. Surg Radiol Anat. 1998;20(5):335–40.
5. Mansour S, et al. Comprehensive and clinical anatomy of the middle ear. Berlin/Heidelberg: Springer; 2013.
6. Hergils L, Magnuson B. Regulation of negative middle ear pressure without tubal opening. Arch Otolaryngol Head Neck Surg. 1988;114:1442–4.
7. Sade J, Luntz M. Gas diffusion in the middle ear. Acta Otolaryngol. 1991;111:354–7.
8. Ars B, Ars-Piret N. Middle ear pressure balance under normal conditions. Specific role of the middle ear structure. Acta Otorhinolaryngol Belg. 1994;48:339–42.

9. Doyle WJ. The mastoid as a functional rate-limiter of middle ear pressure change. Int J Pediatr Otorhinolaryngol. 2007;71(3):393–402.
10. Gaihede M, Dirckx JJJ, Jacobsen H, Aernouts J, Søvsø M, Tveterås K. Middle ear pressure regulation-complementary active actions of the mastoid and the eustachian tube. Otol Neurotol. 2010;31(4):603–11.
11. Alper CM, Kitsko DJ, Swarts JD, et al. Role of the mastoid in middle ear pressure regulation. Laryngoscope. 2011;121(2):404–8.
12. Cinamon U, Sadé J. Mastoid and tympanic membrane as pressure buffers: a quantitative study in a middle ear cleft model. Otol Neurotol. 2003;24(6):839–42.
13. Ars B, Dirckx J, Ars-Piret N, Buytaert J. Insights in the physiology of the human mastoid: message to the surgeon int. J Int Adv Otol. 2012;8(2):296–310.
14. Matanda R, Van de Heyning P, Bogers J, Ars B. Behaviour of middle ear cleft mucosa during inflammation: histo-morphometric study. Acta Otolaryngol. 2006;126(9):905.
15. Klagsbrun M, Soker S. VEGF/VPF: the angiogenesis factor found? Curr Biol. 1993;3: 699–702.
16. Ar A, Herman P, Lecain E, Wassef M, Huy PT, Kania RE. Middle ear gas loss in inflammatory conditions: the role of mucosa thickness and blood flow. Respir Physiol Neurobiol. 2007;155: 167–76.
17. Fink N, Ar A, Sade J, Barnea O. Mathematical analysis of atelectasis formation in middle ears with sealed ventilation tubes. Acta Physiol Scand. 2003;177:493–505.
18. Doyle WJ. Middle ear mechanics in research and otology. In: Rosowski Eiber A, editor. Proceedings of the 4th International Symposium. Singapore: World Scientific Publishing Co. Pvt. Ltd.; 2000. p. 314–21.
19. Pau HW, Sievert U, Just T, Sade J. Pressure changes in the human middle ear without opening the eustachian tube. Acta Otolaryngol. 2009;129:1182–6.
20. Sade J, Ar A. Middle ear and auditory tube: Middle ear clearance, gas exchange, and pressure regulation. Otolaryngol Head Neck Surg. 1997;1997(116):499–524.
21. Tos M, Poulsen G. Attic retractions following secretory otitis. Acta Otolaryngologica. 1980;89:479–86.
22. Maw AR, Bawden R. The long term outcome of secretory otitis media in children and the effects of surgical treatment: a ten year study. Acta Otorhinolaryngol Belg. 1994;48(4):317–24.
23. Stangerup SE, Tos M, Arnesen R, Larsen P. A cohort study of point prevalence of eardrum pathology in children and teenagers from age 5 to age 16. Eur Arch Otorhinolaryngol. 1994;251(7):399–401.
24. Maw AR, Hall AJ, Pothier DD, Gregory SP, Steer CD. The prevalence of tympanic membrane and related middle ear pathology in children: a large longitudinal cohort study followed from birth to age ten. Otol Neurotol. 2011;32(8):1256–61.
25. De Beer BA, Schilder AG, Zielhuis GA, Graamans K. Natural course of tympanic membrane pathology related to otitis media and ventilation tubes between ages 8 and 18 years. Otol Neurotol. 2005;26(5):1016–21.
26. Ars BM, Dirckx JJ, Decraemer WF, Ars-Piret NM. Faulty aeration of the middle ear: repercussion on the tympanic membrane lamina propria. In: Sadé J, editor. The Eustachian tube, basic aspects. Amsterdam: Kugler and Ghedini Publications; 1991. p. 365–71.
27. Sadé J, Berco E. Atelectasis and secretory otitis media. Ann Otol Rhinol Laryngol. 1976;85(Suppl. 25 Pt 2):66–72.
28. Ruah CB, Schachern PA, Paparella MM, Zelterman D. Mechanisms of retraction pocket formation in the pediatric tympanic membrane. Arch Otolaryngol Head Neck Surg. 1992;118(12):1298–305.
29. Danner CJ. Middle ear atelectasis: what causes it and how is it corrected? Otolaryngol Clin N Am. 2006;39(6):1211–9.
30. Zhang Q, Liang J. Transformation of effusion and formation of granulation tissue in the pathologic process of otitis media with effusion. Lin Chuang Er Bi Yan Hou Ke Za Zhi. 1999;13(1):8–11.
31. Marchioni D, Alicandri-Ciufelli M, Grammatica A, Mattioli F, Presutti L. Pyramidal eminence and subpyramidal space: an endoscopic anatomical study. Laryngoscope. 2010;120(3):557–64.

32. Marchioni D, Mattioli F, Alicandri-Ciufelli M, Presutti L. Prevalence of ventilation blockages in patients affected by attic pathology: a case-control study. Laryngoscope. 2013;123(11):2845–53. https://doi.org/10.1002/lary.24165.
33. Aimi K. The clinical significance of epitympanic mucosal folds. Arch Otolaryngol. 1971;94(6):499–508.
34. Aimi K. The tympanic isthmus: its anatomy and clinical significance. Laryngoscope. 1978;88:1067–81.
35. Plava T, et al. Lateral and anterior view to Tensor Tympani Fold and supratubal recess. Am J Otol. 1998;19:405–14.
36. Mansour S, Nicolas K, Naim A, Yamine F, Moukarzel N, Nehme A. Inflammatory chronic otitis media and the anterior epitympanic recess. J Otolaryngol. 2005;34(3):149–59.
37. Morimitsu T, Nagai T, Nagai M, Ide M, Makino K, Tono T, Adachi Y, Kasano F, Fukiyama M, Hayashi A. Pathogenesis of cholesteatoma based on clinical results of anterior tympanotomy. Auris Nasus Larynx. 1989;16(Suppl 1):S9–14.
38. Sade J. Atelectatic tympanic membrane: histologic study. Ann Otol Rhinol Laryngol. 1993;102:712–6.
39. Shunyu NB, Gupta SD, Thakar A, Sharma SC. Histological and immunohistochemical study of pars tensa retraction pocket. Otolaryngol Head Neck Surg. 2011;145(4):628–34.
40. Bremond G, Magnan J, Chays A, Florence A, Gignac D, Lebreuil G. Les poches de retraction, entite pathologique? Ann Oto-laryng (Paris). 1990;107:386.
41. Lennar E. Digital comprehensive summaries of Uppsala dissertations from faculty of Medicine 905. Middle Ear Cholesteatoma: surgical treatment, followup and hearing, restoration, Acta Universitatis, Upsaliensis, Uppsala; 2013.
42. Zhang Q, et al. Identification of Id1 in acquired ME cholesteatoma. Arch Otolaryngol Head Neck Surg. 2008;134(3):306–10.
43. Amioni C, et al. Tympanic atelectasis in children and early surgical approach. Int Adv Otol. 2011;7:293–8.
44. James AL, Papsin BC, Trimble K, Ramsden J, Sanjeevan N, Bailie N, Chadha NK. Tympanic membrane retraction: an endoscopic evaluation of staging systems. Laryngoscope. 2012;122:1115–20.
45. Swartz JD, Berger AS, Zwillenberg S, Popky GL. Ossicular erosions in the dry ear: CT diagnosis. Radiology. 1987;163(3):763–5.
46. Jesic SD, Jotic AD, Babic BB. Predictors for sensorineural hearing loss in patients with tubotympanic otitis, cholesteatoma, and tympanic membrane retractions. Otol Neurotol. 2012;33(6):934–40.
47. SD J, Rovcanin LH, Jovicevic OD, Jotic AD, Slijepcevic NA, Ljubic VR. Pars tensa retractions without cholesteatoma in children: predictors for ossicular chain destruction, air conduction thresholds, and postoperative retractions. Otol Neurotol. 2014;35(6):997–1002.
48. Borgstein J, Gerritsma TV, Bruce IA. Erosion of the incus in pediatric posterior tympanic membrane retraction pockets without cholesteatoma. Int J Pediatr Otorhinolaryngol. 2008;72(9):1419–23.
49. Pothier D, Sadé J, Tos M. Classifications of the tympanic membrane: not reliable? Clin Otolaryngol Allied Sci. 2006;31(3):249.
50. Alzahrani M, Saliba I. Tympanic membrane retraction pocket staging: is it worthwhile? Eur Arch Otorhinolaryngol. 2014;271(6):1361–8.
51. Sade J, Avrham S, Brown M. Dynamics of atelectasis and retraction pockets. Proceedings of the 2nd international conference on cholesteatoma and mastoid surgery. Amsterdam: Kugler Publications; 1982. p. 267–81.
52. Charachon R, Barthez M, Lejeune JM. Spontaneous retraction pockets in chronic otitis media: medical and surgical therapy. ENT J. 1992;71:578–83.
53. Cantering EI, Bluestone CD, Rocketed HE, Beery QC. Effect of decongestant with or without antihistamine on Eustachian tube function. Ann Otol Rhinol Laryngol Suppl. 1980;89(3):290–5.
54. Silverstein H, Light JP, Jackson LE. Direct application of dexamethasone for the treatment of chronic Eustachian tube dysfunction. Ear Nose Throat J. 2003;82(1):28–32.

55. Blanshard JD, Maw AR, Bawden R. Conservative treatment of otitis media with effusion by autoinfl ation of the middle ear. Clin Otolaryngol Allied Sci. 1993;18(3):188–92.
56. Elsheikh MN, Elsherief HS, Elsherief SG. Cartilage tympanoplasty for management of tympanic membrane atelectasis: is ventilatory tube necessary? Otol Neurotol. 2006;27(6):859–64.
57. Dornhoffer J. Cartilage tympanoplasty: indications, techniques, and outcomes in a 1,000-patient series. Laryngoscope. 2003;113(11):1844–56.
58. Blaney SP, Tierney P, Bowdler DA. The surgical management of the pars tensa retraction pocket in the child—results following simple excision and ventilation tube insertion. Int J Pediatr Otorhinolaryngol. 1999;50:133–7.
59. Sharp JF, Robinson JM. Treatment of tympanic membrane retraction pockets by excision. A prospective study. J Laryngol Otol. 1992;106:882–6.
60. Bluestone CD, Cantekin EI, Beery QC. Certain effects of adenoidectomy of Eustachian tube ventilatory function. Laryngoscope. 1975;85(1):113–27.
61. Dempster JH, Browning GG. Eustachian tube function following adenoidectomy: an evaluation by sniffing. Clin Otolaryngol Allied Sci. 1989;14(5):411–4.
62. Honjo I, Tashima K, Mitoma T, Hamada E. Effect of adenoidectomy on Eustachian tube function. Auris Nasus Larynx. 1985;12(Suppl 1):S231–3.
63. Marguet J. Preventive treatment of cholesteatoma. Impharzam Med Forum. 1986;9:23–7.
64. Saliba I, Boutin T, Arcand P, Froehlich P, Abela A. Advantages of subannular tube vs repetitive transtympanic tube technique. Arch Otolaryngol Head Neck Surg. 2011;137(12):1210–6.
65. Jassar P, et al. Long-term ventilation of the middle ear using a sub annular tympanotomy technique: a follow-up study. J Laryngol Otol. 2004;118(12):933–6.
66. McManus LJ. The clinical anatomy of the chorda tympani, a micro CT study. Thesis, Bachelor of Medical Science with Honours. University of Otago; 2012. http://hdl.handle.net/10523/2242.
67. Gopen Q. Surgical procedures. In: Pellet W, Cannoni M, Pech A, editors. Fundamental otology: paediatric and adult practice. New Delhi: Jaypee Brothers Medical Publishers (P) Ltd; 2013. p. 386–7.
68. Couloigner V, Molony N, Viala P, Contencin P, Narcy P, Van Den Abbeele T. Cartilage tympanoplasty for posterosuperior retraction pockets of the pars tensa in children. Ontol Neurotol. 2003;24(2):264–9.
69. Levinson RM. Cartilage-perichondrial composite graft tympanoplasty in the treatment of posterior marginal and attic retraction pockets. Laryngoscope. 1987;97(9):1069–74.
70. Poe DS, Gadre AK. Cartilage tympanoplasty for management of retraction pockets and cholesteatomas. Laryngoscope. 1993;103(6):614–8.
71. Buckingham RA, Stuart DR, Geick MR, Girgis SJ, McGee TJ. Experimental evidence against middle ear oxygen absorption. Laryngoscope. 1985;95(4):437–42.
72. Utech H. Tympanotomy in disorders of sound conduction; its diagnostic and therapeutic possibilities. Z Laryngol Rhinol Otol. 1959;38(4):212–21.
73. Tos M. Cartilage tympanoplasty: classification of methods–techniques–results. Stuttgart, New York: Thieme; 2009. p. I–420.
74. Jansen C. Retraction pocket as a potential for cholesteatoma recurrence. Laryngol Rhinol Otol (Stuttg). 1986;65:499–510.
75. Yanagihara N, Komori M, Hinohira Y. Total mastoid obliteration in staged canal-up tympanoplasty for cholesteatoma facilitates tympanic aeration. Ontol Neurotol. 2009;30(6):766–70.
76. Marchioni D, Alicandri-Ciufelli M, Grammatica A, Mattioli F, Genovese E, Presutti L. Lateral endoscopic approach to epitympanic diaphragm and Prussak's space: a dissection study. Surg Radiol Anat. 2010;32(9):843–52.

Cholesteatoma

8

Contents

S. Mansour et al., *Middle Ear Diseases*,
https://doi.org/10.1007/978-3-319-72962-6_8

8.1 Introduction

Cholesteatoma (synonym: keratoma) is a chronic otitis of the middle ear cleft characterized by "a wrong skin in the wrong place" (Fig. 8.1). It derives from an abnormal proliferation of a keratinizing squamous epithelium.

Cholesteatoma of the middle ear is one of the most complex topics in otology; it has stimulated much research and debates worldwide but still suffers of a lack of consensus regarding most of its aspects.

In this chapter we provide a comprehensive overview of this pathology and the contemporary advances regarding its histopathology, molecular biology, its best evaluation and most adequate management.

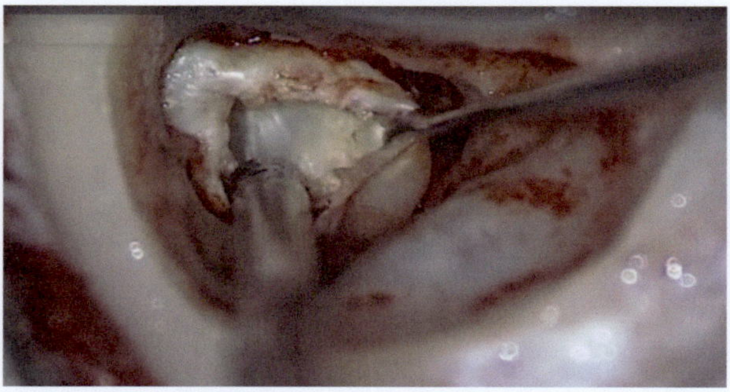

Fig. 8.1 Right ear large cholesteatoma filling the mastoid antrum. Notice that the cholesteatoma is a cystic lesion that consists of an envelope (matrix) and whitish content (keratin)

8.2 Epidemiology

The annual incidence of cholesteatoma is reported to be 9.2 per 100,000 in adults and 3 per 100,000 in children with an overall male predominance of 1.4/1 [1]. The incidence of cholesteatoma varies worldwide. The main factors that contribute to the development and frequency of cholesteatomas are: geography, genetics, sex, age, the environment, and the socio-economic status.

There is a high prevalence in Caucasian populations and it is rare in the Afro-descendants [2].

The incidence of middle ear cholesteatoma peaks in the second and third decade of life.

The mean age in children with cholesteatomatous otitis media is 10 years; the mean age of children with congenital cholesteatoma is 6 years [3].

Association of cholesteatoma in one ear and chronic inflammatory pathology in the contralateral ear is about 50% of cases [4, 5].

8.3 Types of Cholesteatoma

There are two main types of cholesteatoma based on the disease pathogenesis: congenital and acquired [6].

8.3.1 Congenital Cholesteatoma

Congenital cholesteatoma is a benign tumoral process of the middle ear that manifests as a pearly white mass with keratinized stratified squamous epithelium, arising in the middle ear cleft behind an intact tympanic membrane, usually in young ages (Fig. 8.2). Congenital middle ear cholesteatoma is a relatively rare disease representing approximately 2% of the entire cholesteatoma cases [7]. Recently, with the

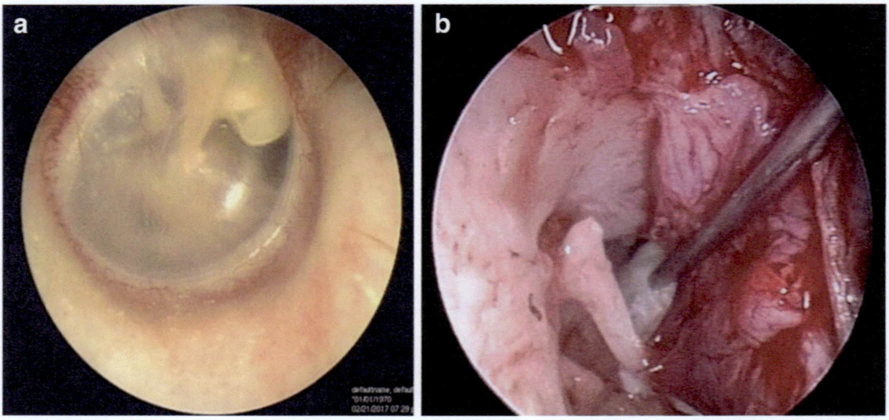

Fig. 8.2 (**a**) Right ear congenital cholesteatoma of the anterosuperior quadrant and (**b**) intraoperative endoscopic removal

Fig. 8.3 Congenital cholesteatoma diagnostic criteria

Congenital Cholesteatoma Diagnostic Criteria

- White mass medial to a normal TM
- No prior history of otorrhea
- No prior history of TM perforation
- No prior history of otologic procedures

increase of interest in this disease, its detection rate is increased, and thus the ratio of congenital cholesteatoma to the entire cholesteatoma has increased to more than 4% [7, 8].

First Derlacki in the sixties and then Levenson in 1989 established a set of criteria for the diagnosis of congenital cholesteatoma in the middle ear (Fig. 8.3). These criteria included:

- A white mass behind a normal tympanic membrane (Figs. 8.2 and 8.4),
- A normal pars flaccida and pars tensa,
- No prior history of otorrhea or perforations, and
- No prior otologic procedures.

Prior bouts of otitis media do not exclude the congenital nature of the disease. Levenson found that the mean age at presentation was 4.5 years with a male preponderance of 3:1.

Two typical sites of origin are described: The most frequent site (two-third of cases) is in the anterosuperior quadrant in the proximity of the Eustachian tube opening, and the second most frequent in the posterosuperior quadrant close to the

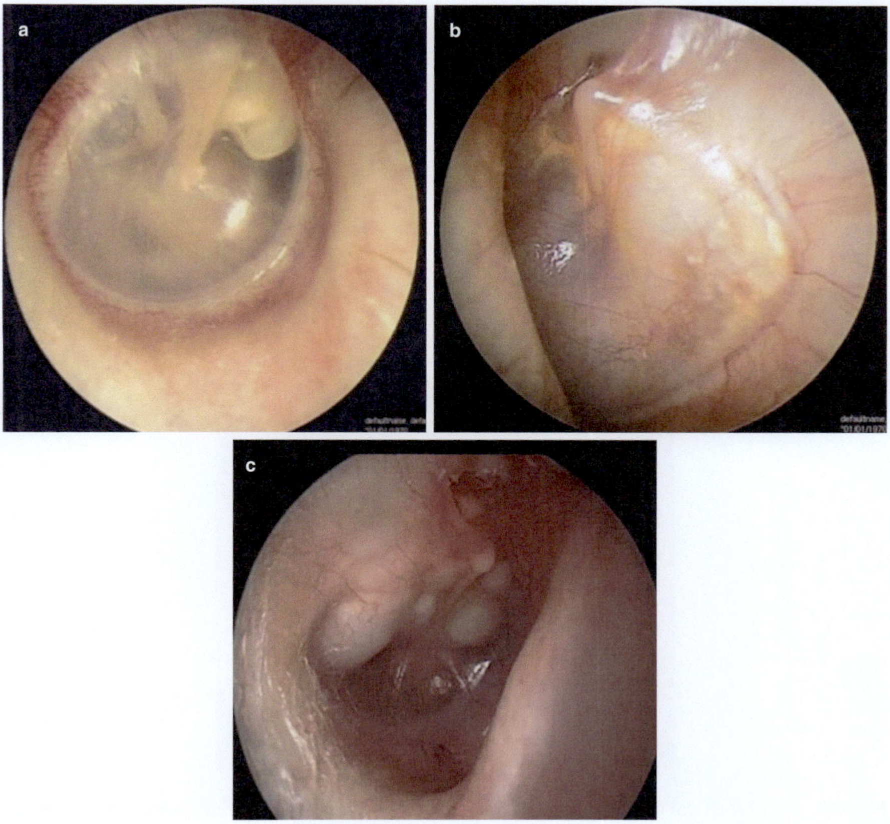

Fig. 8.4 (**a**) Small congenital cholesteatoma in the anterosuperior quadrant of a right ear, (**b**) congenital cholesteatoma of the posterosuperior quadrant of a left ear and (**c**) congenital cholesteatoma of both quadrants: post-sup and ant-sup

incudostapedial joint. In advanced cases, congenital cholesteatoma may involve more than one quadrant of the middle ear (Fig. 8.4).

8.3.2 Acquired Cholesteatoma

Acquired cholesteatoma is a special form of chronic otitis media in which keratinizing squamous epithelium grows from the tympanic membrane or/and the auditory canal skin into the middle ear mucosa. Acquired cholesteatomas of the middle ear are further divided into primary acquired and secondary acquired forms (Shambaugh).

8.3.2.1 Primary Acquired cholesteatoma

The primary acquired cholesteatoma is the most frequent type of acquired cholesteatoma and develops by the progression of an initial retraction pocket into a cholesteatoma. Primary acquired cholesteatomas are named relative to the site of

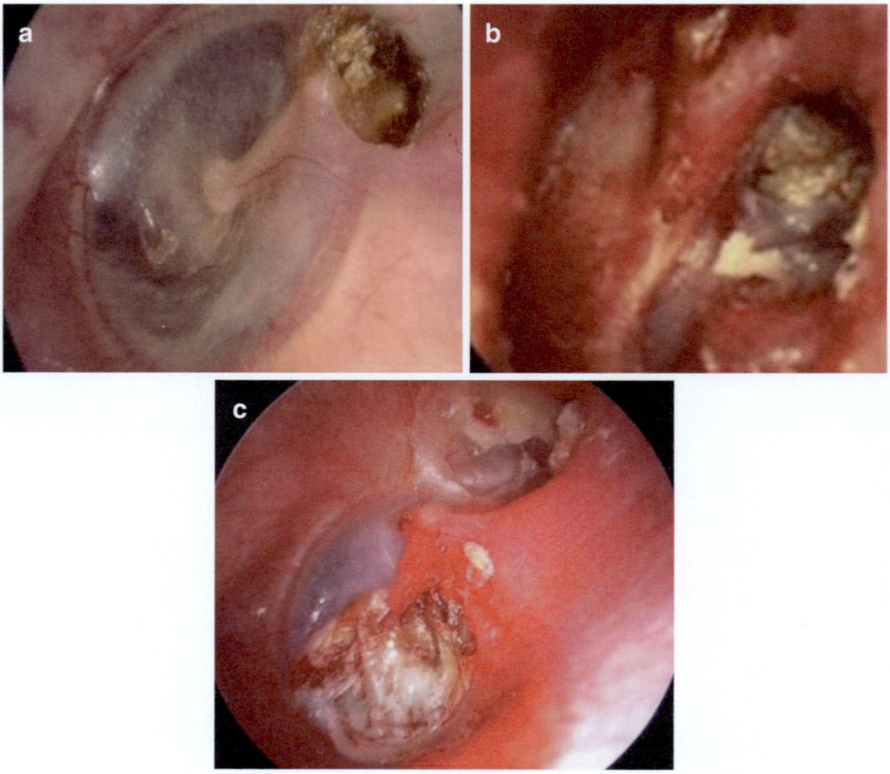

Fig. 8.5 (**a**) Left attical cholesteatoma, (**b**) left ear meso and retrotympanic cholesteatoma and (**c**) left ear double cholesteatomas, attical and mesotympanic

the pocket origin: (1) attic cholesteatoma consecutive to a pars flaccida pocket, (2) mesotympanic cholesteatoma due to a pars tensa pocket, and (3) combined forms, due to double pockets (Fig. 8.5).

The predominant form of acquired cholesteatoma in children develops in 80% from retraction pockets of the pars tensa (especially the posterior sub-ligamentary pars tensa) whereas in adults, this form develops mainly in the pars flaccida (or Shrapnell's membrane).

8.3.2.2 Secondary Acquired Cholesteatoma

Secondary acquired cholesteatoma develops by an epithelial migration from the bottom of the ear canal into the middle ear through a marginal tympanic membrane perforation (Fig. 8.6), which could be due to infection (acute necrotizing otitis media). It could also be due to a trapped skin inside the middle ear following trauma or surgery.

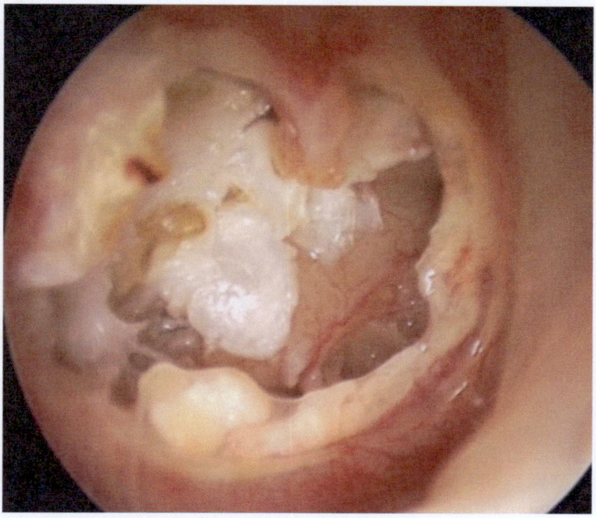

Fig. 8.6 Left ear, cholesteatoma by skin migration through a marginal perforation of right ear

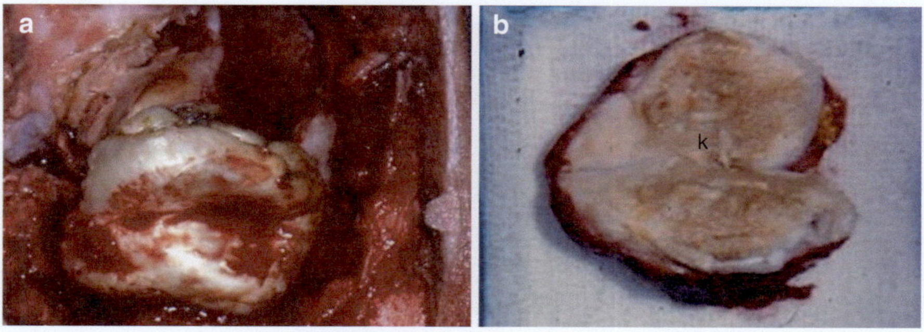

Fig. 8.7 (**a**) Large cholesteatoma with its whitish pearly aspect and (**b**) after removal the cholesteatoma was opened to show its center full with keratin (k) with its greasy aspect, misnamed cholesteatoma

8.4 Histopathology of Cholesteatoma

8.4.1 Macroscopy

In 1829, Cruveilhier [9] described cholesteatoma as a "pearly tumor", due to its whitish pearly appearance (Fig. 8.1). In 1838 Muller [10] gave it the name of "cholesteatoma" due to the greasy aspect of the mass (Fig. 8.7).

8.4.2 Light Microscopy

Light microscopy shows a cyst with three components (Figs. 8.8 and 8.9):

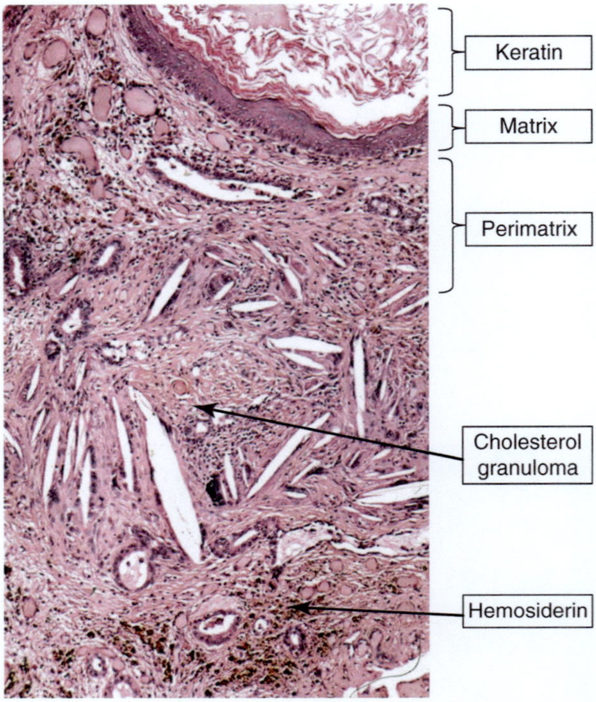

Fig. 8.8 Light microscopy of a cholesteatoma capsule showing the amorphic center made up of squamous keratin debris and matrix made up keratinizing squamous epithelium and perimatrix made up of granulation tissue infiltrated by inflammatory cells and surrounded in this special case by cholesterol granuloma and hemosiderin

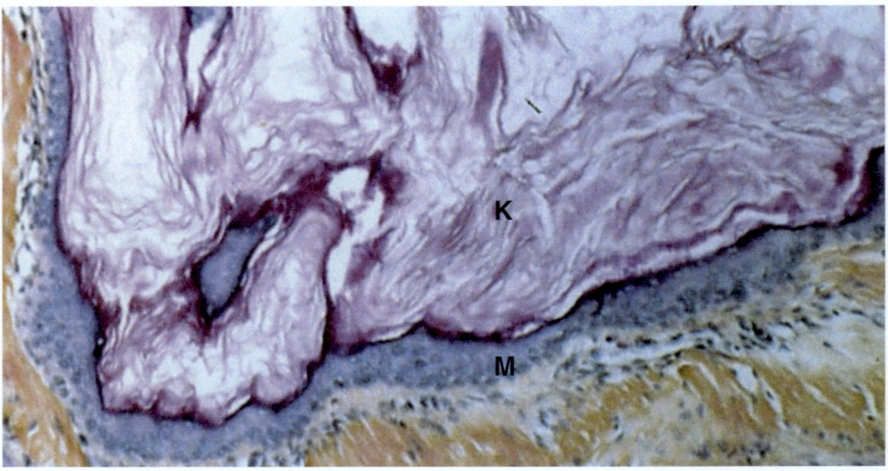

Fig. 8.9 Light microscope: Cholesteatoma with Keratin debris (K), surrounded by keratinizing squamous epithelium; the matrix (M) shows hyperplasia of the basal cell layer

1. The "amorphic center", formed of accumulated desquamated epithelium, enveloped by "the matrix".
2. The matrix is a stimulated proliferative skin with hyperkeratosis desquamation at the surface, hyperplasia of the basal cell layer and deep papillary growing into the subepithelial tissue.
3. The perimatrix is formed of granulation tissue that is the site of an important inflammatory process. The thickness of the perimatrix and the intensity of its inflammatory process determine the aggressiveness of the cholesteatoma.

8.4.3 Electron Microscopy

Electron microscopy studies on cholesteatoma helped to better understand the etiopathogenesis of cholesteatoma. Cholesteatoma consists of an amorphous center containing keratin (made of desquamated keratinocytes of the epidermal layer), the matrix (epidermal layer) and the perimatrix (inflammatory layer) surrounding the matrix (Fig. 8.10). Cholesteatoma matrix has the same histological and cellular structure as the epidermis that is lining the bottom of the external auditory canal. All the maturation stages of the keratinocytes are clearly similar in both structures and demonstrated by electron microscopy of cholesteatoma matrix as the following layers (Fig. 8.11):

- *The stratum corneum* where the cells become dead shells filled with keratin fibers that are electron dense.
- *The stratum granulosum* characterized by keratohyalin grains aligned parallel to the surface.
- *The stratum spinosum* (due to desmosomes attachments) where maturation of the keratinocytes is accompanied by two characteristics phenomena: flattening of the cells and grouping of tonofilaments;
- *The basal stratum:* formed by a unicellular layer, each cell tightly united to the others by desmosomes (tight junctions).

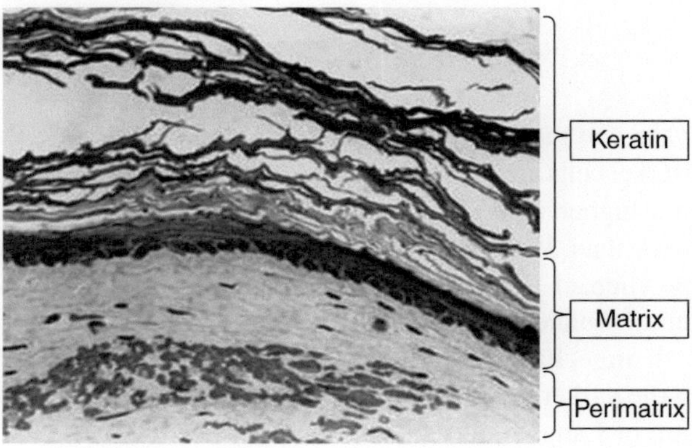

Fig. 8.10 Electron microscope of cholesteatoma with an amorphous center containing Keratin, a squamous stratified epithelium (Matrix) with subepithelial connective tissue containing inflammatory cells (Perimatrix)

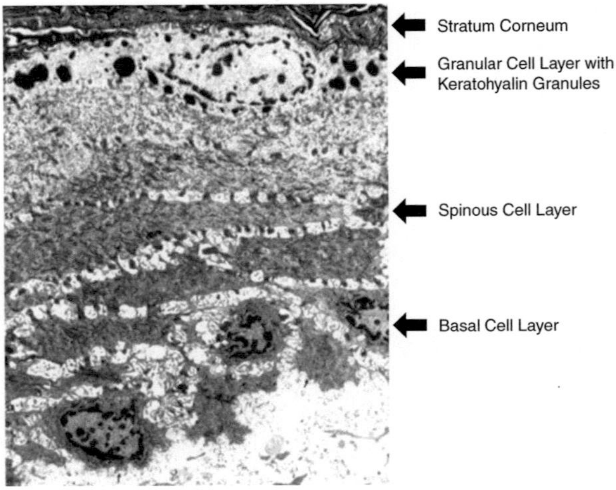

Fig. 8.11 The ultrastructural characteristics of cholesteatomas matrix cell layers are similar to those found in the epidermis; the basal stratum is formed by an unicellular layer. The stratum spinosum (or spinous layer) is the layer found between the *stratum granulosum* and *stratum basale*. Their spiny (Latin, spinosum) appearance is due to shrinking of the microfilaments between desmosomes, this layer is composed of polyhedral keratinocytes that are active in synthesizing fibrillar proteins, known as cytokeratin, which build up within the cells aggregating together forming tonofilaments. The stratum granulosum is characterized by keratohyalin grains. The stratum corneum contains dead keratinocytes that became shells filled with electron dense keratin

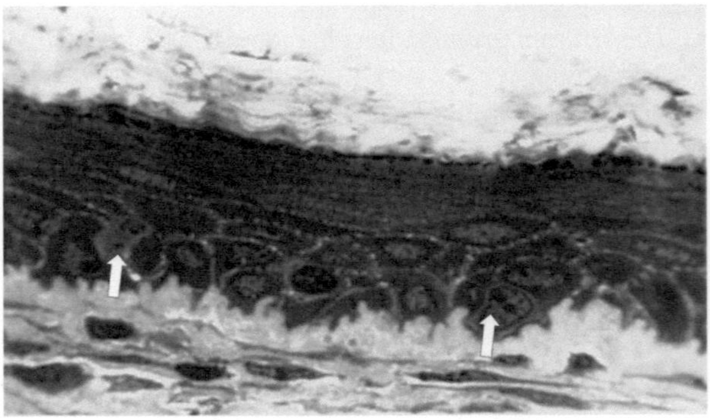

Fig. 8.12 Electron microscope. Between the dark keratinocytes that are linked between themselves by tight junctions, the desmosomes, clear cells are interposed: the Langerhans' cells (arrows)

In contrast to normal epidermis, inflammatory cells, **Langerhans' cells**, and Merkel cells are identified in the stratum spinosum layer of the cholesteatoma matrix in a higher amount compared to the normal epidermis where they never exceed more than 3%. Electron microscopy appearance of Langerhans cells (discovered by Michael Birbeck in 1961) in the cholesteatoma matrix showed characteristic multilobulated nuclei and long cytoplasmic extensions with dendritic expansions.

Langerhans' cells have electron-microscopically a clear appearance in contrast to the darker keratinocytes [11–14] (Fig. 8.12). The key features for the identification of Langherans cells are the presence of Birbeck granules in their cytoplasm,

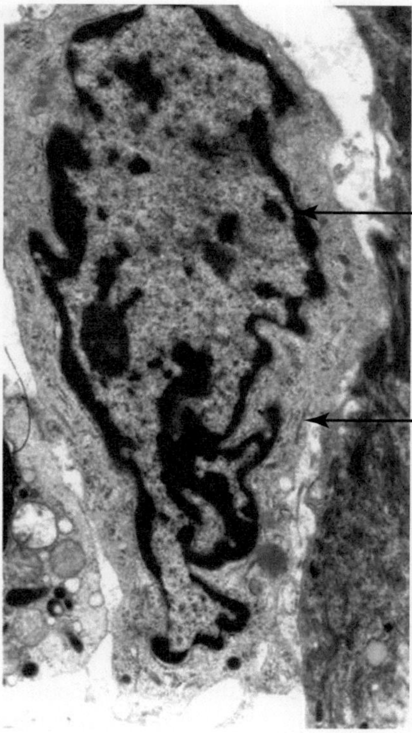

Fig. 8.13 Electron microscopy study of a Langerhans Cell. It exhibits a cleaved or folded nucleus and no tonofilaments or desmosomes. The Birbeck granules are characteristically present in their cytoplasm. These granules are most specific marker for Langerhans Cells. Birbeck granules show a vesicle at one end and sometimes at both ends. In cross sections, the granule with vesicle at one end shows a characteristic appearance, which is termed as 'tennis racket' appearance

they show 200–400 nm in size vesicles, rodlike and tennis racket-shaped structures called Birbeck granules. The nucleus is irregular and the cytoplasm has no tonofilaments. Langerhans' cells are macrophages of the skin with complex biological and metabolic properties due to their relationship with the mononuclear phagocytic system and their immunological response [15, 16] (Fig. 8.13). The function of Birbeck granules could be that they migrate to the periphery of the Langerhans cells and release their contents into the extracellular matrix to enhance their immunologic reaction (Fig. 8.14).

8.5 Pathogenesis of Cholesteatoma

8.5.1 Congenital Cholesteatoma

Several theories emerged in the explanation of congenital cholesteatomas that can be defined as "epithelial inclusions behind an intact tympanic membrane."

1. **Epidermal rest theory**: This theory is based on a finding of cell rests of nonkeratinizing squamous epithelial cells, localized in the lateral wall of the Eustachian tube, close to the tympanic ring. These rests have the potential to become a con-

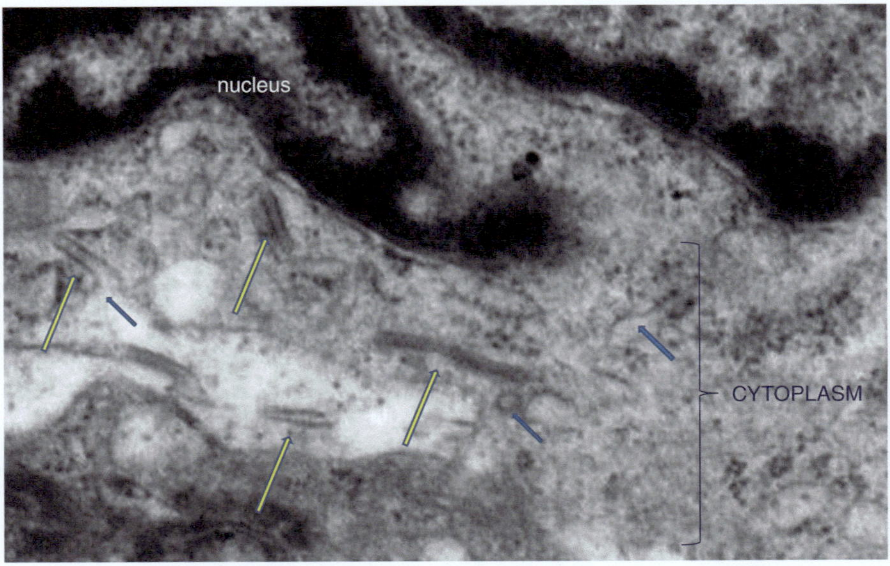

Fig. 8.14 High Magnification of intra- cytoplasm area of Langerhans'cell to identify Birbeck's granules, columnar aspect (yellow arrows) and vesicles (blue arrow)

genital cholesteatoma. This assumption is supported by reports on an increasing number of mesotympanic cholesteatomas originating from the anterosuperior quadrant of the middle ear (Teed-Michael's) [21]. Several arguments and findings published in the literature indicate that the primary origin of the congenital cholesteatoma is from foetal epidermal rests inside the tympanic cavity:

- Histological documentation of congenital cholesteatoma with a squamous epithelial rest in neonatal temporal bone [17].
- Epidermoid tumor arising from ectodermal implants in the fusion plates of the first and second branchial arches [18, 19].
- Conversion of viable squamous epithelial cells of amniotic fluid debris into cholesteatoma [20].
- Congenital cholesteatoma is due to a failure of the inhibitory function of the tympanic ring: ectodermal tissue from the external acoustic meatus may migrate into the middle ear cleft during embryogenesis [22].

2. **Inclusion Theory**: Other authors favor even a way of migration from cells coming initially from the external ear through non evident injuries of the tympanic membrane [23].
   - Inflammatory injury to an intact tympanic membrane results in microperforations in the basal layer that enable the invasion of the squamous epithelium by proliferating epithelial cones through a macroscopically intact but microscopically injured tympanic membrane.
   - "Acquired" inclusion theory, where small residual tears in the tympanic membrane lead to the formation of an inclusion cholesteatoma after healing (Toss) [24].

8.5.2 Acquired Cholesteatoma

Cholesteatoma is a proliferative epithelium with hyperkeratosis, desquamation at the surface, hyperplasia of the basal keratinocytes and deep papillary process growing beneath the neighboring intact mucosa (Fig. 8.21). Between the squamous pluristratified epithelium of the cholesteatoma and the pseudostratified epithelium of the neighboring mucosa, no interjonction is found; there is rather a confrontation line defining a zone of conflicting tissues (Fig. 8.21). This conflict favors a continuous growth and expanding of the epidermal tissue coming from the external auditory canal into the middle ear cavity.

Thus the pathogenic epidermal theory of cholesteatoma origin as from an epidermal layer of the auditory canal bottom into the middle ear—already mentioned in 1888 by Habermann [25])—is definitively confirmed in the 1970s.

Whatever the epidermal proliferation mode would be - tympanic retraction [26, 27], lateral epithelial migration [28], papillary budding [29]—the cholesteatoma corresponds always to Gray's definition [30]: *cholesteatoma is "skin in the wrong place"*.

The common factor for all theories of acquired cholesteatomas is that the keratinizing squamous epithelium has grown beyond its normal limits.

Historically, four theories have been proposed to explain the pathogenesis of acquired cholesteatoma: none is satisfactory by itself for all encountered clinical cases!

1. Invagination theory (retraction pocket theory),
2. Immigration theory,
3. Squamous metaplasia,
4. Basal cell hyperplasia (papillary ingrowth theory).

8.5.2.1 The Invagination Theory

The invagination theory is based on the assumption that the precursors to cholesteatoma are tympanic membrane retraction pockets which are caused by *a dysventilation syndrome of the middle ear compartments* (Figs. 8.15 and 8.16).

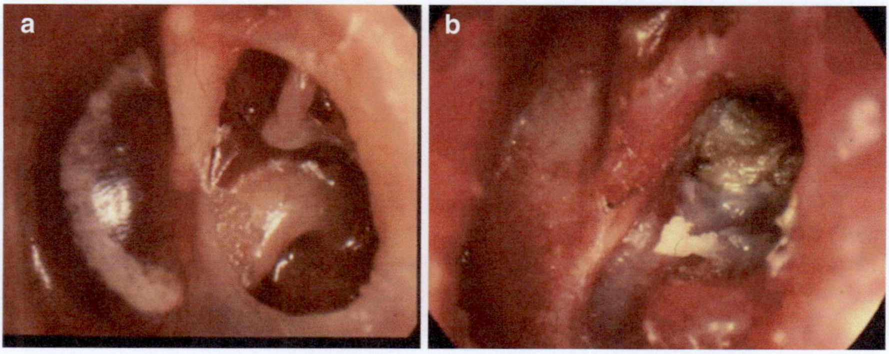

Fig. 8.15 Left ear mesotympanic retraction pocket that evolved into cholesteatoma after 5 years

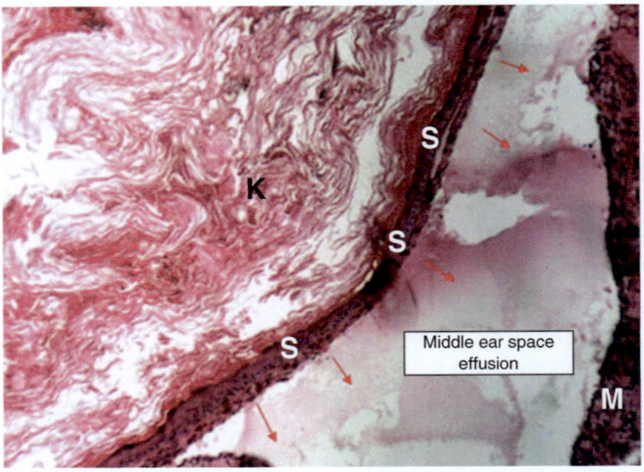

Fig. 8.16 Retraction pocket and its skin (S) invaginating towards the middle ear (small red arrows) with desquamated keratin (K) filling the lumen of the pocket and mucous secretions in the middle ear. The mucosal epithelium medial to pocket retraction is still preserved (M)

1. TM Retraction	Passive process →	Retraction Pocket
2. Epithelial Proliferation	Active process →	Pre–Cholesteatoma
3. Defective Migration	Active process →	Cholesteatoma

Fig. 8.17 From retraction pocket into cholesteatoma

Although the development of a retraction pocket is a passive process, the transformation of a retraction pocket into a pre-cholesteatoma and then into cholesteatoma is a dynamic biologic process along with a dysfunction of the external auditory canal bottom skin immune system (Fig. 8.17).

Two major histological features are present in cholesteatoma and not in retraction pocket: ***Epithelial hyperplasia and defective skin migration***. Epithelial hyperproliferation in the fundus of a retraction pocket and loss of self-cleaning function due to defective skin migration lead to an accumulation of desquamated keratin with subsequent deepening of the retraction pocket resulting in formation of cholesteatoma (Figs. 8.17 and 8.18).

Both, the loss of self-cleaning mechanism and the epithelial proliferation are not a passive phenomenon but enhanced by several immunological factors released through a persistent middle ear inflammatory process. Also an intrinsic dysfunction of the external auditory canal bottom skin immune system intervenes in these phenomena. So the retraction pocket becomes an active invaginating process, leading to a primary acquired cholesteatoma (Fig. 8.19). In Retraction pockets with a narrow neck, there will be inversion of keratin migration and accumulation of keratin inside the pocket with cholesteatoma formation. Two things are present in cholesteatoma and not present in safe retraction pocket: epithelial hyperproliferation and abnormal skin (Fig. 8.19).

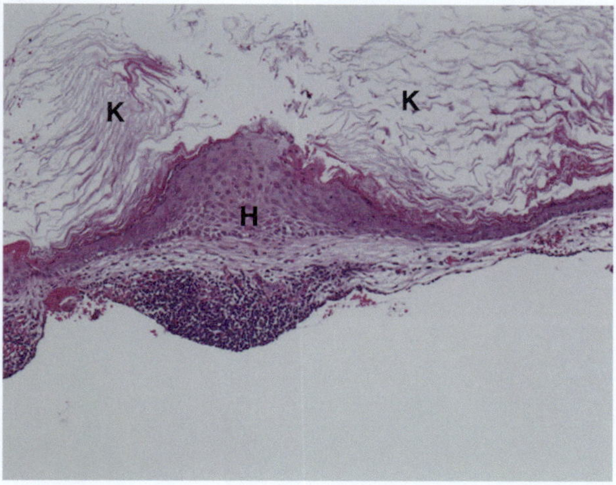

Fig. 8.18 Epithelial hyperplasia (H) with resultant increased production of keratin (K) is an essential step in the development of cholesteatoma. "Courtesy of Pr Moriyama"

Recently, the hypothesis of *mucosal coupling*, thought to be behind the invagination phenomenon in a retraction pocket, is presumed to be one of the main factors behind the arrest of clearance of normal mucosa secretions; consequently it enhances the progress of the retraction mechanism as a pulling effect generated by the mucosal coupling [31].

8.5.2.2 The Migration Theory

The migration theory assumes that the perforation of the eardrum, traumatic or iatrogenic, gives access to the squamous epithelium of the eardrum or of the outer ear canal skin, to invade or migrate into the middle ear leading to the formation of a Secondary acquired cholesteatoma (Fig. 8.20).

In marginal perforations, there is a sharp front line between the skin of the ear canal and the mucosa of the middle ear which is usually respected by the canal skin: so it migrates laterally. However, recurrent ear infections will alter the behavior of the ear canal skin: the stimulated squamous epithelium will invert its migration direction medially into the middle ear cavity. The basal cells of the germinal layer of the skin will proliferate excessively and a keratinizing squamous epithelium will progress into the middle ear cavity through the pre-existing perforation (Fig. 8.21).

Thus the migration of squamous epithelium of the external ear through a tympanic membrane perforation into the middle ear and the excessive production of keratin lead to a cholesteatoma formation.

8.5.2.3 The Squamous Metaplasia Theory

The metaplasia theory stipulated that the epithelium of the middle ear changes into squamous epithelium under the effect of a persistent chronic inflammation. However, there is neither histological nor experimental proof [32, 33]. In fact, middle ear mucosal metaplasia exists but it never transforms into cholesteatoma.

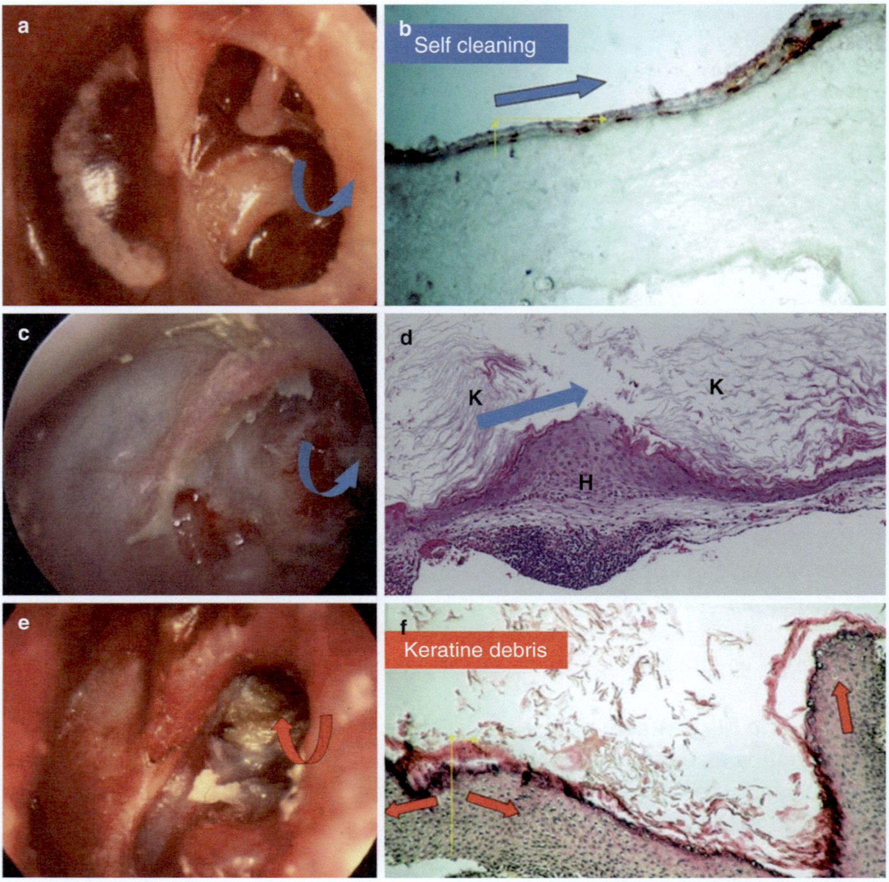

Fig. 8.19 Left ear that progressed from retraction pocket (**a**, **b**) into pre-cholesteatoma (**c**, **d**) and then into cholesteatoma (**e**, **f**). In safe retraction pockets there is active self-cleaning mechanism by lateral migration of the skin without keratin accumulation (**a**, **b**). In precholesteatoma (**c**, **d**) there is hyperplasia of the epithelium of the retraction pocket fundus (**d**), Epithelial hyperplasia (H) with resultant increased production of keratin (K), Courtesy of Pr Moriyama) but the lateral migratory potential of skin is preserved (blue arrow). In cholesteatoma (**e**, **f**), there is both epithelial hyperplasia with defective skin migration (red arrows)

When stimulated by chronic inflammation and irritation, the pseudostratified ciliated columnar epithelium changes progressively into pluri stratified squamous (epidermoid) epithelium, but it stays at the aspect of a "non- squamous non keratinizing epithelium" [34] (Fig. 8.22). In addition, this process is reversible, whereas cholesteatoma is an *irreversible* squamous epidermal disorder. Moreover, the differences observed in the cytokeratin profile between cholesteatoma epithelium and middle ear epithelium are also against this theory [35]. Consequently, the metaplasia theory is not anymore accepted.

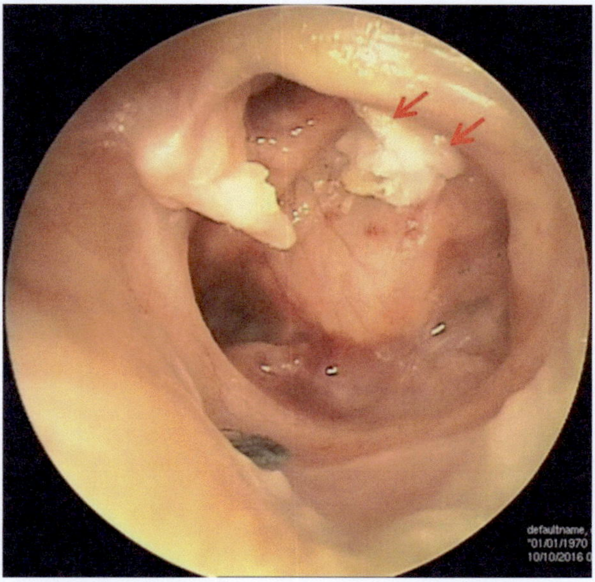

Fig. 8.20 Left ear with marginal perforation with secondary acquired cholesteatoma due to a migration of the skin epidermis on the edge of the perforation inside the middle ear cavity (red arrows)

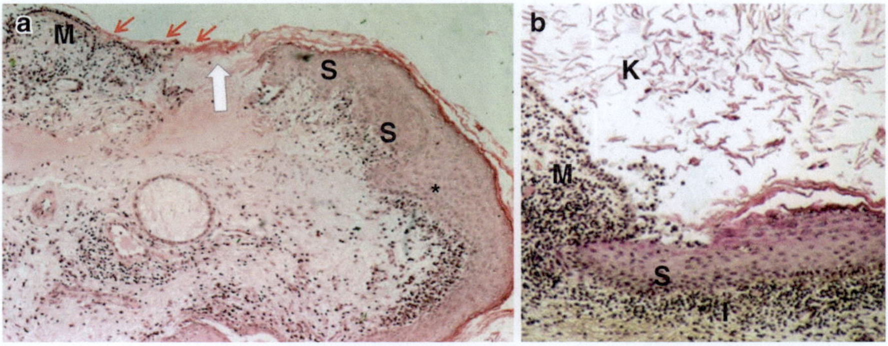

Fig. 8.21 (**a**) Light microscopic examination of the frontier line in a marginal perforation (white arrow) between the skin of the ear canal and the mucosa of the middle ear: the stimulated squamous epithelium of the ear canal skin (S) is very thick (*), excessively proliferative and has inverted its migration direction medially into the middle ear cavity over the middle ear mucosa (M) (red arrows), (b) at higher magnification, excessive keratin formation (K) is seen, due to the inflammatory process (I) present under the epithelium which is responsible for stimulating the ear canal epithelium

8.5.2.4 The Basal Cell Hyperplasia (Papillary) Theory

The basal cell hyperplasia theory postulates that keratin-filled microcysts, buds, or pseudopods formed in the basal layer of the pars flaccida epithelium, invade the sub-epithelial tissue, fuse together, resulting in the formation of cholesteatoma of Prussak's space [36–38].

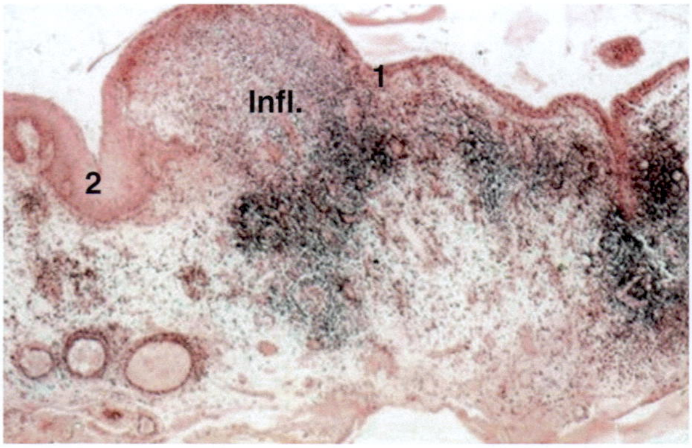

Fig. 8.22 Light microscope: progressive metaplasia of middle ear mucosa from a pseudostratified columnar epithelium (1) to a pluri-stratified squamous epithelium (2) but without keratin formation. Infl.: inflammatory process in the subepithelial layer

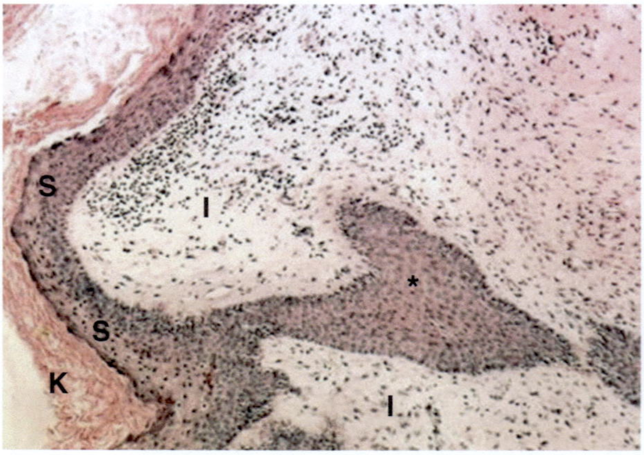

Fig. 8.23 Light microscope showing a pseudopod (*) formed in the basal layer of the pars flaccida epithelium (S) and invading the sub-epithelial tissue which hosts a diffuse inflammatory process (I). K: keratin deposited by stimulated skin (keratosis)

This proliferative behavior of the basal layer is induced by subepithelial inflammatory process (Fig. 8.23) taking place following a Prussak's space dysventilation syndrome.

8.5.2.5 Recent Advances in the Pathogenesis of Cholesteatoma

Current concepts in the pathogenesis of cholesteatoma postulate that cholesteatoma may be the result of a **"defective wound healing process"** where the inflammatory and proliferative stages predominate, but the *maturation end stage* of the wound healing process would never be achieved [39] (*see below*). In addition, the pathogenesis of cholesteatoma does not depend only on the middle ear pathological conditions but, also very probably, on the immunological status of the external auditory bottom skin cells with its specific immune cell potential leading to persistent inflammation process via continuous overproduction of cytokine mediators.

Actually the pathogenesis of the acquired cholesteatoma is a "complex and hybrid process" involving multiple concepts and different findings thanks to the molecular biology studies (see below); thus no single theory alone can fully explain the uncoordinated hyper proliferation, invasion, migration, altered differentiation, aggressiveness, and recidivism of this pathology [40].

8.6 Molecular Biology of Cholesteatoma

The induction of a cholesteatoma formation process seems to be related to both internal molecular dysregulation and some external stimuli in the form of *pro-inflammatory cytokines, growth factors and/or bacterial toxins*. There is an imbalance and a *vicious circle of epithelial proliferation, keratinocytes differentiation and maturation, prolonged apoptosis, and disturbance of self-cleaning mechanisms*. Whatever the exact molecular mechanism may be, cholesteatoma remains a chronic otitis involving both middle ear and external ear canal skin layers.

Histochemical studies lead to understand the more dynamic dimensions of the anatomopathological study of cholesteatoma, especially in regard to **Langerhans'cells**.

Among all cells of a normal external auditory canal bottom epidermis, the number of the Langerhans' cells does not exceed 3%. In cholesteatoma, these cells show quantitative and qualitative modifications. Their number increases significantly and they become grouped into masses at different levels (basal, suprabasal) in the cholesteatoma matrix and perimatrix (Fig. 8.24). Moreover, Langerhans' cells are present at the different stages of **keratinocyte maturation**, confirming their role as *immunological sentinels*.

Langerhans' cells require the cooperation of **activated T-lymphocytes** to become functional. These activated T-lymphocytes (Fig. 8.13) represent the "vital union" of the *immune process* [41]. *Langerhans cells emit long dendritic expansions which create a true network between the neighboring cells: keratinocytes and lymphocytes* (Fig. 8.12). The close contact between these cells is essential for the immune reaction (Figs. 8.25, 8.26 and 8.27).

Langerhans cells seem to play a key role in the proliferative activity of the cholesteatoma, due to their positive tropism towards the keratinized squamous epithelium with its capacity for keratinization. Langerhans' cells maintain this role because of the surrounding inflammatory reaction (induced by lymphocytic activation) and the secretion of osteolytic chemical mediators (*chemical process*) [42].

This inflammatory and immunological duality of Langerhans' cells to stimulate the proliferation of cholesteatoma has a high similarity with lichen planus of the

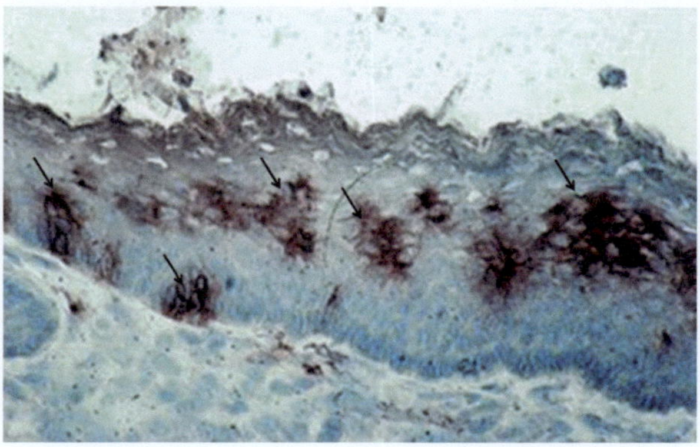

Fig. 8.24 Immunohisto chemical study of the cholesteatoma matrix shows the extensive infiltration with Langerhans' cells (black arrows). Their dendritic expansions create a net for a close contact with neighboring cells

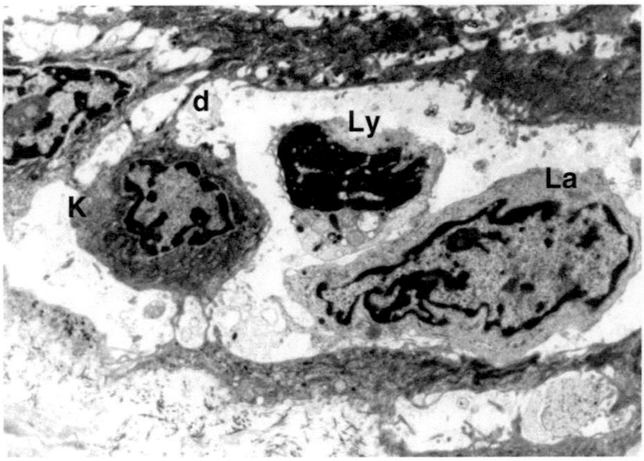

Fig. 8.25 Electron microscopic view showing the "vital union" between Langerhans' cell (La), Lymphocyte-like cell (Ly) and Keratinocytes (K) by desmosomes (d)

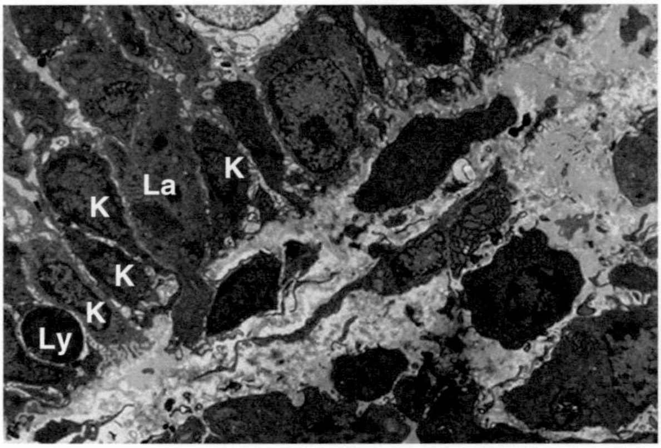

Fig. 8.26 Electron microscopy the inflammatory and immunological process in the matrix of cholesteatoma with interactions between keratinocytes (K), Langerhans cells (La), and lymphocyte-like cells (Ly)

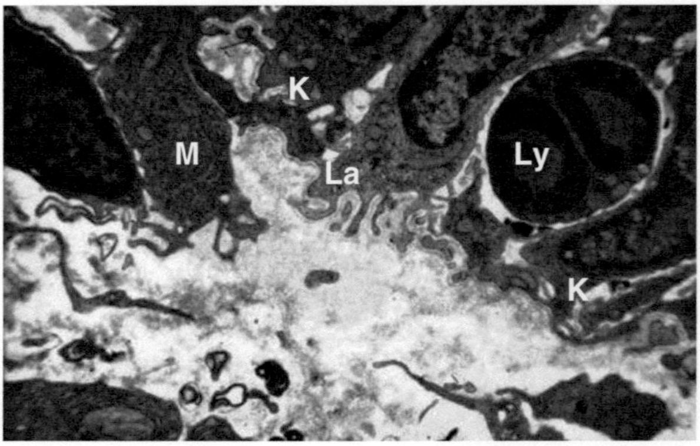

Fig. 8.27 Electron Microscopy: Immune cellular reactions in cholesteatoma. Keratinocyte (K), Langerhans' cell (La), Lymphocyte (Ly), Macrophage (M)

epidermis covering some troublesome mastoid cavities. Lichen planus is characterized by a massive infiltration of the epidermal layer by an infiltrate formed of lymphocytes, macrophages and Langerhans' cells (Fig. 8.28).

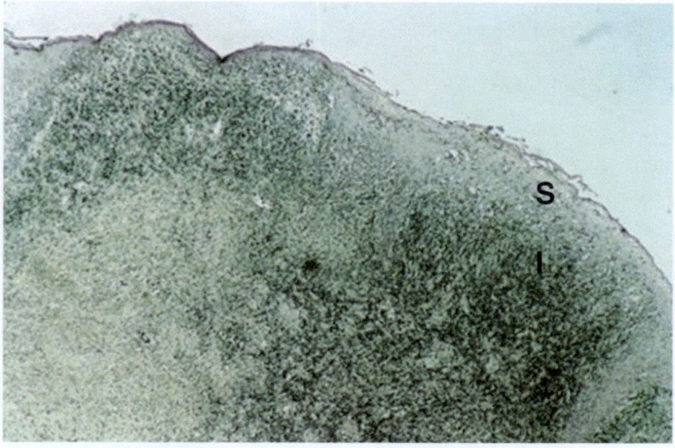

Fig. 8.28 Light microscopy transformation of the epidermic layer in Lichen planus covering a troublesome mastoid cavity. The keratinizing squamous epithelium (S) is infiltrated by lymphocyte cells (I)

8.6.1 Immunohistochemistry of Cholesteatoma

Recent advances in immunohistochemical analysis have revealed an association between the progression of cholesteatoma and excessive host immune response to persisting inflammation in the form of paracrine and autocrine secretions [36, 39, 43–49].

As shown in Fig. 8.29, there are paracrine and autocrine interactions between keratinocytes of the matrix and fibroblasts of the perimatrix that regulate homeostasis and tissue regeneration within a cholesteatoma [36]. In addition, inflammatory cell populations (e.g., lymphocytes, Langerhans cells) in the perimatrix release a variety of growth factors (e.g., IL1, TGFx, cytokeratines,…) (Fig. 8.29). The excessive inflammatory immune response and the release of growth factors in the matrix and perimatrix can lead to an uncontrolled growth and proliferation of keratinocytes and hereby to the cholesteatoma growth and its aggressiveness.

8.6.2 Biochemistry of Cholesteatoma

Keratinocytes are the target cell's receptive to mediator substances that lead to the development of cholesteatoma. Keratinocytes require growth factors to divide and differentiate. *Growth factor polypeptides* as epidermal growth factor (EGF) and transforming growth factor ((TGF-α) play an important role in wound healing, cell regulation and proliferation. Both EGF and TGF-α are upregulated in the cholesteatoma perimatrix (Fig. 8.30) and bind to the upregulated epidermal growth factor receptor (EGFR) on the matrix (Figs. 8.31 and 8.32) [50]. Keratinocytes activation is accomplished by a strong impregnation of ILI, TGF, cytokeratin expression modification and fibroblast activation [39]; *also these factors are the factors encountered in the wound-healing process* (Figs. 8.30, 8.31, and 8.32).

The fundamental difference between the healing process in normal skin and in cholesteatoma, is that in cholesteatoma there is a loss of the growth inhibition by "cell to cell contact". Two factors are involved in this loss of growth control in cholesteatoma:

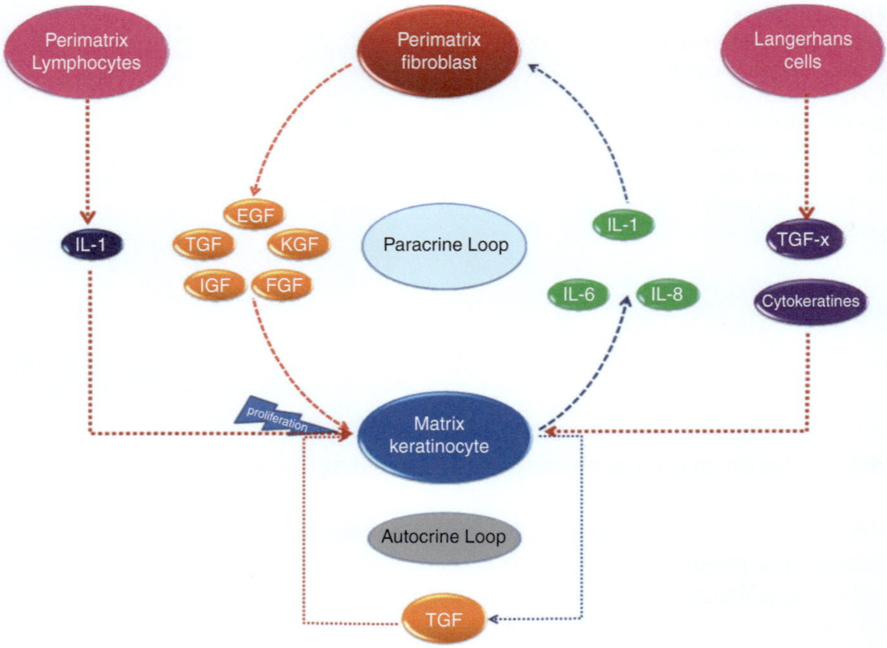

Fig. 8.29 Schematic representation of the paracrine and autocrine interactions between matrix keratinocytes and perimatrix fibroblasts. Keratinocytes release proinflammatory cytokines (e.g., IL-1α, IL-1β, IL-6, PTHrP, and IL-8), which subsequently induce fibroblasts to secrete several cytokines (e.g., KGF, GM-CSF, EGF, TNF-α, PDGF, and TGF-α). These fibroblast-derived cytokines in turn induce the differentiation, proliferation, and migration of matrix keratinocytes. In addition, the TGF-α and TGF-β are upregulated in an autocrine loop, regulating keratinocyte proliferation and differentiation. EGF: epidermal growth factor; GM-CSF: granulocyte-macrophage colony stimulating factor; IL: interleukin; KGF: keratinocyte growth factor; PDGF: platelet-derived growth factor; PTHrP: parathyroid-hormone-related protein; TGF: transforming growth factor; TNF-α: tumor necrosis factor alpha

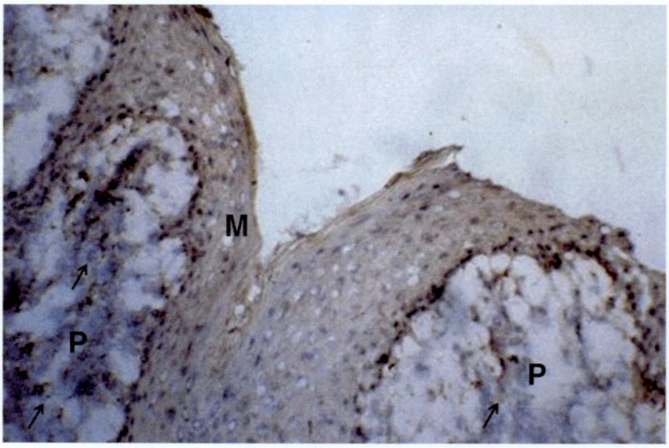

Fig. 8.30 EGF is mainly present (black arrows) in the cholesteatoma perimatrix (P) with medium intensity staining (monoclonal antibody Monosan Mon 8001), whereas the matrix (M) showed very low staining. This means that the origin of EGF is the perimatrix and then diffuse to the matrix to stimulate its proliferation

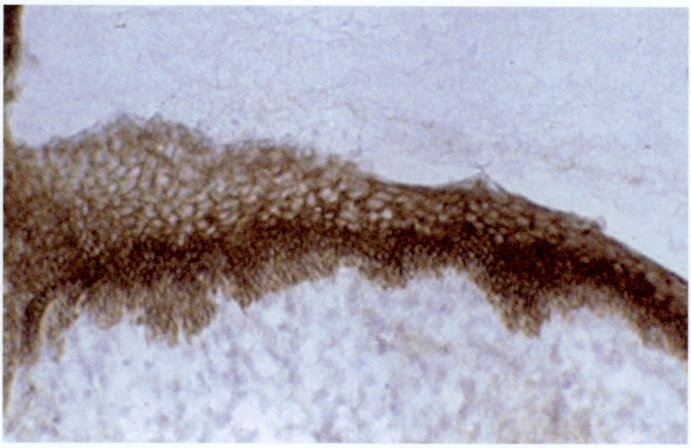

Fig. 8.31 EGF-R AB1 (extracellular epitope of the receptor) is always present in cholesteatoma matrix with a high level of staining (antibody receptor AB1 Oncogene Science)

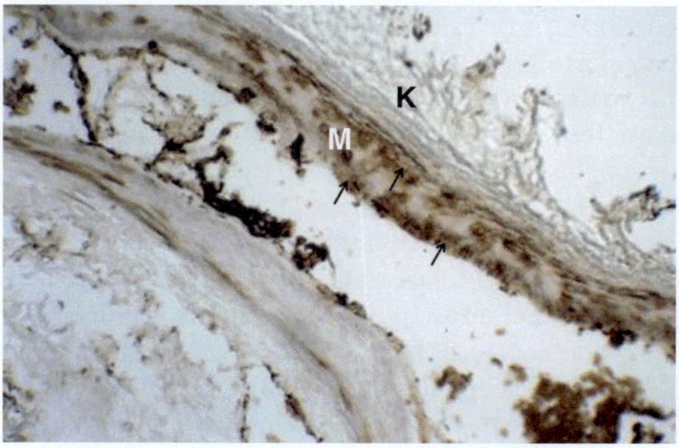

Fig. 8.32 EGF-R AB2 (intracellular epitope of the receptor) is positive (black arrows) in children cholesteatoma matrix (M). Keratin (K)

1. The cholesteatoma develops beyond its normal anatomical site for a "skin". The middle ear environment is not adequate to induce the habitual *cell contact inhibition* to stop the growth, therefore proliferation continues.
2. The inflammatory process produces a *self-maintained immunological cycle* through connective tissue — epithelial reactions in response to the conflict at the level of tissues and cells.

Thus the proliferation of the cholesteatoma matrix is due to an autocrine stimulation circle at the level of the keratinocytes in the matrix and the fibroblasts of the prematrix [51, 52] (Fig. 8.33).

However, this ***theory of a wound healing defect*** cannot explain why many cases of persistent inflammation with granulation tissue formation do not end up with cholesteatoma formation.

8.6.3 Apoptosis and Apoptotic Activity in Cholesteatoma

The loss of balance between apoptotic and antiapoptotic markers (cell death/proliferation) - with the **favorable antiapoptotic activity in cholesteatoma -** favors its

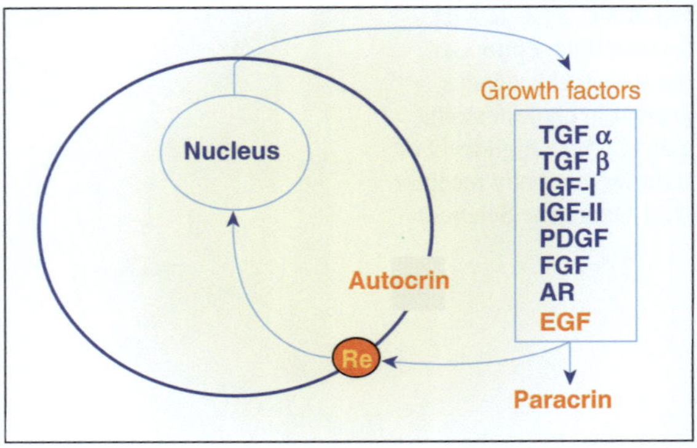

Fig. 8.33 Diagram of hypothetical autocrine (keratinocytes) and paracrine (fibroblasts) dysregulation loop of Keratinocyte cells in cholesteatoma

continuous expansion. It was found that cellular FLICE-like inhibitory protein, an antiapoptotic protein, was upregulated in cholesteatoma epithelium as compared to normal skin without significant changes in p53, (a well-known apoptotic protein) Also, the levels of galectin-3 were found to be significantly correlated with the level of apoptosis and had a protective role against apoptosis activity in recurrent cholesteatoma. Apoptosis was found in the suprabasal layers of cholesteatoma epithelium but not found in the basal layers [53–55].

A recent study showed that "let 7a microRNA" had a vital role in the inhibition of growth and invasion of cholesteatoma keratinocytes via downregulation of miR 21 expression, resulting in a double action: the suppression of proliferation and the induction of apoptotic activity [56]. *These results might pave the way for exploring non-surgical options for cholesteatoma management.*

8.6.4 Biofilms and Cholesteatoma

The keratin layer of cholesteatoma is an ideal environment for biofilm development. The presence of bacterial biofilms in cholesteatoma mediates the host response in a form of chronic inflammation, proliferation, and bone resorption [57]. The presence of antibiotic-resistant bacterial biofilms in cholesteatomas may also explain their aggressiveness.

Bacteria involving the retraction pocket produce some antigens, which will activate different cytokines and lytic enzymes. These cytokines lead to the activation and maturation of osteoclasts with the consequence of degradation of extracellular bone matrix and hyperproliferation, bone erosion and finally progression of the disease [58]. Bacterial biofilms within cholesteatomas may elaborate lipopolysaccharide (LPS) and other bacterial endotoxins that stimulate osteoclastogenesis.

Endotoxin, a component of the bacterial wall, is considered responsible for the initiation of inflammation in the middle ear. It stimulates local macrophages to produce the tumor necrosis factor alpha (TNF-α) and interleukin-1β (IL-1β). Keratinocytes respond to this injury by producing many soluble mediators, including: TNF-α, IL-1β, IL-6, and IL-8, independently from the immune cells (T cells and B cells, macrophages,…) [59].

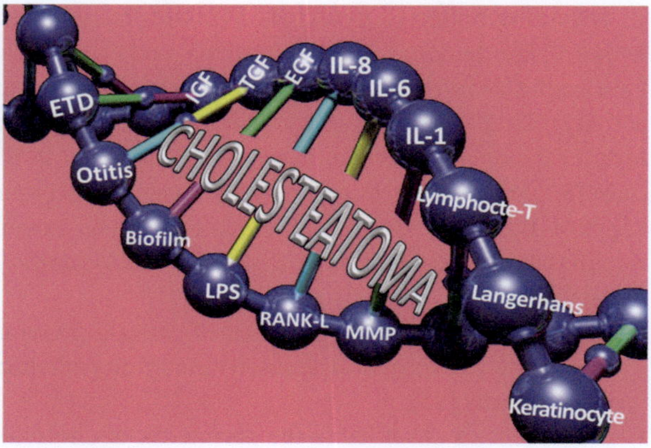

Fig. 8.34 The chain of multiple and complex factors involved in the pathogenesis of cholesteatoma. Most of them are genetically coded

8.7 Genetics of Cholesteatoma

Despite the fact that cholesteatoma is not a tumor, it exhibits clearly clinical features similar to those observed in neoplasms, indicating that the dysregulation of cell growth control may involve *internal genomic alterations.* Nevertheless, the precise underlying genomic mechanisms associated with the formation of cholesteatoma have still to be clarified (Fig. 8.34).

Recent studies have demonstrated a link between pathogenesis and potential genomic alterations in cholesteatoma. The upregulation and activation of epidermal growth factor receptor (EGFR) and its ligand and of transforming growth factor alpha (TGF-α) have been observed in cholesteatoma and in several tumor types [60–62]. Overexpression of EGFR and TGF-α is detected in cholesteatoma indicating that the dysregulation of these genes may be associated with the initiation and progression of cholesteatomas [63, 64]. Finally, alterations in the expression of proto-oncogenes (e.g., c-myc and c-jun) [65–69], upregulation of gap junction beta-2 (GJB2, also known as *connexin 26*) [70–72], and the downregulation of several tumor suppressor genes (e.g., p53, p27, CDH18, 19 and ID4, PAX3, LAMC2, and TRAF2B) [36, 39, 70, 73, 74] have been shown to contribute to the *multifactorial pathogenesis of cholesteatoma.*

8.8 Bone Resorption in Cholesteatoma

In vitro studies revealed that osteoclastic bone resorption could occur in the sites where adequate pressure was induced directly or transmitted to the tympanic cavity with or without the presence of cholesteatoma [75–78].

Despite being the most rigid bone of the human body, the labyrinth can be affected by a variety of factors of bone erosion. Several factors stimulate bone resorption, such as inflammation, local pressure, and specific enzymes [79].

High TNF-α levels stimulate *osteoclasts* that induce bone resorption; also stimulate fibroblasts to secrete collagenase and prostaglandin E which are responsible of necrosis of soft tissues in the middle ear [80].

Several upregulated cytokines in cholesteatoma, including interleukin-1, interleukin-6, interleukin-17, interferon-beta, and parathyroid-hormone-related proteins, have been shown to promote inflammatory bone resorption by promoting osteoclast activity [33, 81, 114]. IL-1 (both IL-1α and IL-1β) was found with an increased level in the epidermis of cholesteatoma compared to the normal squamous epithelium [82, 83]. Recent studies revealed that the receptor activator of nuclear factor kappa-B ligand (RANKL) and matrix-metalloproteinases (MMPs) play a pivotal role in the destruction of bony tissue by cholesteatomas [33, 73, 84].

- Proteolytic inflammatory cytokines (metalloproteinases, MMP2, MMP9) have been shown to have an increased amount in pediatric cholesteatoma in comparison to adults [85].
- Angiogenesis observed in the perimatrix of cholesteatoma is higher in pediatric than adult cholesteatoma [85].

8.8.1 Matrix Metalloproteinases

Recent studies showed that variations in cellular production of matrix metalloproteinases (MMPs) and their specific inhibitors (TIMPs) contribute to the pathophysiology of cholesteatoma, especially in the development of bone erosion. Normally, their activity is tightly controlled, as an increase in their activation would cause a denudement of the extracellular matrix and increased invasiveness by the epithelium. In cholesteatoma, studies have indicated a clear imbalance in the regulation of MMPs, with an overall up-regulation of MMP expression and a decrease in MMP inhibitors resulting in degradation of the extracellular matrix [63, 64, 86, 87].

8.8.2 Collagenase

Collagenase is also involved in the local invasion process by aural cholesteatoma, stimulating the osteoclastic resorption by degrading the osteoid surface of the bone and thus facilitating osteoclastic activity [64].

In conclusion, TNF-alpha [, IL-1α, MMP 9 and tenascin, amphiregulin, MIB1, BMPs and RANKL/OPG ratio are considered to be a reliable index for bone erosion in cholesteatoma [47, 82, 88–93].

8.9 Cholesteatoma Origin and Growth Pathways

On the basis of their site of origin, middle ear cholesteatomas (Table 8.1) can be classified as the following:

- "Pars flaccida (attic) cholesteatomas" (Fig. 8.35a) are located at the upper one-third portion of the tympanic membrane, filling the Prussak space. Initially, pars flaccida cholesteatomas are usually located lateral to the ossicles. On the basis of

Table 8.1 Cholesteatoma origin and growth pathways

Location	Site in the tympanum	Age distribution
(a) Attic/posterior epitympanum (40%)	Pars flaccida	More frequent in adults
(b) Pars tensa/posterior mesotympanum (30%)	Postero-sup. quadrant of pars tensa	More frequent in children
(c) Anterior epitympanum (the least frequent)	Cranially and anteriorly to the malleus head	Mostly in children
(d) Unclassified (about 30%)	Not clearly defined	Includes also two routes cholesteatoma

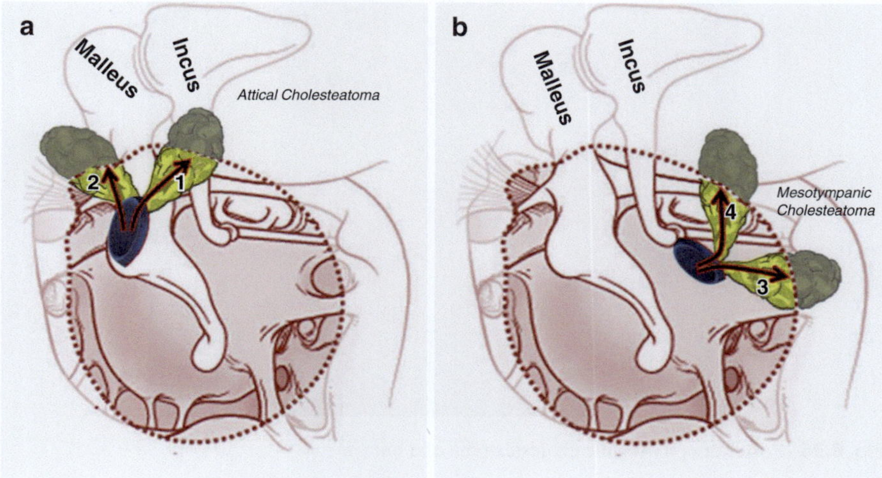

Fig. 8.35 Cholesteatoma origin and spread. (**a**) Attical cholesteatoma usually spreads posteriorly (1) as posterior attical cholesteatoma and rarely anteriorly as anterior attical cholesteatoma (2) and (**b**) mesotympanic cholesteatoma growth pattern into the facial recess and sinus tympani (3); into epitympanum through posterior tympanic isthmus (4)

their extension, they are classified into posterior epitympanic cholesteatoma and anterior epitympanic cholesteatoma.

- "Pars tensa (sinus) cholesteatomas" develop most from the postero-superior part of the pars tensa and most often are localized in the facial recess and sinus tympani of the tympanic cavity and in the mastoid region (Fig. 8.35b). Pars tensa cholesteatomas are mostly located medial to the ossicular chain.
- It is not possible to define the origin of an advanced lesion; hence neither of these classification subgroups is applicable.

The growth pattern of the acquired cholesteatoma is oriented by two main factors: the site of origin of the cholesteatoma and the anatomical compartments in the middle ear cleft.

The ligaments, mucosal folds, ossicles, and walls of the middle ear separating the different compartments do not play the role of barriers but guide the growth of cholesteatoma into distinct pathways throughout the middle ear cleft.

8.9.1 Posterior Epitympanic Cholesteatoma

The most common spread pattern of cholesteatoma originating from the Prussak's space is the posterior epitympanic route (Fig. 8.36) where the cholesteatoma spreads into the superior incudal space (SIS) lateral to the body of the incus and can potentially enter the mastoid through the aditus ad antrum (Fig. 8.37).

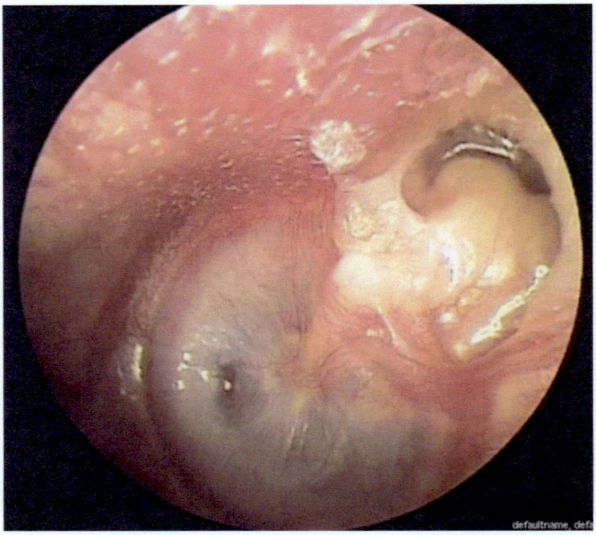

Fig. 8.36 Posterior epitympanic cholesteatoma of a left ear

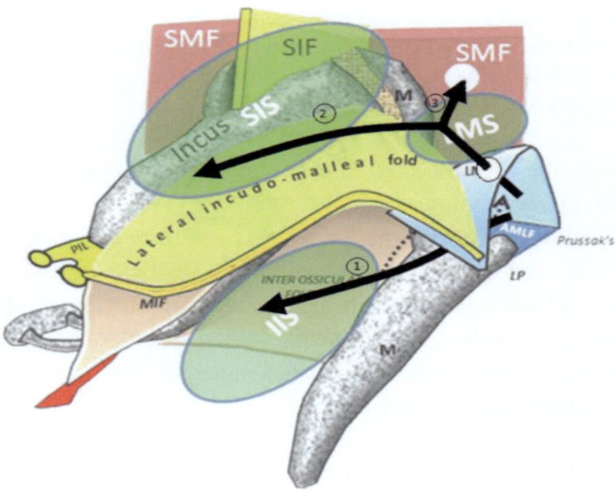

Fig. 8.37 Attical cholesteatoma growth pattern. From the Prussak's space, cholesteatoma can extend through one of the following three tracts. 1: through the posterior pouch of Von Troeltsch to the lower lateral attic (inferior incudal space, IIS). 2: through a defect in the lateral incudal fold (LIF) to the lateral malleal space and then to the superior incudal space (SIS), or 3: from the lateral malleal space through the superior malleal fold defect (SMF) to the anterior attic

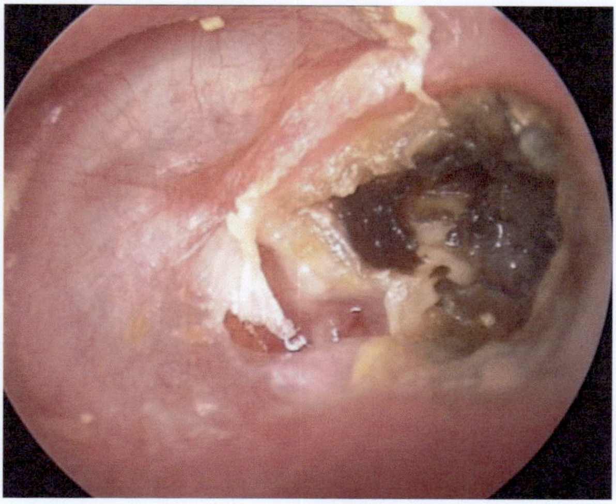

Fig. 8.38 Mesotympanic cholesteatoma of left ear

8.9.2 Mesotympanic Cholesteatoma

The second most common route of cholesteatoma spread is the mesotympanic cholesteatoma through the inferior route, through the *posterior pouch of von Troeltsch* following the embryological course of both the saccus posticus and the saccus superior. It grows medially along the lenticular process and stapes superstructure. Then it may grow upward through the posterior tympanic isthmus toward the posterior epitympanum and then the mastoid antrum or backward directly into the sinus tympani, and may fill the entire middle ear (Figs. 8.35b and 8.38).

8.9.3 Anterior Epitympanic Cholesteatoma

The cholesteatoma reaches the anterior epitympanum through the lateral malleal space beneath the superior malleal fold (following the embryologic saccus anticus trajectory) to enter the anterior epitympanic recess (AER). It may remain in the AER, where the geniculate ganglion is at risk, or progress into the supratubal recess (STR) and the protympanum (Figs. 8.35a and 8.39).

8.9.4 Unclassified Cholesteatomas

Cholesteatomas become unclassifiable according to the previous categories, when they grow beyond the different compartments, involving the middle ear, the epitympanum and the mastoid and their initial origin become unidentifiable or may be the result from two progressing retraction pockets (Fig. 8.40).

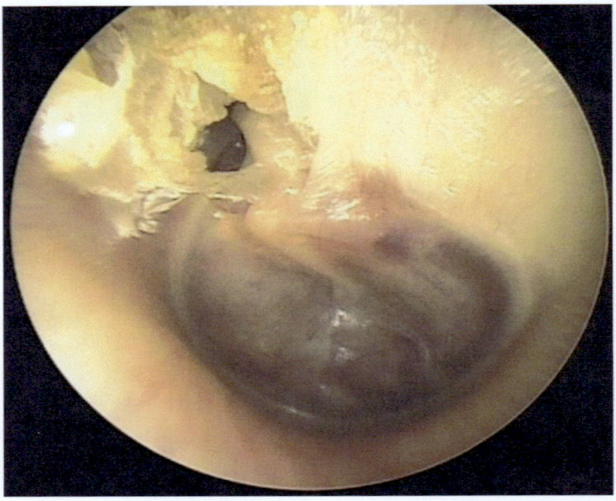

Fig. 8.39 Left ear anterior epitympanic cholesteatoma

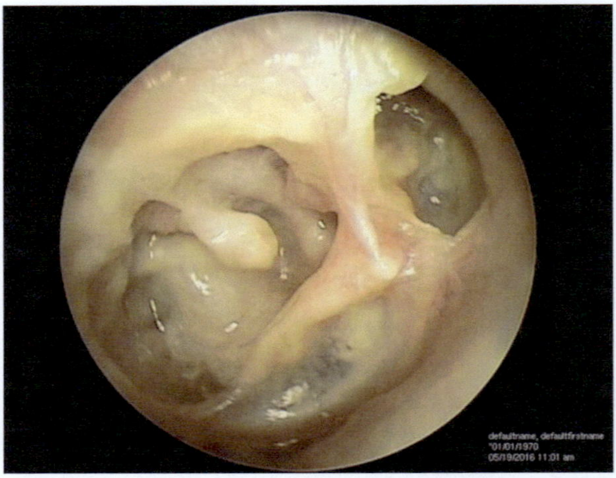

Fig. 8.40 Right ear showing extensive cholesteatoma that involves the attic and the mesotympanum with erosion of head of malleus and incus

8.10 Clinical Manifestations

8.10.1 Symptomatology

Cholesteatomas often progress insidiously, until they become invasive and symptomatic. Occasionally, cholesteatoma manifests by a sudden intratemporal or intracranial complications.

A detailed otologic history should be obtained in order to elicit the early symptoms of cholesteatoma including hearing loss, otorrhea, tinnitus and vertigo. A chronic foul smelling otorrhea and a progressive hearing loss are quasi pathognomonic.

8.10.1.1 Otorrhea

A persistent foul-smelling painless otorrhea is the hallmark of cholesteatoma patients. Unlike simple suppurative otitis media, the otorrhea is not abundant. When the cholesteatoma is infected, it is not responsive to systemic antibiotics. Topical antibiotics may help temporarily. If otorrhea persists for a long duration, polyp formation may occur.

8.10.1.2 Hearing Loss

A conductive hearing loss is a common finding in cholesteatoma, as ossicular chain erosion is common (70%) [94]; however, a relatively good hearing could be present even the ossicular chain is eroded, this is the result of the conductive mass effect of the cholesteatoma itself; *patients should be counseled that there is a possibility of a hearing degradation following the removal of the pathology.*

Evidence of sensorineural hearing loss may indicate an involvement of the labyrinth.

8.10.1.3 Vertigo/Imbalance

A destruction of the bone which overlies the otic capsule, especially the lateral semicircular canal, can trigger vertigo or a balance dysfunction.

8.10.1.4 Facial Nerve Palsy

Facial palsy may be the first sign of a cholesteatoma localized in the anterior epitympanic recess. Violation of the facial nerve bony canal by cholesteatoma rarely manifests by a facial paralysis. Facial nerve palsy with intact tympanic membrane and conductive hearing loss must orient the investigations to a cholesteatoma of the anterior epitympanic recess ethology (See Chap. 10).

Otalgia, headache, vomiting, and fever are not typical presentations of cholesteatoma; however, their occurrence indicates the possibility of impending intratemporal or intracranial complications.

8.10.2 Otomicroscopy

The diagnosis of cholesteatoma is clinical and requires a perfect cleaning of the outer ear canal before inspection of the drum (Fig. 8.41). Typical findings are a marginal tympanic perforation with debris extending into the middle ear (Fig. 8.20) or a retraction pocket filled with keratin. Erosion of the scutum and/or the ossicular chain can be seen. A retraction pocket may be seen, often in the attic and posterosuperior quadrant of the tympanic membrane. Granulation tissue or a polyp may arise from the diseased infected bone of the scutum or the posterior bony wall (Fig. 8.42). Through a transparent tympanic membrane a congenital cholesteatoma in the middle ear can be observed (Figs. 8.4 and 8.6).

Extreme caution should be taken with any polyp removal as it may be adherent to important underlying structures such as the ossicles or facial nerve.

It is of utmost importance to examine the contralateral ear and report the findings.

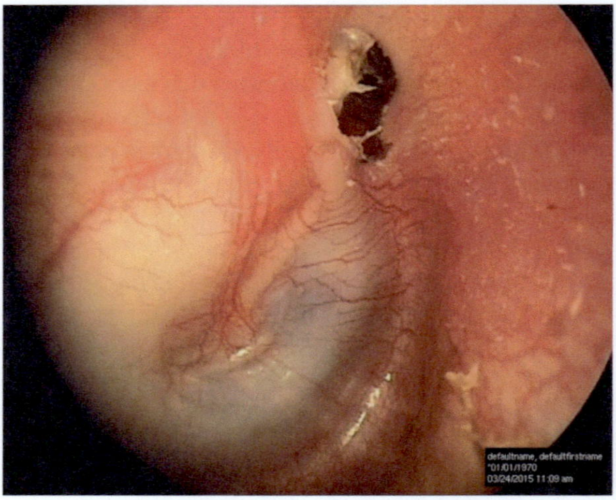

Fig. 8.41 Right ear with attical cholesteatoma. Cholesteatoma visible after ear cleaning

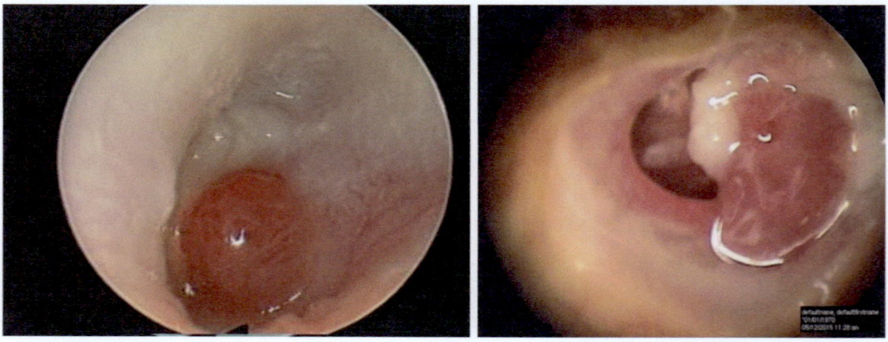

Fig. 8.42 Cholesteatoma with aural polyp

8.10.3 Audiological Evaluation

Pure tone audiometry with air and bone conduction, speech reception thresholds, and word recognition are the basic mandatory audiological assesments for ears with cholesteatoam and they usually reveal a conductive hearing loss with good speech discrimination in the affected ear. The degree of conductive hearing loss will vary considerably depending on the extent of the disease. A conductive deficit more than 40 dB indicates ossicular discontinuity. A drop in bone conduction (BC) level indicates sensorineural hearing loss which could be a sign of labyrinth involvement.

Audiometry results should always be correlated with the 512 Hz tuning fork exam.

8.11 CT-Imaging in Cholesteatoma

The cardinal scanographic sign of cholesteatoma is a soft tissue image, that has characteristically a rounded appearance in early stages (Fig. 8.43).

The cholesteatoma may show initially a slight mass effect on the surrounding structures (Fig. 8.44a), that can become extensive in later stages (Fig. 8.44b).

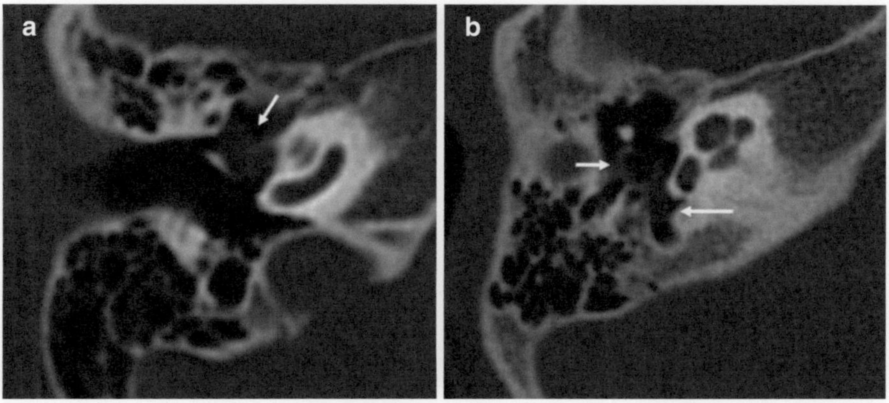

Fig. 8.43 Axial CT image of right ears of different patients: Typical scanographic appearance of a cholesteatoma as a soft tissue mass (arrows), with rounded borders, typically with some air inclusions in an early phase. (**a**) In front of the malleus handle, (**b**) in the posterior mesotympanum (short arrow), and insinuating in the sinus tympani (long arrow)

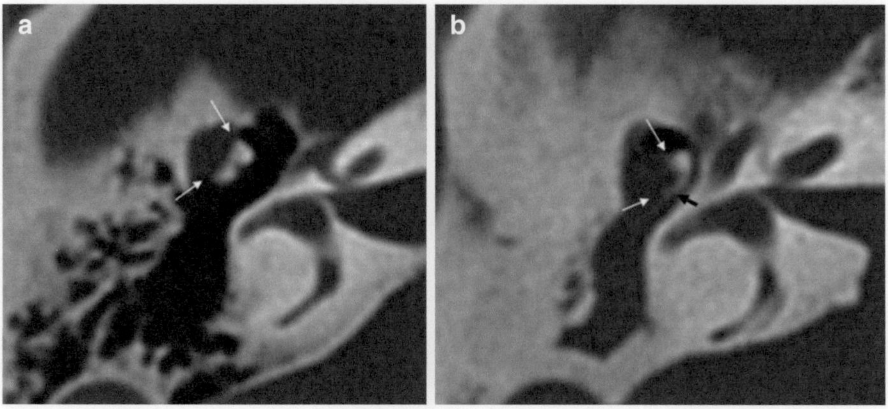

Fig. 8.44 Axial CT-image of a right ear: (**a**) condensation of the lateral attic with slight mass effect on the incudomalleal chain (arrows), (**b**) atticoantral condensation with a prominent mass effect on the incudomalleal chain (white arrows), and advanced lysis of the incus (black arrow)

Cholesteatoma represents the main cause of typical bony erosions and/or ossicular lysis.

8.11.1 Erosion of the Scutum

The erosion of the scutum is suggestive of a pars flaccida cholesteatoma. It may be difficult to assess such bone erosion clinically in an early stage, particularly if a polyp formation is associated (Fig. 8.42). CT-Scan is helpful to detect this early sign, especially in comparing the affected side with the normal aspect of the scutum of the opposite side (Fig. 8.45a, b). Nevertheless lysis of the scutum may be secondary to a Pars Flaccida retraction pocket before its progress to a cholesteatomatous stage (Fig. 8.45c, d).

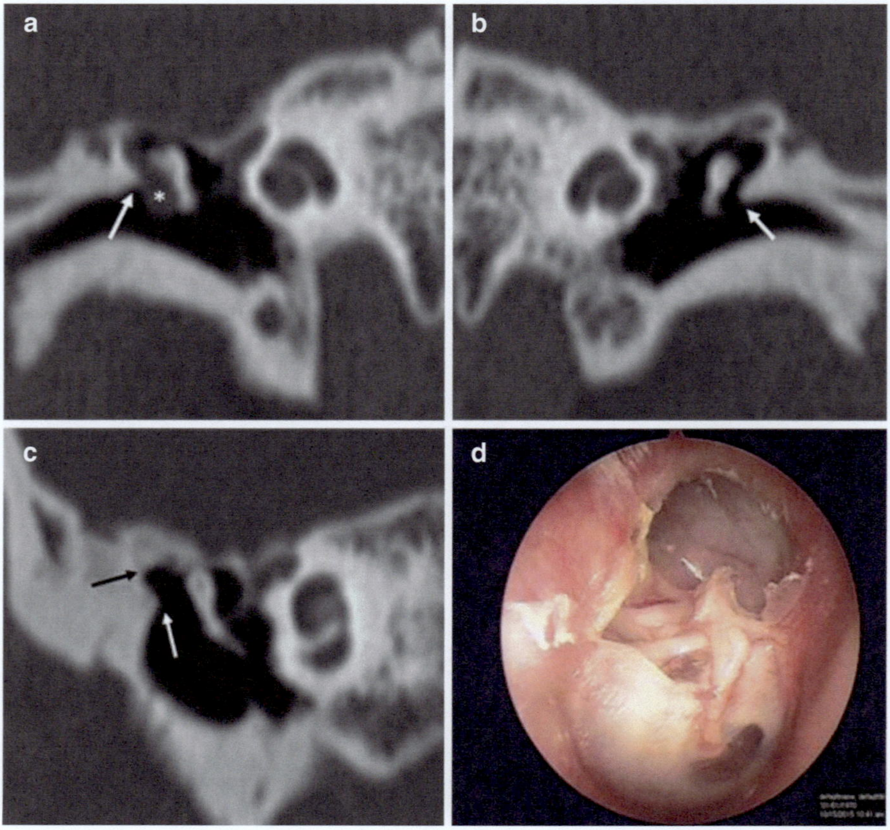

Fig. 8.45 Coronal CT view of (**a**) a right ear with amputation of the scutum (arrow) in contact with a rounded condensation of the lateral attic (*), protruding in the EAC, corresponding to a polype on clinical exam, (**b**) in comparison: the intact scutum (arrow) of the contralateral ear, (**c**) a right ear: amputated scutum (white arrow) due to a retraction pocket, the "virtual" pocket membrane is not individualized on the CT due to its adhesion to the bony attic wall (black arrow) and (**d**) endoscopic view, RP and scutum erosion without cholesteatoma formation

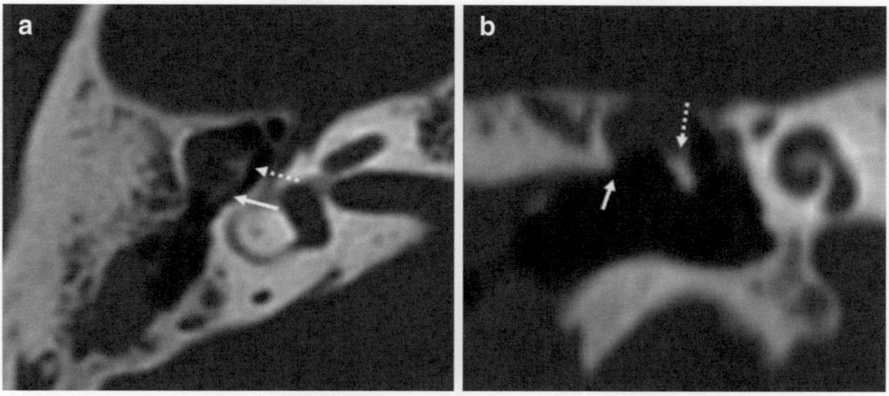

Fig. 8.46 Right ears of two different patients. (**a**) Axial view of a pars flaccida cholesteatoma, that has invaded the malleus head (dotted arrow) and the incus (arrow), (**b**) coronal view of a pars flaccida cholesteatoma, lytic effect on the malleus head (dotted arrow), amputation of the scutum (white arrow)

8.11.2 Erosion of the Ossicles

1. In cases of a *pars flaccida cholesteatoma*, the lytic effect concerns initially the lateral border of the incudomalleolar chain (Fig. 8.46a); the incus being more vulnerable than the malleus, the malleus head is particularly resistant, but it becomes affected by the progress of the cholesteatoma along the anterior malleal ligament which is inserted on the anterior part of the malleus head (Fig. 8.46b).
2. In cases of a *pars tensa cholesteatoma*, the lytic effect involves initially the mesotympanic part of the ossicular chain, first the long process of the incus, then the head of the stapes and more rarely the handle of the malleus (Fig. 8.47).

However, lyses of the long process of the incus or even the stapes can be observed in non- cholesteatomatous inflammatory pathologies, as in pars tensa retraction pocket.

8.11.3 Erosion of the Cog

Sign of a cholesteatomatous process invading the AER is the erosion of the cog; the cog is always preserved in non- cholesteatomatous inflammatory condensations of the AER (Fig. 8.48).

8.11.4 Erosion of the Semicircular Canals (Labyrinthine Fistula)

CT-scan reveals the erosion of the bony wall of the semicircular canals with a sensitivity and specificity up to 100% (see Chap. 9.8) (Fig. 8.49). It may assess the size of the bony defect, that is of concern for its surgical strategy and management.

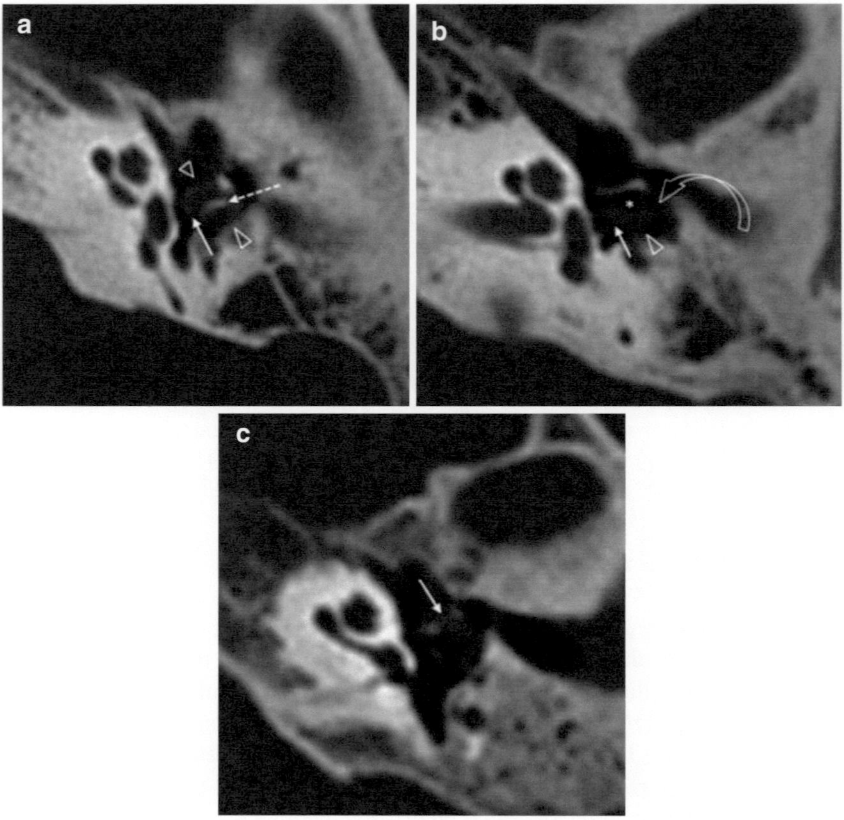

Fig. 8.47 (**a**) Rounded soft tissue image (between the empty arrowheads) causing lysis of the head of the stapes (arrow). The long process of the incus is still present (dashed arrow), (**b**) polylobulated soft tissue mass (empty arrow) of a pars tensa retraction pocket (curved arrow) with lyses of the stapedial head (arrow) and disappearance of the long process of the incus (*) and (**c**) cholesteatoma around the handle of the malleus, with lyses of the malleus handle (arrow)

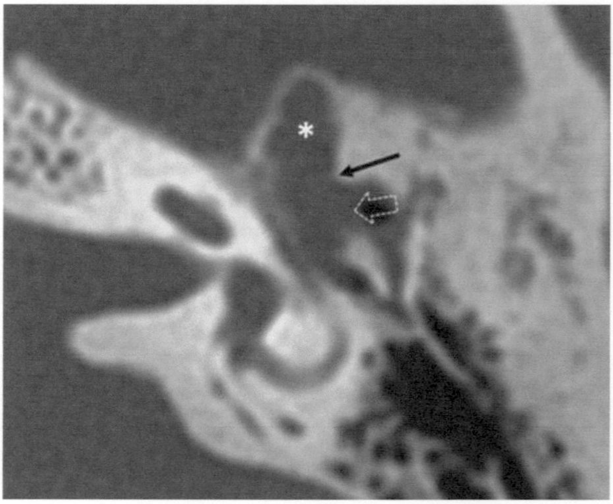

Fig. 8.48 Axial view of a left ear with extended cholesteatoma to the AER (*), the cog is almost completely eroded (black arrow), eroded malleus head (empty arrow)

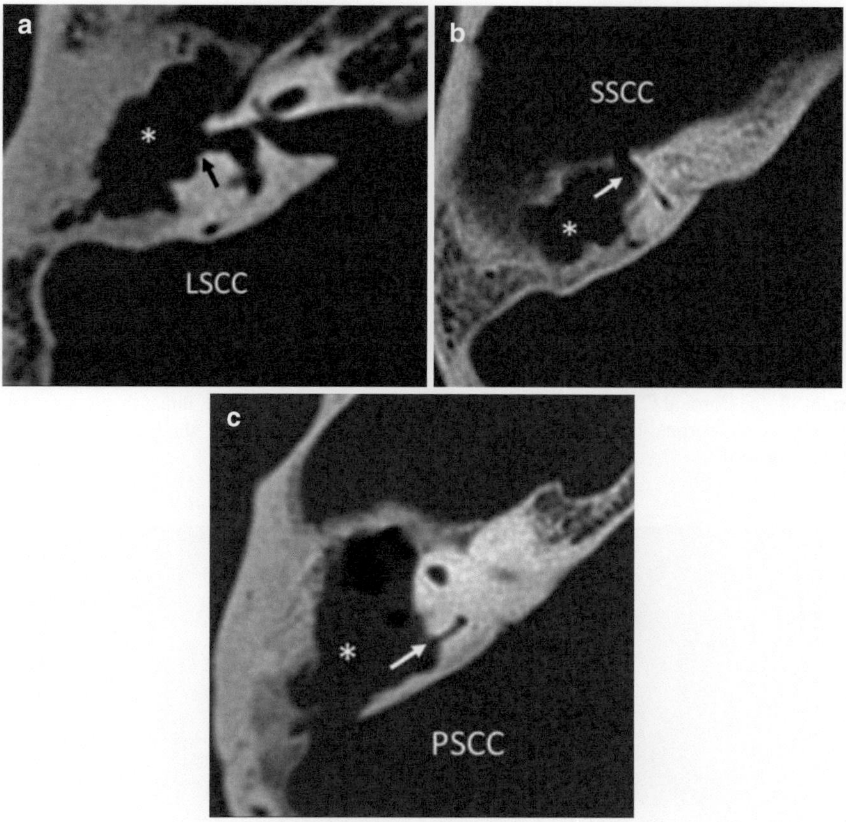

Fig. 8.49 Axial CT images of the right ear of different patients with cholesteatoma of the tympanic cavity (*): (**a**) advanced focal lysis of the bony cover of the lateral semicircular canal (arrow), (**b**) erosion of the superior semicircular canal (arrow) and (**c**) erosion of the posterior semicircular canal (arrow)

8.11.5 Erosion of the of Fallopian Canal

The integrity of the thin bony facial nerve canal is not always easy to confirm scanographically and to differentiate from adjacent soft tissue (Fig. 8.50). Not rarely, the bony canal is spontaneously dehiscent with a slight prominence of the facial nerve, best seen on coronal views. Role of CT Scan is to alert the otosurgeon especially about the anatomical location of the facial nerve in relation to the neighboring soft tissue pathologies.

8.11.6 Erosion of the Tegmen

CT-Scan is specific in confirming the tegmen integrity. The absence of a visible tegmen can be due to a lytic involvement of the tegmen or to a congenital dehiscence: the differential diagnosis is made with the clinical context, comparaison with the controlateral side or associated lytic lesions elsewhere in the middle ear cleft (Fig. 8.51).

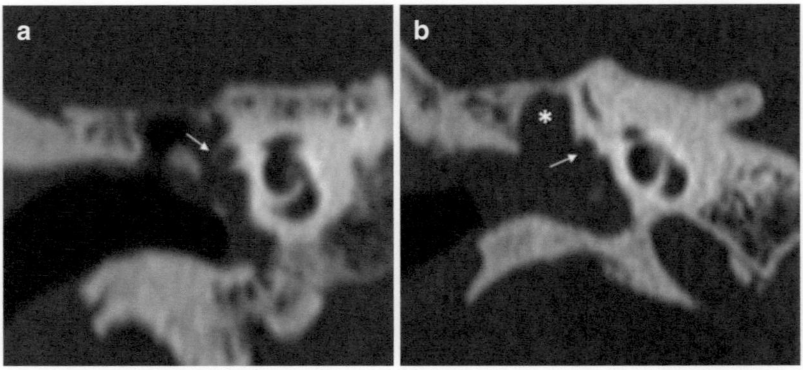

Fig. 8.50 (**a**) Coronal CT on a right ear with pars flaccida cholesteatoma, intact facial nerve canal (arrow) and (**b**) coronal CT of a right ear with a huge cholesteatoma (*), the facial nerve canal is eroded (arrow)

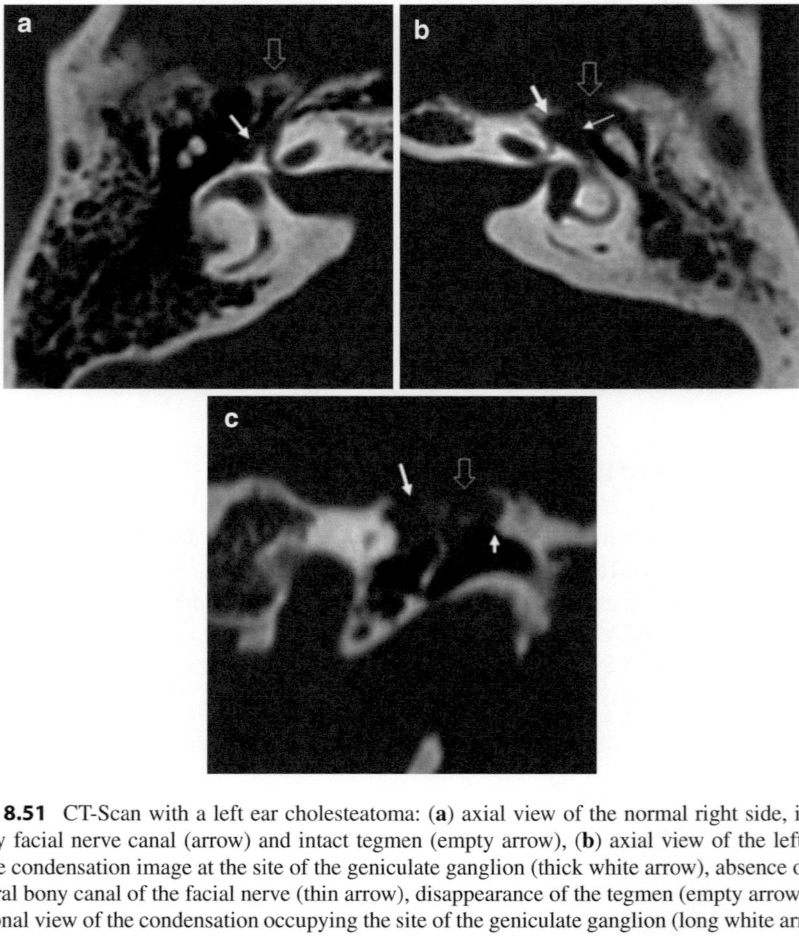

Fig. 8.51 CT-Scan with a left ear cholesteatoma: (**a**) axial view of the normal right side, intact bony facial nerve canal (arrow) and intact tegmen (empty arrow), (**b**) axial view of the left ear: large condensation image at the site of the geniculate ganglion (thick white arrow), absence of the lateral bony canal of the facial nerve (thin arrow), disappearance of the tegmen (empty arrow), (**c**) coronal view of the condensation occupying the site of the geniculate ganglion (long white arrow), disappearance of the tegmen (empty arrow). Amputation of the scutum (short arrow), large opening of the tegmen (empty arrow)

8.11.7 Extension of the Cholesteatoma into the Mastoid

In cases where the antrum is aerated, the negative predictive value is very high that there is no extension of the cholesteatoma into the mastoid (Fig. 8.52a). If the mastoid septa are preserved despite cell condensations, a chronic non-cholesteatomatous infection is the most probable diagnosis (Fig. 8.52b).

CT becomes very indicative of an extension of the cholesteatomatous process to the mastoid, when the mastoid is filled by condensation images with irregular borders (Fig. 8.52c) or the antrum is entirely filled with condensations that have smooth rounded borders (Fig. 8.52d).

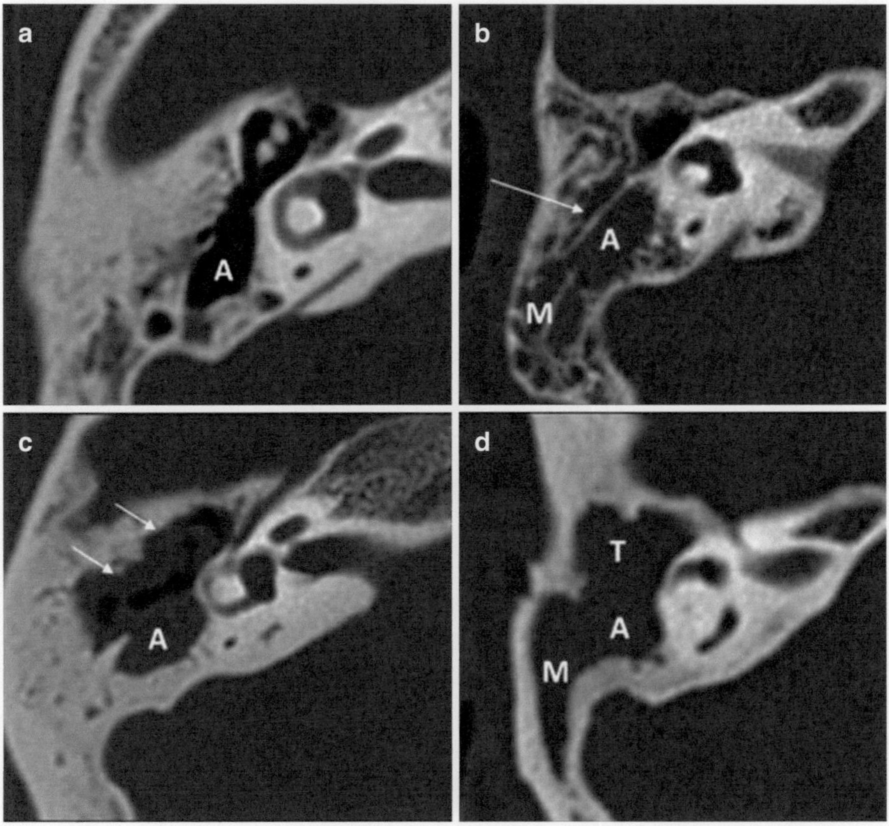

Fig. 8.52 Axial CT-images at the attico-antral level of different patients that presented with attical cholesteatoma, but associated to the following very different aspects of antrum and mastoid: (**a**) a sclerotic mastoid, only the antrum (A) is pneumatized, with regular borders → no extension of the cholesteatoma to the mastoid is suspected, (**b**) antrum (A) and the mastoid cells (M) are completely condensated, but all trabeculations are well preserved → most probably no extension to the antrum/mastoid. Preserved Korner's septum (arrow), (**c**) very thick soft tissue formations with irregular borders (arrows), extending into the antrum (A) highly suspicious for a cholesteatoma extension in a sclerotic mastoid and (**d**) complete disappearance of any mastoid cell with smoothed borders, evident extension of the cholesteatoma to the entire mastoid cavity: T (tympanic cavity), A (antrum), M (mastoid)

8.11.8 External Auditory Canal Lysis

This is a significant CT-scan finding especially when a major part of the posterior bony wall is eroded. This finding is important because of its impact on the selection of the surgical procedure! (see Fig. 8.53).

In some occasions CT may be advantageous over the clinical exam, especially in front of a very dense tympanic membrane after tympanoplasty, with limitation of the otoscopic evaluation (Fig. 8.54).

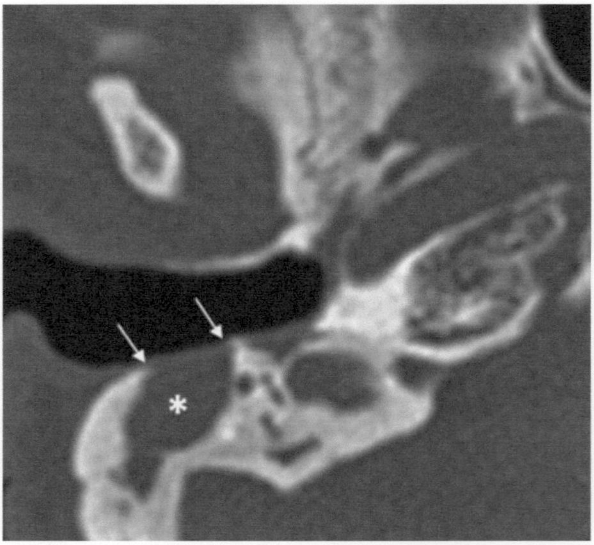

Fig. 8.53 Axial CT image of a right ear with a large defect of the posterior wall of the external auditory canal (between the arrows), due to the bone necrosis by the cholesteatomatous process (*) of the mastoïd

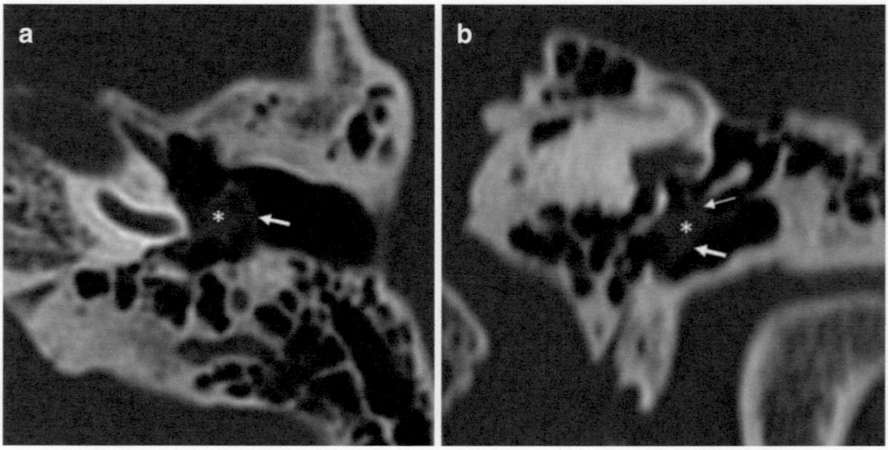

Fig. 8.54 Left ear post tympanoplasty, CHL, behind a thick tympanic membrane on otoscopy, CT revealed (**a**) on the axial CT-image a thickened tympanic membrane (arrow), a retrotympanic round condensation with polylobulated borders, highly suggestive of cholesteatoma (*) and (b) on the coronal reconstruction the thickened tympanic membrane (thick arrow), the condensation image (*) in contact with the incudostapedial joint that starts to be lytic (thin arrow)

Table 8.2 CT-Scan Contribution

Imaging Findings	CT-Scan Value
Well aerated ME cleft spaces	High negative predictive value
Condensation images with rounded borders	Relative high diagnostic value
Diffuse condensations in ME or Mastoid: Granulation tissue? Effusion? Cholesteatoma?	Non-specific value

8.11.9 Limitations of CT Imaging

Condensation images in the tympanic cavity and mastoid are not specific for cholesteatoma and can be also sign of granulation tissue, fibrous tissue, mucosal oedema, effusion or other inflammatory reactions. This is why the cholesteatoma diagnosis is primarily a clinical diagnosis and CT must be read as a complement to the clinical informations. The diagnostic value of CT Imaging is resumed in Table 8.2.

8.12 MRI in Cholesteatoma

MRI offers a very specific diagnostic tool for the detection of postoperative recurrent or residual cholesteatoma: the diffusion weighted imaging. Initially obtained by Echo Planar Imaging (EPI) with 5 mm thickness, it suffered from fair spatial resolution and from susceptibility artefacts. Nowadays, Non-Echo-Planar Diffusion Weighted Imaging (Non EPI-DWI), using turbo spin-echo or multi shot turbo spin echo types of imaging with lesser slice thickness and lesser susceptibility-artefacts, became unanimously the state of the art in MR Imaging for cholesteatoma [95].

Due to the high keratin content of cholesteatoma, both the restricted molecular diffusion and the T2 shine-through effect produce a high signal intensity relative to brain tissue on DW images obtained with b values of 800 or 1000 s/mm^2. The bright signal on b 1000 DW images is evaluated by a subjective qualitative analyses, that can be objectivated by a quantitative analyses of the apparent diffusion coefficient (ADC) in the lesion, that is low in cholesteatoma (values about 700×10^{-6} mm^2/s) but high in non cholesteatomatous tissue that shows values around 1800×10^{-6} mm^2/s. The ADC value is of special interest, when the lesion is of small size and the signal is not very bright on b 1000 mm^2/s. Lingam et al. [95] proposed recently a threshold value of 1300×10^{-6} mm^2/s, ADC values inferior to the threshold being in favor of cholesteatoma, values above of non cholesteatomatous pathologies.

Before the era of the diffusion weighted images, delayed T1 images 30–40 min after injection of Gadolinium have been used for the diagnosis by showing a thin enhancement around the cholesteatoma, that itself does not show any uptake of Gadolinium (Fig. 8.55). However, realization of these delayed sequences is time consuming and today not anymore routinely done, as the diffusion weighted sequences (Fig. 8.56) have proved high sensitivity and specificity.

MRI permits to differentiate other pathologies from cholesteatoma, mainly cholesterol granuloma that has high signal intensity on both T1 and T2 sequences, but no restriction, no contrast enhancement (Fig. 8.57). Granulation tissue, inflammatory

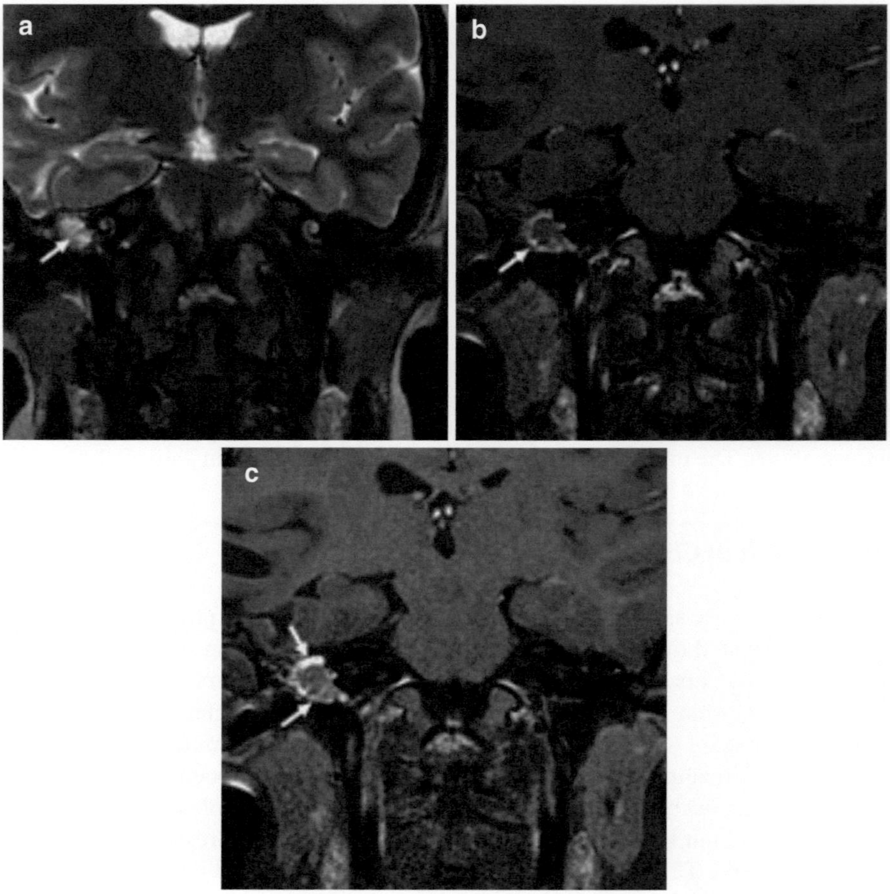

Fig. 8.55 Typical MRI patterns of Cholesteatoma in the right mastoid: (**a**) T2 hyperintense (arrow), (**b**) T1 hypointense (arrow) and (**c**) T1 post Gd delayed images: contrast enhancement around the hypointense cholesteatoma (arrows)

mucosa and scar tissue do not show any restriction, but early Gadolinium contrast enhancement (Fig. 8.58). The main MR findings for the different pathologies are summarized in Table 8.3.

For the primary diagnosis of cholesteatoma, MRI is rarely indicated. Nevertheless, its diagnostic performance in the primary diagnosis has been confirmed with a pooled sensitivity of 92% and a pooled specificity of 97% [96].

However, MRI becomes a precious complementary imaging tool when the clinical presentation and the CT suspect complications and for the postoperative follow up in relation to second look indications.

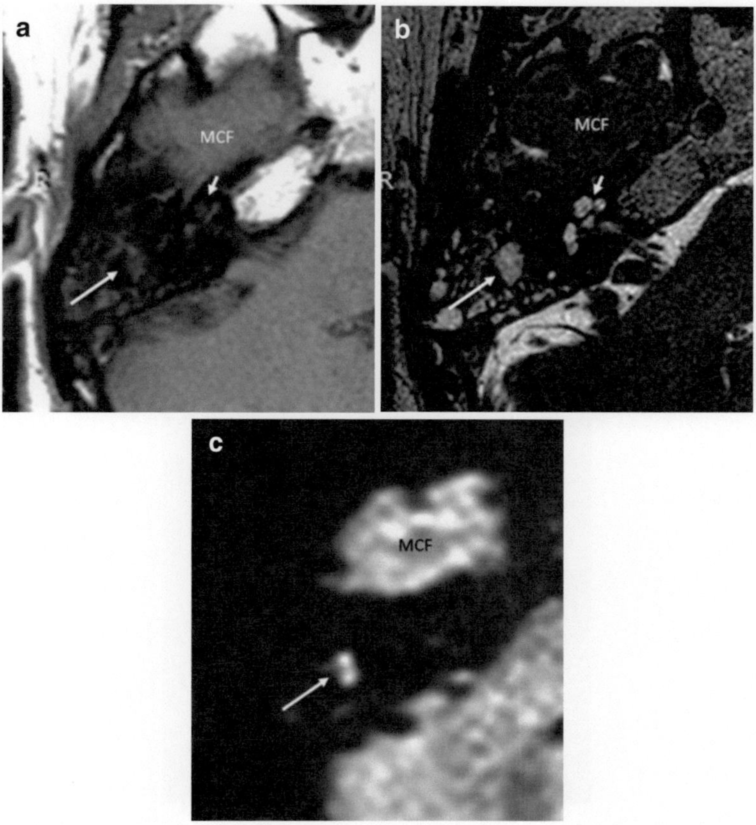

Fig. 8.56 Cholesteatoma of the antrum on the right side, the different slides are taken at the same anatomic level, MCF (middle cranial fossa), the cochlea (small arrow in all slides), (**a**) T1 weighted: hypointense rounded lesion (arrow) surrounded by hypointense mastoid cells, (**b**) T2 slightly hyperintense lesion (arrow) surrounded by condensated mastoid cells, (**c**) Diffusion image b 1000: striking restriction (bright appearance) in this lesion, no restriction elsewhere in the mastoid cells

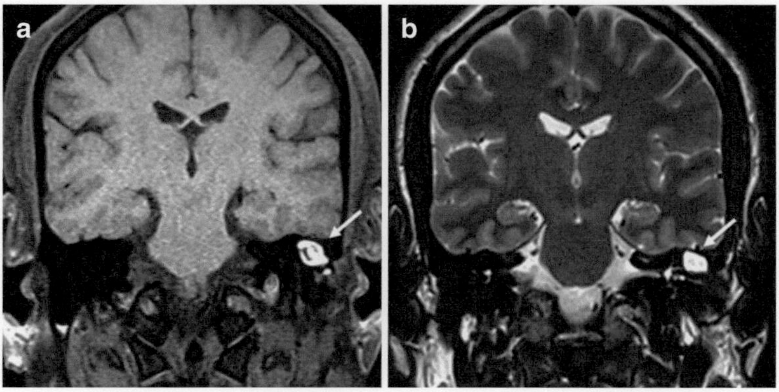

Fig. 8.57 Cholesterol granuloma: *hyper T1, hyper T2* of a left ear. (**a**) coronal T1 weighted image showing a round mass predominantly hyperintense (arrow), containing some central hypointense structures and (**b**) coronal T2 weighted image showing the same hyperintense aspect of the mass lesion (arrow)

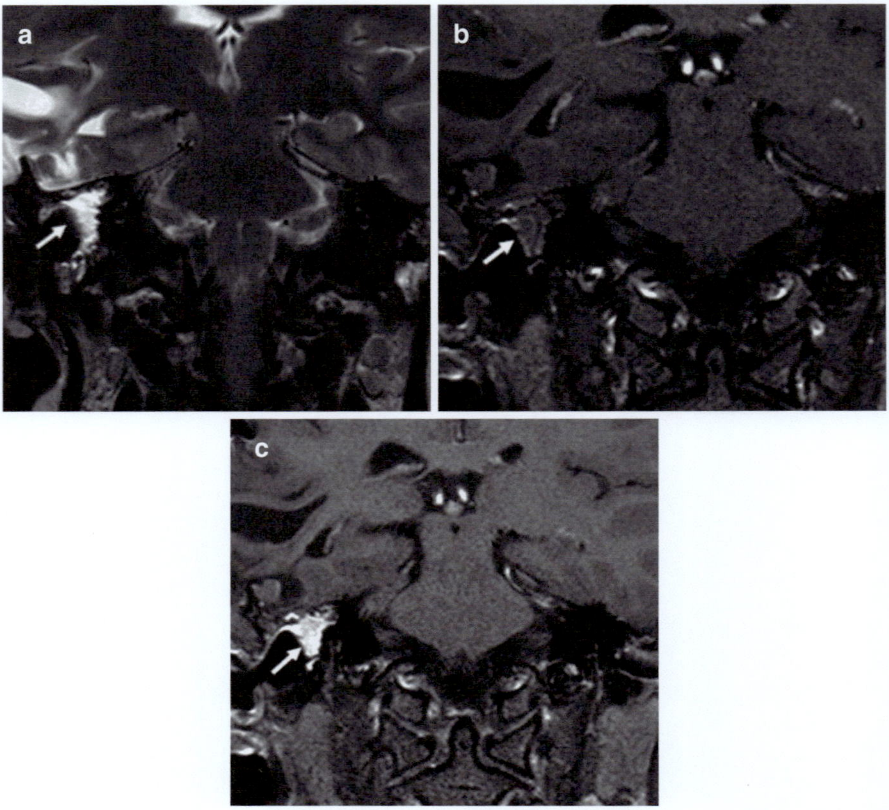

Fig. 8.58 Inflammatory granulation tissues: T2 hyperintense, T1 hypointense, T1 post GD uptake characteristic aspects of inflammatory granulation tissues (white arrow) behind the cholesteatomatous process of Fig. 8.55: (**a**) hyperintense on T2 weighted images, (**b**) hypointense on T1 weighted images and (**c**) with clear contrast uptake on T1 weighted images after Gd administration

Table 8.3 Differential diagnosis by MRI

CHOLESTEATOMA T1: hypointense T2: hyperintense **Diffusion: RESTRICTION** **Gado: no early uptake**	**CHOLESTEROL GRANULOMA** **T1: hyperintense** **T2: hyperintense** Diffusion: no restriction Gado: no uptake
GRANULATION TISSUE T1: hypo/intermediate T2: hyperintense Diffusion: no restriction **Gado: uptake**	**SCAR TISSUE** **T1: hypointense** **T2: hypointense** Diffusion: no restriction **Gado: uptake**

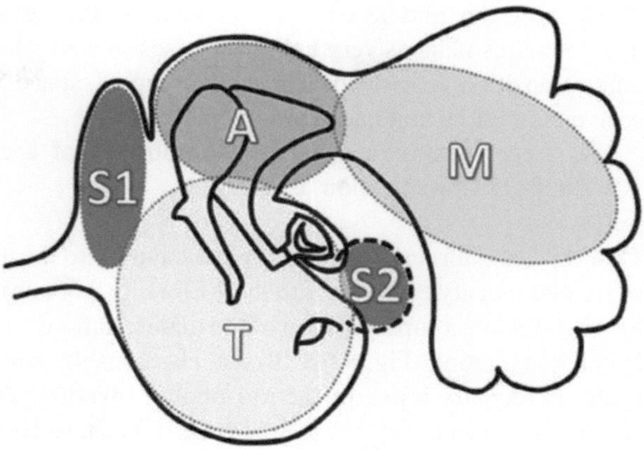

Fig. 8.59 Division of the middle ear spaces using the STAM system as proposed in the EAONO/JOS Classification in 2017

8.13 Staging of Cholesteatoma

Multiple classifications have been proposed (AAO, Lien, Tos, Saleh and Mills, JOS, Telmesani et al., Belal et al.) with the primary aim of comparing results between studies. In addition to the objective of an inter-study comparison of surgical outcomes, a classification system should be able to identify patients who are at risk of cholesteatoma recidivism.

Therefore, the most recent classification proposed by EAONO/JOS in 2017 does not only describe the various localisations of cholesteatoma in the **Attic** (**A**), **Tympanum** (**T**) and **Mastoid** (**M**), but also indicate the sites where the surgery of cholesteatoma meets difficulties for a complete excision hence a high rate of recidivism (**Anterior Epitympanum** (**AER**) **= S1, Sinus tympani = S2**) (Fig. 8.59).

Staging of cholesteatoma according to EAONO/JOS** [97] **is described as follows:

Stage I: ***Cholesteatoma localized at the primary site: in the attic (A) for pars flaccida cholesteatoma, the tympanic cavity (T) for pars tensa cholesteatoma, cholesteatoma secondary to tympanic perforation and congenital chole***

Stage II: ***Cholesteatoma involving two or more sites***

Stage III: ***Cholesteatoma with intratemporal and/or extracranial complications***

Stage IV: ***Cholesteatoma with intracranial complications***

Preoperative CT-Imaging permits to classify the extension of the cholesteatoma correlated to the clinical findings, with a special attention to the anatomical areas of difficult access (S1, S2), which require a planned surgical attention and expertise with a good counseling of the patient. This methodology implies a better compliance for a long follow up.

8.13.1 Clinico-Radiologic Correlations

The scanographic analysis of cholesteatoma can be illustrated according to the schema of the EAONO/JOS Classification, with a special regard to the sites of difficult access (S1 and S2). Sagittal reconstructions along the axis of the incudomalleal chain show the middle ear cleft as seen by the otosurgeon during the surgical approach, this plane is very helpful to assess the S1 space anteriorly and the attico-antral transition posteriorly. The sinus tympani, space S2, however, is much better seen on the initial axial acquisition plane.

Two representative cases of CT-Evaluation of a cholesteatoma according to EAONO/JOS Classification of 2017.

Case 1: Pars tensa retraction from the cavity into the attic, with a rounded process of tissular density extended into the AER (Fig. 8.60a, b). Reconstructions in a sagittal plane enable a superposition of the manifestations to the Schema of the EAONO/JOS Classification (Fig. 8.60c, d) and classifies the cholesteatoma as S1 AM.

Case 2: A pars tensa retraction pocket invading the tympanic cavity adherent to the promontory (Fig. 8.61). On CT, there is a rounded soft tissue mass extended into the sinus tympani (S2) (Fig. 8.62a). Advanced lyses of the incus (Fig. 8.62b). Sagittal reconstruction along the incudomalleal axis show an aerated S1, free attic (A) and mastoid (M) (Fig. 8.62c) .Staging according to EAONO/JOS shows posterior tympanic cavity condensations (T) together with a S2 mass (S2) = stage S2 T.

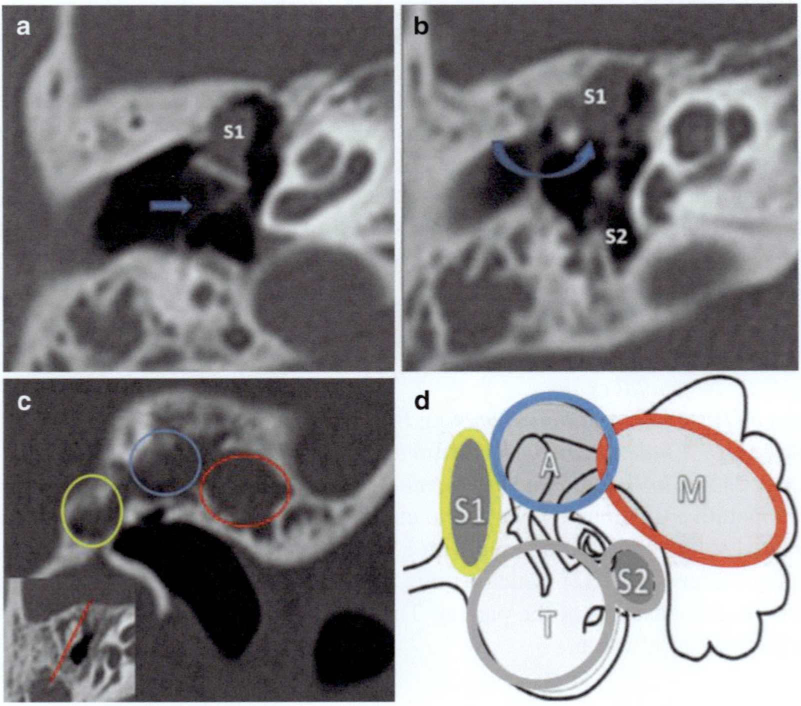

Fig. 8.60 Pars Tensa Retraction Pocket Cholesteatoma: **S1 AM**. Axial CT- image of the right ear: (**a**) retraction of the tympanic membrane (blue arrow), tissue density mass anterior to the malleus handle extending into the anterior epitympanum (S1), (**b**) huge PT retraction pocket (blue arrow) with complete absence of the long process of the incus, soft tissue mass anterior to the malleal neck (S1). Space S2 is free (S2), (**c**) sagittal reconstruction: soft tissue mass in the anterior epitympanum (S1, yellow circle), condensation images of the Attic (blue circle) and the Mastoid (red cercle) and (**d**) Schema of sites according to EAONO/JOS 2017

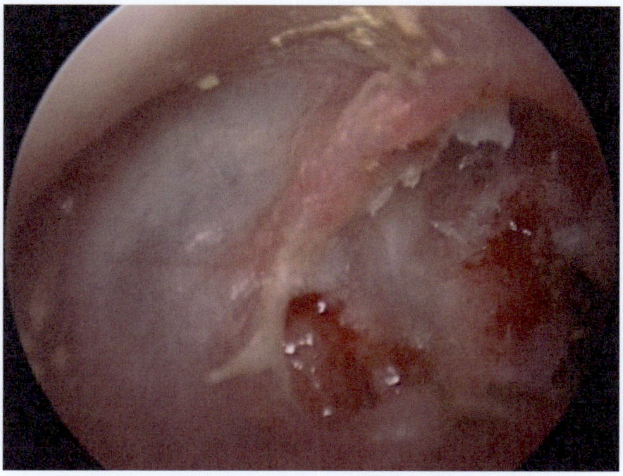

Fig. 8.61 Left pars tensa RP cholesteatoma

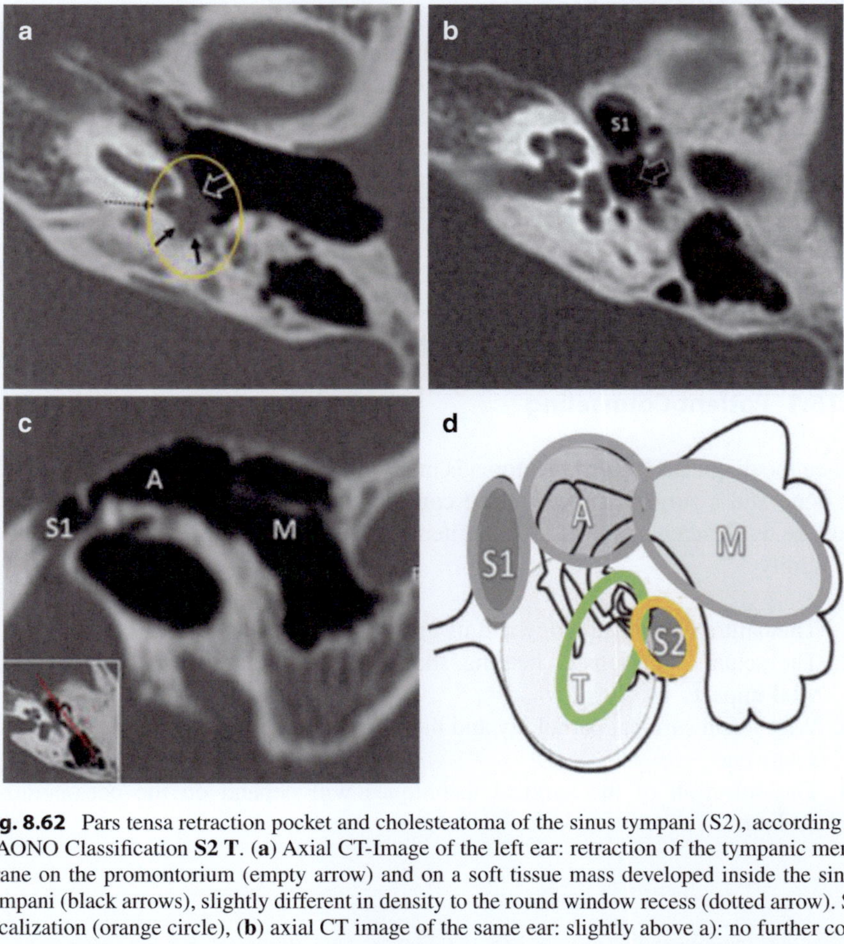

Fig. 8.62 Pars tensa retraction pocket and cholesteatoma of the sinus tympani (S2), according to EAONO Classification **S2 T**. (**a**) Axial CT-Image of the left ear: retraction of the tympanic membrane on the promontorium (empty arrow) and on a soft tissue mass developed inside the sinus tympani (black arrows), slightly different in density to the round window recess (dotted arrow). S2 localization (orange circle), (**b**) axial CT image of the same ear: slightly above a): no further condensation images, but absence of the incus (empty arrow), S1 free, (**c**) sagittal CT-Scan reconstruction along the incudomalleolar axis (red line) showing a aerated AER (S1), free attic (A) and mastoid (M) and (**d**) schema EAONO/JOS 2017

8.14 Management of Cholesteatoma

8.14.1 Medical and Preventive Measures

Until now, no medical treatment is available for cholesteatoma. Research trials for non-surgical treatment of cholesteatoma are limited. New therapeutic approaches should focus on trial of drugs that block the activity of cytokines which are closely related to bone erosion, chiefly TNF-α, MMPs, and IL-1 and IL-6 [98, 99]. In addition, targeted molecules to suppress proliferation and induce apoptotic activity (like 7a microRNA) were proven to have a vital role in the inhibition of the growth of cholesteatoma keratinocytes via downregulation of miR 21 expression [56].

Antimetabolites like topical 5-Fluorouracil act by a downregulation of the keratinocyte growth factor and reduction of proliferative activity and thus curtail the production of keratin debris [100].

Aeration disorders of the middle ear and inflammation are the main predisposing factors for the development of a retraction pocket and cholesteatoma; therefore every mean to improve and optimize the Eustachian tube function must be taken. Special attention must be addressed to the underlying atopy and mucosal disease manifestations which are frequently associated with a dysventilation syndrome, recurrent ME effusions and retraction pocket recidivism.

Retraction pockets have to be identified according to clinico-radiological correlations, that permit their division into stable and unstable pockets, in order to avoid any delay for their surgical therapy and prevent their progress to cholesteatoma (see Chap. 7).

8.15 Surgical Treatment of Cholesteatoma

8.15.1 Patient Counseling

When the diagnosis of cholesteatoma is made, a complete adequate work up should be done and a surgical procedure be considered, a clear and detailed counseling must be undertaken and the following items should be discussed with the patient or his family:

1. The nature of the pathology and its great potential of recurrence.
2. The actual conditions of hearing, the stage of the disease, its functional and vital impacts.
3. Why it is a surgical pathology and the impact of an adequate surgery to insure a safe ear.
4. The selection of the surgical techniques will depend on the per-operative findings.

5. The possible complications of the disease and the possible complications of the surgery.
6. The main objective is to insure a safe ear, hearing rehabilitation may be left to staging.
7. Why second looks must be considered.
8. Why strict care of an open cavity is a need.
9. The great importance of a long term follow up and why it could be for life.
10. Given the disease complexity in the pediatric population, surgeons should provide the comprehensive informations about various surgical strategies to both parents and children in order to avoid any misunderstanding and to ensure a fully informed consent.

8.15.2 Surgical Techniques

Surgery of cholesteatoma implies the following:

1. Total eradication of cholesteatoma to obtain a safe and dry ear.
2. Maintain the best condition for a successful wound healing process in the ear.
3. Restore or maintain the best functional status of hearing.

The essential objective of any surgical technique facing cholesteatoma is to insure at the end of the surgical procedure, that the otologist has done his best to perform, regardless of the applied technique, *a complete removal of the disease*. This is possible to be accomplished whatever the operative time would be. The surgical procedure should be designed for each individual case according to the extent of the disease and his available compliance. Having satisfied this objective, the last step of the surgical procedure is to restore the normal anatomo-physiology of the ear. Whatever the operative procedure would be, the surgery can be divided into two major groups according to the final anatomical aspect:

8.15.2.1 A Closed Technique

It is mainly centered on the respect of the ear canal anatomy or its reconstruction once the complete removal of the disease has been accomplished; this include CWU, CWD with reconstruction of the canal wall, CWD with mastoid obliteration. Each one of these techniques ends up with the *absence of an open mastoid cavity.*

8.15.2.2 An Open Technique

It is mainly centered on the *creation of an open mastoid cavity*. This technique includes the classic CWD, atticotomy without reconstruction or obliteration thus maintaining a communication between the EAC and the operative cavity.

8.15.3 Surgical Procedures

Several clinical considerations must be taken into account when choosing a surgical approach, as each technique has advantages and disadvantages. In addition, the surgeon's expertise of surgical procedures is a major determinant to achieve the main objectives: "***a safe ear and a preserved hearing***".

1) **A CWD mastoidectomy** involves the removal of the posterior bony canal wall.
2) **CWU mastoidectomy** implies the removal of all mastoid air cells while maintaining the integrity of the posterior ear canal wall.
3) **Other procedures:**
   - **Reconstruction** of the ear canal defect which could be partial or total to restore the normal anatomy of the ear canal with the tympanic graft.
   - **Atticoantral mastoid obliteration** can be done after CWU or CWD restoring in both cases the ear canal and thus avoiding an open mastoid cavity.
   - **Ossicular reconstruction** must be decided in relation to the following:
   - The extension of the disease,
   - The hearing level of both ears,
   - The age of the patient,
   - The degree of confidence of the surgeon that he has accomplished a complete removal of the disease (***unthoughtful residual***)

8.15.3.1 Canal-Wall-Down (CWD) Procedure

Indications
- Cholesteatoma of an only hearing ear,
- A major erosion of the posterior bony canal wall,
- A history of vertigo due to a labyrinthine fistula,
- A poor Eustachian tube function,
- A sclerotic mastoid with limited access to the epitympanum (Fig. 8.63).
- Patient non-compliant for follow-up.

Advantages
- Relatively short duration of the surgery despite extensive disease.
- Easy detection of the postoperative residual disease and reduced rate of recurrences; the facial recess is well exteriorized as well as the attic.
- Any postoperative cholesteatoma regrowth can readily be seen and removed as an office procedure (Fig. 8.64).

Disadvantages
- Hearing reconstruction is less successful.
- Open cavity: the mastoid bowl maintenance can be a lifelong problem. Unpleasant appearance of the meatoplasty.

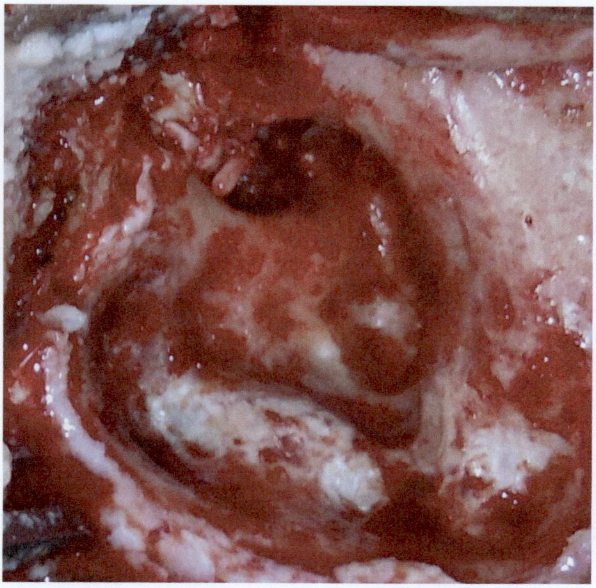

Fig. 8.63 CWD mastoidectomy of left ear

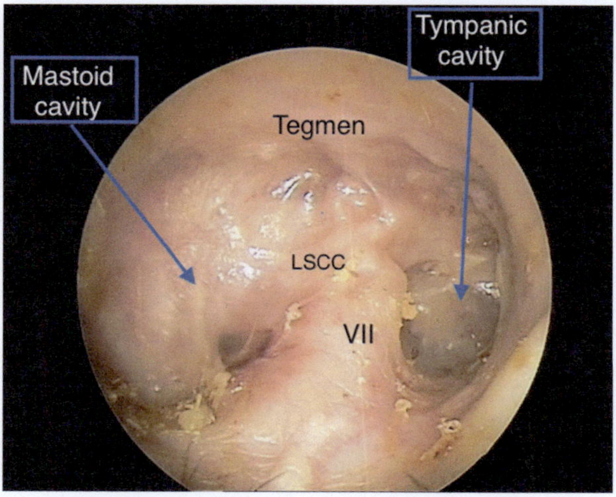

Fig. 8.64 Right ear mastoid cavity of a patient who was operated two years ago for third recurrent cholesteatoma. The cavity is stable and self cleaning. Any residual disease can be easily seen and removed in the office. There are no hidden spaces for the skin to retratct inside it and thus the possibility of recurrent cholesteatoma is very low

- A secondary reconstruction would be less successful.
- Difficulty fitting a hearing aid because of meatoplasty.
- Wet Ear Cavity is the most common reason for revision surgery after CWD mastoidectomy (troublesome mastoid cavity) [101], *due to the following:*
  - Incomplete eradication of the mastoid air-cells disease or inadequate lowering of the facial ridge (85%),
  - Very large cavity or/and inadequate meatoplasty (10%),
  - Recurrent or persistent cholesteatoma (5%) (Fig. 8.65).

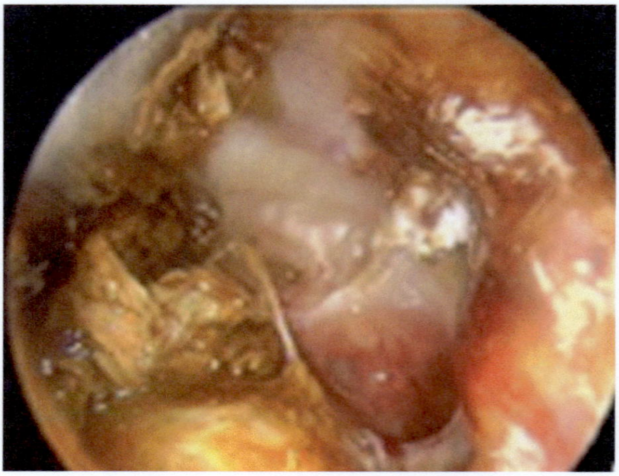

Fig. 8.65 Right troublesome mastoid cavity

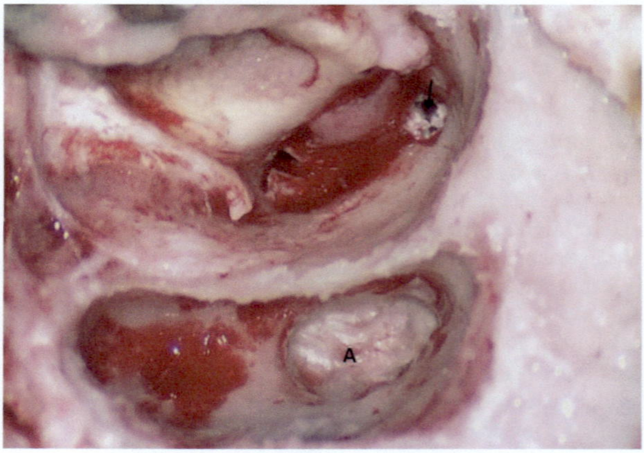

Fig. 8.66 CWU mastoidectomy of left ear. Cholesteatoma originating from Prussak's space (black arrow) and extending into the antrum (A)

8.15.3.2 Canal-Wall-Up (CWU) Procedure

The CWU procedure is recommended to avoid the disadvantages of the CWD.

CWU consists of a preservation of the posterior bony external auditory canal wall during a complete simple mastoidectomy with or without a posterior tympanotomy (Figs. 8.66, 8.67, 8.68).

A staged CWU procedure is often necessary with a scheduled second look operation at 6–18 months for removal of any residual cholesteatoma and for ossicular chain reconstruction, when indicated (Fig. 8.69). In younger children, second-look operations are often scheduled 6–9 months following the primary surgery. In adults, the second look operation is mostly planned after 12 months postoperatively.

Indications

Nowadays a CWU technique is indicated in most cases of cholesteatoma especially for cases with a large pneumatized mastoid. In modern otosurgery, CWU must be the first choice for most cholesteatoma cases.

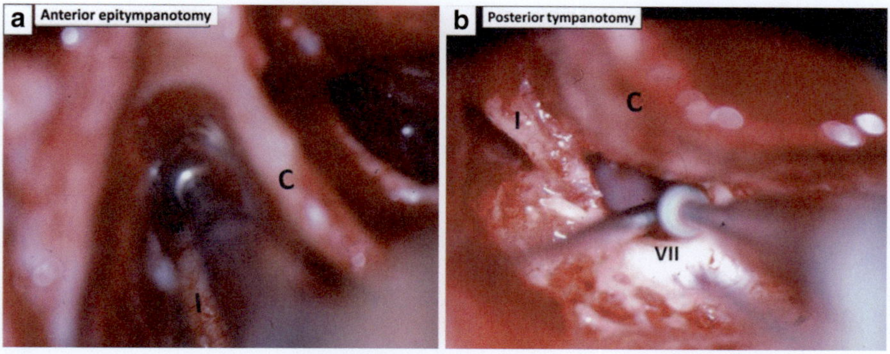

Fig. 8.67 In CWU mastoidectomy, the posterior wall of the ear canal is preserved (C). (**a**) Anterior epitympanotomy is performed to expose the anterior epitympanum and supratubal recess and (**b**) posterior tympanotomy is performed to expose the retrotympanum. M: malleus; I: incus; VII: facial nerve

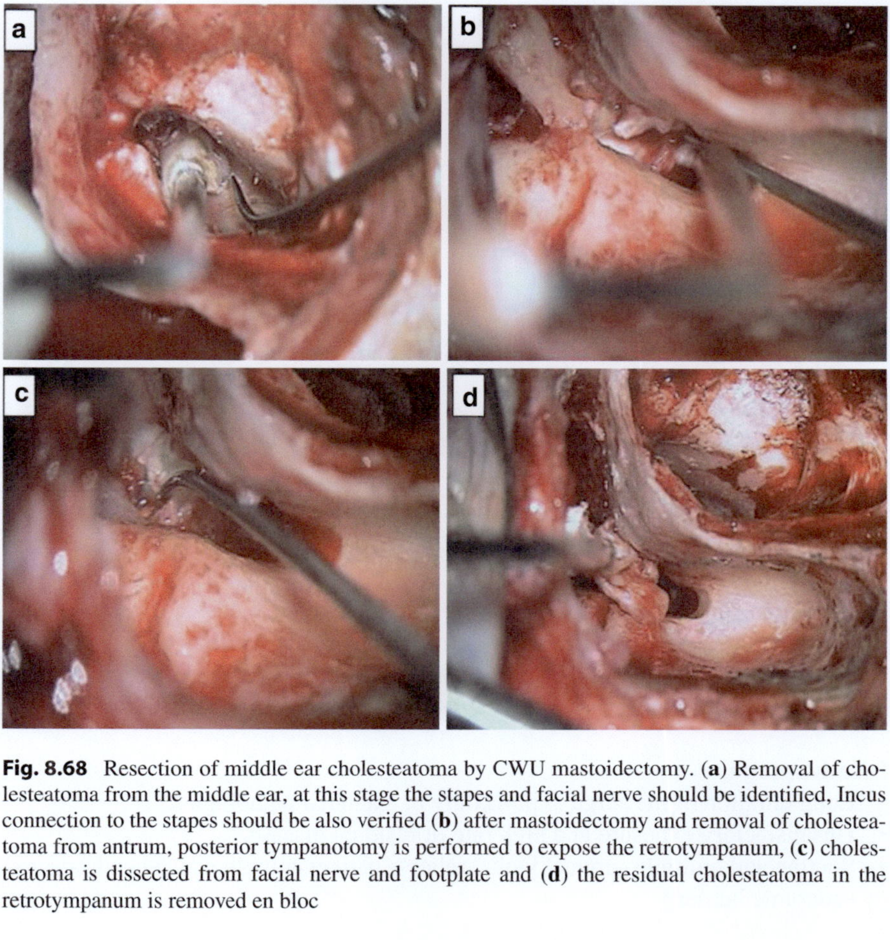

Fig. 8.68 Resection of middle ear cholesteatoma by CWU mastoidectomy. (**a**) Removal of cholesteatoma from the middle ear, at this stage the stapes and facial nerve should be identified, Incus connection to the stapes should be also verified (**b**) after mastoidectomy and removal of cholesteatoma from antrum, posterior tympanotomy is performed to expose the retrotympanum, (**c**) cholesteatoma is dissected from facial nerve and footplate and (**d**) the residual cholesteatoma in the retrotympanum is removed en bloc

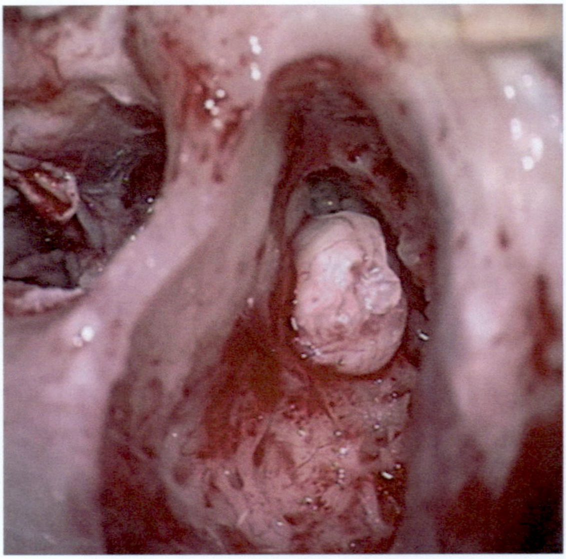

Fig. 8.69 Residual cholesteatoma in a second look surgery after CWU.

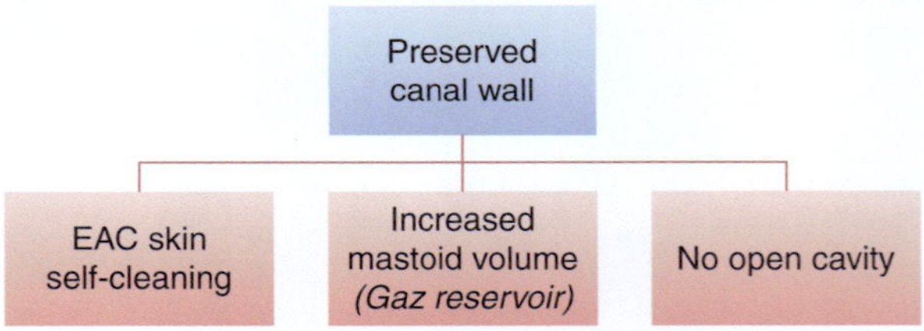

Fig. 8.70 Advantages of CWU procedure

Contraindications

CWU procedures are relatively contraindicated in:

- Only hearing ear,
- A long-standing ear disease after multiple previous procedures and persistent extended pathology,
- A poor Eustachian tube function.
- Extensive lysis of the bony ear canal.

Advantages (Fig. 8.70)

- A more rapid healing with respect of the ear anatomo-physiology.
- A better quality of life for the patient and normal ear contours.
- A better fit of hearing aids when needed.

Disadvantages

- Long duration of the surgical procedure in extended pathologies.
- Unsatisfactory exposure and high rate of residual disease.
- Staging and multiple surgical looks (relative patient compliance dependance and economic burden).

8.15.3.3 Other Surgical Approaches

Various surgical approaches have been developed to address the drawbacks of CWU (high residual rates) and CWD (cavity problems) mastoidectomies. Modified methods include tailor-made tympanomastoidectomy with cartilage reconstruction, transcanal endoscopic management of the cholesteatoma, and laser-assisted cholesteatoma surgery. However, only minimal data related to their outcomes are available. Long-term outcomes require more studies.

(a) Mastoid obliteration

Partial Mastoid obliteration (Fig. 8.71) has been suggested to reduce the size of the open cavity following open technique. Mosher first introduced mastoid obliteration using a pedicle musculoperiosteal flap in 1911 to overcome problems associated with the postoperative mastoid cavity [102]. Since that time, numerous otologists have reported success with mastoid obliteration techniques using alloplastic materials as well as various biogenic implants, such as fat, cartilage, bone paté, bone chips, ceramic powder, Ceravital, and hydroxyapatite [103–105].

The obliteration technique does not confer a great physiological value to the concept of the "mastoid reservoir theory" considered in the CWU technique. Mastoid obliteration reduces the volume of ME cleft cavity, and thereby the amount of gas exchange consumed by the mastoid mucosa; thus the smaller cavity would adapt better to the dysfunction of the Eustachian tube and the aeration deficit. In doing so it reduces a possible dysventilation and secondarily a possible retraction pocket or cholesteatoma recurrences.

(b) Transcanal anterior atticotomy

A transcanal anterior atticotomy is indicated for a cholesteatoma with limited involvement of the middle ear, intact ossicular chain and/or a healthy epitympanum. After removal of the disease, in bloc reconstruction of the resulting cavity is done with cartilage and perichondrium. In such technique the recurrence rate and the probability of a residual tissue are low.

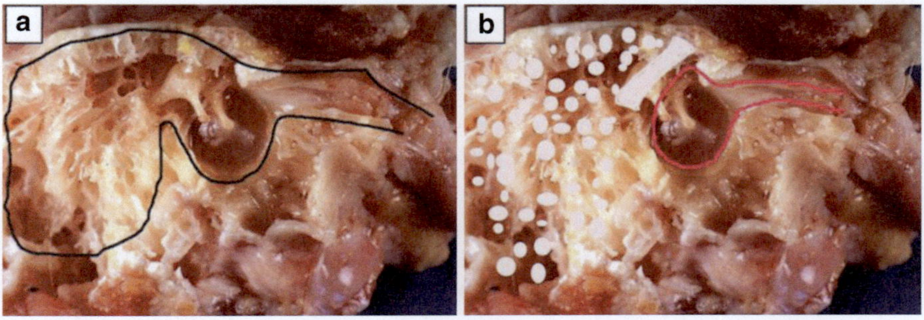

Fig. 8.71 Schema demonstrating the technical concept in mastoid obliteration: Intact canal wall technique with mastoid and attic obliteration, reducing the ME cavity volume in order to adapt the middle ear mucosa gas exchange to the inadequate ET ventilation function

(c) Bondy modified radical mastoidectomy
Although rarely used today, the Bondy procedure is indicated for attic and mastoid cholesteatoma that does not involve the middle ear space and is situated lateral to the ossicles. The Eustachian tube function should be adequate, with an intact pars tensa and well aerated free middle ear spaces.

In conclusion *Facing the duty of any selected technique to secure a perfectly safe ear and exclude any possible residual, surgical expertise is a prerequisite to avoid an unhappy situation when postoperative complications become more frequent or more troublesome than the disease itself. Moreover, if repeated surgeries or multiple looks on the same ear could be the cause of increased surgical risks or patient compliance deficits, it remains that a permanent open mastoid cavity, requiring regular cleaning is not by itself a guaranteed solution for a long term safe ear.*

8.15.4 Endoscopy in Cholesteatoma

The use of endoscopy demonstrated a positive impact on the management of cholesteatoma. Otoendoscopy has the advantages of better visualization of some hidden areas such as: sinus tympani, facial recess, anterior epitympanic space, attic, hypotympanum, medial epitympanum and retrotympanum (Fig. 8.72). The disadvantages of oto-endoscopic surgery are time consuming and "one hand surgery". However endoscope assisted-microsurgery allows the use of the most efficient tools to face difficult sites of localization of the cholesteatoma, and allow its complete removal.

Combined surgeries done with microscope, endoscope or endoscope/microscope [106] should prove their value by confirmed satisfying long term results.

8.15.5 Laser in Cholesteatoma

Some cholesteatoma may be more effectively removed using laser and not by mechanical dissection alone. Using Laser, reduced rates of residual cholesteatoma have been reported with level 2 evidence. This technique permits to maintain hearing when the ossicular chain is still intact. Matrix on the surface of ossicles can be vaporized with laser without the need to manipulate or remove the ossicle.

8.15.6 Surgery of Congenital Cholesteatoma

Congenital cholesteatoma occupies mostly the anterior upper quadrant of the eardrum. When discovered as small as a pearl (Figs. 8.2 and 8.73), complete and in toto excision without opening the capsule of the cholesteatoma is the rule. Extension of such type of congenital cholesteatoma may follow the malleal folds, medial to the

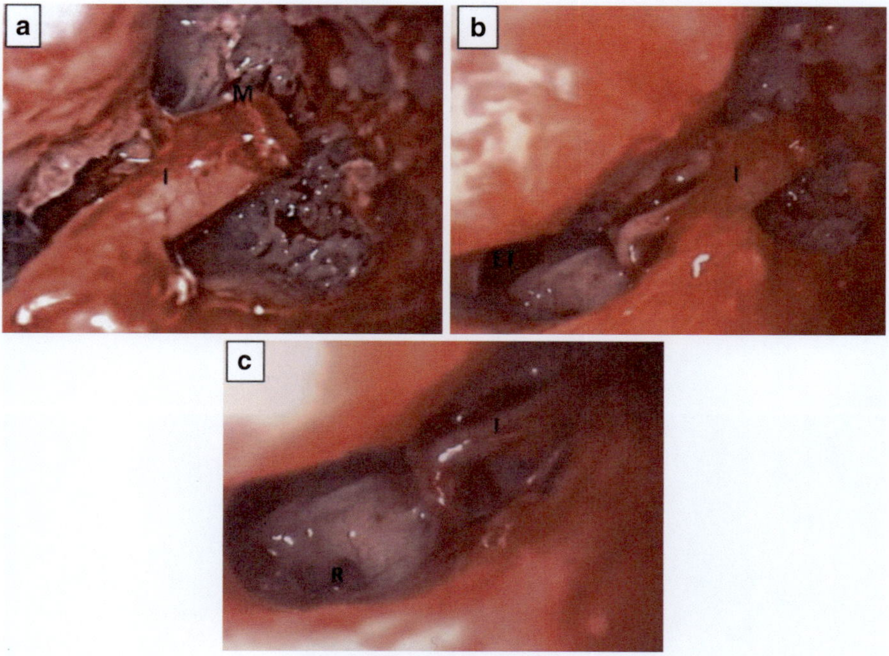

Fig. 8.72 (**a**) Endoscopy of the attico-mastoid area showing the whole epitympanum, (**b**) endoscopy of the middle ear through the posterior tympanostomy showing the Eustachian tube (ET) and (**c**) endoscopy of the retro tympanum using angled scope from the posterior tympanotomy. R: round window; I: incus; M: malleus

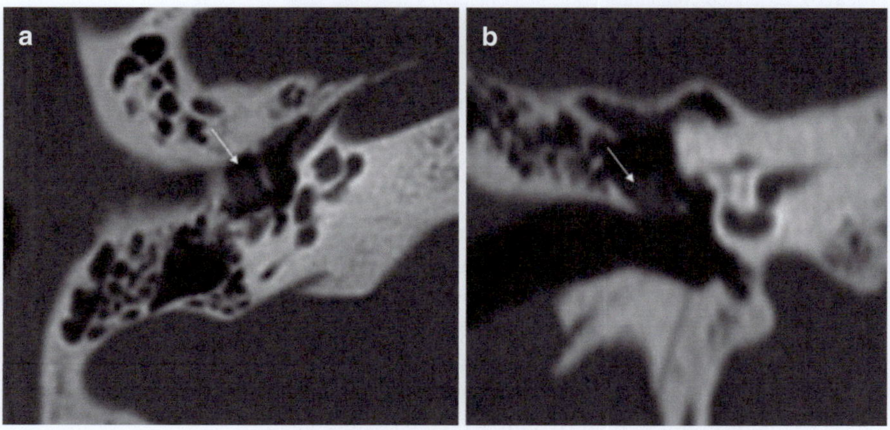

Fig. 8.73 Right ear with a congenital cholesteatoma, localized posterosuperiorly EAONO/JOS stage I. (**a**) axial CT-view and (**b**) coronal reconstruction: small condensation image (arrrow) in the outer attic beside an intact scutum

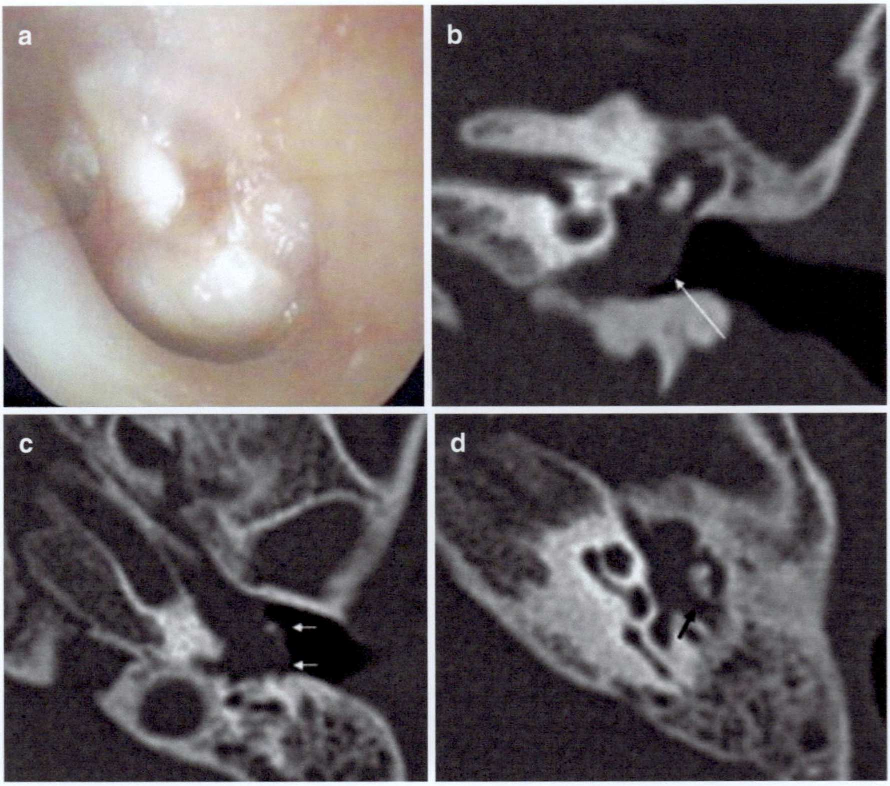

Fig. 8.74 Extended congenital cholesteatoma. (**a**) Otoscopic view of a congenital cholesteatoma bulging behind an intact eardrum, (**b**) corresponding CT view in the coronal plan showing the bulging of the tympanic membrane into the EAC (arrow), (**c**) axial CT-view of the polylobulated bulging (arrows) of the tympanic membrane, that molds an underling polylobated process, even if its density is not specific, (**d**) mass effect on the ossicular chain (arrow), that is pushed laterally and partially lytic

malleus neck, the manubrium and the interosseous fold to reach the incus and the anterior stapes crura. In this case, delicate dissection is required to insure complete excision without opening the capsule or dislocating the ossicles.

Cases of posterosuperior localization of a congenital cholesteatoma are also encountered and may imply an endoscopic removal taking care of a possible extension to the sinus tympani where a residual is feared. In the later situation, Laser surgery is helpful not to disturb a preserved ossicular chain.

When the diagnosis is delayed, congenital cholesteatoma may extend largely and requires the same approaches as in acquired cholesteatoma (Fig. 8.74).

Fig. 8.75 Primary vs. secondary ossicular chain reconstruction (OCR) in cholesteatoma surgery

Primary vs Secondary OCR

- **Primary**
  - Avoid period with CHL
- **Secondary**
  - Permits detection of residual disease
  - Permits ME and TM to heal
  - Motivation for the patient to accept second look
  - Concern for postop. aeration with ET
  - Damaged Mucosa → scaring, fibrosis, retraction

8.15.7 Hearing Rehabilitation in Cholesteatoma Surgery

The second role of surgery in cholesteatoma is to either fix hearing or restore serviceable hearing whenever possible. The management of hearing impairment depends on the type of hearing loss and the possibly reachable degree of hearing recovery.

Hearing results are better with the closed technique than with the open technique, because the tympanic membrane is kept of normal size and position. BAHA offers a viable option to improve hearing outcomes, as long as the bone conduction remains intact.

Ossiculoplasty can be achieved by the placement of an autologous ossicular graft (e.g., bone or cartilage) or a prosthetic device (e.g., partial or total ossicular replacement prosthesis).

The ossicular chain can be restored in one stage surgery when the complete removal of the cholesteatoma is certain. In cases with a potential risk of residual disease, however, ossicular chain reconstruction is often deferred to a second-look operation where a potential residual is anticipated: "safe ear prevails on hearing restoration" (Fig. 8.75).

For surgical technique of ossiculoplasty please refer to Chap. 6.14.2.

8.15.8 Surgery for Cholesteatoma in an "Only Hearing Ear"

In such situation, an utmost surgical expertise must be looked for: cholesteatoma is a much greater risk for hearing loss than a good surgery. Good surgery preserves the present hearing from further deterioration by the cholesteatoma. Careful surgery is expected to insure complete removal of the disease and a satisfactory hearing result. Therefor a transfer of such cases to a tertiary care center is recommended.

8.15.9 Disease Control (Surgery Outcome)

Depending on the procedure, there is a large variation in the postoperative outcomes regarding residuals or recurrences.

It is admitted that the recurrence and residual lesion rates are higher in children: 30% versus 15% in adults. The following factors are incriminated:

1. Sinus tympani invasion and ossicular lysis at the moment of diagnosis
2. An impaired ET function with persistent impaired aeration of the ME
3. A large périmatrix with its more active inflammatory and aggressive mediators.

8.15.10 Follow-Up

Nearly 90% of recurrent disease will appear within 5 years after surgery; however, in a recent long-term study (mean follow-up period of 15.4 years) on cholesteatoma, the mean delay until discovery of the recidivism was found to be 10.4 years. Another long-term study revealed an increase in the rate of recidivism when the follow-up period was extended [107–111]. Thus, it seems imperative that patients undergo periodic follow-up for as long as possible. However, the keys of success to minimize the recidivism rate is the strict and complete eradication of the disease at the initial surgery and the serious consideration of potential recurrence risk factors. Children need more frequently an office follow-up than adults because of their increased likelihood to develop residual cholesteatoma. Pediatric patients are generally followed at least annually until adulthood.

8.15.11 Radiological Follow Up

8.15.11.1 Planned Follow UP During the First Year Postop

Nowadays, MRI imaging can be considered as the first line follow up imaging, because of its lack of irradiation and its superiority to CT-Scan for tissue differentiation. The high negative predictive value of negative diffusion weighted images, reported with up to 100% in early publications [112], raised an enthusiasm among otologists and motivated numerous studies during the last 10 years on this subject. The most recent meta analysis that enrolled 26 postoperative studies over the last 10 years with a series of 1152 patients, confirmed a high pooled sensitivity of 0.93 and specificity of 0.91 for the improved technical conditions by ***non EPI Diffusion weighted sequences*** to detect residual/recurrent cholesteatoma in postoperative middle ear cleft cavities [96].

The PPV was 97.3%, and the NPV 85.2%. *The authors found that cholesteatoma as small as 2 mm could be predictably found.* The use of this imaging modality may help to prevent unnecessary surgery for patients when there is doubt about residual or recurrent cholesteatoma [113].

Nowadays the otologist feels more at ease to perform and promote CWU techniques for most cholesteatoma cases regardless of their location and extension, having in mind that MRI may replace second look surgery, and can even be used repetitively.

However, there is a non-negligible rate of 7.4% of false negative cases found with MRI that turned out to be most often due to the small size of the residual cholesteatoma inferior to 3 mm.

A lack of diagnosis at this stage may give enough time to the growing cholesteatoma to invade once again some challenging areas (S1, S2) before the next imaging control. This dilemma is especially of great concern in pediatric patients and can only be resolved in case by case evaluation of the potential risk of recurrence and realisation of a real second look surgery, that remains the gold standard of diagnostic fiability.

Accordingly and in order to insure a safe ear especially in children, the otologist's attitude would be as the following:

1. *A surgical second-look procedure should be proposed always for patients when a complete removal of the disease during the primary surgery was uncertain to the surgeon and this despite a negative imaging*
2. *MRI evaluation may be appropriate to avoid a surgical second look for patients when the otologist was sure that all the disease has been completely excised by his first surgery and when an unequivocal normal microscopic examination is observed during the first 6 months of the postoperative period.*

8.15.11.2 Postoperative Imaging Longtime After the Initial Surgery in Cases with a "Non-Adequate Follow-Up"

In cases when the clinical diagnosis of a possible residual is doubtful or the surgical procedure has been executed in a different center, CT is the first imaging method to be requested:

1. When CT-Scan demonstrates a complete aeration of the tympanic cavity and the absence of any condensation image in the middle ear cleft, CT alone confirms the absence of any residual or recurrence. In such situation CT has a negative predictive value of almost 100%
2. When CT shows condensation images in the cavity, a high suspicion of a cholesteatoma recurrence is retained if these condensations are:
   - Associated to a recurrent tympanic membrane retraction pocket
   - Associated to smoothed borders of the mastoid septa around the mass
   - Associated to additional bony erosions in comparison with previous CT-Imaging

3. In cases of previous CWU for cholesteatoma, CT can shows a typical aspect of recurrent cholesteatoma hidden in the atticoantral spaces (Fig. 8.76)
4. In cases of an **open mastoid cavity**, and when the otoscopy favors a cholesteatoma recurrence, CT Imaging has an added value (Fig. 8.77)
   - To show erosions of the bony plates: tegmen lysis, sinus plate, LSCC, which are not evident with microscopy
   - To predict the anatomic localization of the sigmoid sinus
   - To assess the sites of predilection for recurrence (S1 and S2).

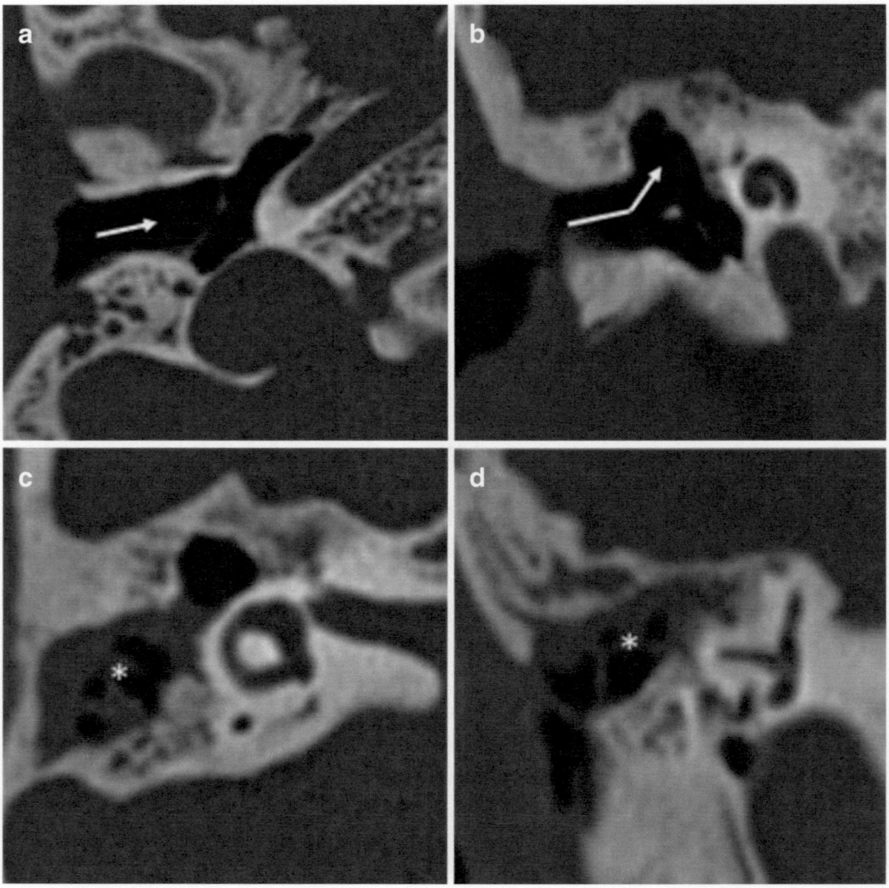

Fig. 8.76 Right ear with recurrence of cholesteatoma in the cavity of mastoïdectomy after CWU. (**a**) A normal thin tympanic membrane, normal EAC, (**b**) amputation of the scutum with a free attic, (arrow) (**c**) axial and (**d**) coronal CT-images show the hidden atticoantral cavity of mastoidectomy, that contains a huge recurrent cholesteatoma (*)

5. If the CT shows a complete condensation of the cavity, it is impossible to distinguish an eventual focal cholesteatoma from surrounding granulation or scar tissue (Fig. 8.78). Complementary MR evaluation can provide differential diagnoses, in case of positive restriction in favour of choelesteatoma (Fig. 8.79); absence of restriction, this is in favour of a non-cholesteatomatous condition (Fig. 8.80).

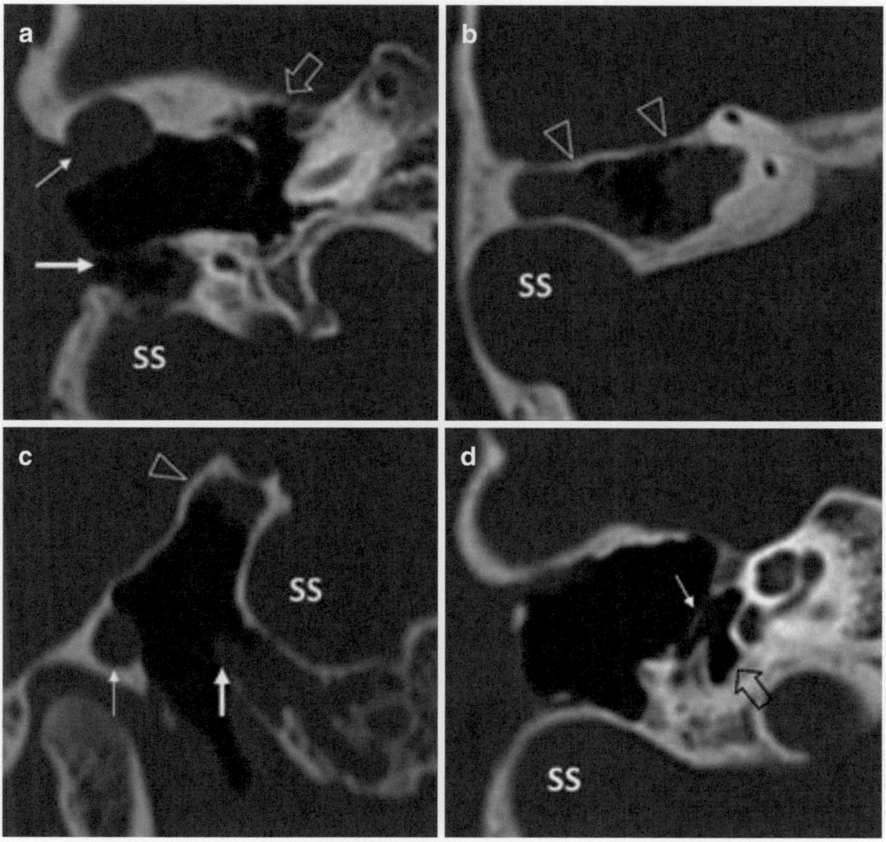

Fig. 8.77 ATCDs of CWD for cholesteatoma. (**a**) Axial CT view of the right ear: rounded tissular masses in the anterior tympanic canal wall (thin arrow) and posterior part of the open cavity (thick arrow), near to the prominent sigmoid sinus (SS in all images), AER free (S1, empty arrow), (**b**) axial CT image passing by the upper attic, with residual cholesteatoma (arrowheads), (**c**) sagittal CT reconstruction showing cholesteatoma anteriorly (thin arrow), in the posterior wall (thick arrow) and in the attic (arrowhead), the prominent sigmoid sinus is lining the whole cavities' height (SS) and (**d**) axial CT image showing the tympanic cavity with a myringostapedopexy (arrow), and a well aerated sinus tympani (S2, empty arrow)

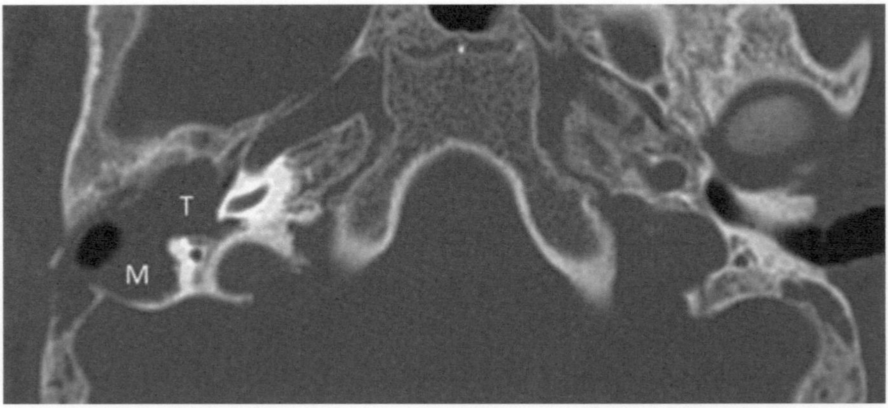

Fig. 8.78 CT follow up with a suspicious otoscopy. The whole middle ear cleft is condensated M: cavity of mastoidectomy, T: tympanic cavity

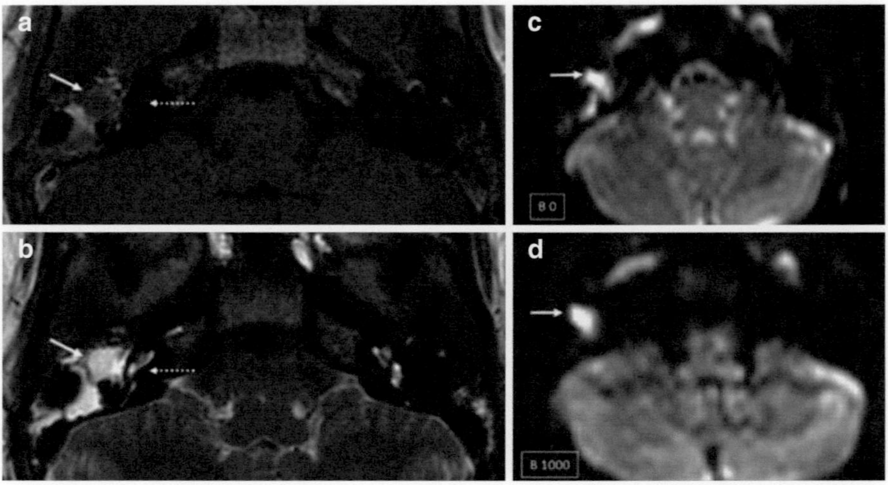

Fig. 8.79 MRI of the temporal bone in the same patient of Fig. 8.76. (**a**) T1 SE weighted image showing a rounded hypointense mass (thick arrow) in the middle ear cavity on the level of the basal turn of the cochlea (dashed arrow), (**b**) T2 TSE weighted image on the same level: the mass is hyperintense (thick arrow), good visibility of the cochlea (dashed arrow) at the same level, (**c**) diffusion weighted image at b = 0: the mass (arrow) is hyperintense due to its T2 effect and (**d**) diffusion weighted image at b = 1000: the mass shows still a high hypersignal that represents restriction and is specific for cholesteatoma at b = 1000

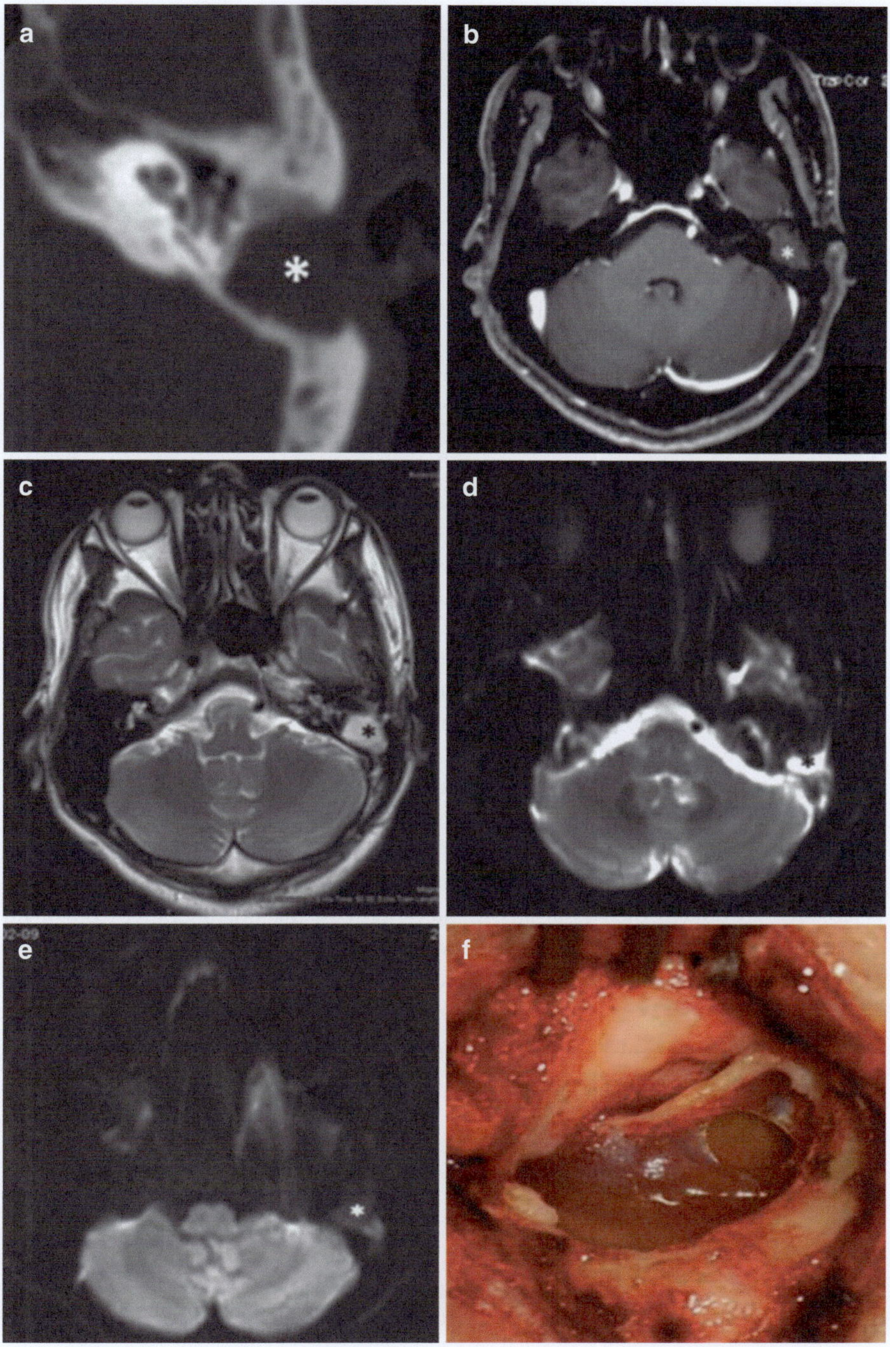

Fig. 8.80 (**a**) After cholesteatoma-surgery, a non specific mastoid opacification (*) is seen on the axial CT-view, (**b**) injected MRI T1 sequence: no enhancement in the corresponding hypointense lesion (*), (**c**) MRI T2 sequence: lesion with homogeneous hypersignal (*), (**d**) diffusion weighted image at b = 0 is very bright (*), and (**e**) diffusion weighted image at b = 1000 is dark for the lesion (*), meaning no restriction; (**f**) surgical exploration reveals only fluid and absence of cholesteatoma

Conclusion

Despite the impressive recent progress concerning cholesteatoma pathology, molecular biology and its immune behavior, its definite pathogenesis remains uncertain. The huge progress in the basic sciences of cholesteatoma was not accompanied by the same level of advances in its surgical therapy. A complete knowledge about the impact of the aeration pathways on the functional anatomophysiology of the middle ear is a prerequisite to deal correctly with its management and better control of its recurrences. All procedures of reconstruction would not control cholesteatoma recurrences if an adequate aeration of the middle ear spaces is not insured and well preserved.

The early diagnosis of a cholesteatoma is the key point to avoid extensive forms and consequently decrease the dilemma of the residual. Advanced Imaging in cholesteatoma pathology enriches its assessment, helps in the clear counseling of the patient and may orient the surgical strategies. An early treatment prevents complications and preserves hearing.

Knowing that the middle ear mucosa cannot generate epidermal tissue as cholesteatoma, a recurrence behind an intact tympanic membrane after a complete removal of cholesteatoma must not exist. Therefore the duty of the otologist is to reach the needed expertise to accomplish the complete and total removal of the cholesteatoma during the first surgery; hereby he decreases greatly the necessity of a systematic second look surgery after a closed technique.

Surgical approaches must be customized to each patient depending on the extent of his disease. The most relevant aim from the surgery is to free the ear from its disease and at the same time to preserve its natural anatomo-physiology.

The otologist must be aware of the serious and potentially life-threatening complications of cholesteatomas especially when preventive medicine is not affordable to all countries.

Nowadays the true rate of recidivism tends to be underestimated or wrongly considered due to the variations in the length of the postoperative follow-up period and the great number of cases which lost compliance to the same otology center. Regarding all surgical techniques it is of utmost importance to screen the correct rate of postoperative "recurrences" in a lifetime follow up duration.

The related advances in the knowledge about its molecular biology and genetic modeling may engender hopefully possible medical therapies of cholesteatoma in the near future.

References

1. Aquino JE, Cruz Filho NA, de Aquino JN. Epidemiology of middle ear and mastoid cholesteatomas: study of 1146 cases. Braz J Otorhinolaryngol. 2011;77(3):341–7.
2. Potsic WP, Korman SB, Samadi DS, Wetmore RF. Congenital cholesteatoma: 20 year experience at the Children's Hospital of Philadelphia. Arch Otolaryngol Head Neck Surg. 2002;126(1):409–14.
3. Nelson M, Roger G, Koltai PJ, Garabedian EN, Triglia JM, Roman S, et al. Congenital cholesteatoma: classification, management and outcome. Arch Otolaryngol Head Neck Surg. 2002;128(1):810–4.

4. Abramson M. Controversies in pediatric otology: point counterpoint. Am J Otol. 1985;6:167–9.
5. Deguine O, Deguine CH. The contralateral ear in cholesteatoma. Cholesteatoma and mastoid surgery. 3rd International Conference of Cholesteatoma, Copenhagen. Amsterdam: Kugler & Ghedine Publications; 1989. p. 393–8.
6. Nevoux J, Lenoir M, Roger G, Denoyelle F, Le Pointe HD, Garabédian E-N. Childhood cholesteatoma. Eur Ann Otorhinolaryngol Head Neck Dis. 2010;127(4):143–50.
7. McDonald TJ, Cody DT, Ryan RE Jr. Congenital cholesteatoma of the ear. Ann Otol Rhinol Laryngol. 1984;93:637–40.
8. Friedberg J. Congenital cholesteatoma. Laryngoscope. 1994;104:1–24.
9. Cruveilher J. Anatomie Pathologie du corps humain. Paris: Bailliere; 1829.
10. Muller J. Uber den feineren Bau and die Formen des krankhaften Geschwulste. Berlin: Reimer; 1838.
11. Ikeda M. Etude en microscopie electronique de la stucture fine du cholesteatoma. J Otorhinolaryngol. 1968;71:84.
12. Bodelet R, Wayoff M. Notes preliminaires sur l'ultrastructure du cholesteatome. Ann Otolaryngol. 1970;87:449.
13. Lim D, Saunders W. Acquired cholesteatoma. Light and electron microscopic observation. Ann Otol. 1972;81:2.
14. Magnan J, Bremond G, De Micco C. Les aspects microscopiques du cholesteatome. Cah ORL. 1975;10:303–11.
15. Vennix P, Kuijpers W, Tonnaer E, Peters TA, Ramaekers FCS. The cytokeratin expression in the normal rat middle ear and during induced OME. In: Tos M, Thomsen J, Peitersen E, editors. Cholesteatoma and mastoid surgery. Amsterdam: Kugler & Ghedini; 1989. p. 111–5.
16. BroeKaert D, Cornille A, Eto H, et al. A comparative immunohistochemical study of cytokeratin and vimentin expression in middle ear mucosa and cholesteatoma and in epidermis. Virchow Arch A Pathol Anat Histopathol. 1988;413:39–51.
17. Karmody CS, Byahatti SV, Blevins N, Valtonen H, Northrop C. The origin of congenital cholesteatoma. Am J Otol. 1998;19(3):292–7.
18. Paparella MM, Rybak L. Congenital cholesteatoma. Otolaryngol Clin N Am. 1978;11:113–20.
19. Sadé J. The etiology of cholesteatoma: the metaplastic theory. In: McCabe B, Sadé J, Abrahamson M, editors. Cholesteatoma: first International Conference. Birmingham, AL: Aesculapius Publishing; 1977. p. 212–32.
20. Piza J, Gonzales M, Northorp CC. Meconium contamination of the neonatal ear. J Pediatr. 1989;115:910–4.
21. Michaels L. An epidermoid formation in the developing middle ear: possible source of cholesteatoma. J Otolaryngol. 1986;15:169–74.
22. Aimi K. Role of the tympanic ring in the pathogenesis of congenital cholesteatoma. Laryngoscope. 1983;93:1140–6.
23. Bennett M, Warren F, Jackson GC, Kaylie D. Congenital cholesteatoma: theories, facts, and 53 patients. Otolaryngol Clin North Am. 2006;39(6):1081–94.
24. Tos M. A new pathogenesis of mesotympanic (congenital) cholesteatoma. Laryngoscope. 2000;110(11):1890–7.
25. Habermann J. Zur Entstehung des Cholesteatoms des Mittelorhes. Arch Otorhinolaryngol. 1888;27:42.
26. Bezold F. Uber das Cholesteatom des Mittelohres. Z Ohrenhk. 1891;21:252–63.
27. Wittmaack K. Wie entsteht ein genuines Cholesteatom? Arch Ohren Nasen Kehlkopfhk. 1933;137:306.
28. Schwartz H, Eysell C. Uber die kunstliche Eroffnung des Warzenfortsatzes. Arch Ohrenheilk. 1873;7:157.
29. Lange W. Uber die Entstrhung des Mittelohre cholesteatoma. Z Hals-Nas-Ohrenhk. 1925;11:250–65.
30. Gray D. The treatment of cholesteatoma in children. Proc R Soc Med. 1964;57:769–71.
31. Jackler RK, Santa Maria PL, Varsak YK, Nguyen A, Blevins NH. A new theory on the pathogenesis of acquired cholesteatoma: Mucosal traction. Laryngoscope. 2015;125(Suppl 4):S1–14.

32. Friedmann I. The comparative pathology of otitis media, experimental and human. II. The histopathology of experimental otitis of the guinea-pig with particular reference to experimental cholesteatoma. J Laryngol Otol. 1955;69(9):588–601.
33. Olszewska E, Wagner M, Bernal-Sprekelsen M, Ebmeyer J, Dazert S, Hildmann H, et al. Etiopathogenesis of cholesteatoma. Eur Arch Otorhinolaryngol. 2004;261(1):6–24.
34. Bremond G, Magnan J, Acquaviva F. Cholesteatoma and epidermoid metaplasia. Differences and similarieties. Acta Otorhinolaryngol Belg. 1980;34(1):34–42.
35. Lepercque S, Broekaert D, Van Cauwenberge P. Cytokeratin expression patterns in the human tympanic membrane and external ear canal. Eur Arch Otorhinolaryngol. 1993;250(2):78–81.
36. Kuo C-L. Etiopathogenesis of acquired cholesteatoma: prominent theories and recent advances in biomolecular research. Laryngoscope. 2015;125(1):234–40.
37. Chole RA, Tinling SP. Basal lamina breaks in the histogenesis of cholesteatoma. Laryngoscope. 1985;95(3):270–5.
38. Yamamoto-Fukuda T, Takahashi H, Koji T. Animal models of middle ear cholesteatoma. J Biomed Biotechnol. 2011;2011. Article ID 394241, 11 pages
39. Albino AP, Kimmelman CP, Parisier SC. Cholesteatoma: a molecular and cellular puzzle. Am J Otol. 1998;19(1):7–19.
40. Kuo CL, Shiao AS, Yung M, Sakagami M, Sudhoff H, Wang CH, Hsu CH, et al. Updates and knowledge gaps in cholesteatoma research. Biomed Res Int. 2015;2015:854024.
41. Magnan J, Chays A, Bremond G, et al. Anatomo-pathologie du cholesteatme. Acta Oto-Rhino-Laryngologica Belg. 1991;45:27–34.
42. Magnan J, Chays A, Bruzzo M, et al. Pathogenesis of cholesteatoma. In: Ars B, editor. Pathogenesis in cholesteatoma. The Hague: Kugler Publications; 1999. p. 105–18.
43. Preciado DA. Biology of cholesteatoma: special considerations in pediatric patients. Int J Pediatr Otorhinolaryngol. 2012;76(3):319–21.
44. Yoshikawa M, Kojima H, Yaguchi Y, Okada N, Saito H, Moriyama H. Cholesteatoma fibroblasts promote epithelial cell proliferation through overexpression of epiregulin. PLoS One. 2013;8(6):e66725.
45. Raynov AM, Choung YH, Park HY, Choi SJ, Park K. Establishment and characterization of an in vitro model for cholesteatoma. Clin Exp Otorhinolaryngol. 2008;1(2):86–91.
46. Cheshire IM, Blight A, Ratcliffe WA, Proops DW, Heath DA. Production of parathyroid-hormone-related protein by cholesteatoma cells in culture. Lancet. 1991;338(8774):1041–3.
47. Yetiser S, Satar B, Aydin N. Expression of epidermal growth factor, tumor necrosis factor-alpha, and interleukin-1alpha in chronic otitis media with or without cholesteatoma. Otol Neurotol. 2002;23(5):647–52.
48. Chung JW, Yoon TH. Different production of interleukin-1α, interleukin-1β and interleukin-8 from cholesteatomatous and normal epithelium. Acta Otolaryngol. 1998;118(3):386–91.
49. Schilling V, Negri B, Bujia J, Schulz P, Kastenbauer E. Possible role of interleukin 1α and interleukin 1 beta in the pathogenesis of cholesteatoma of the middle ear. Am J Otol. 1992;13(4):350–5.
50. Ergün S, Zheng X, Carlsöö B. Expression of transforming growth factor-alpha and epidermal growth factor receptor in middle ear cholesteatoma. Am J Otol. 1996;17(3):393–6.
51. Mayot D, Wayoff M, Bene M, et al. Immunological characteristics of human cholesteatoma matrix. In: Tos M, Thomsen J, Peitersen E, editors. Cholesteatoma and mastoid surgery. Kugler & Ghedini: Amsterdam/Berkley/Milan; 1989. p. 181–2.
52. Bruzzo M, Martin PM, Magnan J. Etude in vitro du systeme EGF-REGF dans le cholesteatome et le conduit auditif externe. J Fr ORL. 1996;45:87–93.
53. Sheikholeslam-Zadeh R, Decaestecker C, Delbrouck C, Danguy A, Salmon I, Zick Y, et al. The levels of expression of galectin-3, but not of galectin-1 and galectin-8, correlate with apoptosis in human cholesteatomas. Laryngoscope. 2001;111(6):1042–7.
54. Olszewska E, Chodynicki S, Chyczewski L. Apoptosis in the pathogenesis of cholesteatoma in adults. Eur Arch Otorhinolaryngol. 2006;263(5):409–13.
55. Chung JH, Lee SH, Park CW, Kim KR, Tae K, Kang SH, et al. Expression of apoptotic vs antiapoptotic proteins in middle ear cholesteatoma. Otolaryngol Head Neck Surg. 2015;153(6):1024–30.

56. Zhang W, Chen X, Qin Z. MicroRNA let-7a suppresses the growth and invasion of cholesteatoma keratinocytes. Mol Med Rep. 2015;11(3):2097–103.
57. Chole RA, Faddis BT. Evidence for microbial biofilms in cholesteatomas. Arch Otolaryngol Head Neck Surg. 2002;128(10):1129–33.
58. Juhn SK, Jung MK, Hoffman MD, Drew BR, Preciado DA, Sausen NJ, Jung TT, Kim BH, Park SY, Lin J, Ondrey FG, Mains DR, Huang T. The role of inflammatory mediators in the pathogenesis of otitis media and sequelae. Clin Exp Otorhinolaryngol. 2008;1(3):117–38.
59. Kupper TS. The activated keratinocyte: a model for inducible cytokine production by non-bone marrow-derived cells in cutaneous inflammatory and immune responses. J Invest Dermatol. 1990;94(6 Suppl):146S–50S.
60. Reinartz JJ, George E, Lindgren BR, Niehans GA. Expression of p53, transforming growth factor alpha, epidermal growth factor receptor, and c-erbB-2 in endometrial carcinoma and correlation with survival and known predictors of survival. Hum Pathol. 1994;25(10):1075–83.
61. Khazaie K, Schirrmacher V, Lichtner RB. EGF receptor in neoplasia and metastasis. Cancer Metastasis Rev. 1993;12(3–4):255–74.
62. Grandis JR, Melhem MF, Gooding WE, et al. Levels of TGF-alpha and EGFR protein in head and neck squamous cell carcinoma and patient survival. J Natl Cancer Inst. 1998;90(11):824–32.
63. Juhász A, Sziklai I, Rákosy Z, Ecsedi S, Adány R, Balázs M. Elevated level of tenascin and matrix metalloproteinase 9 correlates with the bone destruction capacity of cholesteatomas. Otol Neurotol. 2009;30(4):559–65.
64. Laeeq S, Faust R. Modeling the cholesteatoma microenvironment: coculture of HaCaT keratinocytes with WS1 fibroblasts induces MMP-2 activation, invasive phenotype, and proteolysis of the extracellular matrix. Laryngoscope. 2007;117(2):313–8.
65. Shinoda H, Huang C-C. Expressions of c-jun and p53 proteins in human middle ear cholesteatoma: relationship to keratinocyte proliferation, differentiation, and programmed cell death. Laryngoscope. 1995;105(11):1232–7.
66. Holly A, Sittinger M, Bujia J. Immunohistochemical demonstration of c-myc oncogene product in middle ear cholesteatoma. Eur Arch Otorhinolaryngol. 1995;252(6):366–9.
67. Palkó E., Póliska S., Csákányi Z., et al. The c-MYC protooncogene expression in cholesteatoma. Biomed Res Int. 2014;2014:Article ID 639896, 6 pages.
68. Ozturk K, Yildirim MS, Acar H, Cenik Z, Keles B. Evaluation of c-MYC status in primary acquired cholesteatoma by using fluorescence in situ hybridization technique. Otol Neurotol. 2006;27(5):588–91.
69. Ecsedi S, Rákosy Z, Vízkeleti L, et al. Chromosomal imbalances are associated with increased proliferation and might contribute to bone destruction in cholesteatoma. Otolaryngol Head Neck Surg. 2008;139(5):635–40.
70. Klenke C, Janowski S, Borck D, et al. Identification of novel cholesteatoma-related gene expression signatures using full-genome microarrays. PLoS One. 2012;7(12):e52718.
71. Choung YH, Park K, Kang SO, Raynov AM, Chul HK, Choung PH. Expression of the gap junction proteins connexin 26 and connexin 43 in human middle ear cholesteatoma. Acta Otolaryngol. 2006;126(2):138–43.
72. James AL, Chadha NK, Papsin BC, Stockley TL. Pediatric cholesteatoma and variants in the gene encoding connexin 26. Laryngoscope. 2010;120(1):183–7.
73. Maniu A, Harabagiu O, Schrepler MP, Catana A, Fanuta B, Mogoanta CA. Molecular biology of cholesteatoma. Romanian J Morphol Embryol. 2014;55(1):7–13.
74. Bayazít YA, Karakök M, Uçak R, Kanlíkama M. Cycline-dependent kinase inhibitor, p27 (KIP1), is associated with cholesteatoma. Laryngoscope. 2001;111(6):1037–41.
75. Chole RA, McGinn MD, Tinling SP. Pressure-induced bone resorption in the middle ear. Ann Otol Rhinol Laryngol. 1985;94(2 Pt 1):165–70.
76. McGinn MD, Chole RA, Tinling SP. Bone resorption induced by middle-ear implants. Arch Otolaryngol Head Neck Surg. 1986;112(6):635–41.
77. Orisek BS, Chole RA. Pressures exerted by experimental cholesteatomas. Arch Otolaryngol Head Neck Surg. 1987;113(4):386–91.
78. Huang CC, Yi ZX, Yuan QG, Abramson M. A morphometric study of the effects of pressure on bone resorption in the middle ear of rats. Am J Otol. 1990;11(1):39–43.

79. Maranhao A, Andrade J, Godofredo V, Matos R, Penido N. Epidemiology of intratemporal complications of otitis media. Int Arch Otorhinolaryngol. 2014;18(2):178–83.
80. Akimoto R, Pawankar R, Yagi T, Baba S. Acquired and congenital cholesteatoma: determination of tumor necrosis factor-alpha, intercellular adhesion molecule-1, interleukin- 1-alpha and lymphocyte functional antigen-1 in the inflammatory process. ORL J Otorhinolaryngol Relat Spec. 2000;62(5):257–65.
81. Ahn JM, Huang C-C, Abramson M. Interleukin 1 causing bone destruction in middle ear cholesteatoma. Otolaryngol Head Neck Surg. 1990;103(4):527–36.
82. Shiwa M, Kojima H, Kamide Y, Moriyama H. Involvement of interleukin-1 in middle ear cholesteatoma. Am J Otolaryngol. 1995;16(5):319–24.
83. Kim CS, Lee CH, Chung JW, Kim CD. Interleukin-1 alpha, interleukin-1 beta and interleukin-8 gene expression in human aural cholesteatomas. Acta Otolaryngol. 1996;116(2):302–6.
84. Kawai T, Matsuyama T, Hosokawa Y, et al. B and T lymphocytes are the primary sources of RANKL in the bone resorptive lesion of periodontal disease. Am J Pathol. 2006;169(3):987–98.
85. Dornelles Cde C, da Costa SS, Meurer L, Rosito LP, da Silva AR, Alves SL. Comparison of acquired cholesteatoma between pediatric and adult patients. Eur Arch Otorhinolaryngol. 2009;266(10):1553–61.
86. Schönermark M, Mester B, Kempf HG, Bläser J, Tschesche H, Lenarz T. Expression of matrix-metalloproteinases and their inhibitors in human cholesteatomas. Acta Otolaryngol. 1996;116(3):451–6.
87. Visse R, Nagase H. Matrix metalloproteinases and tissue inhibitors of metalloproteinases: structure, function, and biochemistry. Circ Res. 2003;92(8):827–39.
88. Sastry KV, Sharma SC, Mann SB, Ganguly NK, Panda NK. Aural cholesteatoma: role of tumor necrosis factor-alpha in bone destruction. Am J Otol. 1999;20(2):158–61.
89. Juhasz A, Sziklai I, Rakosy Z, Ecsedi S, Adany R, Balazs M. Elevated level of tenascin and matrix metalloproteinase 9 correlates with the bone destruction capacity of cholesteatomas. Otol Neurotol. 2009;30(4):559–65.
90. Macias MP, Gerkin RD, Macias JD. Increased amphiregulin expression as a biomarker of cholesteatoma activity. Laryngoscope. 2010;120(11):2258–63.
91. Mallet Y, Nouwen J, Lecomte-Houcke M, Desaulty A. Aggressiveness and quantification of epithelial proliferation of middle ear cholesteatoma by MIB1. Laryngoscope. 2003;113(2):328–31.
92. Oger M, Alpay HC, Orhan I, Onalan EE, Yanilmaz M, Sapmaz E. The effect of BMP-2, BMP-4 and BMP-6 on bone destruction of cholesteatoma presence. Am J Otolaryngol. 2013;34(6):652–7.
93. Jeong JH, Park CW, Tae K, Lee SH, Shin DH, Kim KR, et al. Expression of RANKL and OPG in middle ear cholesteatoma tissue. Laryngoscope. 2006;116(7):1180–4.
94. Haidar H, Sheikh R, Larem A, Elsaadi A, Abdulkarim H, et al. Ossicular chain erosion in chronic suppurative otitis media. Otolaryngol (Sunnyvale). 2015;5:203.
95. Lingam RK, Khatri P, Hughes J, Singh A. Apparent diffusion coefficients for detection of postoperative middle ear cholesteatoma on non–echo-planar diffusion weighted images. Radiology. 2013;269(2):504–10.
96. Lingam RK, Bassett P. A meta-analysis on the diagnostic performance of non-echoplanar diffusion-weighted imaging in detecting middle ear cholesteatoma: 10 years on. Otol Neurotol. 2017;38(4):521–8.
97. Yung M, Tono T, Olszewska E, Yamamoto Y, Sudhoff H, Sakagami M, Mulder J, Kojima H, İncesulu A, Trabalzini F, Özgirgin N. EAONO/JOS joint consensus statements on the definitions, classification and staging of middle ear cholesteatoma. J Int Adv Otol. 2017;13(1):1–8.
98. Vitale RF, Ribeiro Fde A. The role of tumor necrosis factor-alpha (TNF-alpha) in bone resorption present in middle ear cholesteatoma. Braz J Otorhinolaryngol. 2007;73(1):117–21.
99. Schonermark M, Mester B, Kempf HG, Blaser J, Tschesche H, Lenarz T. Expression of matrix-metalloproteinases and their inhibitors in human cholesteatomas. Acta Otolaryngol. 1996;116(3):451–6.

100. Yamamoto-Fukuda T, Terakado M, Hishikawa Y, Koji T, Takahashi H. Topical application of 5-fluorouracil on attic cholesteatoma results in downregulation of keratinocyte growth factor and reduction of proliferative activity. Eur Arch Otorhinolaryngol. 2008;265(10):1173–8.
101. Li S, Meng J, Zhang F, Li X, Qin Z. Revision surgery for canal wall down mastoidectomy: intra-operative findings and results. Acta Otolaryngol. 2016;136(1):18–22.
102. Mosher HP. A method of filling the excavated mastoid with a flap from the back of the auricle. Laryngoscope. 1911;21(12):1158–63.
103. Kuo C-L, Lien C-F, Shiao A-S. Mastoid obliteration for pediatric suppurative cholesteatoma: long-term safety and sustained effectiveness after 30 years' experience with cartilage obliteration. Audiol Neurotol. 2014;19(6):358–69.
104. Singh V, Atlas M. Obliteration of the persistently discharging mastoid cavity using the middle temporal artery flap. Otolaryngol Head Neck Surg. 2007;137(3):433–8.
105. Palva T. Operative technique in mastoid obliteration. Acta Otolaryngol. 1973;75(4):289–90.
106. Hunter JB, Zuniga MG, Sweeney AD, Bertrand NM, Wanna GB, Haynes DS, Wootten CT, Rivas A. Pediatric endoscopic cholesteatoma surgery. Otolaryngol Head Neck Surg. 2016;154(6):1121–7.
107. Austin DF. Single-stage surgery for cholesteatoma: an actuarial analysis. Am J Otol. 1989;10(6):419–25.
108. Cody TR, McDonald TJ. Mastoidectomy for acquired cholesteatoma: follow-up to 20 years. Laryngoscope. 1984;94(8):1027–30.
109. Vartiainen E, Virtaniemi J. Findings in revision operations for failures after cholesteatoma surgery. Am J Otol. 1994;15(2):229–32.
110. Lau T, Tos M. Cholesteatoma in children: recurrence related to observation period. Am J Otolaryngol Head Neck Med Surg. 1987;8(6):364–75.
111. Roger G, Denoyelle F, Chauvin P, Schlegel-Stuhl N, Garabedian E-N. Predictive risk factors of residual cholesteatoma in children: a study of 256 cases. Am J Otol. 1997;18(5):550–8.
112. Dubrulle F, Souillard R, Chechin D, Vaneecloo FM, Desaulty A, Vincent C. Diffusion-weighted MR imaging sequence in the detection of postoperative recurrent cholesteatoma. Radiology. 2006 Feb;238(2):604–10.
113. Jindal M, Riskalla A, Jiang D, Connor S, O'Connor AF. A systematic review of diffusion-weighted magnetic resonance imaging in the assessment of postoperative cholesteatoma. Otol Neurotol. 2011;32:1243–9.
114. Haruyama T, Furukawa M, Kusunoki T, Onoda J, Ikeda K. Expression of IL-17 and its role in bone destruction in human middle ear cholesteatoma. ORL J Otorhinolaryngol Relat Spec. 2010;72(6):325–31.

Complications of Chronic Otitis Media

9

Contents

9.1 Introduction

Chronic suppurative otitis media (CSOM) is a common disease that should be carefully treated, as severe complications can develop. Better control of the superimposed infection in CSOM, since the introduction of antibiotics, explains the recent decrease of CSOM-related complications. Nevertheless, these complications remain

S. Mansour et al., *Middle Ear Diseases*,
https://doi.org/10.1007/978-3-319-72962-6_9

a serious concern, often life threatening, particularly in developing countries and socioeconomically unfavorable regions. The intimate proximity of the middle ear and mastoid air cells to the extracranial and intracranial compartments makes them vulnerable to the spread of infection from the middle ear cleft. The emergence of multidrug-resistant pathogens in CSOM and acquired immunodeficiency diseases (such as AIDS…) made these complications again more prevalent.

This chapter is dedicated to study the main complications related to CSOM in safe *and* unsafe ears.

Complications of CSOM are divided into intratemporal and extratemporal:

- ***Intratemporal complications (ITC)*** include: labyrinthine fistula, facial nerve paralysis (FNP), mastoid abscess, petrositis, labyrinthitis.
- ***Extratemporal complications (ETC)*** can be *intracranial (ICC)* such lateral sinus thrombophlebitis, meningitis, intracerebral abscesses and meningo-encephaloceles or *extracranial (ECC)* mainly as subperiosteal abscess and Bezold's abscess.

Thirty percent of complications of CSOM are intracranial, among them 5–26% result in mortality [1–3]. ICCs of AOM usually develop rapidly and are often recognized and treated promptly, with a reasonable recovery of function. Conversely, unrecognized CSOM, often neglected, could take years to develop complications, which are often severe, life-threatening and somehow difficult to diagnose or treat.

9.2 Historical Perspective

Hippocrates stated in 460 BC that "acute pain in the ear with continued high fever is to be dreaded for; the patient may become delirious and die." In the pre antibiotic era, complications from otitis media occurred abundantly and was accompanied by a high morbidity and mortality rate. This was recognized by the Roman physician Celsus (25 AD) and the Arabian physician Avicenna (980–1037 AD).

It was Morgagni (1682–1771 AD) who recognized that the ear infection came first and the brain abscess takes place secondly.

Brain abscess: It was in 1768 that Morand reported a successful operation for a brain abscess.

In 1881 MacEwen reported a successful series of brain abscesses that were operated on by him [4]. Körner, in 1908, was able to find 268 reported operations with 137 recoveries [5].

Meningitis: Sulfonamides started to be used for acute otitis media in 1935 and penicillin was introduced in 1942. Despite these advances, meningitis remained the most frequent cause of death in otitis media, and otitis media was by far the most frequent cause of meningitis not due to *Neisseria meningitidis*.

Lateral sinus thrombosis: First mentioned in 1826, but 30 years later, Lebert accurately described the pathology of otitic sinus thrombosis [6].

***Petrositis*:** In 1904 Gradenigo described the syndrome of persistent aural discharge, severe fifth cranial nerve pain, and sixth nerve paralysis caused by infection of pneumatic cells in the petrous portion of the temporal bone with adjacent meningitis [7]. Kopetsky and Almour [8] in 1930 and Eagleton [9] in 1931 described the first attempts to drain an abscess of the petrous apex.

Although the incidence of the complications of otitis media has declined and a whole new range of antibiotics has been introduced, complications have not been eradicated.

9.3 Epidemiology

The prevalence of otogenic complications ranges between 0.3 and 5% and depends on the socioeconomic level of the country and its health system [3, 10–15]. Complications are more frequent in young and middle-aged adults, they occur predominantly in males. Extracranial complications (EC) occur more often than intracranial complications (IC): ***Mastoid abscess is the most common intratemporal complication and Meningitis is the most common intracranial complication*** [3, 10, 16].

Kangsanarak et al. [12] found in a study of 17,000 patients 102 cases with IC and/or EC complications (prevalence of complications of 0.69%). In another study of 24,321 patients collected over 13 years, there were 87 cases with IC complications, with a prevalence of 0.36% for IC complications [17]. Mustafa et al. [16] found in a study of 1803 patients (1994–2004) in Kosovo 91 patients (5%) with complications. Osma et al. [3] reported in a study of 2890 patients during a 9-year period (1990–1999), 93 patients (3.22%) with complications.

Reports emanating from some developing countries indicated the persistence of a high prevalence of complications of CSOM, particularly intracranial.

The drop in the prevalence of CSOM complications in developed countries can be attributed to the major development of antibiotherapy as well as to the recent advances made in the diagnostic imaging (CT and MRI).

The life-threatening intracranial complications such as brain abscesses and meningitis dropped from 22% in the two last decades to 6% in the recent years [10]. The current mortality rates in patients with intracranial complications of CSOM have dropped to almost 0% [1, 12, 16–18]. This decrease in mortality may be attributable to improvements in the surgical techniques and advances in critical care.

Surgical findings revealed most often the presence of ***cholesteatoma in both EC and IC complications***; this *explains why ears with cholesteatoma are considered as "unsafe" ears.* Kangsanarak et al. found that 80% of patients had complications due to chronic otitis media associated with a cholesteatoma [12]. Osma et al. reported that 78.5% of patients had a cholesteatoma, while 21.5% showed only inflammatory granulation tissues [3].

9.4 Pathophysiology of Complications

- The tendency of middle ear infections to spread beyond the limits of the middle ear is influenced by numerous factors including: the unrecognized or neglected pathology, the virulence of the infecting organism, the host resistance, the adequacy of antibiotic therapy, the anatomic pathways and barriers to spread, and the drainage of the pneumatic spaces wether natural or surgical.
- Immunocompromised individuals are at higher risk to develop not only otitis media but also complications of otitis media.
- The bony barriers of the ME cleft may be eroded by osteitis, granulation tissue, or cholesteatoma, thus allowing infection to spread into the cranial cavity from the middle ear.
- The pathways of EC and IC complications include: thrombophlebitis of the venules of the adjacent cranial bones, bone erosion by pressure or enzymatic actions, preformed pathways and hematogenous spread (Fig. 9.1).

9.4.1 Complication Through Bone Erosion

In CSOM, the most frequent pathway for the extension of infection beyond the ME cleft is bone erosion. Bone erosion is usually caused by cholesteatoma; less often by chronic osteitis. The bone eroding suppurative process is initially surrounded by a protective granulation formation as a last line of defense. However, after a period of

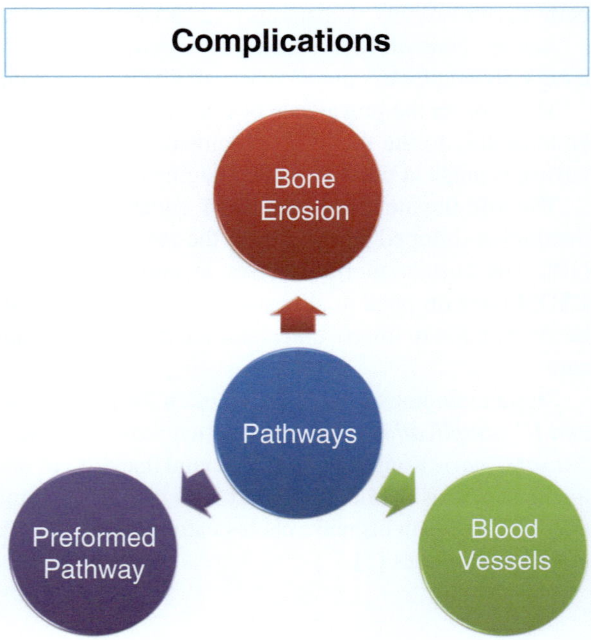

Fig. 9.1 The three possible pathways for spread of infection in chronic otitis media leading to otogenic complications

time of resistance, the pus, under pressure, penetrates the wall of protective granulations by pressure necrosis leading to spread of infection beyond the middle ear.

bone necrosis → granulations → pus → penetration

Bone erosion as the pathway of spread presents the following characteristics:

1. The complication occurs several weeks or more after an exacerbation of the infection in chronic otitis media of long duration.
2. A prodromal period of partial or intermittent involvement of the structure frequently precedes the diffuse involvement:
   - A milder, intermittent facial weakness may precede complete facial paralysis,
   - Recurrent mild vertigo may precede diffuse purulent labyrinthitis,
   - Localized meningismus may precede diffuse purulent meningitis.
3. At operation, a dehiscence of the bony barrier is found between the suppurative focus and the neighboring structure. A layer of granulations covers the exposed soft tissue of the noble neighboring structure.

The treatment of a complication by bone erosion is directed towards the complication and always includes surgical removal of the suppurative, bone-eroding focus in the temporal bone. If such removal is omitted, the complication is likely to recur or to respond poorly to treatment.

9.4.2 Direct Extension Through Preformed Pathways

The preformed pathways may be:

- A normal anatomic opening in the bony wall, such as the oval or round window, internal auditory canal, cochlear aqueduct, or endolymphatic duct and sac.
- A developmental dehiscence such as a patent suture (fistulae) or a dehiscent floor of the hypotympanum over the jugular bulb or a congenital dehiscence of the tegmen.
- The result of a skull fracture or previous surgery.

The extension by preformed pathways may occur in either acute exacerbations of chronic suppurative otitis media or acute otitis media.

The diagnosis is suggested by the following characteristics:

1. History of repeated episodes of meningitis, of a skull fracture, or of an operation on the temporal bone
2. The complication occurs early in the exacerbation of acute infection
3. At operation, a dehiscence of the bone barrier is found.

The treatment of complications by a preformed pathway is directed towards the complication along with closure of the fistula and surgical evacuation of any collection of pus within the temporal bone.

9.4.3 Complication by Thrombophlebitis

There is a rich network of small venules within the temporal bone that creates a communication between the extracranial, intracranial, and cranial diploic veins. Infection can spread from the mucosa of the middle ear and mastoid through intact bone by means of a progressive thrombophlebitis of these small venules. Progressive retrograde thrombophlebitis is the usual route for the formation of an otogenic brain abscess.

The extracranial and intracranial venous system anastomoses with the mastoid emissary veins that enter the sigmoid sinus, which drains the superior and inferior petrosal sinuses. All dural venous sinuses are interconnected. Thus, sigmoid sinus thrombophlebitis can lead to thrombophlebitis of other sinuses as well.

Thrombophlebitis as the pathway of spread of infection in CSOM may present the following characteristics:

1. The complication occurs early in the acute infection, sometimes within a day or two of the onset, usually within the first 10 days.
2. At operation, the bony walls of the middle ear and mastoid cells are intact, no bony dehiscence, no mastoid abscess formation.
3. Whereas venous thrombophlebitis usually leads to cerebellar abscess, arterial spread of the infection leads to temporal lobe abscess. Diffuse septicemia and hematogenous spread of infection usually result in meningitis.

Treatment of complication by thrombophlebitis is directed toward the complication itself along with the surgical evacuation of any collection of pus within the temporal bone.

9.5 Prodromal Symptoms and Signs of Complications

The most frequent symptoms of the patients with complications are otalgia, otorrhea, headache, and fever [1, 12, 16, 17]. In patients with CSOM, the following symptoms are prodromal signs of complications:

- **Earache**, when pus becomes under pressure in the middle ear cleft, must alert the clinician that an intracranial complication may be impending.
- **Headache** and drowsiness are alarming symptoms.
- **Visual field defect is** one of the earliest signs of brain abscess.
- **Fever** suggests meningitis or sinus thrombosis.

Clinical suspicion of complications is relevant when there is:

- Fever, increased otorrhea, associated with inferolaterally displaced pinna,
- Retro-orbital pain on the side of an infected ear,

- Vertigo or nystagmus in a patient with an infected ear,
- Facial paralysis on the side of an infected ear,
- Headache or lethargy, papilledema, meningism, or focal neurological signs or seizures.

Due to the common use of antibiotics, only 20% of patients have a positive bacterial culture of the pus sample and cultures are often negative.

9.6 Diagnostic Imaging

- **CT scan** with injection is the first diagnostic method of choice to evaluate the temporal bone when infectious complications of CSOM are suspected. CT may show signs of an extended cholesteatoma inside the cavity and/or bony erosions of the walls of the cavity or a possible IC or EC collection.
- **MRI** is the complementary imaging study of choice for locating otogenic intracranial complications, with a higher diagnostic accuracy, increased sensitivity and specificity than CT especially for infectious complications beyond the osseous **extratemporal** limits of the cavities that can appear even without bony lysis.
- **MR venography** is the most valuable method to diagnose lateral sinus thrombophlebitis (LST).

Due to the high probability of coexistence of several complications in the same patient, the combination of CT and MR Imaging is recommended in every patient with a suspected CSOM complication.

9.7 Types of Complications

Complications of CSOM are often encountered in an unfavorable milieu or in developing countries where cholesteatoma manifests sometimes by a complication before the discovery of the original pathology (Table 9.1).

Table 9.1 Complications of Chronic Otitis Media

Intratemporal	**Extratemporal**	
	Intracranial	*Extracranial*
Labyrinthine fistula	Lat. sinus thrombosis	Sub-periosteal abscess
Facial paralysis	Meningitis	Bezold's abscess
Petrositis	Extradural abscess	
Labyrinthitis	Subdural abscess	
	Cerebral abscess	

9.8 Intratemporal Complications of CSOM

9.8.1 Labyrinthine Fistulae

Labyrinthine fistulae continue to be among the most common complications of chronic suppurative otitis with cholesteatoma.

9.8.1.1 Diagnosis

- **Clinically** a labyrinthine fistula may be silent. Periodic vertigo or significant disequilibrium is found in about 60% of patients with fistula. The ***fistula test*** is positive only in 32–50% of patients. Although sensorineural hearing loss is found in most of these patients (68%), it is not a sensitive indicator of a fistula [19, 20].
- **Preoperative CT**: Sensitivity and specificity of a HRCT with cuts of 0.5 mm thickness have reached more than 90% [21] (Figs. 9.2 and 9.3).
- **MRI can demonstrate in large labyrinthine fistulae** the loss of the high T2 signal of the liquid canal content when the cholesteatoma has invaded the lumen of this canal. However the definitive diagnosis of a fistula, especially its type and size is confirmed during prudent and delicate surgical exploration.

9.8.1.2 Management

According to the **size and extent of the fistula** as visualized on the preoperative CT (Figs. 9.2 and 9.3), the surgical maneuver is planified. Multiple studies showed that larger fistula have worse hearing results postoperatively than smaller ones [22, 23]. The outcome of fistula reparation at surgery depends on

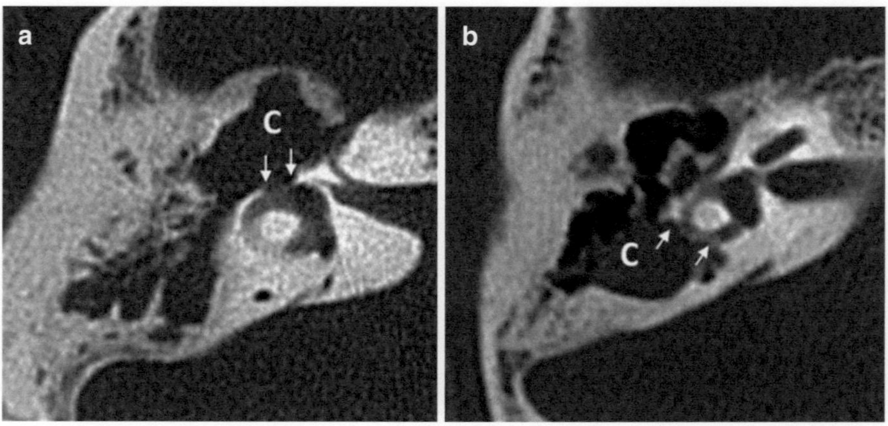

Fig. 9.2 Axial CT images of the right ear of two different patients with cholesteatoma (C) of the tympanic cavity: (**a**) focal lysis of the bony canal wall of the LSCC less than 2 mm (between the two arrows) and (**b**) extended erosion of the bony canal wall of the LSCC about 5 mm of length (between the two arrows)

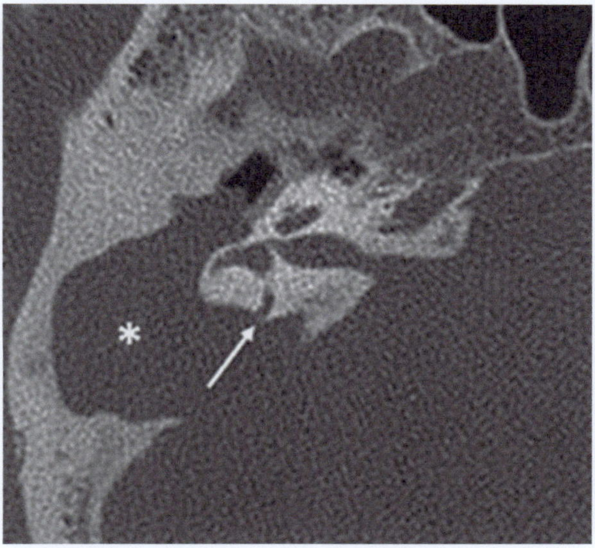

Fig. 9.3 Axial right CT image with a huge cholesteatoma (*) of the atticoantral cavity, having eroded a part of the posterior arc of the PSCC (arrow)

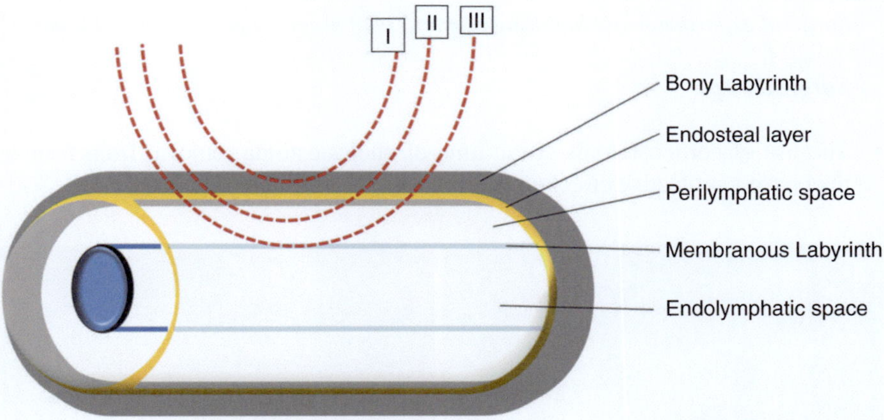

Fig. 9.4 A fistula staging system according to Dornhoeffer and Milewski [19]

its size and the violation of the endosteum [42]. Dornhoffer and Milewski [19] introduced a staging system for fistulae (Fig. 9.4) depending on the involvement of the underlying labyrinth.

- Type I: bony erosion but intact endosteum.
- Type II: the endosteum is violated.
- Type IIa: with preservation of the perilymphatic space.
- Type IIb: with violation of the perilymphatic space (by the disease itself or by surgical manipulations).
- Type III: the matrix is in intimate contact with the membranous labyrinth.

Dornhoffer and Milewski [19] demonstrated that no hearing loss resulted from removal of matrix in type I or IIa fistulae where the endosteum was violated but the perilymphatic space was not disrupted; in contrary when the perilymph or the endolymph was involved or violated significantly (type IIb and type III), almost half of the patients experienced significant hearing loss postoperatively. Intraoperatively steroids reduce significantly the risk of post-op hearing deterioration. In fact, the most common side effect after surgery is not the risk of hearing loss but the risk of residual vertigo [19].

The anatomic location of the fistula also has a significant impact on the hearing results: A 35% rate of profound deafness has been reported with fistulae, that involve the promontory (Fig. 9.5), compared with 3% rate of deafness with semicircular canal fistulae [20]. In consequence, fistulae involving the cochlea should be approached with more caution because of the greater risk for iatrogenic sensorineural hearing loss.

Complete removal of the matrix from the fistula site can be performed in a single setting, or in a staged approach with a second-look procedure. A recent review of the literature found that hearing preservation for patients who underwent complete removal was equivalent to patients where the matrix was left over the fistula [20].

Surgical expertise while handling a fistula is of major impact on the outcome.

Surgical steps

- The use of corticosteroids at the time of cholesteatoma removal from fistulae may have a protective effect on hearing.

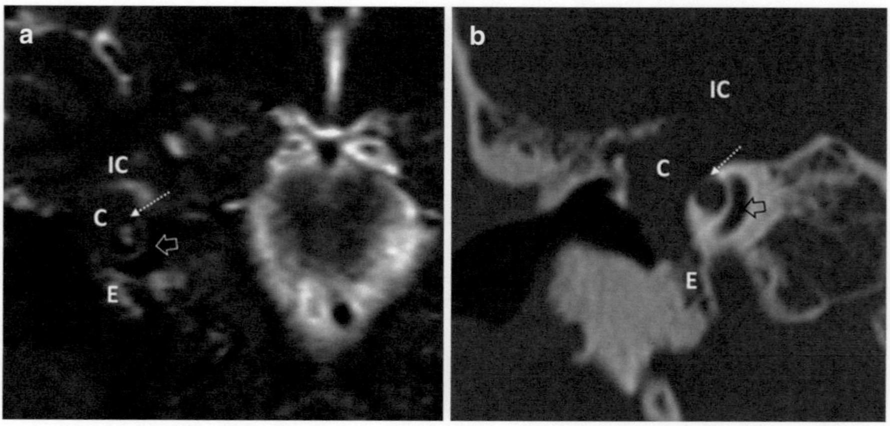

Fig. 9.5 (**a**) Coronal T2 weighted MR image showing a cholesteatoma (C) extended through a dehiscent tegmen into the middle cerebral fossa (IC), with lyses of the promontory and a denuded third turn of the cochlea (dashed arrow). Basal turn of the cochlea (empty arrow). E = effusion in the inferior mastoid. (**b**) The corresponding coronal CT image: cholesteatoma (C), effusion (E) and the intracerebral structures (IC) have all the same imaging aspect on CT-Scan in this window. Denuded third turn of the cochlea (dashed arrow). Basal turn of the cochlea (empty arrow)

- Removal of the cholesteatoma from the middle ear and mastoid must be completed before dealing with the fistula surgery.
- Small fistula involving the labyrinth can be removed safely in a primary setting.
- Large fistula involving the labyrinth can be treated by careful removal of the cholesteatoma matrix and covering the defect with bone pate and fascia (Fig. 9.6).
- *In large fistula, if the matrix is very adherent to the endosteum, it is recommended to leave the matrix and come back after 6–12 months later rather than to violate the endosteum and perilymph which could lead to devastating sensorineural hearing loss and vertigo. The Zini' technique using irrigation with Mesna (a mucolytic solution) is useful and safer facilitating the elevation of the cholesteatoma matrix from the membranous labyrinth.*
- *Fistula involving the cochlea should be approached preferably by exteriorization of matrix remaining on the fistula.*
- *The materials used to cover the fistula site can be fascia/périchondrium/bone "pate."*

During revision of troublesome mastoid cavities, the surgeon should be very careful to the high probability of LSCC fistula (12–15%) and should be prudent during elevation of the mastoid epithelium not to violate the endosteum (Figs. 9.7 and 9.8).

9.8.2 Facial Palsy

Otogenic causes of facial nerve paralysis include AOM, COM without cholesteatoma, and cholesteatoma. In AOM, facial paralysis usually occurs with a dehiscent

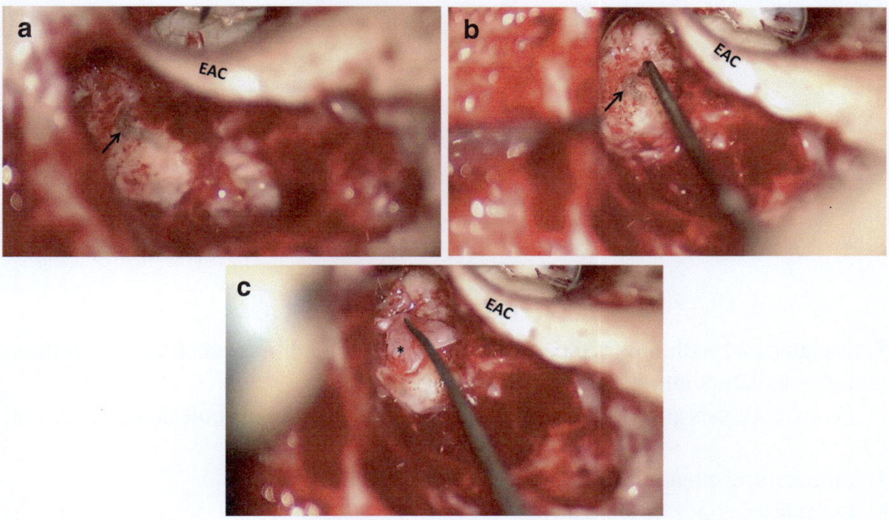

Fig. 9.6 Right ear LSCC. CWU mastoidectomy. (**a**) LSCC fistula (black arrow); (**b**) the bone around the fistula should be scratched to remove mucosa and necrotic bone; (**c**) fistula is covered by bone pate and fascia (*)

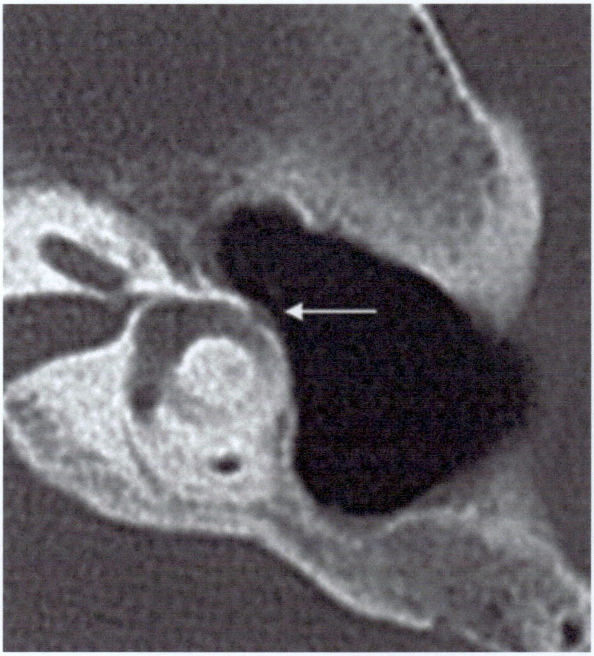

Fig. 9.7 Axial CT-view of an open mastoid cavity of a left ear showing a fistula of the LSCC (arrow) developed under the epithelium of the skin coverage and in the absence of any infection or cholesteatoma recurrence (skin contact)

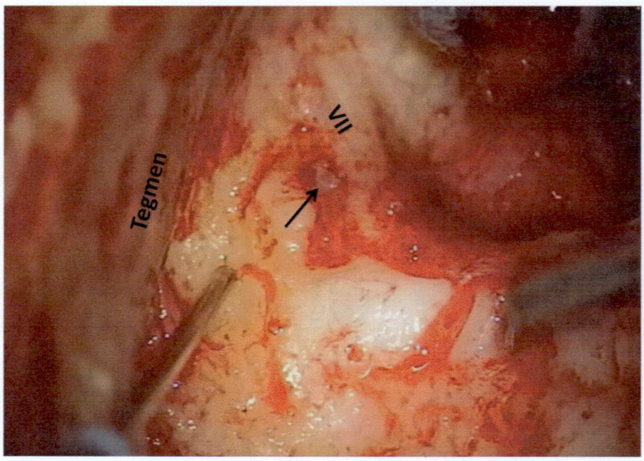

Fig. 9.8 Right ear mastoid cavity revision showing large LSCC fistula (black arrow). VII: tympanic segment of facial nerve

Fallopian canal within its tympanic segment, allowing direct penetration of inflammatory mediators into the facial nerve itself.

Facial paralysis as a CSOM complication, mostly found in cholesteatoma, is due:

- to infection spread through a canal dehiscence (neuritis),
- to toxic enzymes of the matrix,
- or to ischemia due to direct nerve compression by the cholesteatoma.

Spread of the infection along the nerve tissue, rather than compression atrophy, may be the major factor in most cases of FNP resulting from CSOM. In contrast to facial palsy secondary to acute otitis media which is of rapid onset and carries a good prognosis after adequate treatment, facial nerve paralysis secondary to cholesteatoma develops often in a slowly progressive way and has worse prognosis.

Cholesteatoma was observed in 80% (51/64 patients) with chronic otitis media causing facial paralysis in a study by Savić and Djerić [25], in 70% (14/20 patients) by Altuntas et al. [26], in 67% (16/24 patients) by Yetiser et al. [27], and in 59% (27/46 patients) by Kim et al. [28]. However facial nerve paralysis could be secondary to granulation tissue associated with non-cholesteatoma CSOM or to acute infectious exacerbation superimposed on the COM.

Cholesteatoma erodes the Fallopian canal and the matrix comes in direct contact with the facial nerve. It is thought that bacteria and neurotoxic substances secreted from the cholesteatoma matrix adherent to facial nerve cause direct inflammation of the nerve, leading to a deterioration of the facial nerve function.

Historically, the incidence of iatrogenic FNP associated with ear surgery has been estimated to be 0.6–3.7% [29]. In revision mastoid surgery, the frequency may be as high as 4–10% [30]. These historical numbers are very high; nowadays, with the advancement of surgical microscopes, surgical instruments, and facial nerve monitoring, iatrogenic facial nerve palsy became very rare.

9.8.2.1 Diagnosis of Facial Palsy

The diagnosis of otogenic facial paralysis is made on clinical grounds. Facial nerve paralysis due to COM may be either abrupt or of gradual onset. Abrupt onset results from an acute infectious exacerbation superimposed on the COM, while gradual onset is typically due to the compression from a cholesteatoma or granulation tissue.

The most common site of facial nerve involvement is at the geniculate ganglion due to disease in the anterior epitympanum followed by the tympanic segment (Fig. 9.9) and second genu (Fig. 9.10).

CT-Imaging demonstrates a facial nerve canal dehiscence in 67/75 to 89% of cases [31]. The sensitivity and specificity of CT were 69% and 87%, respectively [32]. Recent data confirm a rising tendency for the positive predictive value of the CT with modern acquisition techniques and multi dimensional reconstructions, whereas former studies did state only a poor radiosurgical agreement for the facial canal dehiscence [33].

9.8.2.2 Management of Facial Palsy

Whereas treatment of facial palsy in AOM requires immediate myringotomy, antibiotherapy and corticotherapy, the treatment of facial paralysis in CSOM cases requires immediate surgical intervention to remove the **cholesteatoma** or **granulation tissue** in contact with the facial nerve. The nerve is approached on both sides of the involvement, and a diamond burr is used to decompress the nerve and expose the epineurium for 1 cm on both sides of the diseased segment. Once the proximal and distal segments of the Fallopian canal have been opened, blunt dissection is used to remove the disease from the epineurium. The nerve sheath does not have to be incised unless the cholesteatoma has invaded the nerve itself. Administration of intravenous antibiotics and high-dose steroids are also helpful.

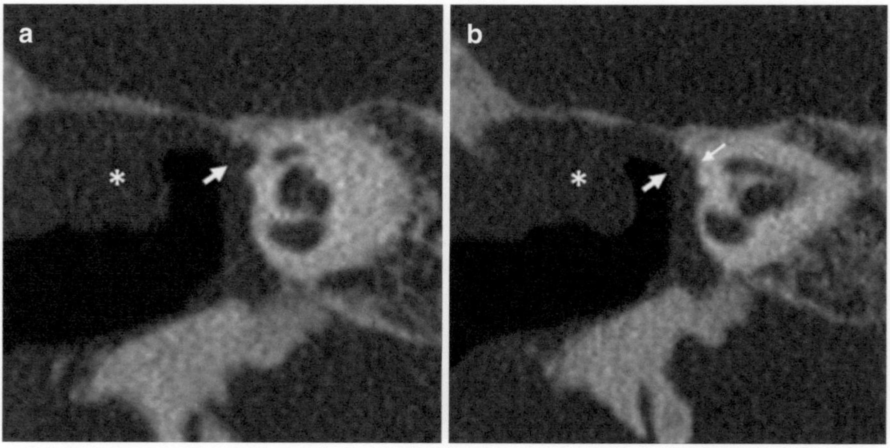

Fig. 9.9 Patient with a FNP in CSOM: coronal CT reconstructions of the right ear show lysis of the scutum and replacement of the whole superior auditory canal wall by a huge polypoid soft tissue mass (*), with prolapse in the EAC. (**a**) Lysis of the bony canal of the facial nerve in its tympanic segment (arrow) and (**b**) slightly more posteriorly: complete disappearance of the bony canal of the VII (between the thick and thin arrow), that is not anymore distinguished from the surrounding soft tissue mass

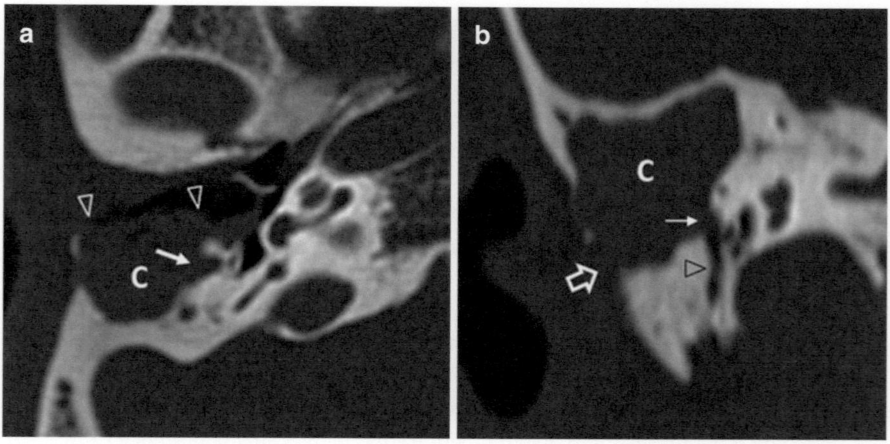

Fig. 9.10 CT images of a right ear with extended cholesteatoma (C) to the mastoid. (**a**) Axial view showing a huge cholesteatoma inside the mastoid cavity with a large lysis of the posterior tympanic wall (between the two arrowheads). Erosion of the facial nerve canal (arrow) of the third portion immediately inferior to the second genu and (**b**) coronal CT-reconstruction showing erosion of the bony canal of the second genu (white arrow) and the third portion of the VII on the coronal image (arrowhead). In addition, focal lysis of the lateral wall of the mastoid (empty arrow)

The presence of cholesteatoma decreases the effectiveness of surgical gain and indicates a poor prognosis after surgery. Post operative recovery of the facial nerve function is seldom the case. The duration of onset of facial paralysis prior to its surgery is an important factor. Longer durations can cause more severe deterioration of the facial nerve and poor surgical outcomes. Patients with facial paralysis due to COM should be operated on as early as possible, regardless of the severity or degree of facial function impairment, the presence of cholesteatoma, type of onset, age and any previous otologic surgical history.

Iatrogenic injury to the nerve during surgery should be recognized and immediately repaired by a decompression of the nerve proximal and distal to the site of injury. Following ear surgery, facial palsy may present immediately post-op or it could develop with delayed onset. There may be complete paralysis or partial loss of function. In general, facial nerve exploration with decompression or restoration of the continuity of the nerve is performed when there is immediate complete facial nerve injury after mastoidectomy. In case of complete or near complete transection, primary anastomosis or cable grafting should be done. When the palsy is incomplete, a wait-and-see policy is generally indicated. It is recommended to proceed to exploration surgery within 3 weeks when clinical and neurophysiological observations predict an unfavorable prognosis.

9.8.3 Petrous apicitis

Petrous apicitis occurs when the infection extends beyond the confines of the middle ear and mastoid into the petrous apex. Patients may present with **Gradenigo syndrome,** when the clinical symptoms of retro-orbital pain, aural discharge, and abducens (CN VI) palsy are present. Some patients may present with isolated petrositis after resolution of otitis media (Fig. 9.11). MRI and CT help to define the extent of the disease, to assess any intracranial spread, and planify the surgical approach.

Treatment includes systemic antibiotics with petrous apicectomy in cases that do not respond to medical therapy.

9.8.4 Labyrinthitis

Infection spreads to the inner ear through the round and oval windows or through one of the semicircular canals fistulae secondary to bony erosion.

There are four categories of labyrinthitis: Acute serous, acute suppurative, chronic, and labyrinthine sclerosis (Table 9.2).

9.8.4.1 Acute Serous Labyrinthitis

Serous labyrinthitis occurs when bacterial toxins and host inflammatory mediators, such as cytokines, enzymes cross the round window membrane, causing inflammation of the labyrinth in the absence of direct bacterial contamination. This condition is associated with acute or chronic middle ear disease: Toxins, enzymes, and other inflammatory products infiltrate the scala tympani, forming a fine precipitate just medial to the round window membrane. Penetration of the inflammatory agents into the endolymph at the basilar turn of the cochlea results in a mild to moderate, high-frequency SNHL.

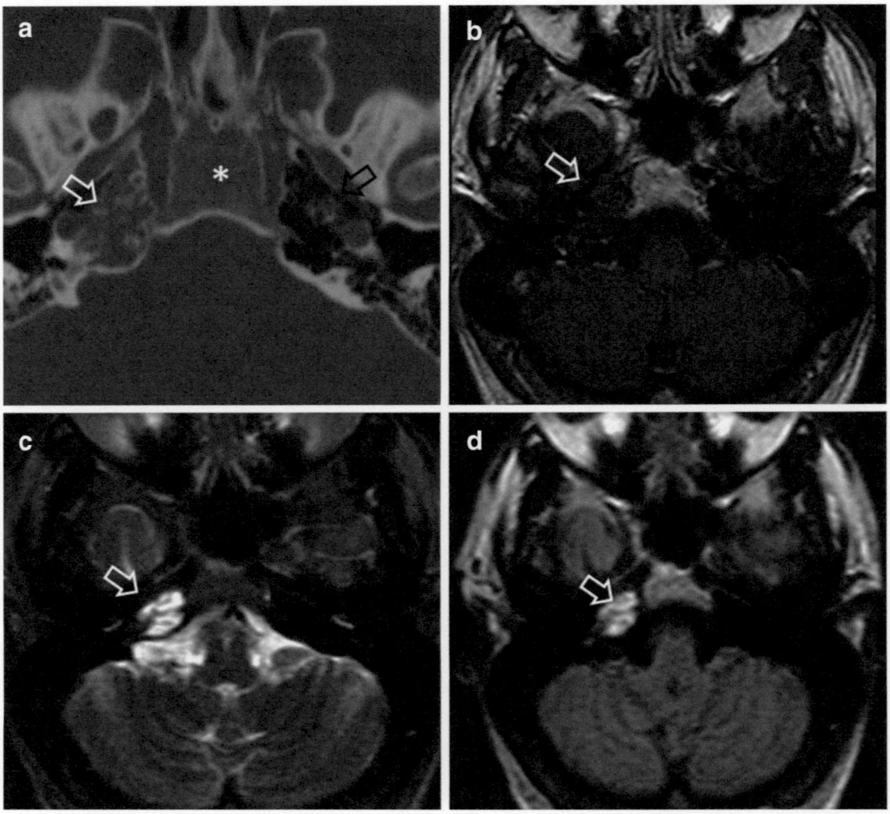

Fig. 9.11 Patient with petrositis after resolution of otitis media. (**a**) Axial CT-image: completely condensated right petrous apex (white empty arrow) with disappearance of several trabeculations. The left petrous apex (black empty arrow) is entirely pneumatized. Clivus (*), (**b**) axial T1 weighted MRI: the petrous apex condensations are hypointense on T1 and (**c**) axial T2 weighted and (**d**) Flair MRI: hyperintense petrous apex on the right side (white empty arrow)

Table 9.2 Different stages of labyrinthitis with symptoms, diagnosis, imaging and treatment

Labyrinthitis	Symptoms	Nystagmus	Imaging	Treatment
Acute serous	Acute onset of vertigo and HL	Nystagmus beating towards the affected ear	MR T1-Gd: uptake of Gd in the semicircular canals	Early ME surgery
Acute suppurative	Profound SNHL, tinnitus, vertigo, vomiting	Nystagmus beating away from the affected ear	MR T1-Gd: uptake of Gd in the semicircular canals	Aggressive debridement labyrinthectomy + broad spectrum AB
Chronic fibrous	Anacusis		MR: attenuation of T2 signal inside the canals (fibrosis)	Treat underlying ME disease if indicated
Ossificans	Anacusis		CT: ossified labyrinth, MR: disappearance of the canals on T1 + T2	Treat underlying ME disease if indicated

Clinical examination demonstrates a *nystagmus* with the rapid component directed *towards the affected ear.*

Treatment: Early surgical exploration, to remove the infection source in the middle ear and mastoid, and reduce the irritation and damage of the labyrinth.

9.8.4.2 Acute Suppurative Labyrinthitis

When suppurative labyrinthitis occurs (Fig. 9.12), it is almost always associated with cholesteatoma. It presents with profound hearing loss, tinnitus, and severe vertigo with associated ataxia, nausea and vomiting. Patients initially demonstrate a nystagmus, at the beginning with a rapid component directed toward the affected ear; rapidly later due to the destruction of the membranous labyrinth, by a nystagmus beating away from the affected ear.

Treatment: Treatment of acute suppurative labyrinthitis includes aggressive surgical debridement (including labyrinthectomy, to prevent possibly lethal intracranial complications of meningitis or encephalitis), along with the administration of broad-spectrum antibiotics of good cerebrospinal fluid penetration. Culture and sensitivities should direct the definitive antibiotic regimen.

9.8.4.3 Chronic Labyrinthitis

It is characterized by unsteadiness and hearing loss. Most commonly, the infection reaches the labyrinth through the lateral semicircular canal.

Treatment: The treatment involves mastoidectomy to clear the primary disease.

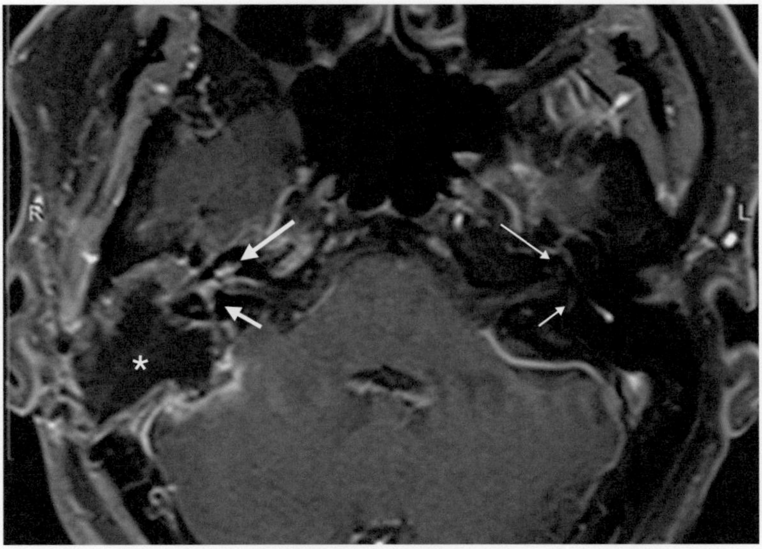

Fig. 9.12 Post right subtotal petrosectomy with fat obliteration for extensive cholesteatoma complicated by acute suppurative labyrinthitis. Axial T1 weighted image with Gd: important uptake of the contrast in the cochlea (long thick arrow) and the labyrinth (short thick arrow) on the right side, huge abscess in the mastoid (*) to compare with a normal faint signal of the labyrinth on the left (cochlea long small arrow, vestibule and canals short thin arrow)

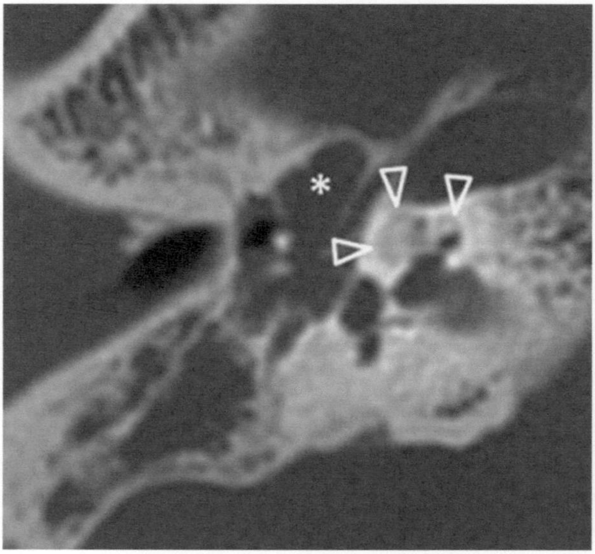

Fig. 9.13 Axial CT-image of a right ear with condensation images in the AER (*), the tympanic cavity and the mastoid. Almost completely calcified cochlea (surrounded by the empty arrows) due to postinfectious sclerotic labyrinthitis

9.8.4.4 Labyrinthine Sclerosis or Labyrinthitis Ossificans

Calcification in the fluid-filled spaces of the inner ear can be the end stage of the infectious process and manifest as profound hearing loss and vestibuloplegia. The clinical presentation becomes mostly silent due to the adaptation phenomenon secondary to a replacement of the membranous labyrinth by fibrous tissue and later on by new bone formation (Fig. 9.13). Such pathology could be a major problem for cochlear implant rehabilitation.

9.9 Extratemporal Intracranial Complications

Intracranial or intracerebral complications of CSOM are potentially life-threatening. However, infections such as a periosteal abscess, lateral sinus thrombosis or intracranial abscess occur in less than *1%* of all cholesteatomas. Symptoms suggesting an impending intracranial complication include suppurative malodorous otorrhea, usually with chronic headache, otalgia and/or fever. The presence of mental status changes with nuchal rigidity or cranial neuropathies warrant neurosurgical consultation with urgent intervention.

Epidural abscess, subdural empyema, meningitis and cerebral abscesses should be treated immediately prior to the definitive otologic management of the ear disease.

9.9.1 Lateral Sinus Thrombophlebitis (LST)

Lateral sinus thrombophlebitis occurs when the infection extends through the mastoid bone into the sigmoid sinus. The infected thrombus may release septic emboli, causing distal infarcts. Patients may present with an altered mental status, headaches, retroauricular pain, postauricular edema, and fever.

LST is generally considered as the third or fourth most common IC complication and often associated with other IC and EC complications (Fig. 9.14). However, Mostafa et al. reported LST as the most common IC complication [13]. The apparent increase in the incidence of LST in patients with intracranial complications of CSOM in developing countries may be the result of the better detection nowadays, owing improved imaging facilities.

9.9.1.1 Diagnosis

The classic clinical presentation of sigmoid or lateral sinus thrombosis is the presence of high spiking fever in a "picket fence" pattern, often seen with headaches and alteration of the general conditions.

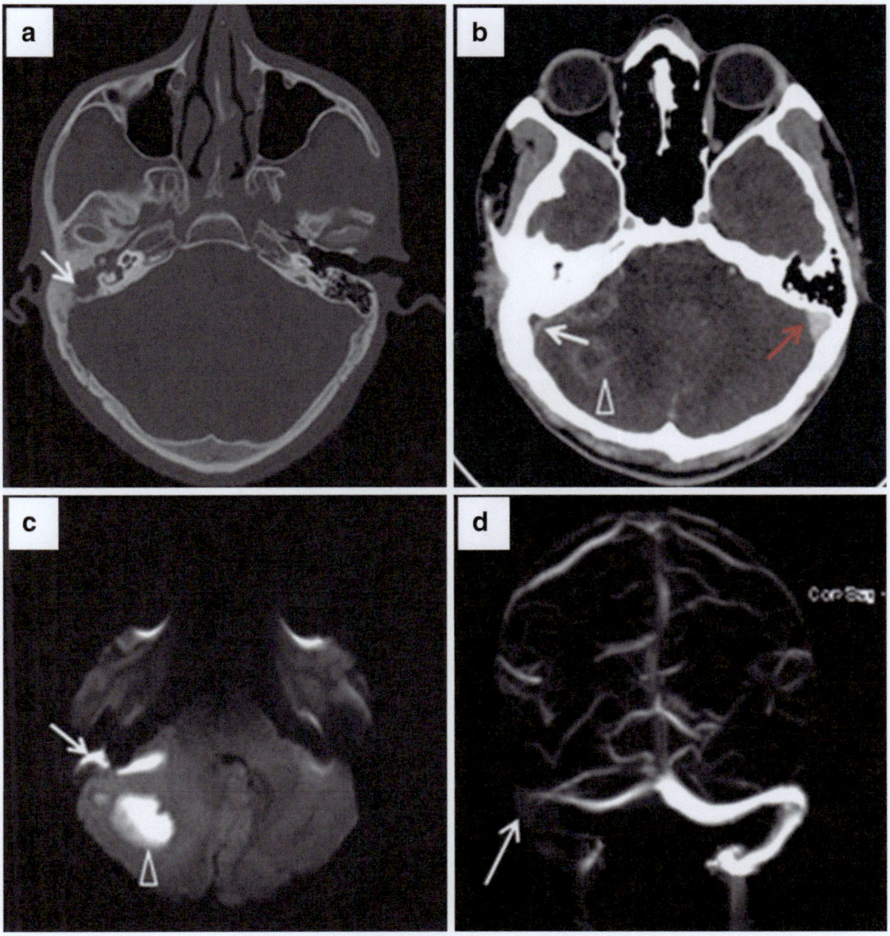

Fig. 9.14 Right ear cholesteatoma complicated by sigmoid sinus thrombophlebitis and multiple cerebellar abscesses. (**a**) Axial CT in the bone window showing enlarged and condensated antrum with smoothed bony borders (arrow), (**b**) injected CT in brain window: non opacified right sigmoid sinus (white arrow) compared to the normal sigmoid sinus contrast uptake on the left side (red arrow); cerebellar abscess (triangle), (**c**) diffusion image with B1000 s/mm^2: the white lesion (arrow) is a typical restriction image of cholesteatoma in the antrum (arrow). Cerebellar abscess (triangle) also with restriction and (**d**) MRV confirms the thrombosis of the right sigmoid sinus (arrow)

Imaging:

On contrast enhanced CT-Scan, the thrombus inside the sigmoid sinus can be seen as a lack of contrast uptake after i.v. iodine contrast injection, in contrast to the slim contrast uptake in the sinus wall whereas the opposite side is well perfused (Fig. 9.14a). Confirmation of the diagnosis by MRI venography is very reliable (Figs. 9.14d and 9.15c), using 2D time of flight sequences, with no

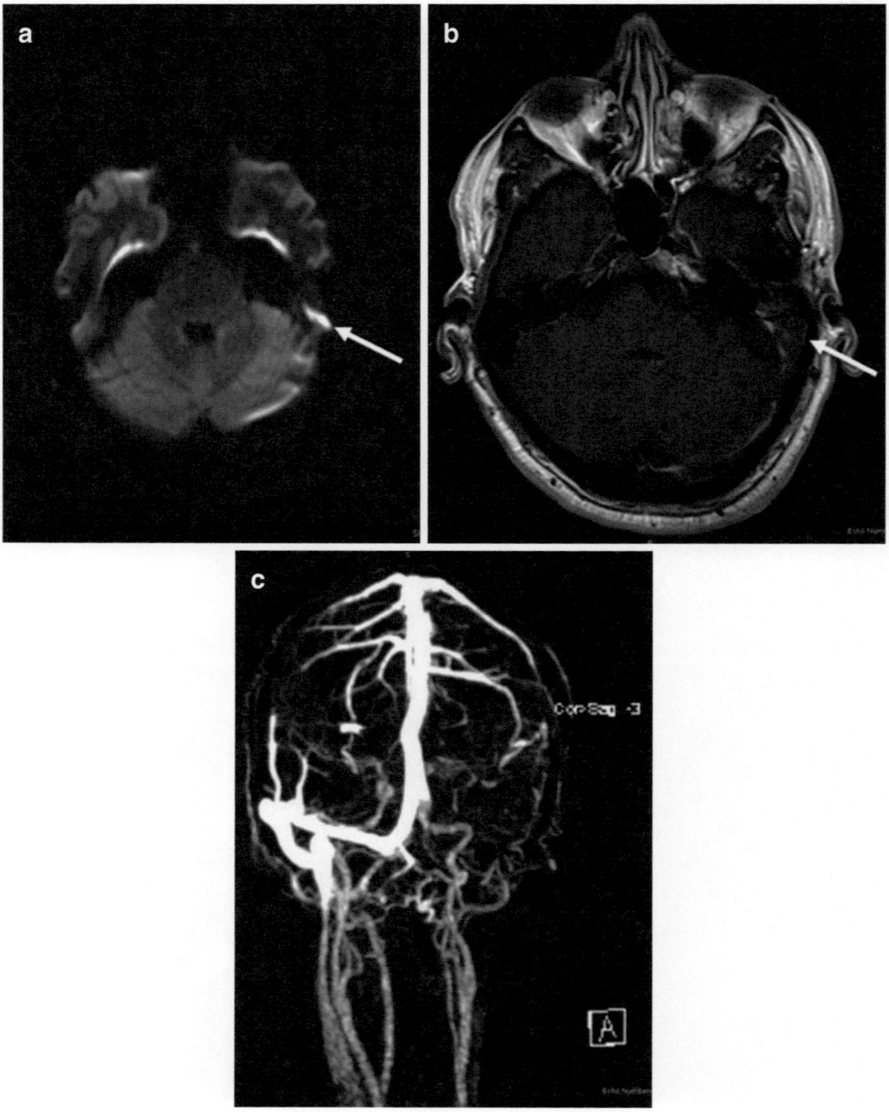

Fig. 9.15 Left ear cholesteatoma complicated by SS thrombophlebitis. (**a**) Diffusion weighted image B1000 s/mm^2 with positive restriction in the mastoid corresponding to the cholesteatoma, (**b**) injected T1, large hypointense filling defect inside the sigmoid sinus (arrow) and (**c**) MRV: no visibility of the left sigmoid sinus: extended sinus venous thrombophlebitis

need of injection of Gadolinium, or with a comparable high sensitivity CT-venography after iodine contrast injection. The MR technique offers in addition the possibility for a detailed follow up to evaluate clot propagation or resolution.

9.9.1.2 Management

- **Culture-directed antimicrobial treatment** is the first step in the management of sinus thrombophlebitis. A debate still exists on the necessity of anticoagulation and its efficacy in establishing recanalization of the sigmoid sinus.
- **Mastoidectomy** with drainage of perisinus purulence is indicated in patients who do not respond to systemic antibiotics. Removal of the entire thrombus until bleeding starts may be done but is not necessary and may result in additional complications, including intracranial hemorrhage. Ligation of the internal jugular vein is rarely required for patients with progressive septic emboli who do not respond to systemic therapy.

9.9.2 Meningitis

Meningitis develops as a consequence of a direct or hematogenous spread of the infection. If meningitis is suspected, a lumbar puncture (after fundoscopy) is the initial diagnostic step to recover the causative organism for culture and sensitivity. When stable, the patient should have mastoid surgery to clear the source of infection.

9.9.3 Intracranial Abscesses

Depending of the progressive intracranial spread of the infection, abscesses can form in the extradural or subdural space or later even intraparenchymal.

9.9.3.1 Brain Abscesses

After meningitis, brain abscesses represent the second most common intracranial complication of chronic otitis media (COM) [15] with a widespread associated mortality rate ranging between 7% and 61% in most large series [15, 34]. Roughly 50% of brain abscesses in adults and 25% in children are believed to stem from otogenic infections [35, 36]. Otogenic brain abscesses are often located in the adjacent temporal lobe (almost arterial spread) (Fig. 9.16) or in the cerebellum (Fig. 9.17) (almost due to a veinous spread of the infection), with the middle segment of the temporal lobe and lateral lobe of the cerebellum most frequently affected. The infection spreads intracranially through bony defects in the tegmen tympani (Fig. 9.16c) or Trautmann's triangle or via spread of an infected clot within small emissary veins of the skull to the venous sinuses.

Their presentation may be indolent, as they grow initially in "silent" areas of the brain.

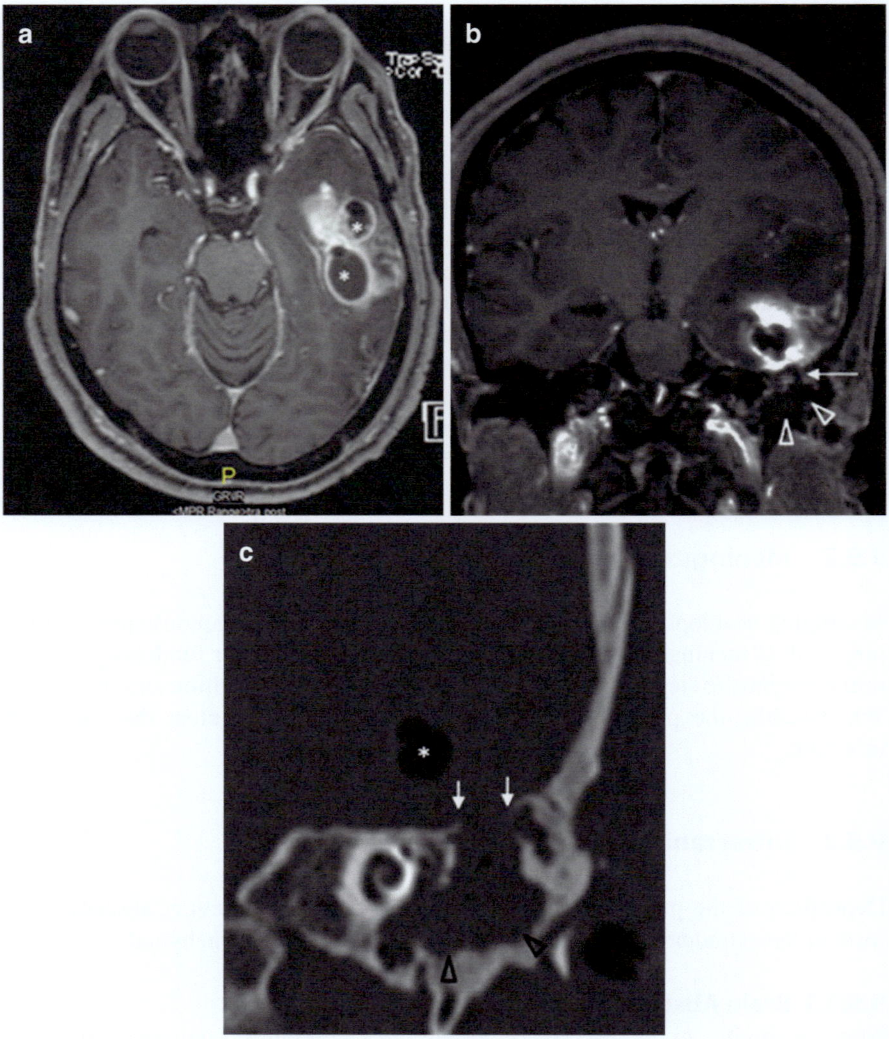

Fig. 9.16 Intracerebral abscesses in the temporal fossa due to superinfection of cholesteatoma extending from the middle ear cleft through a large defect in the tegmen into the mid cerebral fossa. (**a**) Axial T1 weighted image after Gd: two abscess formations (*) are seen in the temporal parenchyma, surrounded by an important Gd uptake, (**b**) the middle ear cavity is filled up with cholesteatoma (triangles), that is extending (white arrow) into the mid cerebral fossa and (**c**) the corresponding coronal CT-reconstruction shows a complete lysis of the tegmen between the arrows and signs of superinfection in the mid cerebral fossa by the pathologic inclusion of air in this region (*)

(a) **Imaging:**

On non enhanced images, brain abscess can be suspected by diffuse free air inside the brain parenchyma (Fig. 9.16c). Brain abscesses can be easily seen as hypodense collections inside the brain parenchyma with peripheral rim enhancement after iodine contrast injection. MRI with i.v. injection of

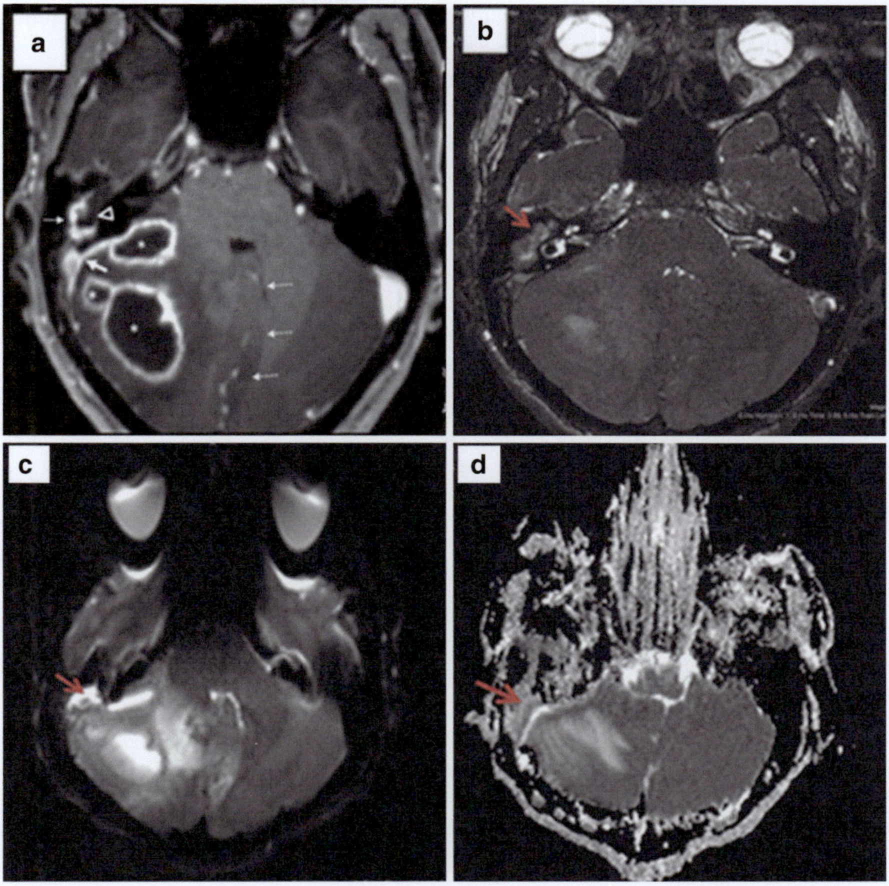

Fig. 9.17 Emergency consultation of an unrecognized cholesteatoma in a patient with seizures and subcoma. (**a**) Axial MRI, T1 weighted sequence fat sat after injection de Gd: Several right cerebellar abscesses (*) associated to a linear enhancement of the dura (small thick arrow). Contrast uptake inside the attic (thin arrow), surrounding a hypointense nonenhancing mass (empty arrowhead). Note the important mass effect of the abscesses on the midline structures, that are deviated to the left side (dashed arrows), (**b**) T2 showing a large hypointense mass in the tympanic cavity and the mastoid, (**c**) diffusion weighted image showing restricted diffusion of the mastoid lesion, confirming cholesteatoma (red arrow), the intracerebellar abscesses show also restriction and (**d**) the corresponding ADC map confirms the cholesteatoma in the ME cavity by a typical dark signal (red arrow)

Gadolinium is the most accurate imaging modality, especially for the associated meningeal enhancement, and the relation to the neighboring cerebral structures (Figs. 9.16 and 9.17).

(b) **Management:**

Neurosurgical drainage, and antibiotic therapy are the standard of care.

Typically, treatment of otogenic brain abscesses first involves aspiration of the pus or complete excision of the abscess, after which parenteral antibiotic therapy is initiated to eradicate the primary nidus of infection. However, recent evidence shows that small abscesses up to 2 cm can be treated with parenteral antibiotic therapy alone, and cases of multiple abscesses respond similarily best to parenteral antibiotic therapy after the largest lesion has been aspirated [37, 38].

The most appropriate way to treat the otologic component is somewhat controversial.

In the presence of CSOM with or without cholesteatoma, a mastoidectomy is required to eradicate the source of infection. The most appropriate time to perform the mastoidectomy is controversial. It has been conventional teaching that a mastoidectomy is performed in a delayed manner after the patient had recovered from the abscess and neurosurgical drainage.

However current recommendations advise to perform a mastoidectomy at the time of abscess drainage to remove the infectious focus, provided that the patient is stable enough to tolerate this additional surgery [15].

9.9.3.2 Epidural Abscesses

Epidural abscess may present with meningitic signs and symptoms or may be asymptomatic.

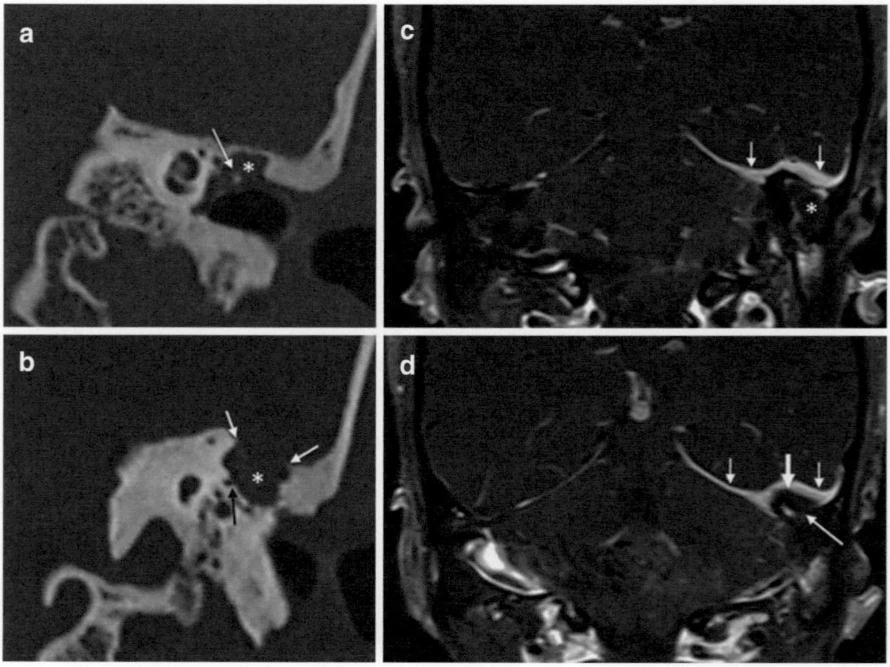

Fig. 9.18 23-year-old man. (**a**, **b**) Coronal CT reconstructions of the left ear are suggestive of a large cholesteatoma in the ME cavity (*), (**a**) with an advanced ossicular lysis (*arrow*), (**b**) with a large lysis of the tegmen (*between the white arrows*) and lysis of the bony wall of the PSCC (*black arrow*). (**c**, **d**) Coronal T1 weighted images with fat sat after Gd injection: (**c**) the cholesteatoma appears as a non-enhancing hypointense mass inside the ME cavity (*), thick enhancement of the dura (*small white arrows*) above the tegmen, (**d**) hypointense formation (thick white arrow) immediately above the tegmen: epidural abscess, surrounded by a thick meningeal enhancement (small white arrows). The tegmen is focally interrupted (long white arrow)

(a) **Imaging:**
Abscesses and their intracranial extension are best shown on MRI, especially on T1 weighted images after injection of Gadolinium with saturation of the fat. The abscess can develop on an underlying cholesteatoma (Fig. 9.18) or as a purely infectious complication (Fig. 9.19).

(b) **Management:**
Treatment consists of a mastoidectomy to clear up the primary disease followed by transmastoid drainage of the abscess (the bone overlying the dura is removed to evacuate the pus and granulation until normal dura is reached).

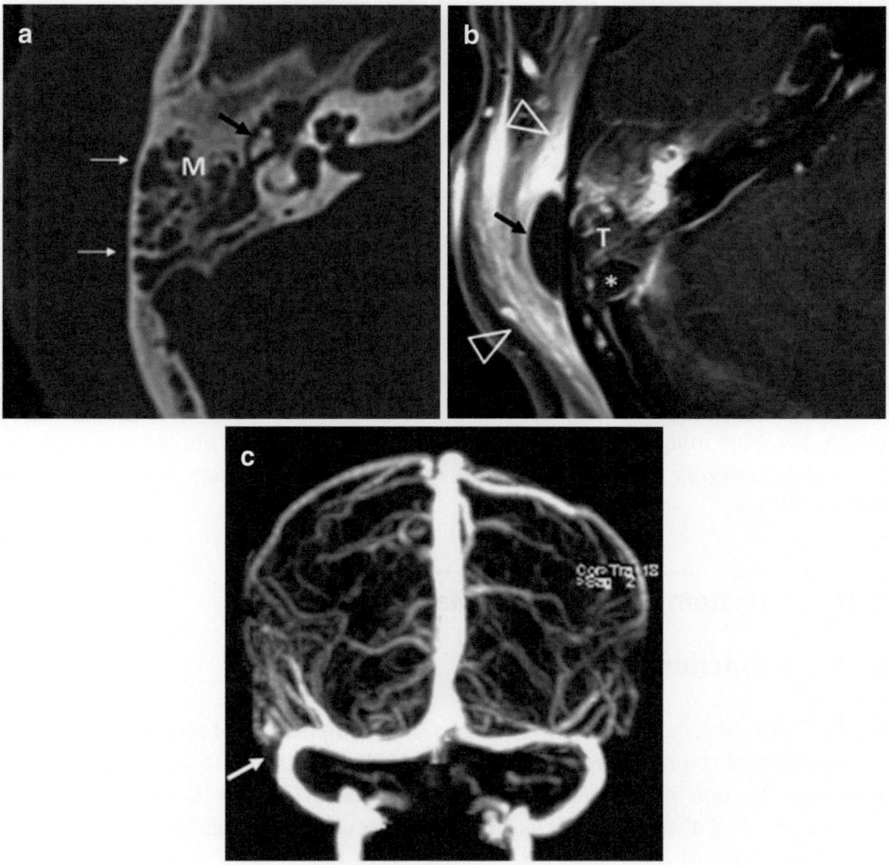

Fig. 9.19 30-year-old patient presented with fever, pain and retroauricular swelling. (**a**) Axial CT-image of the right ear showing a diffuse soft tissue swelling laterally to the mastoid (M), that is completely condensated, also the tympanic cavity, but no lysis. The lateral cortical wall is intact (white arrows). The ossicular chain is intact (black arrow), (**b**) axial T1 weighted MR image with fat sat post Gd: subperiosteal abscess (black arrow) in the soft tissues over the mastoid, surrounded by a huge peripheral soft tissue contrast uptake (empty arrowheads). A second abscess (*) is situated posterior to the tegmen (T) in the epidural space = extradural abscess, *mimicking an eventual thrombus of the LSS* and (**c**) the MR venography sequence demonstrates bilateral symmetrically well permeable lateral sinuses (so no LST) at the level of the epidural abscess (white arrow)

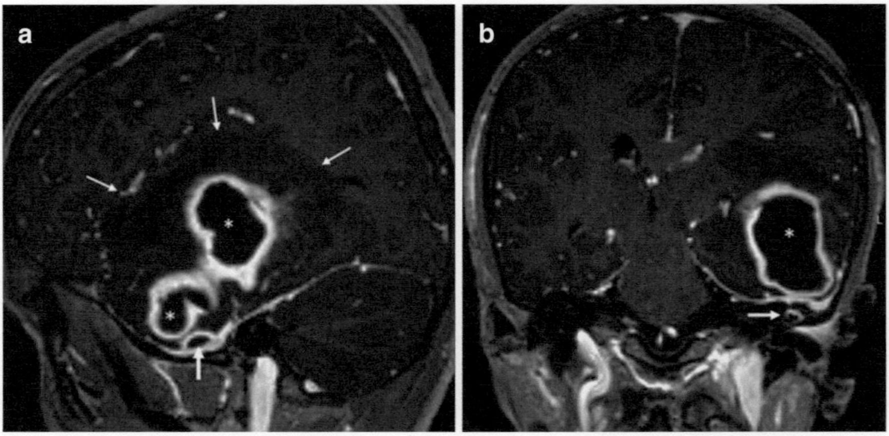

Fig. 9.20 20-year-old man who presented to the emergency for ear pain, fever, headache and vomiting. (**a**) Sagittal T1 weighted TSE fat sat post Gd showing a subdural abscess (thick white arrow) with adjacent strong meningeal enhancement, and several intracerebral abscesses (*). Important mass effect of the perilesional oedema (small white arrows) and (**b**) coronal T1 weighted TSE fat sat post Gd shows a ringlike contrast uptake inside the attic (white arrow) in favor of an intratemporal abscess, meningeal enhancement along the tegmen and a large intracerebral abscess (*)

9.9.3.3 Subdural Abscesses

Patients with a subdural abscess (see example in Fig. 9.20) are very ill and exhibit meningeal signs, eventually seizures, and hemiplegia. Prompt neurosurgical consultation, adequate imaging, drainage, and antibiotics are the appropriate treatment.

Otologic surgery to remove the nidus of infection is necessary once the patient has stabilized.

9.10 Extratemporal Extracranial Complications

9.10.1 Subperiosteal Abscess

Mastoid abscess is the most common extracranial complication of chronic otitis media and is frequently complicated by a subperiosteal abscess, the most common extratemporal complication that occurs with chronic otitis media (Figs. 9.19 and 9.21).

Subperiosteal abscess occurs as a result of vascular extension secondary to phlebitis of the mastoid veins or by direct extension of the purulent material through an erosion of the septa and the cortex secondary to an acute or coalescent mastoiditis [39]. Subperiosteal abscesses are seen more commonly in young children with AOM, but are also found in chronic otitis with and without cholesteatoma [1].

9.10.1.1 Diagnosis

Often, the diagnosis of a subperiosteal abscess is made on clinical grounds:

- systemic symptoms, including fever and irritability

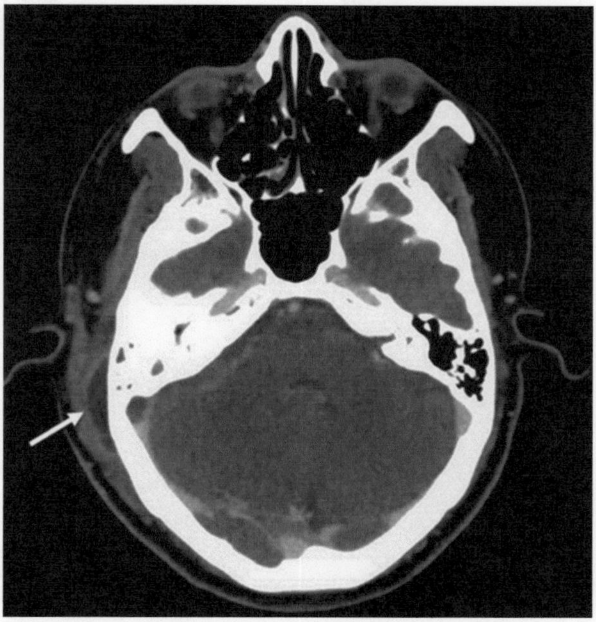

Fig. 9.21 Injected axial CT-scan in a patient with right ear CSOM complicated by subperiosteal abscess (arrow) and also a small perisigmoid collection

- local signs, including a protruding auricle that is laterally and inferiorly displaced, and the presence of a fluctuant, erythematous, tender area behind the ear

When the diagnosis is not certain on clinical evaluation, a contrasted CT scan can demonstrate the abscess and the cortical defect in the mastoid. [40].

9.10.1.2 Management

Conventional teaching and current literature advocate draining the abscess, in conjunction with a cortical mastoidectomy [3, 4]. Lately, less invasive treatment options have emerged, as abscess poncture, myringotomy and IV antibiotics. When associated to cholesteatoma, surgical intervention is warranted and conservative alternatives are not advised.

The skin incision for the mastoidectomy should be modified to incorporate the abscess cavity for an adequate drainage. Once the abscess is drained, a mastoidectomy is performed and the cholesteatoma is managed in the standard manner.

If not treated, subperiosteal abscess may erode the skin and drain spontaneously leading to the development of a postauricular fistula (Fig. 9.22). This complication disappeared in developed countries but is still present in some developing countries with poor health system.

9.10.2 Bezold's Abscess

In the presence of coalescent mastoiditis, if the mastoid cortex is violated at its tip, as opposed to its lateral cortex, an abscess will develop in the neck, deep in the sheat

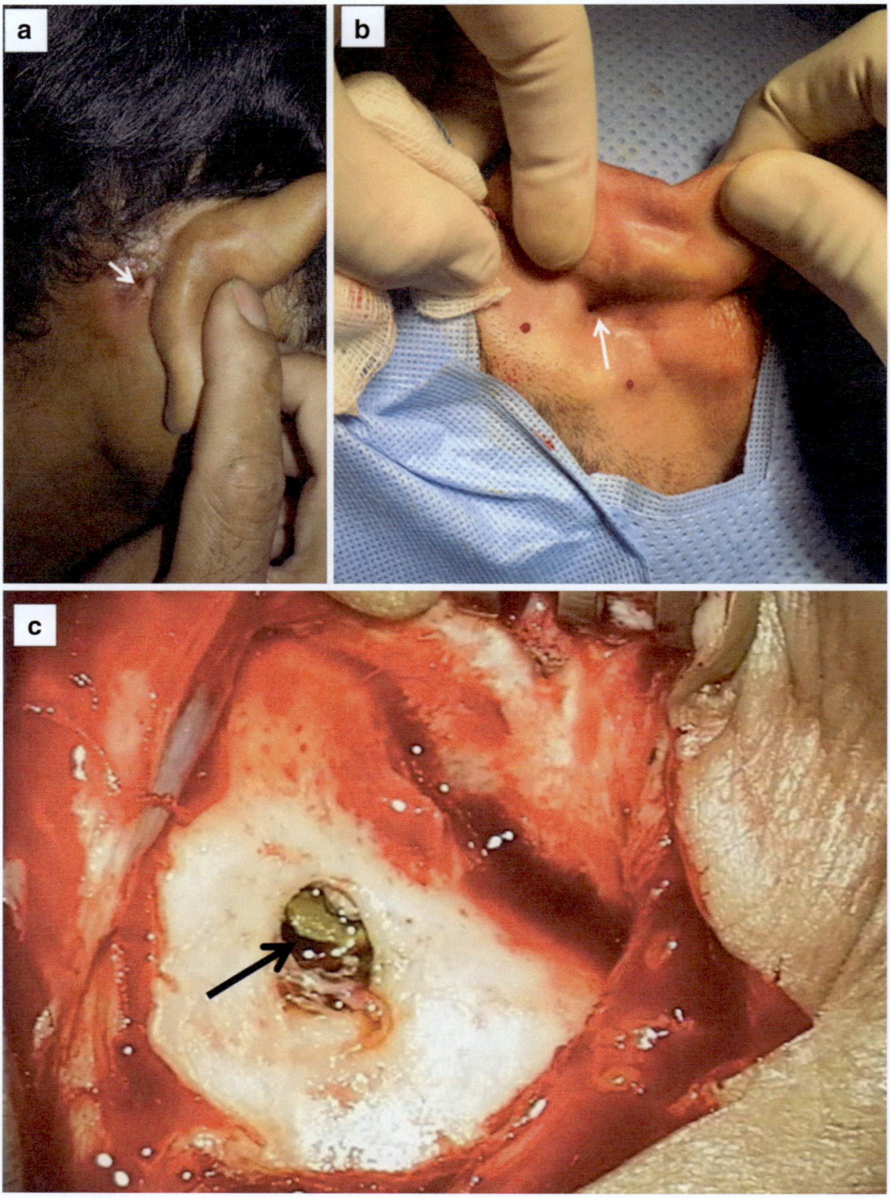

Fig. 9.22 Right ear mastoid fistula as shown by white arrow in (**a**) and (**b**). (**c**) Peroperative view after raising the musculoperiosteal flap, the mastoid cortex has an evident defect (black arrow), mastoid cholesteatoma is clearly visible through the defect

of the sternocleidomastoid muscle. Cholesteatoma mass obstruction of the aditus increases the possibility of infectious progression through the mastoid cortical tip, presenting clinically as a subperiosteal or Bezold's abscess. This abscess will present as a tender, deep, poorly defined mass in level II of the neck. Because the abscess develops from air cells at the tip of the mastoid, it is found in older children and

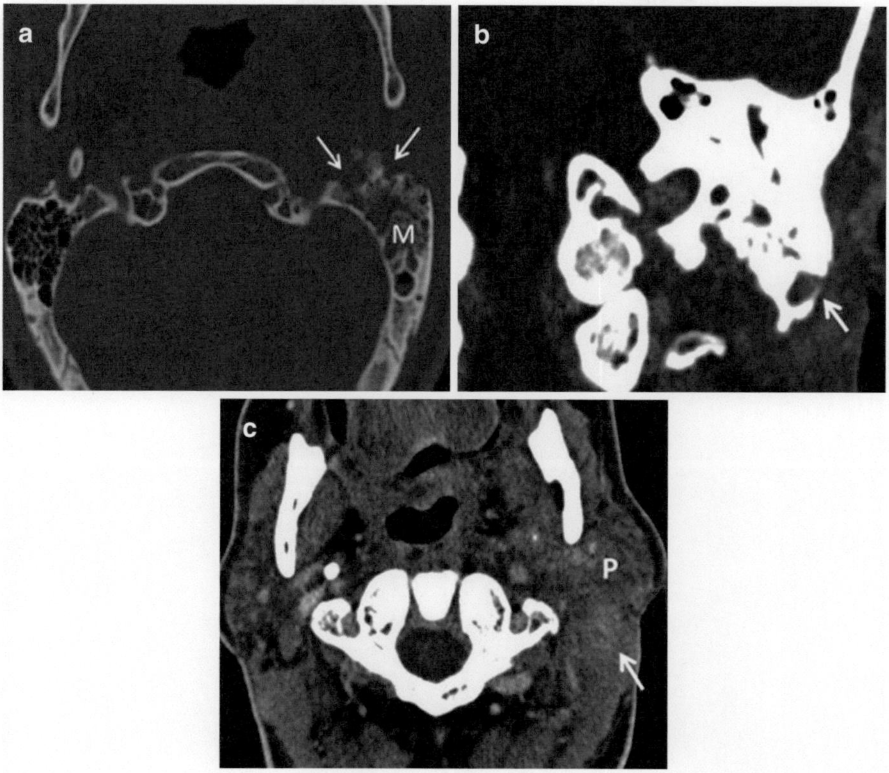

Fig. 9.23 CT Imaging of a Bezold abscess: (**a**) axial CT-image: the left mastoid (M) is almost completely condensated, with lytic signs of the cortex of its anterior wall (white arrows), (**b**) coronal CT-reconstruction of the left mastoid with an evident erosion on the tip of the mastoid (arrow) and (**c**) axial CT-image below the level of the mastoid tip: diffuse infiltration of the soft tissues of the level II cervical space, with a slight mass effect on the parotid gland (P). Slight contrast enhancement in the center of the abscess (arrow)

adults, where pneumatization of the mastoid has extended largely to the tip. Most of these abscesses result from direct extension through the cortex, but transmission through an intact cortex by way of mastoid vein phlebitis is also known to occur [3].

Although Bezold's abscess is more commonly a complication of AOM with mastoiditis in children, it is also known as a complication of COM with cholesteatoma [41].

9.10.2.1 Diagnosis

The presentation of an enlarged, tender, deep neck mass must be differentiated from inflammatory cervical lymphadenopathies, which is difficult by clinical means alone.

CT-Imaging: A contrasted CT scan of the neck and mastoid is recommended to make the diagnosis of a Bezold's abscess [42]: it consists in a rim-enhancing abscess with a surrounding inflammation regarding a bony dehiscence in the tip of the mastoid (Fig. 9.23).

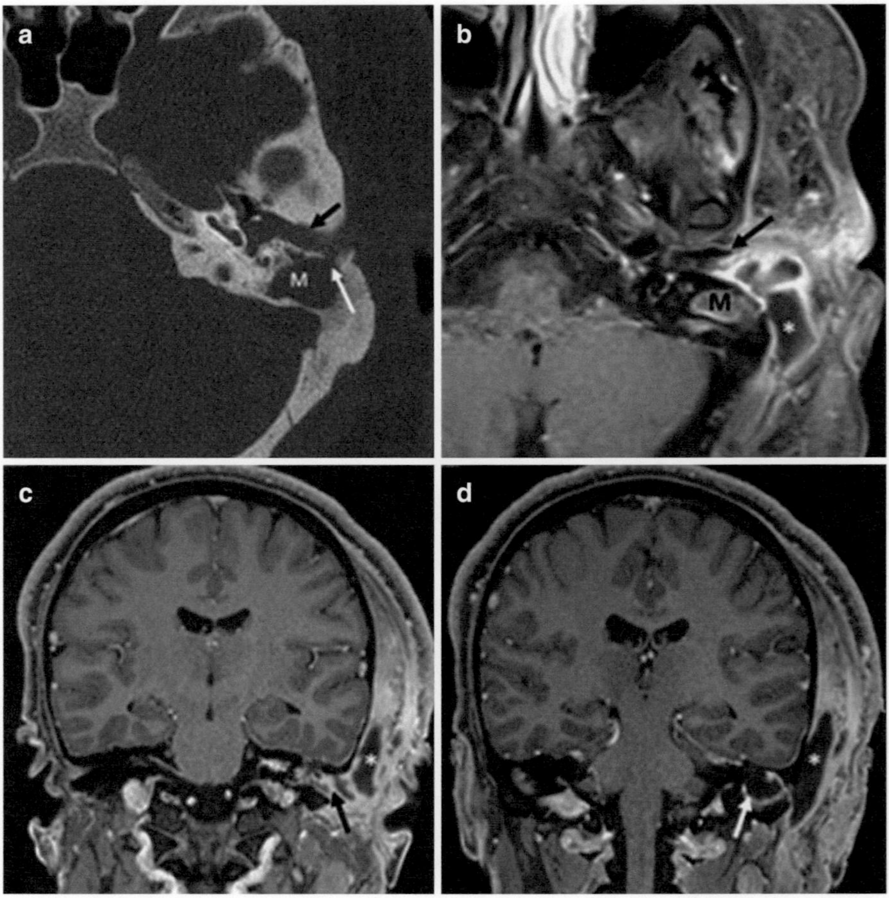

Fig. 9.24 Left ear cholesteatoma complicated by Luc's abscess. (**a**) Axial CT image showing the defect in the posterior wall of the ear canal (white arrow) allowing the pus to spread from the mastoid (M) to the ear canal (black arrow). (**b**) Injected T1 MRI showing the meatal abscess (black arrow) extending into the cervical space (*). (**c, d**) Coronal injected T1 weighted MRI showing the spread of pus from the ear canal (black arrow in **c**) to the temporal space (* in **c** and **d**). Cholesteatoma in the mastoid (white arrow in **d**)

9.10.2.2 Management

Open incision and drainage of the cervical abscess through a *transcervical approach (for adequate drainage) combined with a mastoidectomy* to address the mastoiditis and the cholesteatoma.

9.10.3 Other Extra Temporal Extracranial Abscesses

Other very rare abscesses are encountered which are managed in the same manner such as Luc's abscess (Fig. 9.24) (an infection tracking along EAC and collecting deep to the temporalis muscle), Mouret's abscess (when the pus extends into the parapharyngeal and retropharyngeal space with resultant trismus) and Citelli's abscess (it occurs when pus from the mastoid tip trickles down along the posterior belly of the digastric muscle to the occipital and cervical region). These abscesses are mentioned for their historical description.

Conclusion

With the advances of vaccination, applied genetics and ambitious public health care systems, the complete control of CSOM is reachable. The continuous improvement in its early diagnosis and prompt management permit the avoidance of complications.

Public health measures and the accurate medical assistance facilities are the prime responsibility of every nation. Medical expertise must be shared between developed and developing countries in order to eradicate life-threatening complications of the disease.

The burden of their socio-economic costs is a strong motivation for such efforts.

References

1. Yorgancılar E, Yildirim M, Gun R, Bakir S, Tekin R, Gocmez C, et al. Complications of chronic suppurative otitis media: a retrospective review. Eur Arch Otorhinolaryngol. 2013;270:69–76.
2. Manzar N, Manzar B, Kumar R, Bari ME. The study of etiologic and demographic characteristics of intracranial brain abscess: a consecutive case series study from Pakistan. World Neurosurg. 2011;76:195–200.
3. Osma U, Cureoglu S, Hosoglu S. The complications of chronic otitis media: report of 93 cases. J Laryngol Otol. 2000;114:97–100.
4. Macewen W. Pyogenic Infective Disease of the Brain and Spinal Cord. Glasgow, James Maclehouse & Sons, 1893.
5. Korner O. Otitischen Erkrankungen des Hirns, de Hirnaute und der Blutleiter. Wiesbaden. 1908.
6. Lebert. Ueber Gehirnabscesse. Virchows Arch 1856;10:78.
7. Gradenigo G. Über die Paralyse des Nervus abducens bei Otitis. Arch Ohrenheilkunde. 1907;774:149–87.
8. Kopetzky SJ, Almour R. The suppuration of the petrous pyramid: pathology, symptomatology and surgical treatment (part III). Ann Otol Rhinol Laryngol. 1931;40:396–414.
9. Eagleton WP. Unlocking of the petrous pyramid for localized bulbar (pontile) meningitis secondary to suppuration of the petrous apex. Arch Otolaryngol. 1931;13:386–422.
10. Rupa V, Raman R. Chronic suppurative otitis media: complicated versus uncomplicated disease. Acta Otolaryngol. 1991;111(3):530–5.
11. Dubey SP, Larawin V. Complications of chronic suppurative otitis media and their management. Laryngoscope. 2007;117:264–7.
12. Kangsanarak J, Fooanant S, Ruckphaopunt K, Navacharoen N, Teotrakul S. Extracranial and intracranial complications of suppurative otitis media: report of 102 cases. J Laryngol Otol. 1993;107:999–1004.
13. Mostafa BE, El Fiky LM, El Sharnouby MM. Complications of suppurative otitis media: still a problem in the 21st century. ORL J Otorhinolaryngol Relat Spec. 2009;71(2):87–92.
14. Dubey SP, Larawin V, Molumi CP. Intracranial spread of chronic middle ear suppuration. Am J Otolaryngol. 2010;31(2):73–7.
15. Sennaroglu L, Sozeri B. Otogenic brain abscess: review of 41 cases. Otolaryngol Head Neck Surg. 2000;123:751–5.
16. Mustafa A, Heta A, Kastrati B, Dreshaj S. Complications of chronic otitis media with cholesteatoma during a 10-year period in Kosovo. Eur Arch Otorhinolaryngol. 2008;265(12):1477–82.

17. Kangsanarak J, Navacharoen N, Fooanant S, Ruckphaopunt K. Intracranial complications of suppurative otitis media: 13 years' experience. Am J Otol. 1995;16(1):104–9.
18. Greenberg JS, Manolidis S. High incidence of complications encountered in chronic otitis media surgery in a U.S. metropolitan public hospital. Otolaryngol Head Neck Surg. 2001;125:623–7.
19. Dornhoffer JL, Milewski C. Management of the open labyrinth. Otolaryngol Head Neck Surg. 1995;112(3):410–4.
20. Copeland BJ, Buchman CA. Management of labyrinthine fistulae in chronic ear surgery. Am J Otolaryngol. 2003;24(1):51–60.
21. Meyer A, Bouchetemblé P, Costentin B, Dehesdin D, Lerosey Y, Marie JP. Lateral semicircular canal fistula in cholesteatoma: diagnosis and management. Eur Arch Otorhinolaryngol. 2016;273(8):2055–63. https://doi.org/10.1007/s00405-015-3775-6.
22. Magliulo G, Terranova G, Varacalli S, et al. Labyrinthine fistula as a complication of cholesteatoma. Am J Otol. 1997;18(6):697–701.
23. Gacek RR. The surgical management of labyrinthine fistulae in chronic otitis media with cholesteatoma. Ann Otol Rhinol Laryngol. 1974;83(Suppl 10):1–19.
24. Stephenson MF, Saliba I. Prognostic indicators of hearing after complete resection of cholesteatoma causing a labyrinthinefistula. Eur Arch Otorhinolaryngol. 2011;268(12):1705–11. https://doi.org/10.1007/s00405-011-1545-7.
25. Savić DL, Djerić DR. Facial paralysis in chronic suppurative otitis media. Clin Otolaryngol Allied Sci. 1989;14:515–7.
26. Altuntas A, Unal A, Aslan A, Ozcan M, Kurkcuoglu S, Nalca Y. Facial nerve paralysis in chronic suppurative otitis media: Ankara Numune Hospital experience. Auris Nasus Larynx. 1998;25:169–72.
27. Yetiser S, Tosun F, Kazkayasi M. Facial nerve paralysis due to chronic otitis media. Otol Neurotol. 2002;23:580–8.
28. Kim J, Jung G-H, Park S-Y, Lee WS. Facial Nerve Paralysis due to Chronic Otitis Media: Prognosis in Restoration of Facial Function after Surgical Intervention. Yonsei Medical Journal. 2012;53(3):642–48.
29. Schuring AG. Iatrogenic facial nerve injury. Am J Otol. 1988;9:432–3.
30. Wiet RJ. Iatrogenic facial paralysis. Otolaryngol Clin N Am. 1982;15:773–80.
31. Yu Z, Wang Z, Yang B, Han D, Zhang L. The value of preoperative CT scan of tympanic facial nerve canal in tympanomastoid surgery. Acta Otolaryngol. 2011;131(7):774–8.
32. Magliulo G, Colicchio MG, Appiani MC. Facial nerve dehiscence and cholesteatoma. Ann Otol Rhinol Laryngol. 2011;120(4):261–7.
33. Chee NW, Tan TY. The value of pre-operative high resolution CT scans in cholesteatoma surgery. Singapore Med J. 2001;42(4):155–9.
34. Nalbone VP, Kuruvilla A, Gacek RR. Otogenic brain abscess : the Syracuse experience. Ear Nose Throat J. 1992;71:238–42.
35. Ludman H. Complications of suppurative otitis media. In: Scott-Brown WG, Kerr AG, Groves J, editors. Scott-Brown's otolaryngology. 5th ed. London: Butterworths; 1987. p. 264–91.
36. Syal R, Singh H, Duggal KK. Otogenic brain abscess : management by otologist. J Laryngol Otol. 2006;120:837–41.
37. Basit AS, Ravi B, Banerji AK, Tandon PN. Multiple pyogenic brain abscesses : an analysis of 21 patients. J Neurol Neurosurg Psychiatry. 1989;52:591–4.
38. Moorthy RK, Rajshekhar V. Management of brain abscess : an overview. Neurosurg Focus. 2008;24:e3.
39. Harker LA, Shelton C. Complications of temporal bone infections. In: Cummings CW, editor. Cummings otolaryngology head and neck surgery. 4th ed. Philadelphia: Elsevier Mosby; 2005. p. 3013–38.
40. Hashisaki GT. Complications of chronic otitis media. In: Canalis RF, Lambert PR, editors. The ear: comprehensive otology. Philadelphia: Lippincott Williams & Wilkins; 2000. p. 433–6.
41. Furukawa K, Arai E, Kobayashi T, et al. A case of Bezold's abscess associated with cholesteatoma. Nippon Jibiinkoka Gakkai Kaiho. 1992;95(12):1901–5.
42. Castillo M, Albernaz VS, Mukherji SK, et al. Imaging of Bezold's abscess. Am J Roentgenol. 1998;171(6):1491–5.

Diagnosis and Clinico-Radiologic Correlations in Conductive Hearing Loss with a Normal Appearing Tympanic Membrane

10

Contents

S. Mansour et al., *Middle Ear Diseases*,
https://doi.org/10.1007/978-3-319-72962-6_10

10.1 Introduction

Conductive hearing loss with a normal appearing tympanic membrane occurs when acoustic signals are attenuated during their transmission from the external environment to the inner ear. In most cases, conductive hearing loss results from a blockage of the sound conduction by diseases, abnormalities or any damage to the middle ear structures.

The diagnostic pathway starts with a good history taking, a good otoscopic examination and a complete audiologic evaluation. We will emphasize on the high value of clinico-radiologic correlations and their impact on the decision making of the best therapeutical approach.

We present in this chapter the different causative groups and sub-groups of pathologies, from otosclerosis to the sequelae of ignored previous episodes of infection, trauma, ossicular anomalies, third window phenomenon, hidden retrotympanic effusions or masses, and mainly congenital ossicular anomalies as fixation or discontinuity.

10.2 Clinico-Radiologic Exploration

10.2.1 History Taking

History taking must be accurate and complete (Table 10.1). Important facts to reveal are the duration, the progression, and the laterality of the deafness. Former episodes

Table 10.1 History clues

History details	Indicative for
• Hearing loss + family history + tinnitus in adult	Otosclerosis
• Presence of vertigo	Third window phenomena
• History of recurrent otitis media	Incus necrosis, tympanosclerosis
• History of head trauma	Ossicular chain discontinuity
• Unilateral pulsatile tinnitus	Paraganglioma
• Young patient	Glue ear or middle ear anomaly

of ear discharge or head injury must be well recognized. A detailed family history is of importance, especially when other members of the family report the same complaints:

- a bilateral progressive conductive hearing loss, frequently associated with tinnitus, in a young adult patient with positive family history is highly indicative for otosclerosis.
- a non-progressive hearing loss in the first decade of life is suggestive of congenital middle ear anomalies, because juvenile otosclerosis is rarely detected before the age of 10 years.
- In the presence of vertigo and Tullio phenomenon (vertigo associated with loud noise), a third window pathology should be suspected.
- A history of recurrent otitis media during childhood suggests a sequela of chronic otitis media. A well healed tympanic membrane of normal appearance can cover an ossicular discontinuity due to incus necrosis or an ossicular chain fixation due to a hidden intratympanic tympanosclerosis.
- A history of head trauma suggests the possibility of a post-traumatic ossicular chain dislocation or discontinuity behind an intact tympanic membrane.
- Paget disease can be considered, involving the temporal bone or the ossicles
- Similarly osteogenesis imperfecta with a progressive hearing loss is diagnosed on the basis of associated symptoms (eg, blue sclera or multiple fractures).

10.2.2 Physical Examination

The examination of the tympanic membrane should include careful microscopic inspection of its four quadrants at rest and after inflation of the Eustachian tubes by a Valsalva maneuver (Fig. 10.1a). In the majority of children, the microscopic examination can be adequately done following a good communication with the child. However, all means must be used to perform an adequate examination of the ear, even if this would require a general anesthesia. A pneumatic otoscope (Siegel's maneuver) can be used to evaluate the mobility of the intact tympanic membrane. Pressure-induced vertigo and nystagmus may be present in ears with third-window lesions, most likely superior semicircular caused by a canal dehiscence. A very

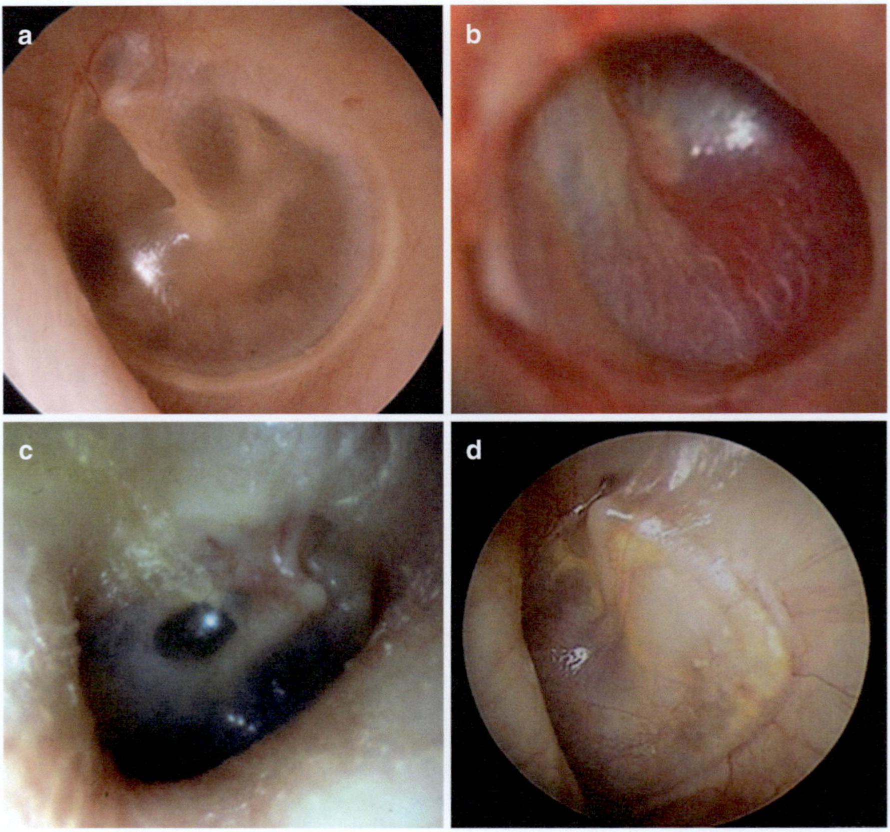

Fig. 10.1 Different aspects of the tympanic membrane. (**a**) Normal left ear otoscopy. (**b**) Red color of an intact tympanic membrane: tympanic paraganglioma. (**c**) Blue tympanic membrane in otitis media with effusion (long term standing bluish fluid). (**d**) Congenital cholesteatoma behind a normal tympanic membrane

delicate manipulation of the manubrium under microscope with a smooth pick may inform about malleus fixation.

After careful inspection of the tympanic membrane, the middle ear cavity should be carefully inspected through the transparent tympanic membrane (Fig. 10.1a). Behind a normal tympanic membrane, several discolorations can be seen:

- A red mass of the tympanic floor may suggest a tympanic glomus. (Fig. 10.1b).
- A blue discoloration suggests a hemotympanum or a chronic form of middle ear effusion (Fig. 10.1c).
- A white mass suggests a congenital cholesteatoma (Fig. 10.1d).

Tuning fork test, that is not at all an "old fashioned" method, is still essential and mandatory. It reveals the conductive type of hearing loss (Rinne and Weber). It can be very helpful to localize the affected side. In patients with superior canal dehiscence, a tuning fork held on the ankle may travel up the body, and be heard in the affected ear. This is generally best tested with a 128 Hz tuning fork.

10.2.3 Audiometric Testing

10.2.3.1 Pure Tone Audiometry

A thorough audiometric evaluation is essential in establishing the diagnosis and must be done in appropriate settings with accurate masking.

The audiogram pattern may give clue to the underlying disease (Fig. 10.2):

- Low frequency ABG is a sign of ossicular chain fixation.
- The presence of a Carhart notch (a dip of BC of 20–30 dB at 2-kHz) suggests stapes fixation mainly by otosclerosis or tympanosclerosis [1].
- An air bone gap (ABG) above 30 dB over all the frequencies suggests an ossicular chain discontinuity.
- High frequency ABG is in favor of an erosion of the long process of the incus with a residual fibrous band connecting the incus to the stapes head.
- A low-frequency air-bone gap with bone conduction thresholds that are better than 0 dB (−5 to −20 dB) is suggestive of a third window lesion [2].

10.2.3.2 Objective Audiometry: Stapedial Reflex, Tympanometry, VEMP

Stapedial reflex and tympanometry should be included in every audiological evaluation to establish the differential diagnosis of the conductive hearing loss.

Stapedial Reflex

Usually absent in CHL that is due to middle ear diseases; but it is commonly present in CHL due to inner ear diseases (third window phenomenon) [3–6] (Fig. 10.6) (see Chap. 1).

Tympanometry

Usually the peak of the tympanogram is evident at a normal pressure level. The height of the peak for otosclerosis is often normal or below the normal range. A high peak of compliance is not compatible with a diagnosis of otosclerosis.

The following display of curves is reported to help interpreting the tympanograms in the possible underlying etiologies of the conductive hearing loss with normal appearing tympanic membrane (Fig. 10.3):

VEMP (Cervical or Ocular)

The vestibular evoked myogenic potentials (VEMP) is a test used to measure vestibular response to sounds transmitted through the ear canal and middle ear. VEMP responses could be affected by diseases of the middle ear.

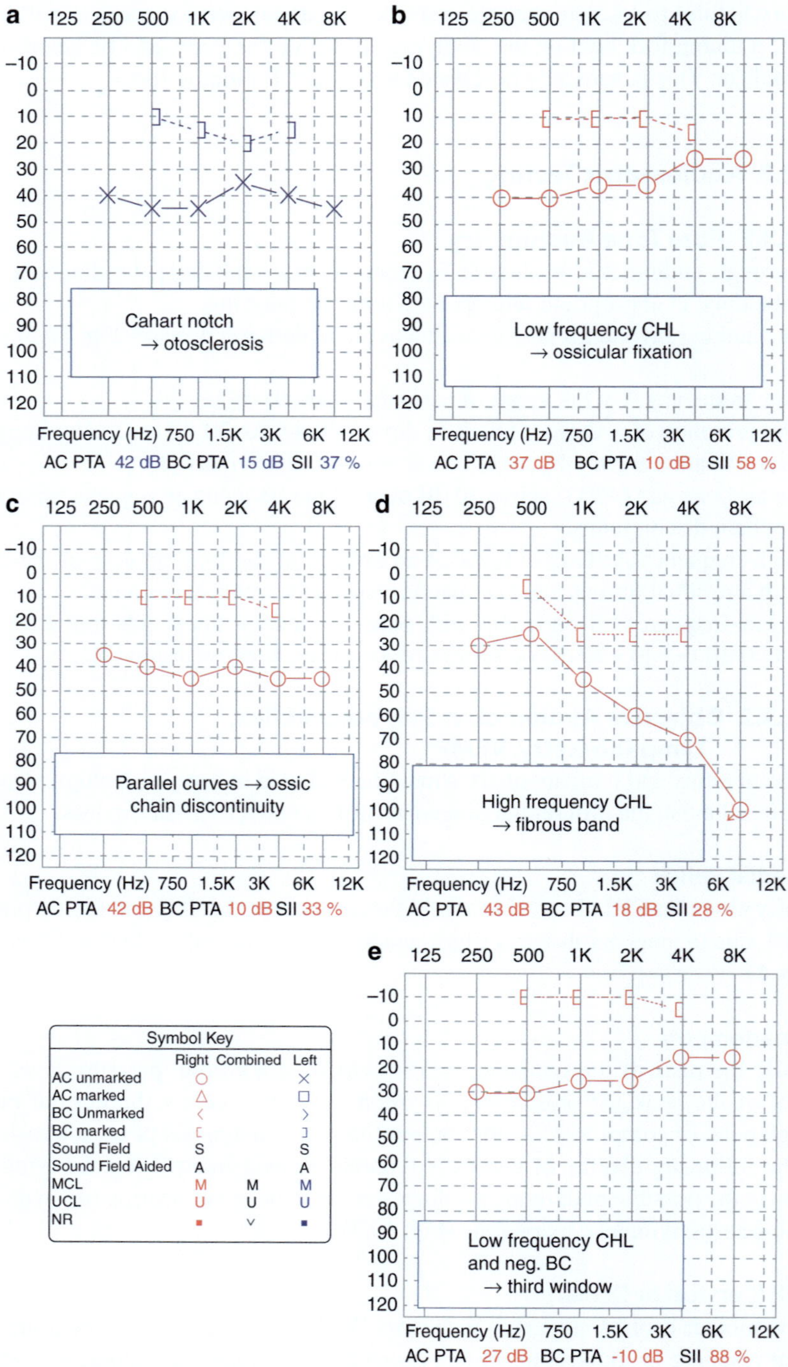

Fig. 10.2 (**a**) Audiogram with Carhart notch suggestive of otosclerosis; (**b**) Audiogram with low frequency CHL suggestive of ossicular fixation; (**c**) Audiogram with parallel curves suggestive of ossicular chain discontinuity; (**d**) Audiogram with high frequency CHL suggestive of fibrous band; (**e**) Audiogram with low frequency CHL and negative BC is suggestive of a third window lesion

In case of suspicion of a third window, VEMP should be done.

1. **VEMP** is usually abolished or attenuated in middle ear diseases responsible of CHL (Fig. 10.4).
2. **VEMP** is usually exaggerated and hypersensitive in inner ear (third window) origin of CHL (Figs. 10.5 and 10.6).

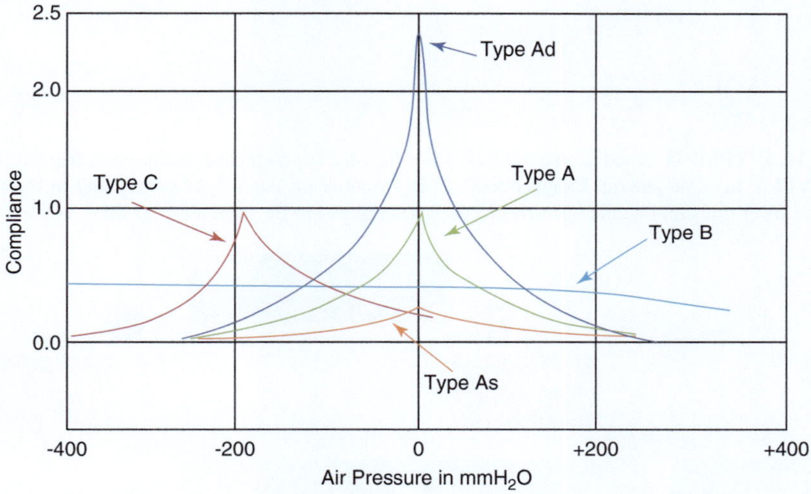

Fig. 10.3 Different types of tympanogram: Type A: normal tympanic compliance, *Type As:* increased stiffness of the tympano-ossicular system indicative of ossicular fixation, *Type Ad*: hypermobile drum indicative of ossicular discontinuity. Type B: suggestive of a glue ear. Type C: negative pressure in the middle ear space (nasal congestion, or ear infection)

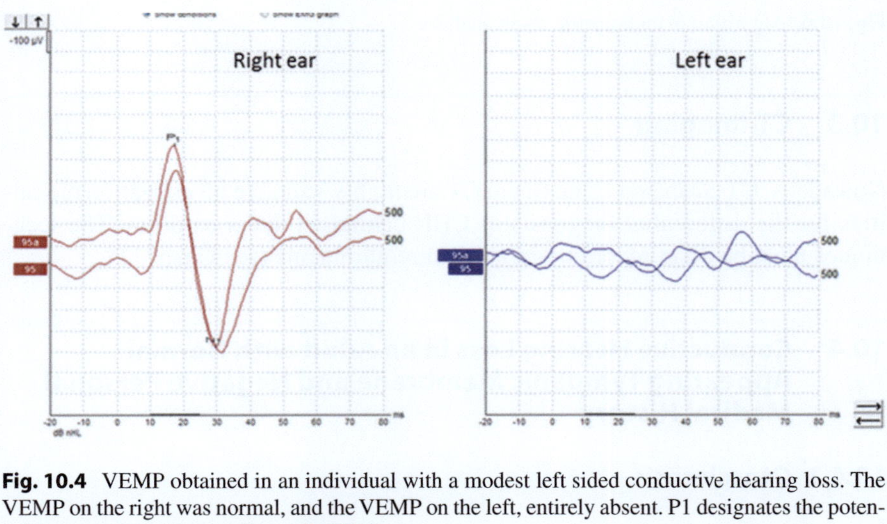

Fig. 10.4 VEMP obtained in an individual with a modest left sided conductive hearing loss. The VEMP on the right was normal, and the VEMP on the left, entirely absent. P1 designates the potential that occurs at 13 ms (often called P13)

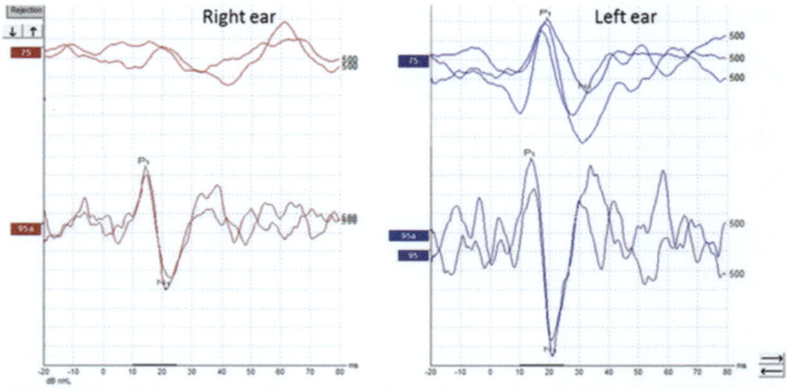

Fig. 10.5 VEMP obtained in an individual with left sided superior canal dehiscence. Right threshold VEMP in same person. Exaggerated VEMP response on the left side compared to the right side; Lower threshold on the left side (75 dB) as compared to the right side (95 dB)

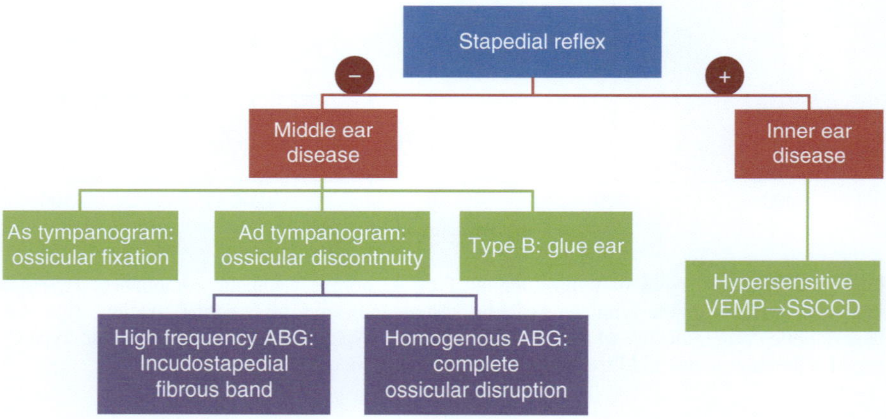

Fig. 10.6 Algorithm of audiometric result analysis

10.3 CT-Imaging

Nowadays, CT-Scan and Cone Beam CT are highly valuable investigation modalities for the differential diagnosis of CHL behind an intact eardrum. The techniques must be done according to modern requirements (see Chap. 11).

10.4 Conductive Hearing Loss in an Adult with Normal Appearing Tympanic Membrane and Negative Personal Medical History

10.4.1 Otosclerosis

Otosclerosis is the most frequent cause for a conductive hearing loss with an intact tympanic membrane. The hearing loss starts usually in the second or third decade of life and

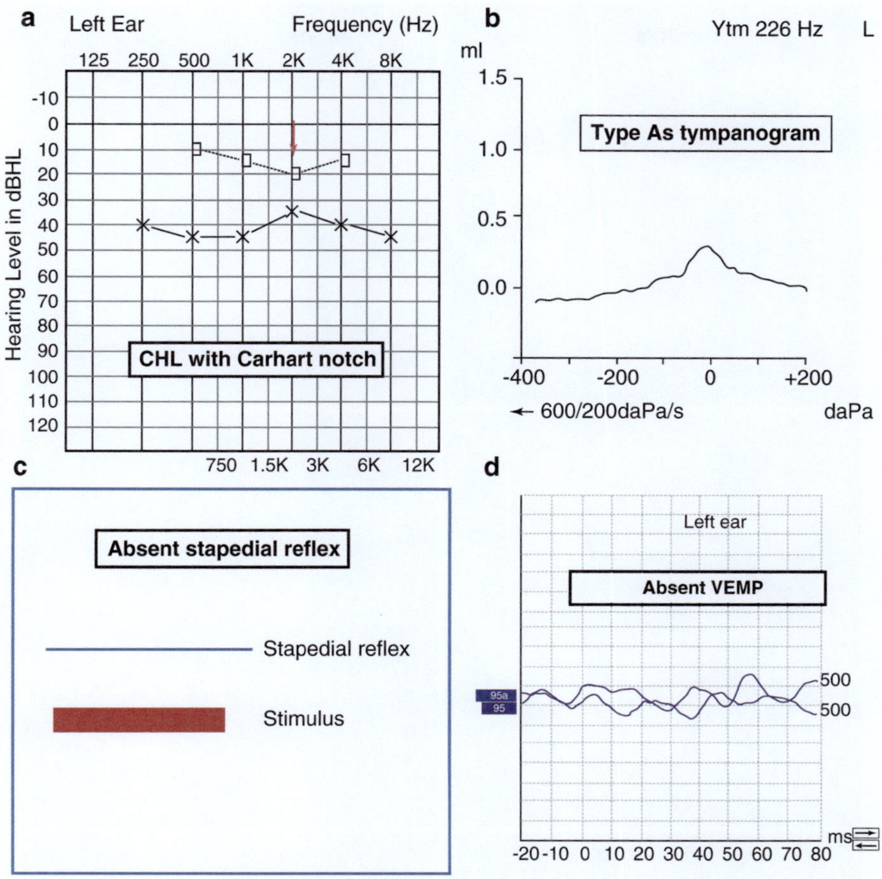

Fig. 10.7 Typical audiological studies in a patient with otosclerosis. (**a**) Audiogram with conductive hearing and Carhart notch (red arrow). (**b**) As pattern tympanometry. (**c**) Absent stapedial reflex. (**d**) VEMP reduced response

it could be the main clinical symptom. Otosclerosis is more common in female patients and bilateral in approximately 80% of cases. Its site of predilection is the fissula ante fenestram, where a cartilaginous tissue is present embryologically and becomes progressively ossified. Bilateral involvement and the presence of tinnitus, Carhart notch on the audiogram, and negative stapedial reflex, support the diagnosis of otosclerosis (Fig. 10.7).

In the presence of unilateral disease with **As** tympanogram, palpation of the malleus under microscope is helpful to check its mobility and thus to rule out a malleus fixation (see Chap. 1).

10.4.1.1 CT-Imaging

A typical hypodense pre vestibular focus more or less extended to the footplate is diagnostic for a fenestral manifestation of otosclerosis (Fig. 10.8a–c). This is the most frequent manifestation (about 75% of cases with otosclerosis). Round window manifestation (Fig. 10.8d) is less frequent, but not rare (9–13%) [7, 8], retrocochlear otosclerosis with more extensive peri cochlear manifestations (Fig. 10.8e, f) affects 10–20% of cases [9] (see Chap. 1).

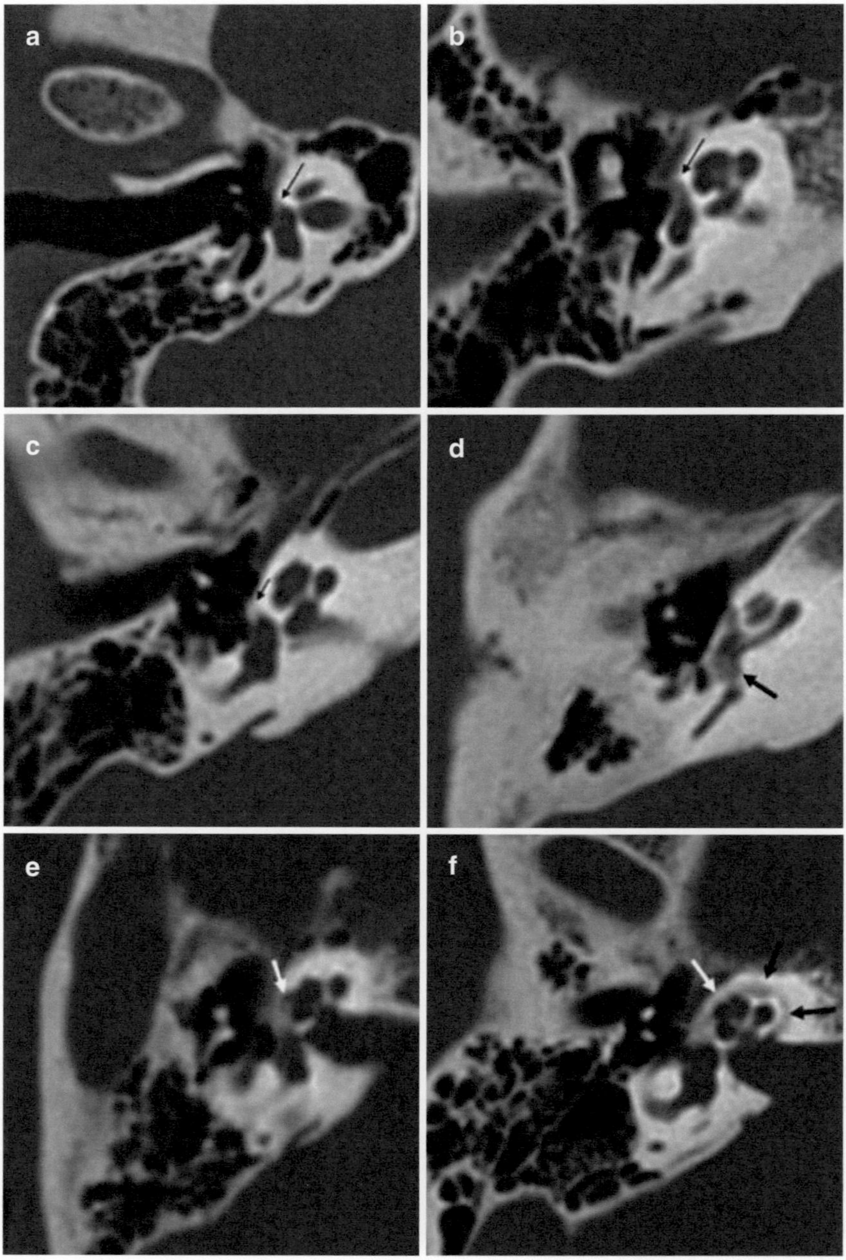

Fig. 10.8 Axial images of right ears, with different typical manifeations of otosclerosis: (**a**) typical small prevestibular focus in the fissula ante fenestram, (**b**) large hypodense focus >1 mm (arrow), their hypodensity is in favor of active foci; (**c**) hyperdense focus (arrow): inactive otosclerosis, difficult to distinguish from the adjacent otic capsule density, (**d**) round window otosclerosis: the entire window (black arrow) is obliterated (RW4), (**e**) large antefenestral focus of otosclerosis, coming in intimate contact with the endosteum of the cochlea (white arrow) (**f**) extended otosclerotic foci as an hypodense rim around the cochlea laterally with deep contact to the endosteaum of the cochlea (white arrow), medially the hypodense otospongiotic rim does not come in contact with the cochlea (black arrows)

10.4.2 Idiopathic Malleus Fixation

10.4.2.1 Clinics

An isolated malleus head fixation (MHF) was first described by Goodhill in 1966 [10]. An acquired malleus fixation occurs most commonly in the later decades of life and it is frequently associated with presbycusis. Clinically, the disease is usually unilateral or more rarely bilateral and manifests by a progressive conductive or mixed hearing loss with an intact tympanic membrane. It could be associated to otosclerosis; therefore it is a rule to check the mobility of the malleus before engaging into a stapedectomy in patients with otosclerosis.

10.4.2.2 CT-Imaging

A preoperative CT may show, with a high sensitivity, a close contact between the malleus head and the attic wall, or a tissue band between the head and the attic wall that covers more than half of the diameter of the malleus head; this is considered to be very indicative of fixation (Fig. 10.9).

Ossification of the anterior malleal ligament has only a minor impact on hearing, almost 5 dB of conductive hearing loss [11] (Fig. 10.10).

10.4.2.3 Treatment

The preoperative suspicion of malleus head fixation allows the surgeon to obtain a clear consent from the patient and permits the selection of a more adequate surgical approach [12]. Nevertheless the definitive diagnosis of MHF is mostly confirmed at the time of surgery. In most cases, the surgical treatment either with mobilization or bypass technique could offer a satisfactory recovery of the hearing loss although complete closure of the ABG is often not achieved.

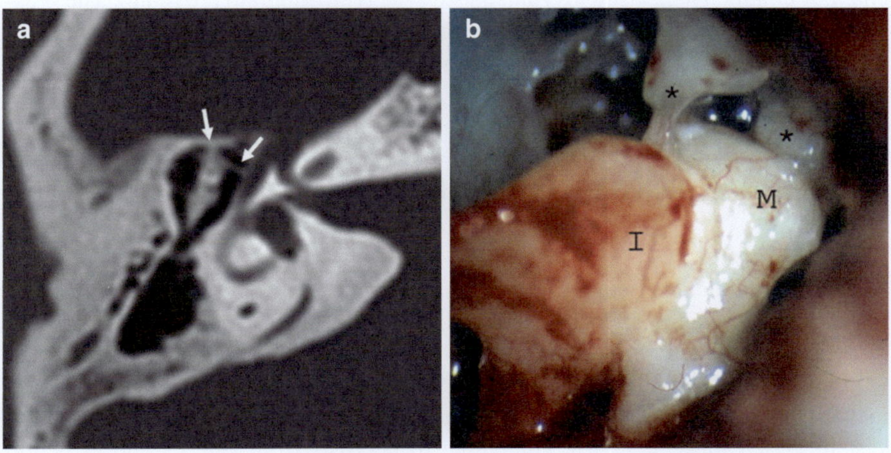

Fig. 10.9 (**a**) Preoperative coronal CT of a right ear: large calcified band between the malleus head and the tegmen (arrows), covering a large part of the malleus head, indicative of fixation. (**b**) Peroperative view: Fixed malleus head of the right ear: superior and anterior bony fixation (*) of the head of malleus (M); incus (I)

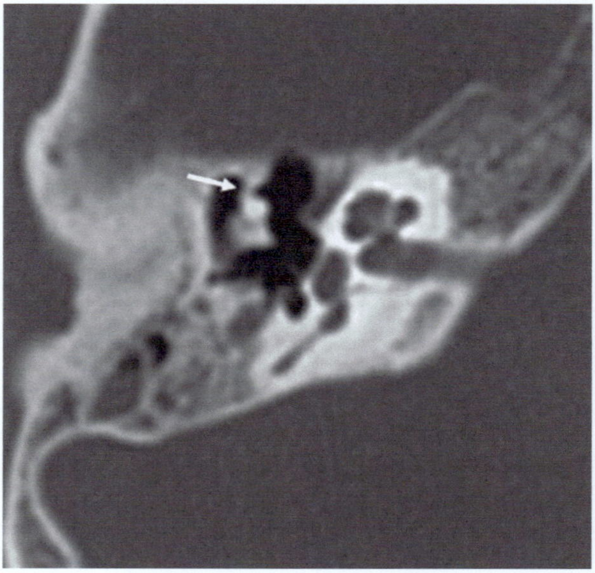

Fig. 10.10 Axial CT-image of right ear showing an ossification of the anterior malleal ligament (arrow)

10.5 Conductive Hearing Loss in the Adult with Normal Appearing Tympanic Membrane and a Past History of Recurrent Ear Infection

Conductive hearing loss in a patient with a past history of recurrent ear infections is most likely due to ossicular chain dysfunction (discontinuity or fixation) behind a well healed tympanic membrane. Recurrent infections may lead to osteitis of the long process of the incus with subsequent necrosis and discontinuity of the ossicular chain. A conductive hearing loss and an Ad type tympanogram are found. The presence of myringosclerosis should evoke the diagnosis of ossicular chain tympanosclerotic fixation; however, it is possible to have middle ear tympanosclerosis behind a normal tympanic membrane.

10.5.1 Ossicular Chain Discontinuity

10.5.1.1 Clinics

In case of ossicular chain interruption, pneumatic otoscopy can show a hypermobile intact tympanic membrane which is usually atrophic. In case of complete ossicular discontinuity, the conductive hearing loss is generally of more than 40 dB over all the frequencies, with a type Ad tympanogram. Necrosis of the long process of the incus is frequent, due to its thin diameter and its own particular fragile vascular system which make it highly vulnerable to necrosis from osteitis and ischemic changes. The ossicular defect is some times replaced by a fibrous band. In such condition, the audiogram is characteristic and shows conductive hearing loss with an ABG more important on high frequencies (Fig. 10.11).

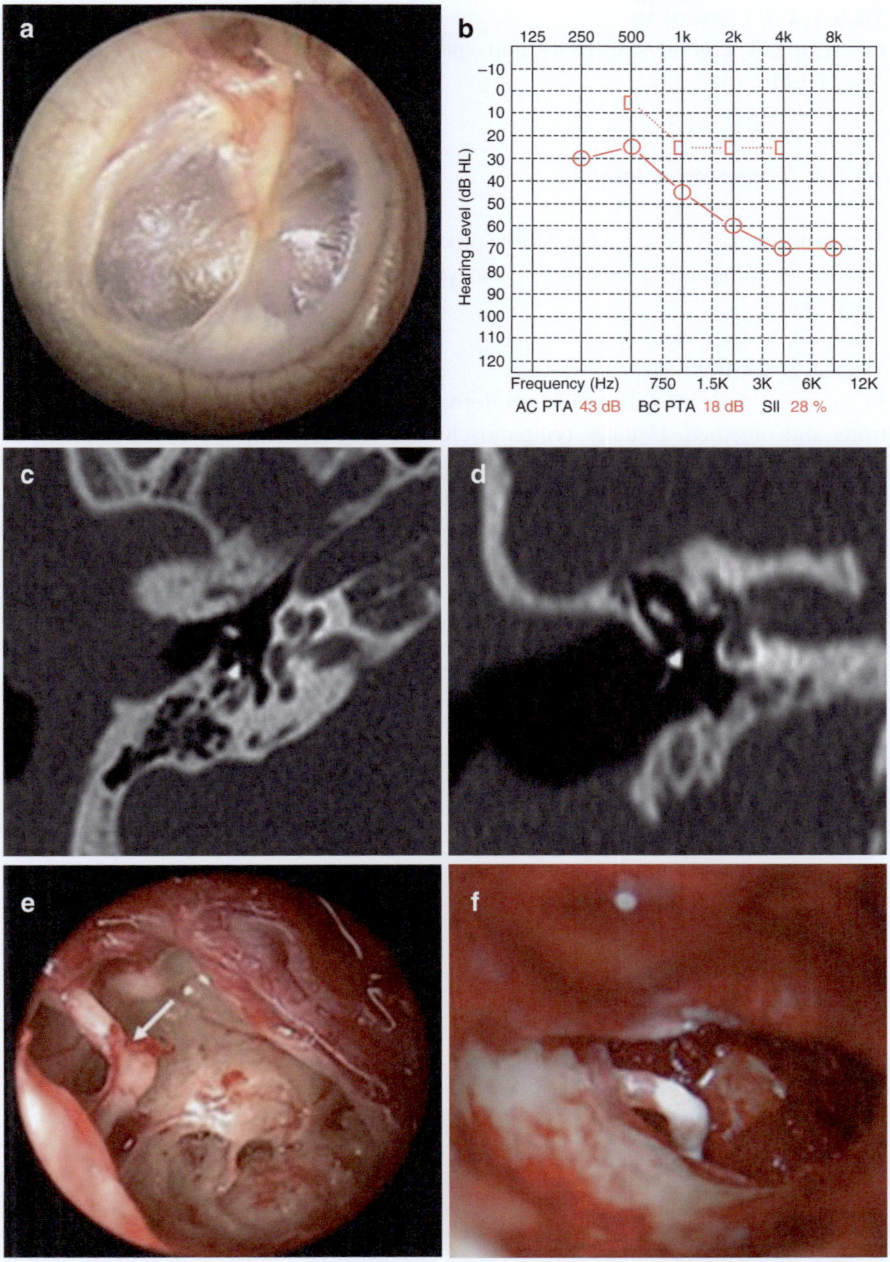

Fig. 10.11 (**a**) Otoscopy of a right ear with incudostapedial chain interruption showing intact but atrophic ear drum, (**b**) audiogram: mostly high frequencies gap, (**c**) axial CT-Image and (**d**) coronal CT image showing the interruption between the long process of the incus and the stapes head (arrow), (**e**) per-operative findings: bony defect of lenticular process of the incus replaced by a fibrotic tissue around the incudostapedial articulation (arrow). (**f**) Ossicular reconstruction by bone cement

10.5.1.2 CT-Imaging

CT-Scan has a good sensitivity and specificity to demonstrate the incus defect (Fig. 10.11c, d).

10.5.2 Tympanosclerosis

Tympanosclerosis is a hyalinization process of middle ear mucosa secondary to chronic inflammation, and may involve ligaments, tendons and ossicles (see Chap. 5).

10.5.2.1 Clinics

Most of the patients with tympanosclerosis report a history of recurrent ear infections and otorrhea. Usually tympanosclerosis leaves white patches on the drum which could be intact or perforated. Tympanosclerosis may result in a severe conductive hearing loss if the deposits immobilize the whole ossicular chain.

Clinically, it may mimic otosclerosis especially when the tympanic membrane looks intact without myringosclerosis: this could result in a diagnostic dilemma regarding the etiology of the conductive hearing loss. Tympanometry will show a reduction of the mobility of the tympanic membrane.

10.5.2.2 CT-Imaging

CT will demonstrate focal or linear condensation images within the middle ear (Fig. 10.12a), with or without calcifications. In case of non-calcified images, specificity of the CT-Scan is low. When the tympanosclerosis becomes extensive enough,

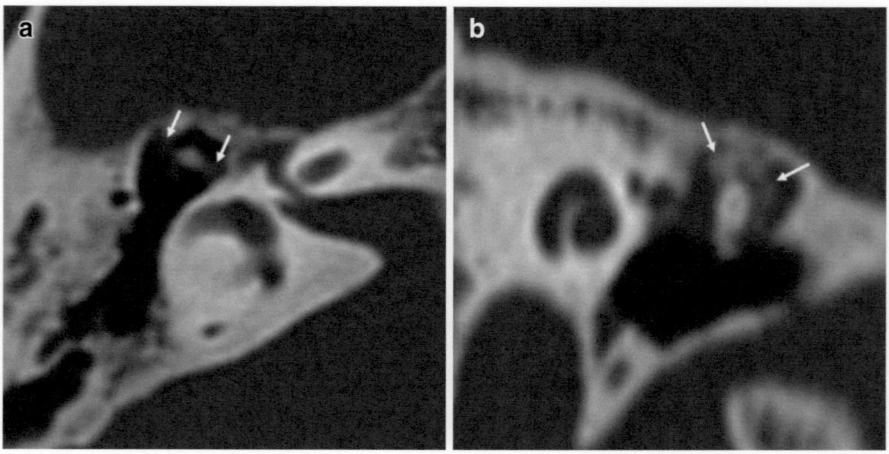

Fig. 10.12 (**a**) Axial CT-image of a right ear: bands of hypodense tissue extended between the malleus head and the attic wall (arrows). Tympanosclerosis intraoperatively. (**b**) Coronal image of a left ear: numerous calcifications are situated in the attic around the malleus—a typical image of tympanosclerosis

the deposits can appear like an ill-defined mass with heterogeneous calcifications (Fig. 10.12b) like large calcified blocs, which are easily identified on CT scan (Various examples are illustrated in chapter 5, Figs. 5.19–5.24).

10.6 Conductive Hearing Loss with a Normal Appearing Tympanic Membrane and a Past History of Head Trauma

Trauma of the temporal bone can cause neurological deficits, facial paralysis and a hemotympanum or CSF leak. ***Longitudinal temporal bone fractures*** after a temporo-parietal trauma are associated with a high incidence of conductive deafness secondary to ossicular disruption. These varieties of fractures typically spare the otic capsule, so that a sensorineural hearing loss is unusual. In contrast, transverse ***temporal bone fractures*** of the temporal bone secondary to fronto-occipital trauma often involve the inner ear and cause sensorineural hearing loss. However, they can also separate the ossicles and spare the otic capsule.

A conductive hearing loss can manifest at a later stage after a sudden disruption of the previously injured ossicular chain. Also the trauma event could be forgotten by the patient and the symptom of hearing loss could be reported long time after the event. In many adults with traumatic ossicular dsruptions, the trauma actually ocuured in childhood. Such an ear injury may not be detected because most small children do not compain of the resulting hearing loss. Tympanometry is of importance in the diagnosis of these lesions and it will show an absent stapedial reflex, an abnormal compliance and a low impedance system.

There are two types of ossicular injuries:

- ***Dislocation*** (incudostapedial and incudomalleolar joint separation, stapedio-vestibular dislocation)
- ***Fracture*** (fracture of the malleus, incus, and stapes).

Of the three middle ear ossicles, the incus is the most vulnerable to traumatic injuries because it is suspended between two stable bones, the malleus and stapes, with only one firm point of attachment—the posterior incudal ligament. The vulnerability of the incus is compounded by the contraction of the middle ear muscles. A traumatic blow causes an abrupt severe reflex muscle contraction. The stapedius muscle rotates the stapes posteriorly and laterally out of the oval window. The tensor tympani muscle contraction simultaneously pulls the malleus handle medially towards the promontory. After a severe blow, the reflex muscle contractions make the incus, and more specifically the incudostapedial joint, the most vulnerable link in the ossicular chain. Incudomalleal dislocation is also common injury, whereas stapedio-vestibular dislocation and ossicular fractures are rare (Table 10.2).

The CT-Scan has a high sensitivity and specificity for temporal bone fractures (Fig. 10.13). Even years after the trauma, the fracture line will remain visible on the scan.

Table 10.2 Ossicular chain trauma

Incidence of ossicular chain trauma
1. Incudostapedial joint separation is the most common ossicular injury
2. Incudomalleal dislocation is the second most common ossicular injury
3. Stapes superstructure`s fracture is the third most common ossicular injury
4. Fracture of the malleus is the least common

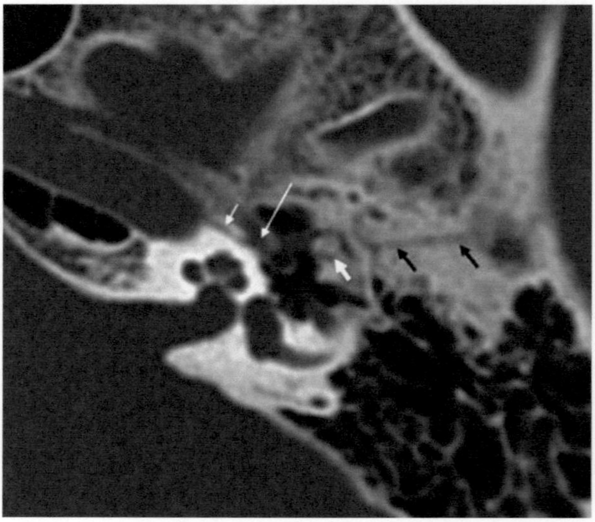

Fig. 10.13 Axial image of a left ear: longitudinal fracture line (black arrows) passing through the incudo-malleal joint space (white arrow) with separation of the incus head and the malleus head, then typically passing through the facial nerve canal (slim long arrow) and irradiating into the petrous carotid canal (small arrow)

10.6.1 Incudostapedial Dislocation

10.6.1.1 Clinics

Incudostapedial dislocation is the most common post-traumatic abnormality of the ossicular chain owing to the tenuous suspension of the incus between the firmly anchored malleus and stapes [13, 14].

Another mechanism for disruption of the incudostapedial joint has been postulated: The stapedius tendon most often attaches to the neck of the stapes near the incudostapedial joint, the tendon for the tensor tympani muscle is fixing the neck of the malleus, a tetanic contraction of these tendons as a result of severe head injury causes medial thrust traction of the incus and concomitant posterior puffing of the head of the stapes, resulting in incudostapedial joint disruption [15].

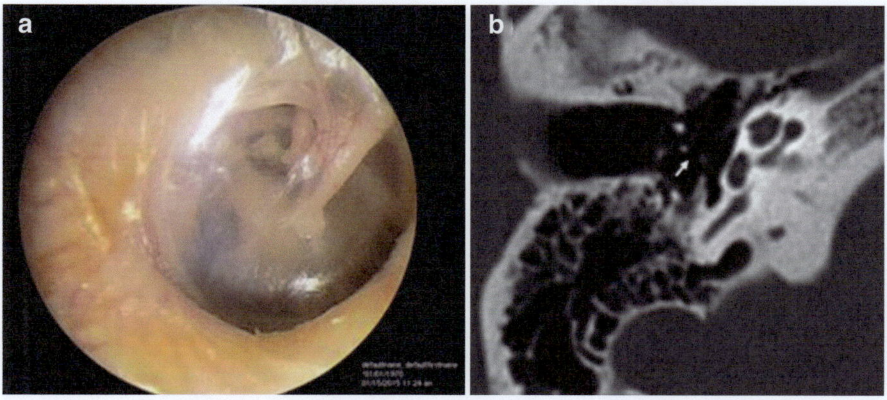

Fig. 10.14 (**a**) Right ear otoscopy showing discontinuity of the incudostapedial joint (arrow). (**b**) Axial CT-image: large diastasis of the incudo-stapedial joint (arrow)

At surgical exploration, Hough and Stuart found incudostapedial joint separation in 82.3% of cases of ossicular chain traumatic injuries [14].

10.6.1.2 CT-Imaging

On axial CT scans or oblique reconstructions, disruption of the incudostapedial joint appears as an abnormal enlargement of the dark cleft between the head of the stapes and the long process of the incus (Fig. 10.14).

10.6.2 Incudomalleolar Discontinuity

10.6.2.1 Clinics

The incudomalleolar joint, a saddle-shaped diarthrodial articulation, is protected in the epitympanum. The malleus is the most firmly attached ossicle; it is secured by the tympanic membrane, anterior and lateral malleal ligaments, and tensor tympani muscle and tendon. In cases of trauma, the malleus usually stays in place or moves slightly. On the contrary, the incus, which is the heavier ossicle (25 mg), has no muscular anchor and has the weakest soft-tissue attachment of the ossicles. The displacement of the incus can be moderate or severe.

10.6.2.2 CT-Imaging

The incudomalleolar disarticulation is well visualized on axial CT images, that show the diastasis between the head of the malleus (the "scoop of ice cream") and the body and short process of the incus (the "cone", Fig. 10.15a), or even a complete luxation of the head of the malleus out of the articulation (Fig. 10.15b).

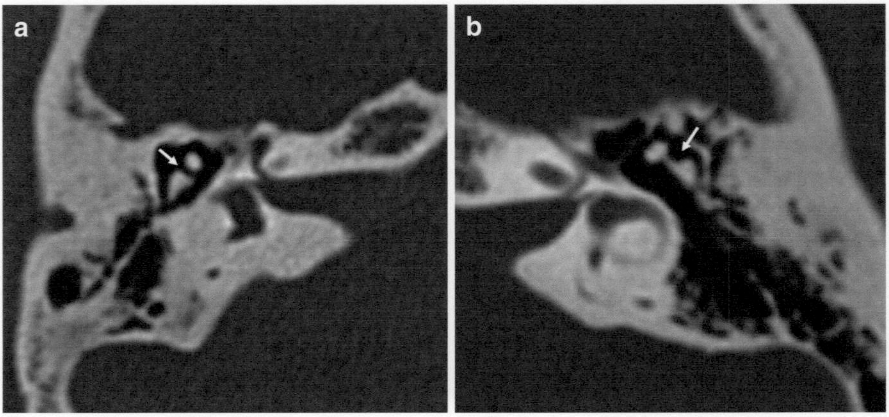

Fig. 10.15 Axial images of the (**a**) right ear and (**b**) left ear: (**a**) Post-traumatic diastasis of the incudomalleal joint (arrow). (**b**) Post-traumatic incudo-malleolar joint disjunction with luxation

10.6.3 Dislocation of the Incus

10.6.3.1 Clinics

The position of the heavy, weakly anchored incus between the firmly anchored malleus and the stapes, makes it relatively more vulnerable to traumatic dislocation [14]. After severe skull trauma, the incus may be dislocated due to its inertia [16], when incudomalleolar joint separation is associated to incudostapedial joint separation or a fracture of the stapes.

The incus may be displaced into the epitympanic recess or prolapsed into the lower part of the tympanic cavity (Fig. 10.16).

10.6.4 Stapedio-vestibular Dislocation

10.6.4.1 Clinics

Stapedio-vestibular dislocation is an uncommon injury because the annular ligament attaches firmly the stapes to the oval window. This happens frequently with associated lesion of the eardrum secondary to a strong hand splash trauma and a stapedio-vestibular joint dislocation; a perilymph fistula may result.

10.6.5 Fracture of the Malleus

Fracture of the malleus is rare, usually situated at the neck or the manubrium due to a direct traumatic impact; this fracture is usually associated with other severe damages. Depending of the fracture site, oblique reformations through the long axis of the malleus may demonstrate the fracture line (Fig. 10.17).

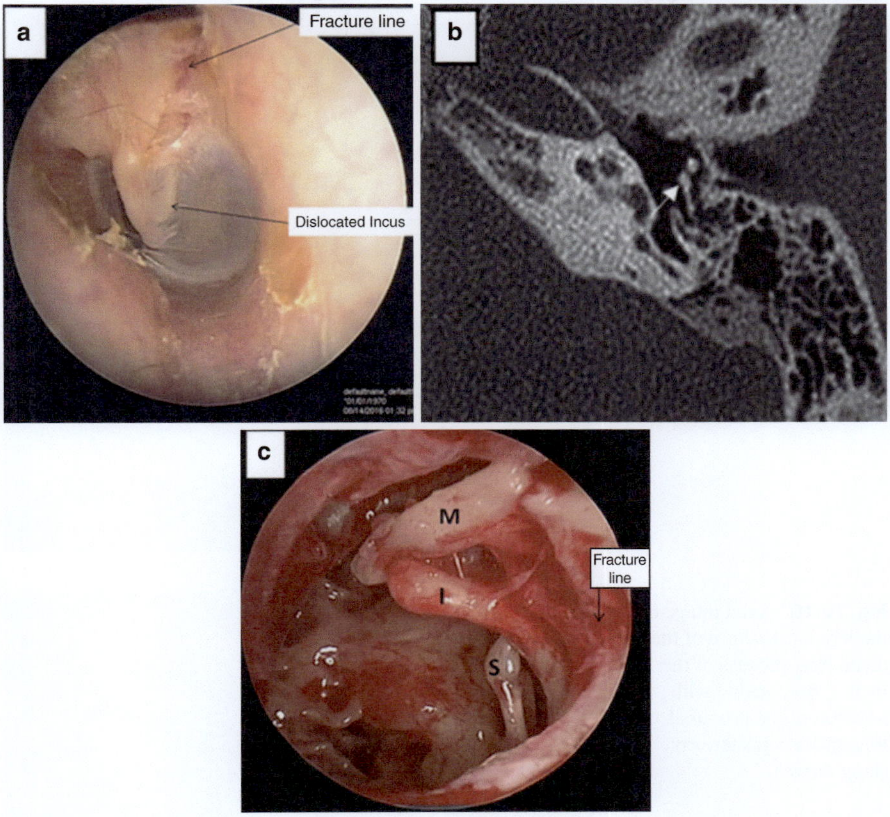

Fig. 10.16 (**a**) Left ear otoscopy showing traumatic luxation of the incus; (**b**) axial CT-image of a left ear with incus luxation (white arrow) posteriorly fallen in the facial nerve recess and incudomalleolar disarticulation. (**c**) Intraoperative view showing luxation of incus (I) which is prolapsed into the tympanic cavity. *M* malleus; *S* stapes

10.6.6 Fracture of the Incus

The fracture affects mainly the long or lenticular process. Axial, coronal, or reformatted images through the axis of the long process allow the diagnosis of this injury, often with luxation of the broken part (Fig. 10.18).

10.6.7 Fracture of the Stapes

10.6.7.1 Clinics

Fracture of the arch of the stapes occurs secondary to torsion. Fracture of the footplate mainly occurs secondary to transverse fractures (translabyrinthine fractures) passing

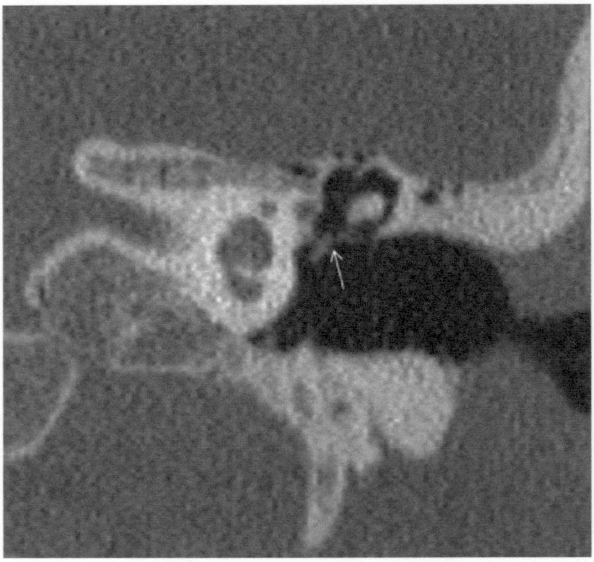

Fig. 10.17 Fracture of the malleus neck (arrow)

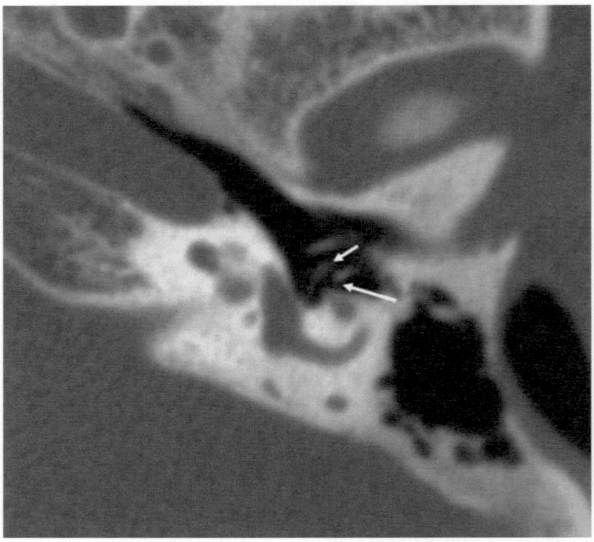

Fig. 10.18 Axial image of the left ear: fracture of the distal long process of the incus (short arrow) with luxation of the proximal long process posteriorly (long arrow)

through the oval window (Fig. 10.19). A fracture of the footplate (with or without displacement of the fragments) may cause a perilymph fistula with pneumolabyrinth.

10.6.7.2 CT-Imaging

Fracture of the crura is often difficult to visualize due to the tiny aspect of the crura (Fig. 10.20). The best plane to analyse the crura and the footplate is on the reconstructed stapes plan (see Chap. 11). In cases of fracture of both crura, the footplate stays in place, but there is a loss of continuity between the crura and the footplate.

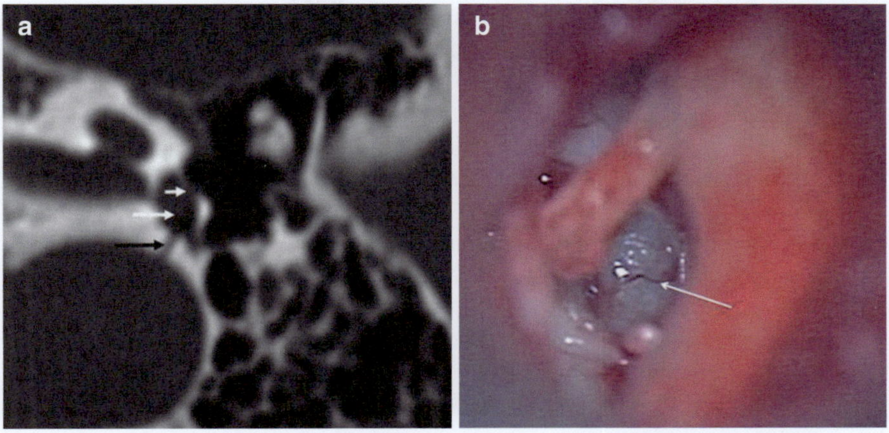

Fig. 10.19 Transversal fracture through the left ear: (**a**) on a reconstructed CT-image the fracture line is crossing the anterior bony ridge of the jugular foramen (black arrow), passing by the round window (long white arrow) and the oval window (short white arrow) (**b**) middle ear exploration showing fracture of the footplate (white arrow)

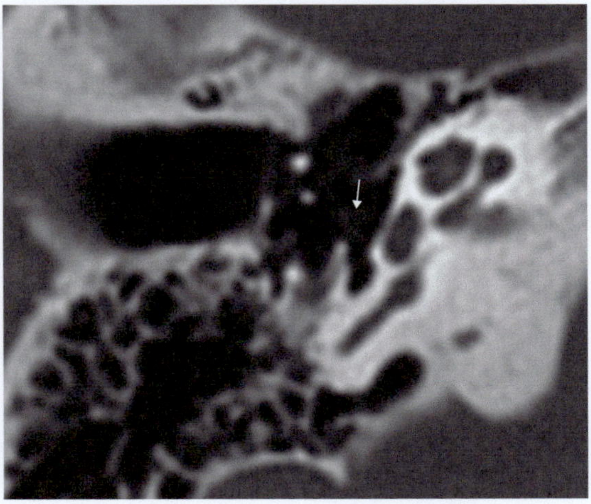

Fig. 10.20 Fracture of the anterior stapedial crus (arrow)

This may be difficult to be recognized in an acute trauma, when the fracture is most often associated to a hemotympanum.

10.6.7.3 Surgery

During middle ear exploration, the ossicular chain and the footplate are mobile and the crura fracture can be difficult to identify. In such cases, endoscopy or anteroposterior palpation of the crura are helpful for the diagnosis.

10.7 Conductive Hearing Loss with a Normal Appearing Tympanic Membrane and Vertigo and Tullio Phenomenon

Conductive hearing loss in a patient with vertigo and Tullio phenomenon should evoke the diagnosis of third window pathology.

The cochleovestibular system has 2 functional windows. The oval window, which houses the footplate of the stapes and allows sound to enter the scala vestibuli and the round window which allows release pressure and mechanical energy from the scala tympani.

Stapes movements normally would cause pressure in the scala tympani. This would be transmitted across the basilar membrane to be relieved at the round window membrane. With a third window connected to the scala vestibuli, for example by superior canal dehiscence, stapes movement induced perilymph pressure becomes instead channeled through this low impedance pathway.

This results in pressure release through the third window, with less energy left to move the basilar membrane with resultant hearing loss. This fluid flow also results in the movement of the SCC cupula, and in an inappropriate stimulation of the rotation sensing vestibular structure by this acoustic energy.

This is why third-window lesions must be considered in the differential diagnosis of CHL with an intact tympanic membrane. They can mimic otosclerosis and may lead to an incorrect diagnosis and even to a non-successful stapedectomy [3]. CT is the first method of choice to search for the bony dehiscence. MRI is valuable to demonstrate the contact of the dura with the labyrinthine membrane.

10.7.1 Dehiscence of the Superior Semicircular Canal (SSCD)

Superior semicircular canal dehiscence (SSCD) is a bony defect of the otic capsule at the apex of the superior semicircular canal (SSC). Whilst such a defect is identifiable in up to 9% of temporal bones on CT, it is estimated that only 0.1% of the general population have symptoms or signs related to it.

The true aetiology remains unknown; originally it was thought to be triggered by trauma or barotrauma but it is now thought to be related to gradual thinning of bone of the middle cranial fossa over the SSC, although in most patients there is no definite date of onset. SSCD affects both ears in about 25% of patients, also consistent with congenital predisposition [17].

10.7.1.1 Physiopathology and Biomechanics

The contact between middle cranial fossa dura and the inner membranous tissue of the SSC results in a lower impedence in the vestibular system allowing for vestibular stimulation following pressure and sound transmission in addition acoustic energy is lost via the SSC dehiscence thus it is shunted away from the cochlea with a resulting loss of conductive hearing. Also pressure difference across cochlear partition is more than normal results in an improved threshold of bone conduction. This is called ‘pathologic third window’ in the otic capsule.

10.7.1.2 Clinics

The clinical features associated with SSCD were described for the first time in 1998 by Minor et al. [18]. This syndrome of 'pathologic third window' in the otic capsule manifests by:

- *Vestibular manifestations*: Most commonly seen are oscillopsia or true vertigo following loud noises (Tullio phenomenon) or pressure in the ear canal (Hennebert's sign). Some patients present with a chronic dysequilibrium that does not appear to be the result of sound or pressure. Pressure difference across cochlear partition is more than normal.
- *Auditory manifestations*: Autophony or unusual awareness of sounds such as one's heel strike, teeth brushing, chewing, heartbeat or even eye movements. Typically patients with cochlear manifestations of SSCD hear internal body sounds but don't hear external sounds (hearing loss). Also pulsatile tinnitus is reported.
- *Clinical examination* reveals normal otoscopy. Valsalva may result in nystagmus and acute vertigo. The nystagmus is usually in the direction of stimulation of the SSC and is usually torsional and in an upward direction. Rinne test is negative and Weber lateralizes to affected ear. A tuning fork held on the ankle may travel up the body, and be heard in the affected ear. This is generally best tested with a 128 Hz tuning fork.
- *Audiogram* shows a mild ABG predominantly in the low frequencies. SSCD patients will have bone conduction thresholds at -5 or -10 dB HL (Fig. 10.2e). Audiologist must look for when the diagnosis is suspected. Preservation of the acoustic reflex in an ear with conductive hearing loss, provides a useful test for differential diagnosis of CHL due to third window pathology: most middle ear pathologies with CHL result in the loss of the acoustic reflex.
- *VEMP testing*: SSCD syndrome may lower the thresholds for VEMP in the affected ear. In SSCD syndrome, there is a 'path of at least resistance' that shunts acoustic energy through the vestibular labyrinth rather than through the cochlea. This typically yields a 20 dB lowered VEMP threshold (70 dB compared with 95 dB) (Fig. 10.5). Moreover, VEMP thresholds are concordant with symptoms, therefore helping in the differential diagnosis in selecting the most affected ear for surgery in cases of bilaterally SSCD.
- *Electrocochleography (ECoG)*: Arts et al. identified that patients with SSCD consistently have elevations in the summating potential (SP) to action potential (AP) ratio, and that this abnormality corrects after surgical plugging of the affected canal [19].

10.7.1.3 CT-Imaging

The SSCD syndrome is the best documented and most investigated third-window lesion of the inner ear. CT scan has a sensitivity and negative predictive value of 100% for SSCD, independent of the CT techniques used (former 1 mm collimation versus newer 0.5 mm collimation). The advanced 0.5 mm collimation raises the specificity up to 96% and the positive predictive value up to 93% for SSCD [20].

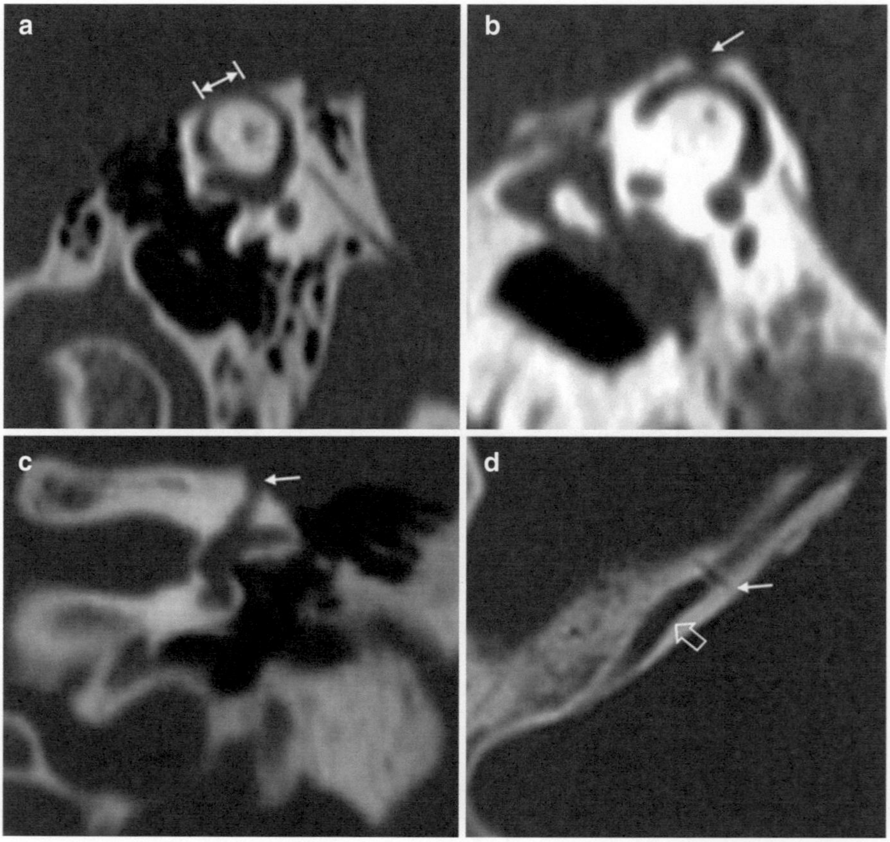

Fig. 10.21 (**a**) CT reconstruction along the Poeschl plane (see Chap. 11), showing the whole SSCC on one image and permit to measure the length of the dehiscence. (**b**) Same reconstruction plane as in a), dehiscence of the SSCC into the superior petrous venous sinus (SPVS) (arrow) (**c**) in this patient, a simple coronal reconstruction is already diagnostic for the SSCC (arrow) (**d**) typical aspect on the axial image of the dehiscence of the SSCC (arrow) in the SPVS (empty arrow)

A SSCD is characterized by a focal loss of bone that covers the superior canal, creating a close contact between the lumen of the canal and the cranial cavity, or between the canal and the sinus of the superior petrous vein (SPVS) (see Fig. 10.21) [21].

On routine CT-Scan, the SSCC is first analyzed on the standard coronal plane: if the bony coverage is visible, the diagnosis of dehiscence is excluded with a negative predictive value of 100%; no supplementary reconstructions are needed.

When axial and coronal views suggest a possible dehiscence, complementary reconstructions are needed along *the Poeschl plan* parallel to the SSCC, that reduce the partial volume effects and allow in optimized conditions visualization of layers of bone as thin as 0.1 mm [22, 23]. The perpendicular plane, *the Stenvers plan* displays the superior cortex of the SSCC in a perfect cross-section (see Chap. 11). It has also a negative predictive value of 100%, when the bony coverage is well visualized in this plane [24].

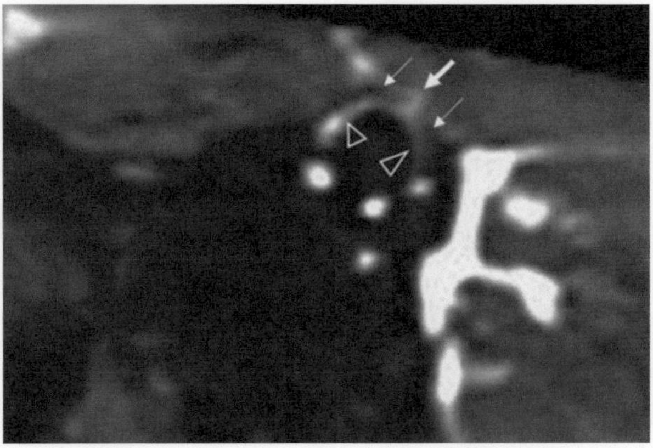

Fig. 10.22 T2 weighted CISS MRI with reconstruction in the plane of the superior semicircular canal (empty arrowheads): absence of bone and a close contact between the dura and the labyrinthine membrane (thick white arrow), in contrast to the adjacent labyrinthine bone wall (thin arrows)

If the supplementary reconstructions confirm a dehiscence, the length of the deficient bony cover should be measured to be able to differentiate between an insignificant dehiscence (inferior to 2 mm) and a relevant dehiscence above 6 mm that may eventually be the subject for a surgical repair (Fig. 10.21a, b).

When SSCD dehiscence is diagnosed by CT, MRI is used to confirm the intimate contact between the Dura and the labyrinthine membrane (Fig. 10.22).

10.7.1.4 Management

Management depends on the type of symptoms and their severity.

Most patients have mild symptoms and may be managed conservatively in the knowledge that there is no serious pathology present.

In patients with disequilibrium related to loud sounds, avoidance and the use of earplugs is recommended.

Only when patients are severely affected by disabling vestibular symptoms or severe autophony should surgery be contemplated:

Canal Plugging and Resurfacing:

- The aim of surgery is to either cover the defect or to obliterate the SSC. Resurfacing consists of covering the defect by a cartilage or a ship of bone, however such montage may migrate under the pulsation of the brain and symptoms may recur after few months. Obliteration consists of plugging of the two arms of the canal by bone wax and is safe for inner ear function and give long lasting stable resolution of symptoms.
- The best approach to the SSC is through middle cranial fossa which offers better visualization and obliteration of the deshisence (Fig. 10.23).
- The transmastoid approach is an alternative when the tegmen is high, such situation is an exception because in most of the SSCD cases the tegmen hangs low.
- Postoperatively, resolution of symptoms is immediate and is achieved in more than 90% of cases. SSC surgery is associated with a low risk of sensorineural hearing loss.

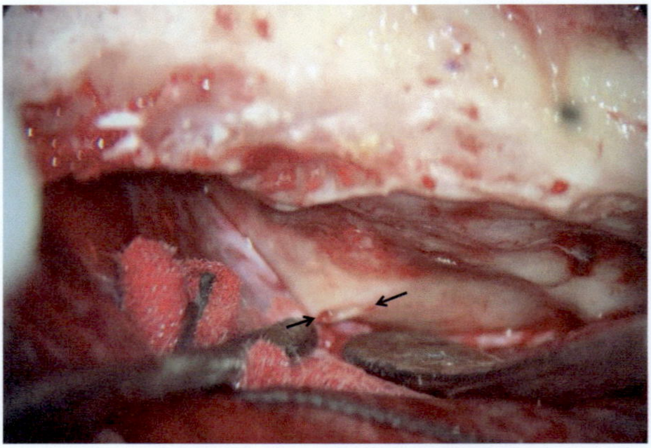

Fig. 10.23 Left side middle cranial fossa approach showing significant dehiscence of the left superior semicircular canal (between the two black arrows)

Round Window Procedures:

– Consists of a procedure to reinforce the round window membrane by a variety of methods as an attempt to dampen SSCD symptoms [25] Nevertheless, inner ear biomechanics would suggest, that these approaches should exacerbate vertigo, by shunting acoustic energy preferentially across vestibular sensory epithelia. The reported relief was transient; furthermore, occlusion of the round window is thought to induce a hearing loss [26].

10.7.2 Dehiscence of the PSCC and LSCC

Dehiscence of the PSCC follows the same pathophysiology as SSCD. The dehiscence in these cases is observed between the canal and the posterior cranial cavity or the jugular bulb [20, 27–29]. It could be an unnoticed complication of an endolymphatic sac decompression surgery.

Dehiscence of the LSCC is much more frequently observed in the presence of an eroding pathology of the middle ear cavity (cholesteatoma) where other causes for a conductive hearing loss are more obvious (see section 9.8.1 in chapter 9).

10.7.3 Large Vestibular Aqueduct

The enlarged vestibular aqueduct was first discovered by Mondini in 1791, during a temporal bone dissection [30].

The enlarged vestibular aqueduct syndrome is associated with Pendred's syndrome and with mutations in the SLC26A4 (PDS) gene.

The enlarged vestibular aqueduct is the most common inner ear anomaly found on radiographic evaluation of children with hearing loss.

10.7.3.1 Clinics

The spectrum of enlarged vestibular aqueduct hearing loss ranges from complete deafness in early childhood to stable hearing well into adult life.

All three types of hearing loss (sensorineural, mixed, and conductive) have been reported in the condition.

Pure conductive hearing loss is by far the least common type in all studies reported.

Although some investigators describe sensorineural hearing loss in the majority of patients, some believe that nearly all patients with enlarged vestibular aqueduct have an airbone gap, particularly at the lower frequencies [31–33]. The conductive component of the hearing loss observed in ears with an enlarged vestibular aqueduct is thought to be due to a decompression of the energy through the enlarged connection between the aqueduct and the vestibule [34].

Many investigators have noted that a significant number of enlarged vestibular aqueduct patients lose some or all of their hearing with certain events, mainly head trauma. The head trauma need not to be severe. In addition to head trauma, some investigators have also linked barotrauma (including Valsalva), upper respiratory tract infections, noise trauma, and physical exercise to hearing loss.

The natural history of the acute trauma induced hearing loss is quite variable, with some patients having full recovery while other patients have persistent hearing loss without improvement.

Currently, there is no valid method to predict what a patient's hearing will be in the years to come.

10.7.3.2 Imaging

The vestibular aqueduct is large, when its mid portion shows a diameter superior of 2 mm. The origin of the vestibular aqueduct is almost always thin (Fig. 10.24).

The large vestibular aqueduct may be an isolated finding in patients with conductive hearing loss, or can be part of a Mondini malformation mainly of type IP II (Fig. 10.25a). Exceptionally there may be coexistence between Mondini and otosclerosis (Fig. 10.25b).

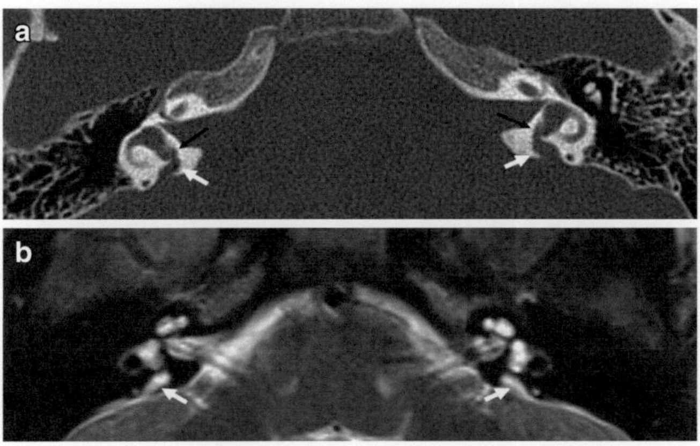

Fig. 10.24 (**a**) Axial CT-image showing a bilaterally symmetrically enlarged vestibular aqueduct (white arrows); the origin of the vestibular aqueduct on the lateral border of the vestibule is always thin (black arrows). (**b**) The corresponding T2 weighted CISS MR-image on an axial plane, showing the bilateral dilatation of the mid and distal portion of the vestibular aqueducts on both sides

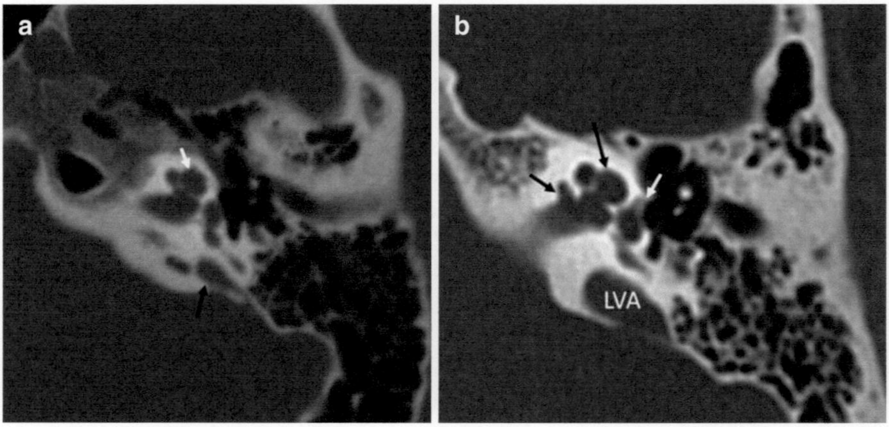

Fig. 10.25 Axial images of ears with conductive hearing loss. (**a**) Mondini malformation type IP II with lack of **partition** between the 2nd and third cochlear turn (white arrow) and LVA (black arrow). (**b**) Mondini malformation IP II with lack of partition of the 2nd and third cochlear turn (long arrow) with LVA, associated to otosclerosis with a typical fenestral focus (white arrow) and a typical focus in contact with the anterior border of the internal auditory canal (short black arrow)

10.7.3.3 Management

We recommend for LVA patients avoiding contact sports and avoiding activities that might provoke a barotrauma such as scuba diving, sneezing with the nose pinched closed, straining when going to the bathroom, weight lifting, and other similar activities. The natural history of the disease is known to have a high incidence of spontaneous recovery after fluctuations in hearing. Corticosteroids are often used to treat sudden drop in hearing in patients with LVA. Endolymphatic sac surgery has been attempted to improve or even stabilize hearing in patients with enlarged vestibular aqueducts. In 1989, Jackler reviewed this very supposition and concluded that endolymphatic sac shunt surgery is contraindicated in the disorder after four of seven patients he operated on had a significant early decline in hearing thresholds on postoperative follow-up evaluation [35]. Welling, in 1999, had similar results, performing endolymphatic sac occlusion on 10 patients, with 9 patients having some degree of additional hearing loss after the procedure [36]. Hearing rehabilitation with hearing aids or cochlear implantation remain the mainstays of treatment.

10.7.4 Dehiscence Between Cochlea and Carotid Canal

Kim and Wilson [37] described a patient with an air-bone gap that persisted after uneventful stapedectomy and even after revision; this patient was found to have a dehiscence between the cochlea and the carotid canal on retrospective reexamination of his CT-images. They concluded that the present dehiscence between the cochlea and the carotid canal may act as a third window, dissipating the acoustic energy away from the cochlear partition [37] (Fig. 10.26).

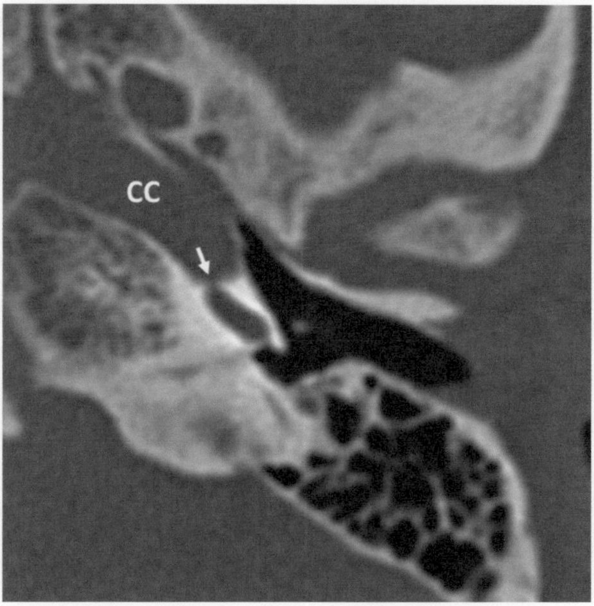

Fig. 10.26 Axial image of the left ear, showing a dehiscence of the basal cochlear turn (arrow) into the carotid canal (CC)

10.7.5 Paget Disease of the Temporal Bone and Third Window Phenomenon

This is rare. Patients with extensive Pagetic involvement of the otic capsule typically present a mixed hearing loss with an air-bone gap in the lower frequencies. It is hypothesized that the microfractures and/or Pagetic bone surrounding the cochlea act as a third window dissipating the sound energy transmitted through the stapes footplate away from the cochlea. [38, 39].

10.8 Conductive Hearing Loss with a Retrotympanic Effusion or a Mass behind a Normal Appearing Tympanic Membrane

Any fluid or soft tissue formation in the middle ear can affect the columellar effect of the ossicular chain and lead to a conductive hearing loss.

10.8.1 Middle Ear Effusion

10.8.1.1 Clinics

In certain cases, serous otitis media could be missed despite a good microscopic otoscopy. The most common cause of fluid in the middle ear is secretory otitis media, a common condition that induces a conductive hearing loss (tympanogram shows a type B curve) (Fig. 10.27).

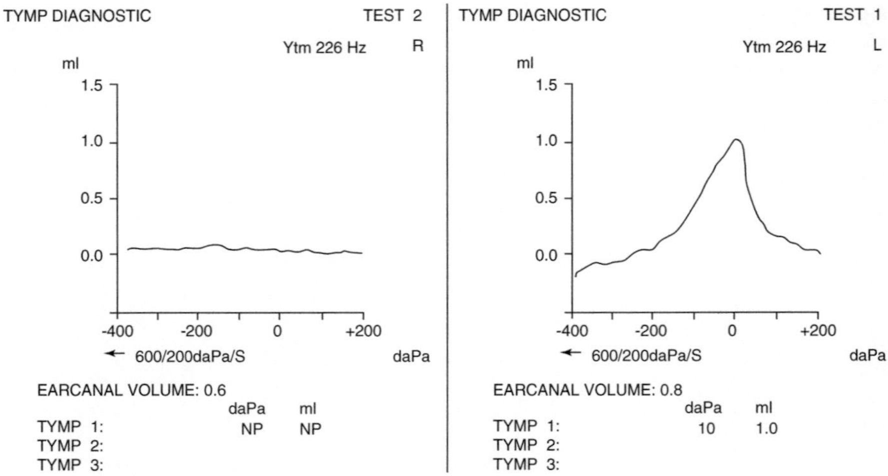

Fig. 10.27 Patient with a right glue ear, left ear is normal; Tympanometry showing curve type B in the right ear and curve type A in left ear

Careful examination of the tympanic membrane shows a mildly retracted ear drum with loss of translucency, and fluid may, or may not be seen and some times air-fluid level or air bubbles (Fig. 10.35). This is why in cases of CHL the tympanogram is very helpful to do the positive diagnosis.

10.8.1.2 CT-Imaging

In some occasions with suspected CSF fluid filling the middle ear cavity, presenting the same clinical picture as ME effusion, CT imaging is valuable to look for the etiological diagnosis.

10.8.2 Masses in the Middle Ear

A soft tissue mass can develop in the epitympanum or the hypotympanum behind a normal eardrum and progress to affect the columellar effect of the ossicular chain causing CHL. At the beginning, this mass can be hidden in the Middle Ear and it may not be easily seen on otomicroscopy through a normal tympanic membrane.

At this stage, CT scan is the only tool to show the existing mass causing the CHL. Some associated symptoms such as pulsatile tinnitus may orient the clinical suspicion of the diagnosis. Nevertheless when the mass becomes visible behind an intact eardrum, its aspect becomes more indicative for the cause of the CHL

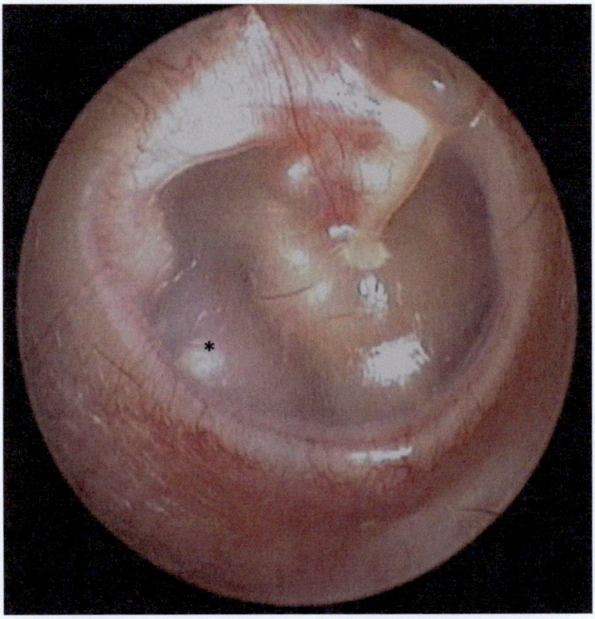

Fig. 10.28 Right ear otoscopy showing high jugular bulb (*) obliterating the round window and causing mild conductive hearing loss

Table 10.3 Typical locations of different ME masses

Retrotympanic mass	Indicative for
Anterosuperiorly	Congenital cholesteatoma
Posteroinferiorly	Paraganglioma or high jugular bulb
Posterosuperiorly	Meningoencephalocele or facial nerve schwannoma

(Fig. 10.28). The most common pathologies that are expected, depending on their location behind the tympanic membrane, are shown in Table 10.3:

10.8.3 Congenital Cholesteatoma

10.8.3.1 Clinics

Congenital cholesteatoma is most frequently arising from residual embryogenic epidermoid formations in the anterior mesotympanum. It is more frequently seen behind an intact antero-superior quadrant of the tympanic membrane (Fig. 10.29). But a congenital cholesteatoma may occupy the anterior epitympanic recess being not visible behind a normal appearing tympanic membrane and causing conductive hearing loss when it comes in contact with the ossicular chain or after eroding parts of the ossicles (Fig. 10.30).

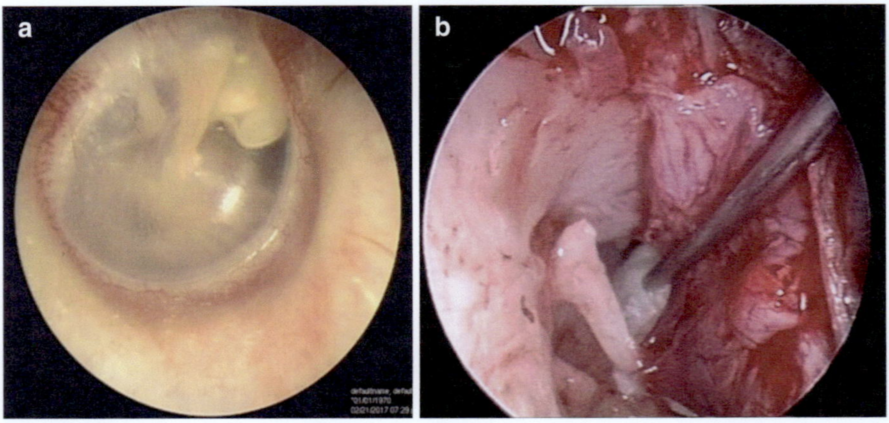

Fig. 10.29 (**a**) Right ear congenital cholesteatoma of the anterosuperior quadrant, (**b**) Intraoperative endoscopic removal

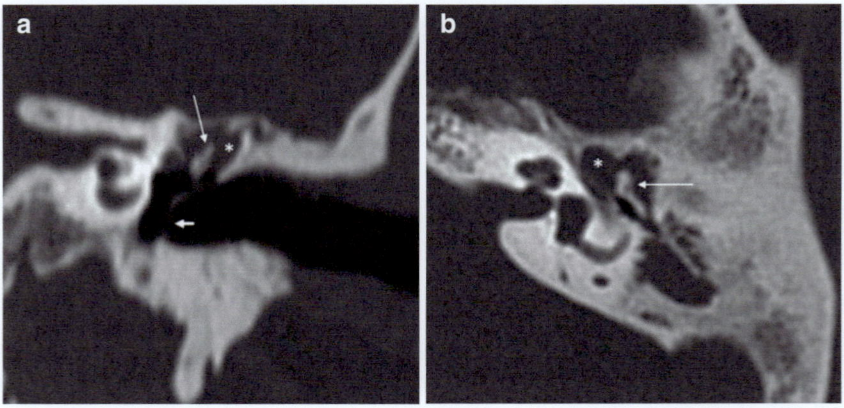

Fig. 10.30 Congenital cholesteatoma: (**a**) coronal CT reconstruction showing an intact tympanic membrane (short arrow), attic condensation (*) and advanced erosion of the incus (long arrow). (**b**) Axial CT image showing a completely condensated AER (*), absence of the cog and lytic signs of the incus (long arrow)

The diagnosis should be done before its aggressive extension that may later invade the facial nerve causing facial palsy with an unfavorable prognosis and an absence of recovery even after adequate surgical treatment (see chapter 8).

10.8.3.2 CT-Imaging

On CT-Scan, cholesteatoma is always suspected whenever there is erosion of the cog, the ossicles or the different osseous borders of the cavity (Fig. 10.30).

10.8.4 Paraganglioma

10.8.4.1 Clinics

A glomus tympanicum is classically seen along the fibers of the tympanic plexus on the cochlear promontory (Fig. 10.31). When it is still small in size, it may stay confined to its initial localisation, however with time it comes into contact with the ossicular chain and causes CHL.

10.8.4.2 CT-Imaging

On CT, paragangliomas are strongly enhancing, when injected (Fig. 10.32).

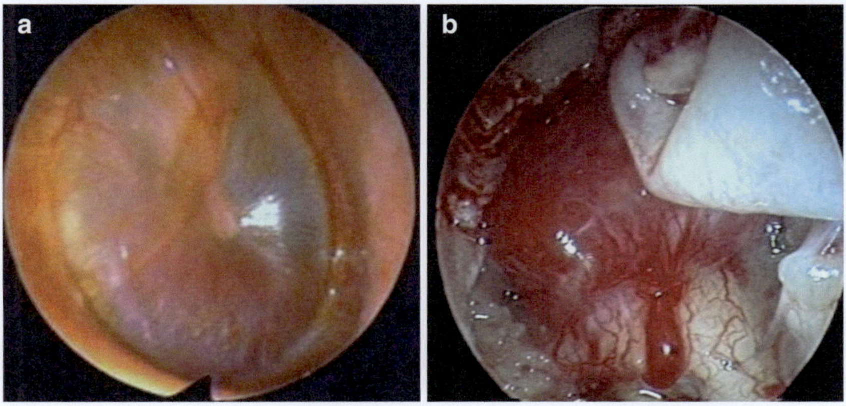

Fig. 10.31 (**a**) Right ear retrotympanic reddish mass in the postero-inferior quadrant suggestive of glomus tumor. (**b**) Intraoperative view of a glomus tympanicum in another patient

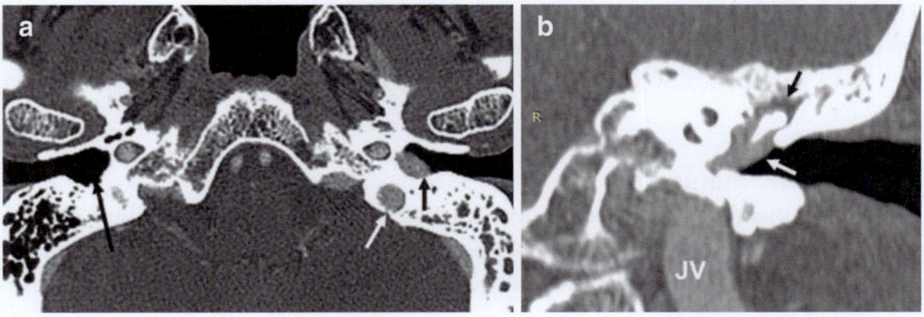

Fig. 10.32 Left glomus tumor. (**a**) Injected axial CT images showing a strongly enhancing hypotympanic mass in the left ear (black short arrow), with a similar enhancement to the jugular vein (white arrow). Normal aerated hypotympanum on the right side (long black arrow) (**b**) injected coronal reconstructions showing the enhancing mass behind the tympanic membrane (white arrow) surrounding the long process of the incus—notice the lower density in the epitympanum corresponding to fluid retention (black arrow)

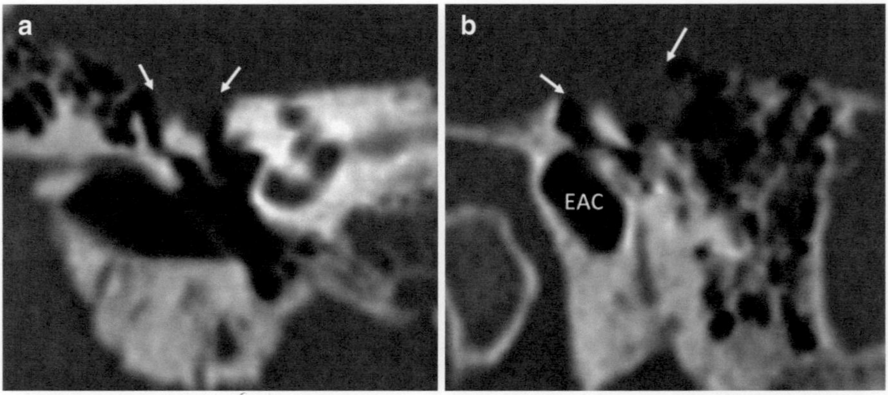

Fig. 10.33 CT scan with coronal reconstruction: (**a**) large dehiscence of the tegmen with herniated soft tissue coming into close contact to the ossicular chain. (**b**) Sagittal reconstruction: the dehiscence of the tegmen is large in the antero-posterior diameter (between the arrows), the herniated tissue comes into close contact to the ossicular chain

10.8.5 Meningoencephalocele

10.8.5.1 Clinics

A dehiscence of the tegmen may be congenital or acquired; the latter being spontaneous or secondary to trauma, infection, cholesteatoma, and/or previous surgery. One complication of the tegmen dehiscence is a meningoencephalocele, a condition that leads to a hearing loss due to the mass effect of herniated tissue onto the ossicles (Figs. 10.33 and 10.34).

10.8.5.2 CT-Imaging

On CT both sagittal and coronal oblique reformats are helpful for assessment of the degree of dehiscence of the tegmen, as well as the mass effect of herniated tissue (Fig. 10.33).

10.8.5.3 MR Imaging

An MRI is mandatory to characterize showing isointense signal with the cerebral tissues in continuity with the cerebral cavity the content of the herniated tissue, that is almost always a meningoencephalocele, and to assess its limits relative to the middle ear structures (Fig. 10.34).

10.8.6 Schwannoma of the Facial Nerve

10.8.6.1 Clinics

A facial nerve schwannoma can expand the canal and impinge on the stapes resulting in a conductive hearing loss [40, 41]. Facial paralysis will raise suspicion of the

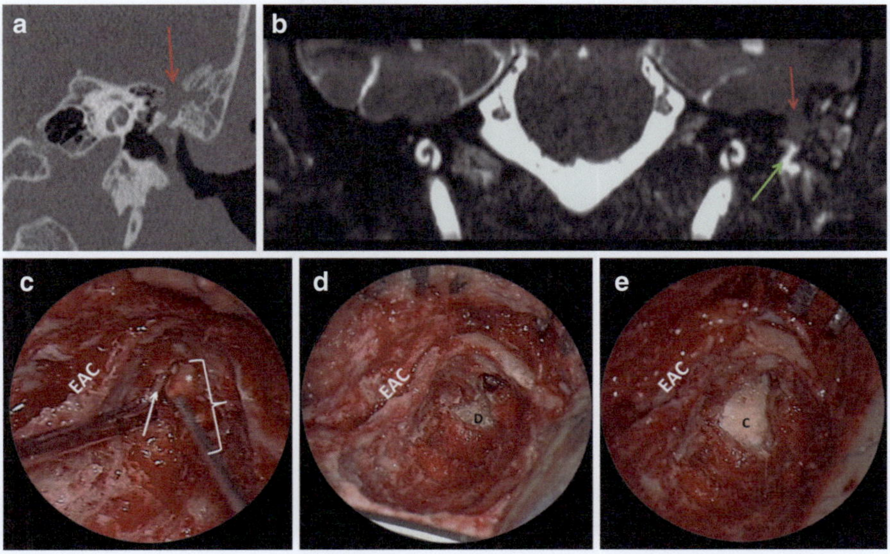

Fig. 10.34 A case of left ear menigoencapholcele in a patient who presented with CHL and normal tympanic membrane. (**a**) CT scan in coronal plane showing the defect in the tegmen and non specific condensation images (red arrow). (**b**) MRI with coronal reconstruction of CISS sequence showing the encephalocele (red arrow) with equal signal to the cerebral tissue above and fluid in the middle ear (green arrow). (**c**) Intraoperative view during the separation of the encephalocele (*asterisks*) from the incus body (white arrow). (**d**) after reduction of encephalocele the dura is reinforced by a dura patch (D), (**e**) the tegmen defect is reconstructed with cartilage (c) in underlay technique. EAC: external auditory canal.

diagnosis, but facial weakness is not always present with a facial nerve schwannoma; conductive hearing loss may be the only finding.

10.8.6.2 CT-Imaging

CT-Scan is often the first method that may demonstrate a mass effect along the facial nerve (Fig. 10.35). MRI with injection of Gadolinium shows generally a homogeneous uptake after contrast injection.

10.9 Conductive Hearing Loss with a Normal Appearing Tympanic Membrane in Children

The most frequent cause of conductive hearing loss in children is a chronic otitis media with effusion (Fig. 10.36). When hardly recognized by otoscopy, tympanometry is strongly suggestive.

Otherwise a *non-progressive* conductive hearing loss in children detected in the first decade with *normal* tympanometry is mostly often due to congenital anomalies of the middle or inner ear. In contrary, a *progressive* conductive hearing loss reported

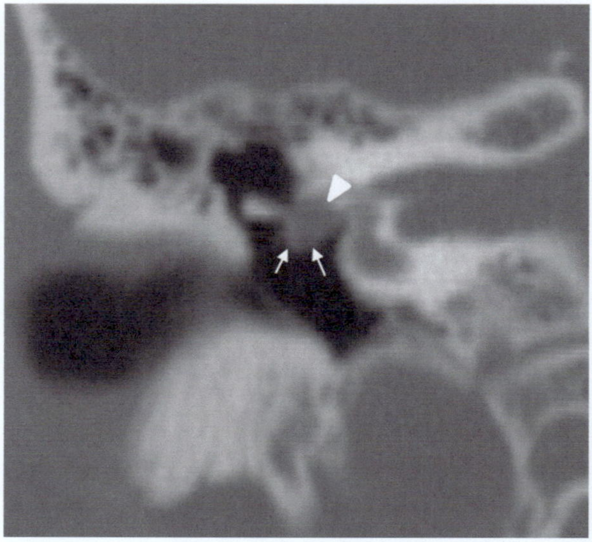

Fig. 10.35 CT with coronal reconstruction of the right ear showing a mass of the tympanic segment of the facial nerve (white arrowhead), with mass effect on the incudostapedial chain (white arrows)

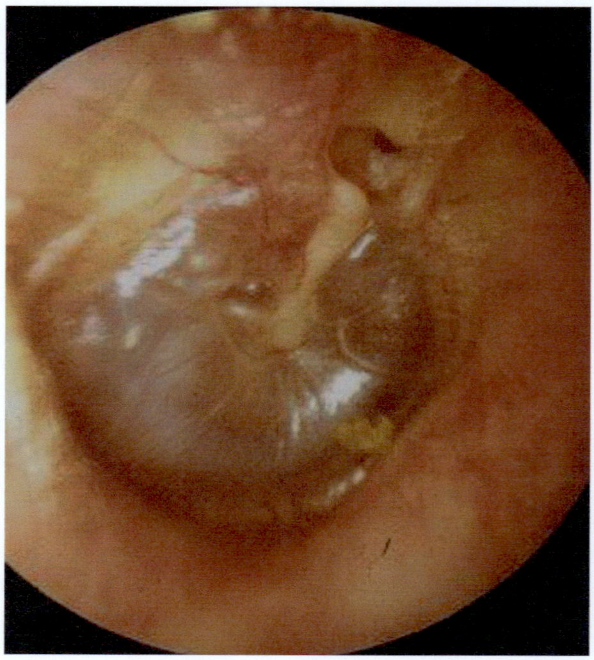

Fig. 10.36 Right middle ear effusion

at the second or third decade of life is mostly due to otosclerosis. Congenital ossicular anomalies can either be isolated or combined with other ear anomalies. In 25% of cases, they are associated to a first or second branchial arch anomalies [42].

The most common isolated ossicular anomalies are stapes ankylosis [43] and incudostapedial discontinuity [44, 45]. In case of fixations, a pneumatic otoscopy may demonstrate a less mobile eardrum, and audiometry may show an absent stapedial reflex and type As tympanometry.

10.9.1 Congenital Stapes Fixation (Stapedio-vestibular Ankylosis)

10.9.1.1 Clinics

Isolated congenital stapes fixation represents 20–35% of ossicular malformations [46–48]. Congenital stapes fixation is due to the absence of development of the annular ligament with a resultant fixation between the peripheral lamina stapedius and the oval window border [49]. The non-progressive nature of conductive hearing loss is an essential clinical argument in favour of the diagnosis.

Clinically, the differential diagnosis of congenital stapes fixation includes other ossicular malformations, congenital otosclerosis, oval window atresia or congenital cholesteatoma [50].

10.9.1.2 CT-Imaging

The annular ligament is not visible on CT-Scan, therefore CT-Scan may be reported completely negative in absence of any otosclerotic focus. In certain cases, congenital stapes fixation can be associated to other ossicular malformations, minor inner ear malformations, especially to anomalies of the semicircular canals (Fig. 10.37).

10.9.2 Congenital Ossicular Discontinuity

10.9.2.1 Clinics

During microscopic otoscopy, when the eardrum is transparent, a defect of the long process of the incus must be always looked for.

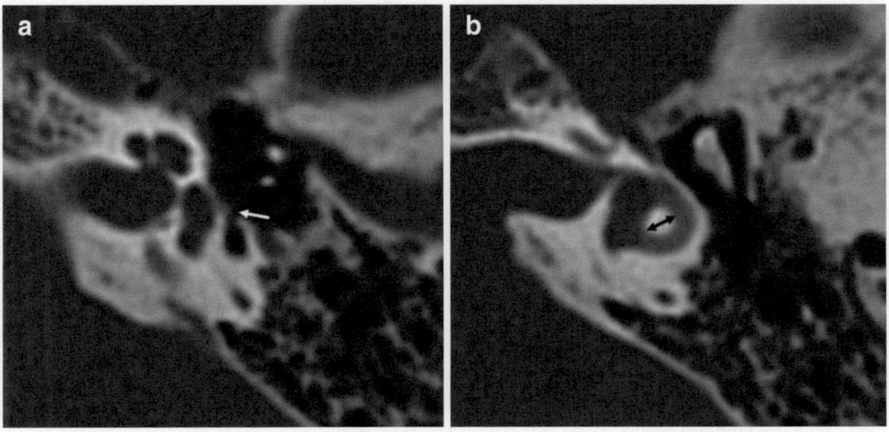

Fig. 10.37 Axial CT images of the left ear: (**a**) Typical posterior thickening of the footplate (white arrow), associated in (**b**) to a minor malformation of the LSCC with a too small bony island (arrow with two heads)

Congenital discontinuity shows most frequently a thin fibrous continuity between the incus and the stapes (Figs. 10.38 and 10.39), in absence of any sign of retraction of the tympanic membrane or an inflammatory process inside the middle ear cavity.

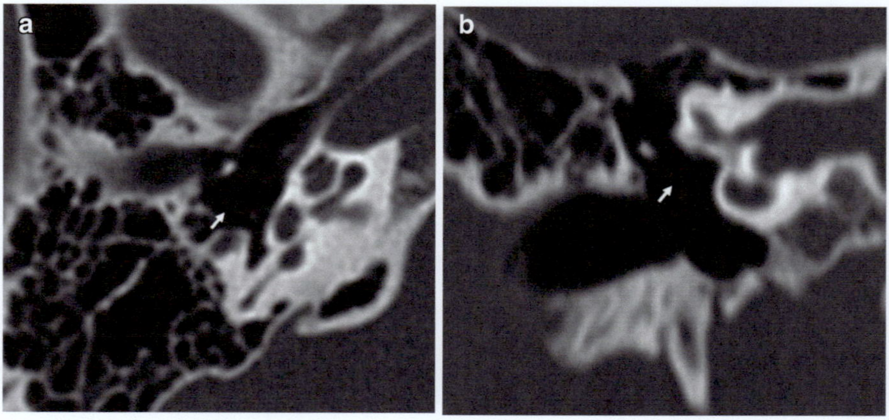

Fig. 10.38 (**a**) Axial CT image of the right ear: Missing long process of the incus (arrow). (**b**) Coronal reconstruction of the right ear: missing long process of the incus (arrow), visibility of a very thin structure in place of the incudostapedial joint

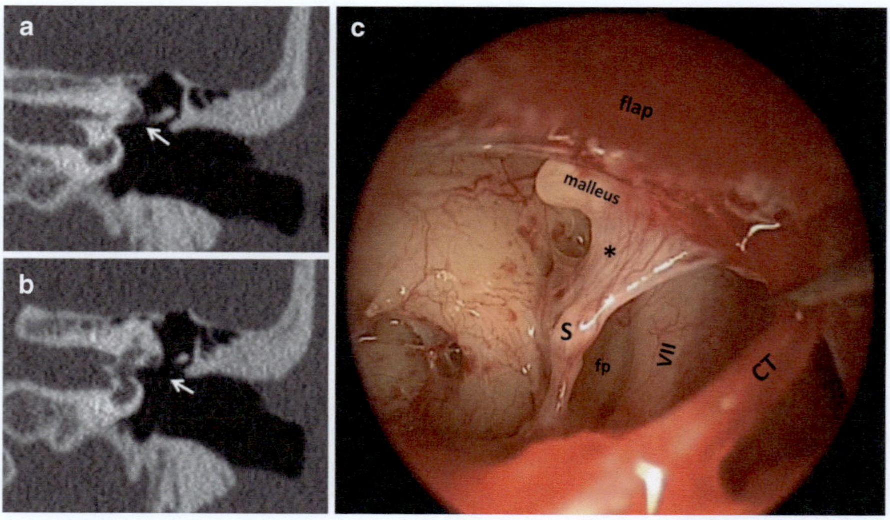

Fig. 10.39 A case of left CHL with normal tympanic membrane. (**a**, **b**) Coronal CT scan shows the absence of the long process of incus. (**c**) Intraoperative view showing the complete absence of the incus which is replaced by a fibrotic band (*) connecting the head of stapes (S) to the malleus; notice that the chorda tympani (CT) is unusually large: Second arch anomaly. VII: facial nerve; *fp* footplate

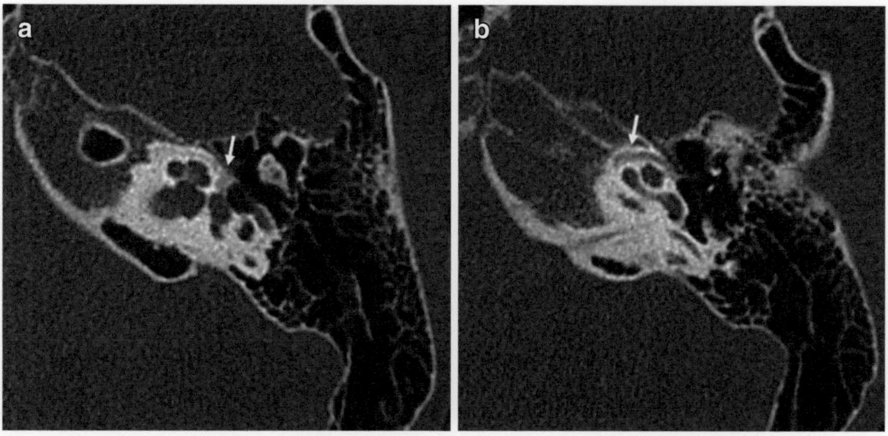

Fig. 10.40 8 years old girl with bilateral conductive hearing loss: axial CT-images of the left ear show (**a**) a typical focus of pre vestibular otosclerosis (arrow), (**b**) a typical peri cochlear hypodensity manifestation of otosclerosis (arrow)

10.9.3 Juvenile Otosclerosis

The most important characteristics of juvenile otosclerosis in children is the *progressive type* of the conductive hearing loss associated to a positive family history (Fig. 10.40), in contrary to the congenital stapes ankylosis with a stable non-progressive deafness.

It is important to differentiate preoperatively between otosclerosis and congenital stapedial fixation, because the postoperative results tend to be inferior in congenital stapedial fixation because of the usually associated minor anomalies of other ear structures. Juvenile otosclerosis in young children has a tendency to progress rapidly to even obliterative forms. Moreover, after stapedotomy and successful closure of the AB Gap, the disease may regrow rapidly and again immobilize the prosthesis in a short or medium period of time postoperatively.

10.9.4 Congenital Ossicular Chain Anomalies

10.9.4.1 Congenital Malleus Fixation

A congenital malleus fixation results from a fusion of the petrosquamous and petrotympanic sutures. The congenital malleus fixation consists in a close bony contact between the malleus or incus and the attic wall (Fig. 10.41a). The impact on hearing of such a malleus head fixation is around 20–25 dB conductive hearing loss. Often the tegmen appears to be abutting the head of the malleus on the axial images; however this relationship is optimally defined in the sagittal plane (Fig. 10.41b).

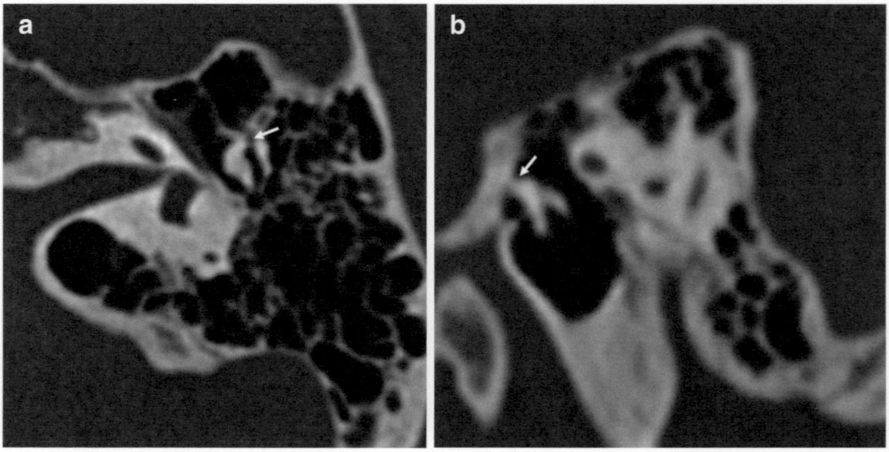

Fig. 10.41 17 years old patient with no previous history of ear drainage or infection who presented with left CHL and normal tympanic membrane. (**a**) Axial CT image of a left ear showing a large and very dense and bar-like fixation of the malleus head to the attic wall (arrow): congenital malleus fixation (**b**) sagittal reconstruction along the malleus axis showing a dense contact between the malleus head and the anterior attic wall (arrow)

Rarely, the fixation contact is established by a persistent bony bridge that connect the malleus handle to the posterior tympanic sulcus; this condition was first described by Nomura in 1998 as the ***malleus bar*** [51].

10.9.4.2 Congenital Incus Fixation

It is a rare finding, the least common congenital ossicular anomaly that may be found during intervention for CHL. There have been few reports in the literature that describe an isolated congenital incus fixation. The incus was reported to be in synostosis to the scutum, to the epitympanum or to the tympanic segment of facial nerve [52–56].

During development of the three ossicles, the incus is the first to start ossification followed by the malleus, and finally the stapes. Its outer endochondral ossification is completed when the Fallopian canal begins its ossification process. Delay in the ossification of the incus may explain the possible fixation of the incus to the tympanic segment of the Fallopian canal during development (Fig. 10.42).

10.9.4.3 Triple Ossicular Fixation

Triple ossicular fixation is per se a very rare entity. Further, association of triple ossicular fixation and inner ear malformations are rarely reported [42] (Fig. 10.43).

The association of ossicular fixation and semicircular canal malformation is reported but the pathogenesis not yet clearly explained, because they do not come from the same embryological origin, but they develop almost at the same time around 6–7 weeks of gestation.

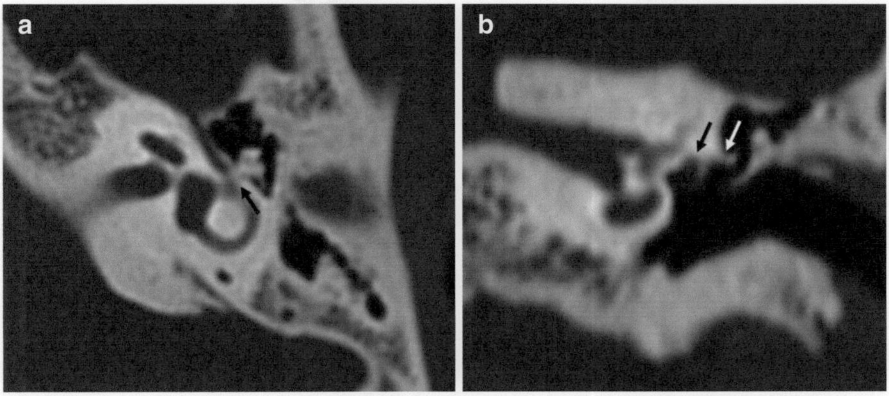

Fig. 10.42 (**a**) Axial CT image of the left ear: fixity of the incus onto the Fallopian canal (arrow). (**b**) Coronal reconstruction left ear: showing the attachment of the incus to the medial attic wall (white arrow) and the Fallopian canal, 2nd portion of the facial nerve (black arrow)

10.9.4.4 Congenital Morphological Anomalies of the Stapes

An increasing number of recent publications report morphologic stapes anomalies other than footplate fixation to be the cause of conductive hearing loss with normal appearing tympanic membrane; nevertheless these dysmorphic stapes are almost always associated with footplate fixation (Figs. 10.44 and 10.45). In the study from Hun Park et al., the authors found numerous malformed shapes of the stapes with a bilaterality in 54% of cases (66 ears); 80% of them were associated to a fixed footplate [57].

10.9.4.5 Congenital Atresia of the Oval Window (CAOW)

Clinics

The oval window is a junctional zone during ear development forming the interface between the middle ear and the inner ear. The embryology of oval window atresia is related directly to the development of second branchial arch structures [58]. When the primitive stapes fails to fuse with the primitive vestibule, the oval window formation is not sufficiently induced, resulting in a congenital absence or aplasia of the oval window (CAOW) and an anomalous stapes is found that is either partial, rudimentary, or even absent [59, 60].

CT-Imaging

On temporal bone HRCT, there is only a very small or even absent opening in the bony plate at the site of the footplate. This may be associated to an anomalous trajectory of the horizontal segment of the facial nerve canal [61] (Figs. 10.46 and 10.47 and 10.48). This entity counts for about 0.5–1.2% of causes for congenital conductive hearing loss [62].

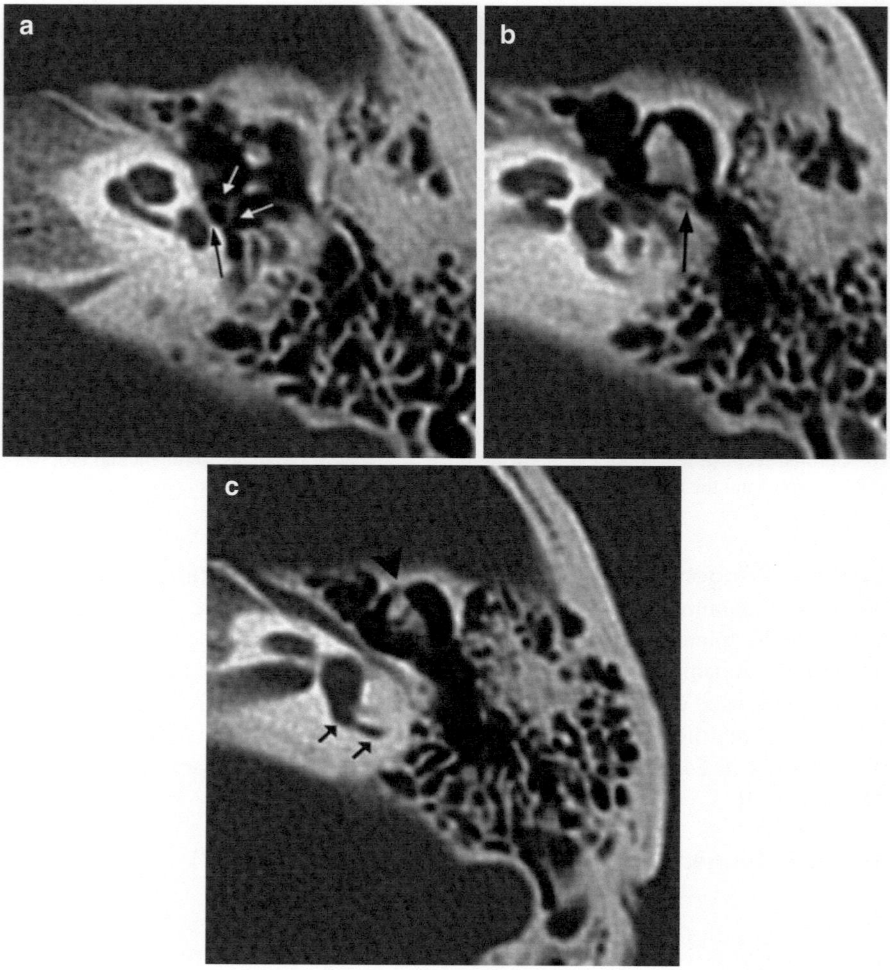

Fig. 10.43 Axial images on the left ear with intraoperatively confirmed triple ossicular fixation. (**a**) a dense and thickened stapes (white arrows) and a dense footplate (black arrow). (**b**) A thick sclerotic plaque on the medial attic wall fixing the incus. (**c**) A thickened ligament fixing the malleus head (arrow head) to the antero-superior attic wall. Notice the associated very small PSCC (small arrows)

10.9.5 DFN-3 (X-Linked Deafness with Stapes Gusher) and Third Window Phenomenon

10.9.5.1 Clinics

DFN-3, a rare pathology selective to male, is characterized by a mixed hearing loss with the occurrence of a **perilymph gusher** upon attempted fenestration of the footplate [37, 63–66]. The air-bone gap is greater in the lower frequencies, and the stapedial reflex may be preserved. Gusher occurs due to the congenital absence of the

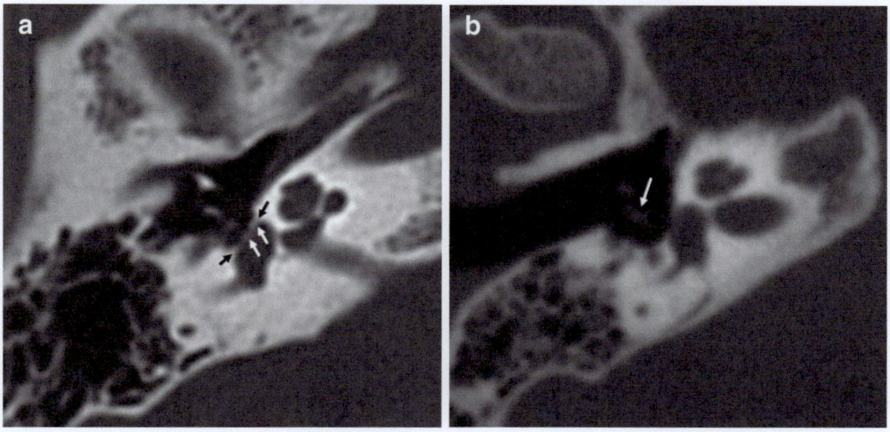

Fig. 10.44 Axial CT images of the right ear of two different patients (**a**) Large oval window (between 2 black arrows), small and tiny stapes crura, inserting in proximity to each other on the footplate (between the two white arrows); (**b**) enlarged stapes head (arrow)

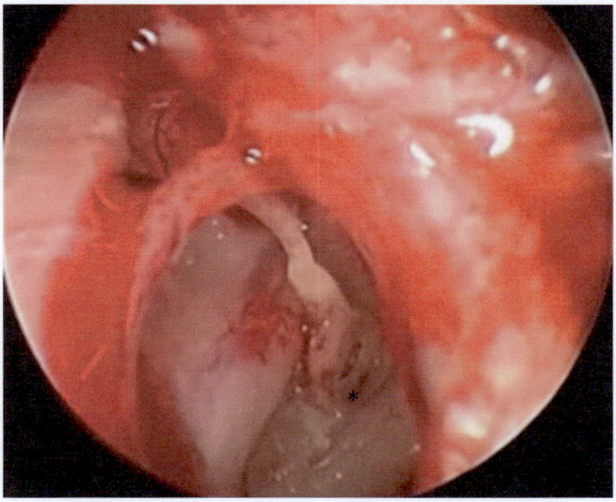

Fig. 10.45 Dysmorphic small stapes, absent stapedial tendon, oval window (*) in a right ear

cochlear modiolus and of the lamina cribrosa at the fundus of internal auditory canal which allows a direct communication between the CSF in the internal auditory canal and the perilymph of the inner ear. The high pressure in subarachnoid space is transmitted to the inner ear and blocks the footplate from movement leading to the conductive element in hearing loss as well as progressive cochlear nerve dysfunction affecting the sensorineural component of hearing. These findings are usually bilateral. Some of the obligate female carriers had milder forms of the same anomaly associated with milder hearing loss [67]. Recognition of congenital X-linked mixed hearing loss is important because it changes the treatment and precludes stapedectomy.

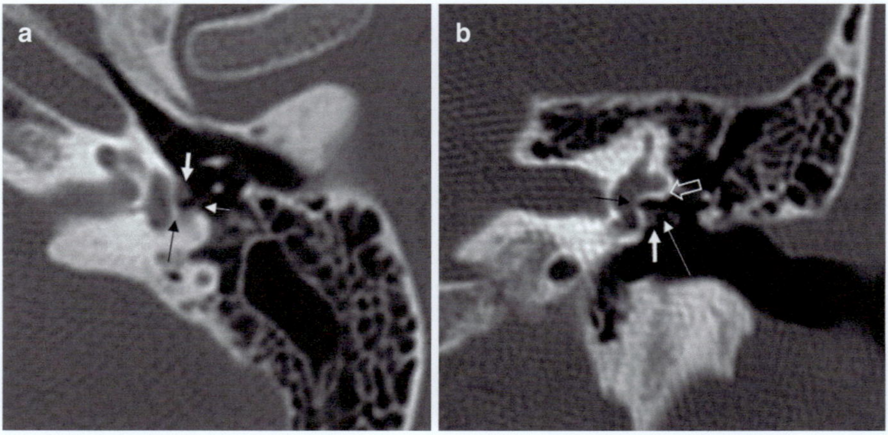

Fig. 10.46 (**a**) Axial CT-image showing a dense inferior border of the oval window (black arrow), small stapes (thin white arrow), abnormal facial nerve in front of the anterior part of the oval window (thick white arrow) (**b**) coronal CT-reconstruction showing the empty space of the normal facial nerve place (empty arrow), the facial nerve is located inferiorly to the oval window niche (short white arrow), coming in contact with the small stapes (long white arrow). The oval window opening is hypoplastic (black arrow)

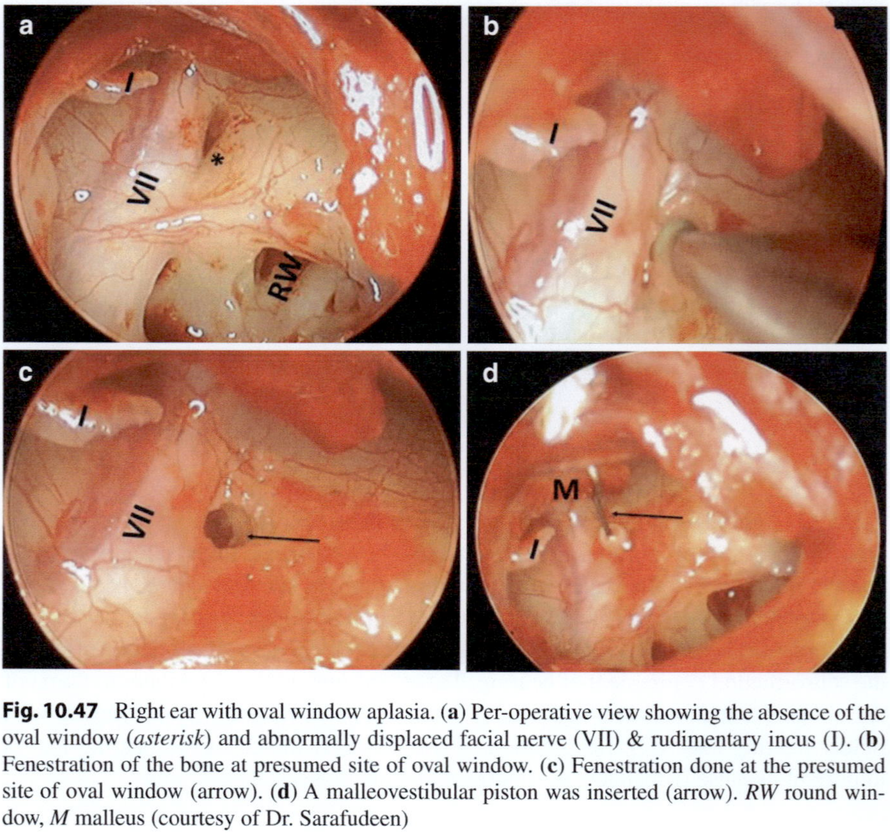

Fig. 10.47 Right ear with oval window aplasia. (**a**) Per-operative view showing the absence of the oval window (*asterisk*) and abnormally displaced facial nerve (VII) & rudimentary incus (I). (**b**) Fenestration of the bone at presumed site of oval window. (**c**) Fenestration done at the presumed site of oval window (arrow). (**d**) A malleovestibular piston was inserted (arrow). *RW* round window, *M* malleus (courtesy of Dr. Sarafudeen)

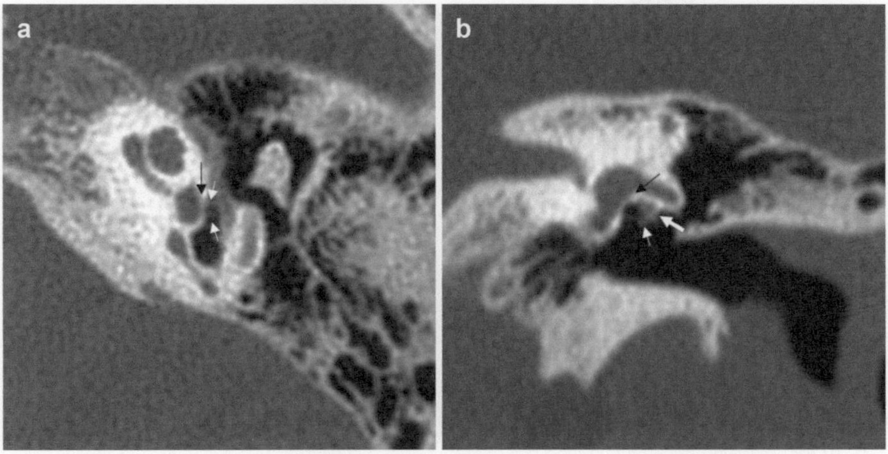

Fig. 10.48 14 years old boy with Fallot`s tetralogy and important CHL of -65 dB on the left side. (**a**) Axial CT-image of the left ear shows two small stapes branches inserting in an hypoplastic oval window (black arrow) (**b**) Coronal CT reconstruction: the facial nerve is completely procident (thick white arrow), in close contact to the head of the stapes (small white arrow). Hypoplasia of the oval window (black arrow)

10.9.5.2 CT-Imaging

The most frequent imaging finding in X-linked stapes fixation is a bulbous internal auditory canal and an incomplete separation of the basal turn of the cochlea from the fundus of the internal auditory canals.

The pathological widening concerns also the Fallopian canal. The widened angle between the first and the second segment of the facial nerve is highly suggestive of the Gusher syndrome, enabling the preoperative diagnosis of this pathology [68–70] (Figs. 10.49 and 10.50).

10.9.5.3 Management

Regarding treatment of patients with stapes gusher, the first step is to avoid surgery in those with only conductive hearing loss. Conductive hearing loss may be treated with external hearing aids. If the patients have profound sensironeural hearing loss, cochlear implantation is a viable option. During surgery, a round window gusher may develop but may be easily controlled after continuous suctioning for few minutes giving time for for CSF to drain through the round window. Because there is a risk of advancing the electrode into the internal auditory canal, intra-operative telemetric measurement and postoperative confirmation of its position first with radiographs and, if needed, afterward with CT is necessary.

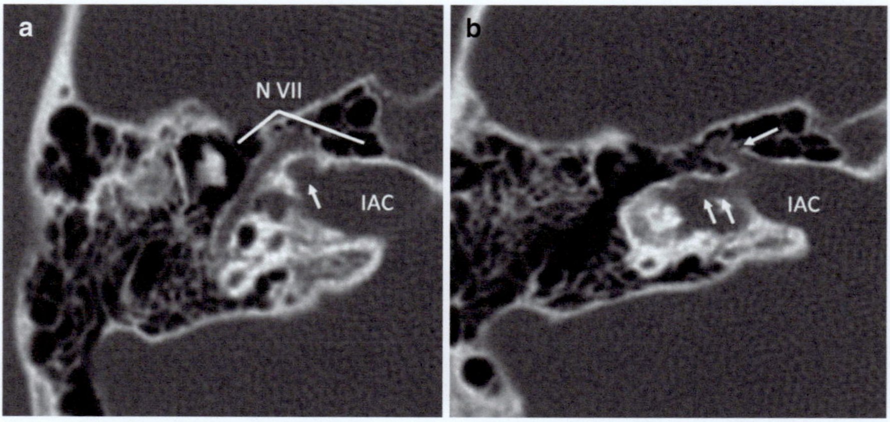

Fig. 10.49 A young male patient who has a right conductive hearing loss suspicious of otosclerosis. Axial image of the right ear: typical scanographic signs of Gusher syndrome: (**a**) Enlarged communication between the IAC and the cochlea (white arrow). Widened angle between the first and second portion of the facial nerve (angle). (**b**) Very large appearance of the first portion of the facial canal (one arrow) and the superior vestibular canal (two arrows). The IAC = internal auditory canal is globulus

Fig. 10.50 Gusher after footplate fenestration during stapedectomy in a right ear (Courtesy of Dr. Robert Vincent)

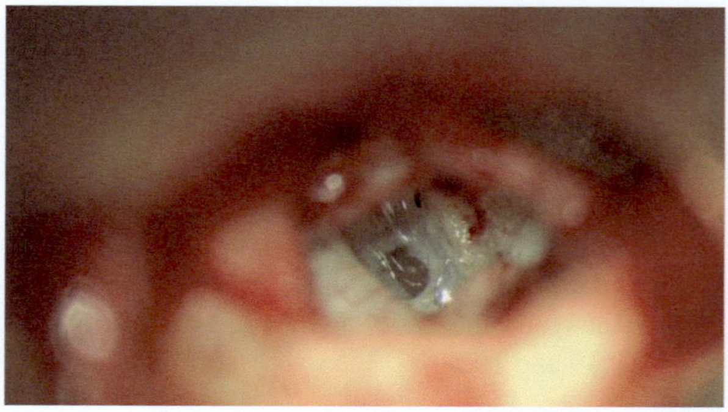

10.9.6 Other Inner Ear Malformations

Some inner ear malformation (like anomalies of SCC, LVA, Mondini, micro cochlea) (Fig. 10.51) may manifest by a conductive hearing loss.

The most accepted proposed theory of CHL in inner ear malformation is that the conductive component of the hearing loss can be explained by a back pressure of perilymphatic fluid which results in decreased stapes mobility. The evidence is an increased rate of perilymphatic gushers and oozers encountered when the inner ear is opened, either during stapedotomy or cochleostomy [71–74].

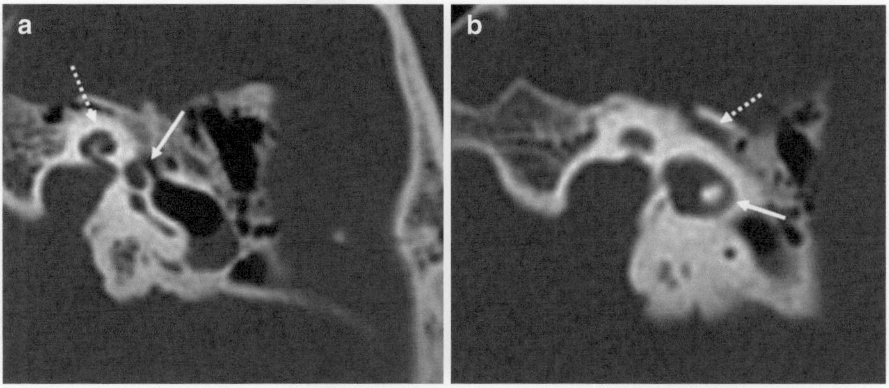

Fig. 10.51 Male child with CHL: axial CT-Imaging reveals middle and inner ear malformations: (**a**) micro cochlea (dotted arrow), oval window difficult to assess (white arrow) due to malformed middle ear cavity (**b**) malformed LSCC with a small bony island (white arrow), large 2nd portion of the facial nerve (dotted arrow)

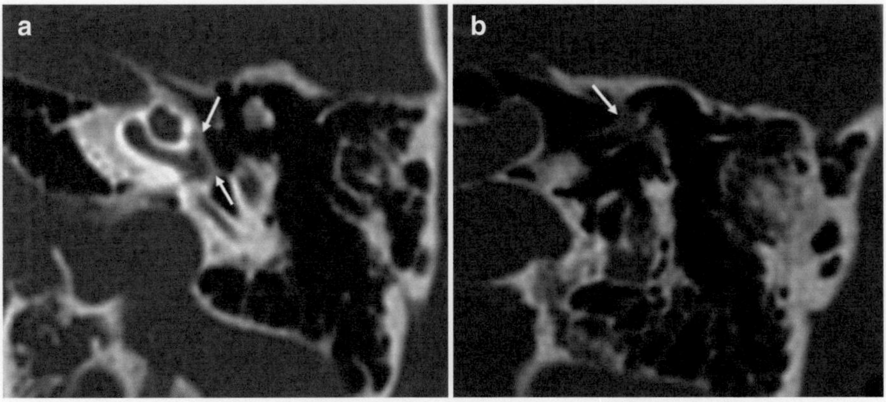

Fig. 10.52 Axial images of the left ear in osteogenesis imperfecta: (**a**) typical hypodense foci of the pre vestibular region and the footplate (between the arrows), mimicking otosclerosis; (**b**) extensive demineralization of the ossicles (arrow)

10.9.7 Osteogenesis Imperfecta OI

10.9.7.1 Clinics

Osteogenesis imperfecta (OI), or brittle bone disease is an autosomal-dominant connective-tissue disorder with deficiency of type I collagen and predominantly characterized by fragile bone and sometimes blue sclera. Conductive hearing loss develops in half of the OI patients and often progresses to a mixed hearing loss.

Tympanometry shows absence of the acoustic reflex with a very high compliance value (type Ad tympanogram) (Fig. 10.52).

10.9.7.2 CT-Imaging

CT shows extensive hypodense areas around the cochlea and the osseous labyrinth; even the ossicles may show a complete demineralization (Figs. 10.52 and 10.53).

10.9.7.3 Management

The conductive hearing loss of osteogenesis imperfecta may be treated by stapedotomy. A high incidence of floating footplate could be found at operation, with an increased likelihood of sensorineural deafness after surgery.

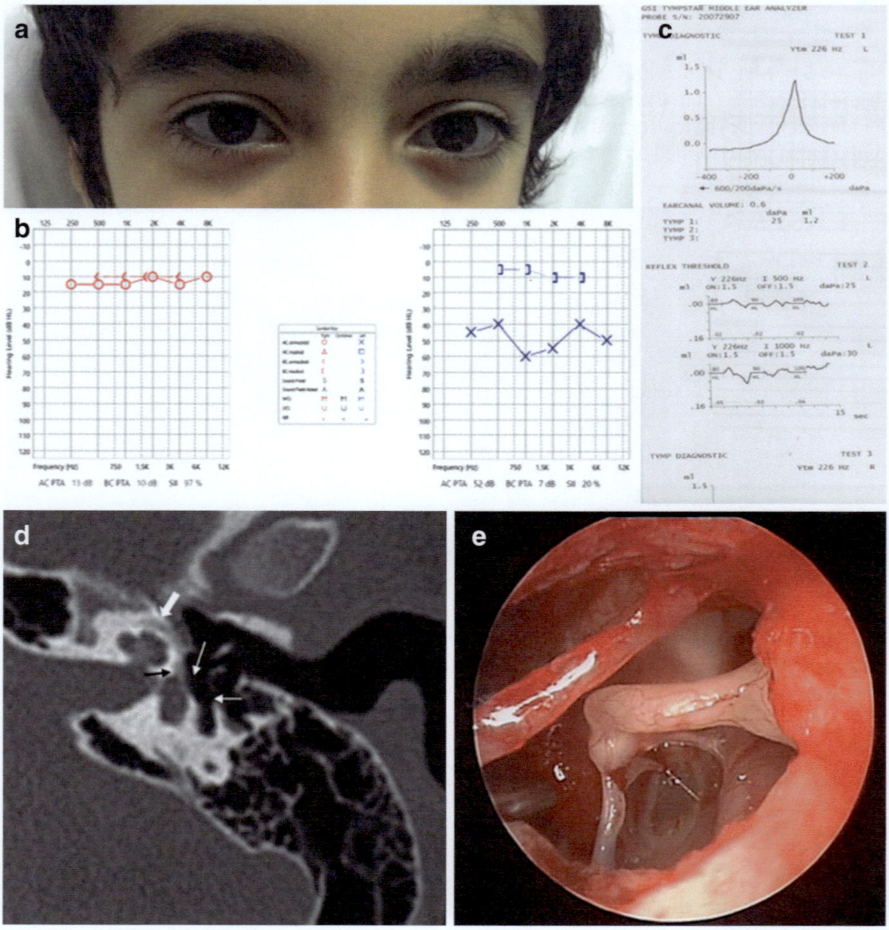

Fig. 10.53 (**a**) 9 years old boy with blue sclera. (**b**) Audiogramme: left open ABG (suggestive of ossicular discontinuity). (**c**) Type Ad tympanogram; (**d**) axial image of the left ear with fracture of the two branches of the stapes (white thin arrows), foci of demineralization around the cochlea (thick arrow) and pre vestibular (black arrow), as in otosclerosis; (**e**) endoscopic exploration showed fractured crura and fixed footplate

10.10 Conductive Hearing Loss with a Normal Appearing Tympanic Membrane and Negative Temporal Bone Computed Tomography

There are several reasons why a CT Scan in a patient with normal appearing tympanic membrane and conductive hearing loss, may come out negative:

10.10.1 Unreliable CT Scan

The technical details must be respected according to state of the art recommendations (see Chap. 11)

- Inframillimetric slice thickness, small intervals, convenient windowing and respect of the standardized plan passing by the LSCC on the axial plane.
- the patient must be cooperative and the images must not suffer from motion artefacts
- CT must be read by a trained and experienced radiologist for this complex anatomical area
- Cone-beam is becoming a complementary tool for radiologic diagnostic investigations in stapes malformations, SSCC dehiscence

Despite recent advances of specific technology regarding diagnostic imaging of the temporal bone, and their careful applications, the CT-Scan may come back negative for an obvious form of otosclerosis or any other hidden differential diagnosis.

Therefore another algorithm of possible infra radiologic pathologies must be considered.

10.10.2 Infra Radiologic Otosclerosis

- *False negative CT*-Scan may occur in the early phase of the disease when the sclerotic focus did not reach yet a significant size to be radiologically evident.
- *False negative CT* may be due to complete mature sclerotic changes of the otosclerotic focus that may become hardly differentiated from the contiguous normal bone (see Chap. 1). Therefore the otosclerotic patient suffering from conductive or even mixed hearing loss since a long time and having a normal tympanic membrane could present a negative CT-Scan. Explorative tympanotomy will give the diagnosis. It is admitted that the otospongiosis phase of the disease (immature stage of otosclerosis) is less probable in late adult age.

10.10.3 Third Windows

Despite the fact that CT-Scan has a 100% negative predictive value for common third window pathologies, we have to consider that some uncommon third window pathologies may be missed during the radiologic analysis such a very rare carotid cochlear dehiscence or posterior semicircular canal dehiscence!

A study [75] done on 15 patients who suffered from a conductive hearing loss with normal appearing tympanic membrane and who did have a negative preoperative CT-Scan, showed during surgery the following percentage of the etiological diagnosis:

- 10 patients had infra-radiologic otosclerosis,
- 4 patients had ossicular chain ankylosis
- 1 patient had a fracture of the stapes.

Thus additional and larger studies based on clinico-radiological correlations must be accomplished, possibly with more coordinated efforts between multiple oto-radiologic centers, to evaluate the actual rate of the different pathologies, mentioned above, which *can be* missed by the preoperative CT-Scan and how to improve the way to reach preoperatively the causative diagnosis. More the CT analysis of this condition is routinely requested and adequately done before surgery, more the clinico-radiologic correlations should improve and more the otologist and his patients will benefit from a better care and postoperative results.

Conclusion

Nowadays, in front of a conductive hearing loss with normal appearing tympanic membrane, a complete workup is a must before any surgical exploration. An accurate clinical evaluation, improved audiology tests and preoperatve CT-Scan are prerequisites to find out the causal diagnosis. Clinico-radiological correlations are important to perform an adequate differential diagnosis, which influences greatly the outcome of the management and follow up. In some cases, the imaging may fail to demonstrate a preoperative diagnosis, in such situation and after a good counseling of the patient, an explorative tympanotomy remains the only way to find out the underlying pathology.

References

1. Yasan H. Predictive role of Carhart's notch in pre-operative assessment for middle-ear surgery. J Laryngol Otol. 2007;121:219–21.
2. Rosowski JJ, Songer JE, Nakajima HH, Brinsko KM, Merchant SN. Clinical, experimental, and theoretical investigations of the effect of superior semicircular canal dehiscence on hearing mechanisms. Otol Neurotol. 2004;25(3):323–32.
3. Minor LB, Carey JP, Cremer PD, Lustig LR, Streubel SO, Ruckenstein MJ. Dehiscence of bone overlying the superior canal as a cause of apparent conductive hearing loss. Otol Neurotol. 2003;24:270–8.
4. Halmagyi GM, Aw ST, McGarvie LA, et al. Superior semicircular canal dehiscence simulating otosclerosis. J Laryngol Otol. 2003;117:553–7.

5. Mikulec AA, McKenna MJ, Ramsey MJ, et al. Superior semicircular canal dehiscence presenting as conductive hearing loss without vertigo. Otol Neurotol. 2004;25:121–9.
6. Modugno G, Brandolini C, Savastio G, Ceroni AR, Pirodda A. Superior semicircular canal dehiscence: a series of 13 cases. ORL J Otorhinolaryngol Relat Spec. 2005;67:180–4.
7. Veillon F, Cassleman JW, Meriot PH, Cahen-Riehm S, Sick H. Imagerie de L'Oreille et de L'os temporal (vol. 6). Lavoisier MSP, Collection Imagerie Médicale; 2013.
8. Mansour S, Nicolas K, Ahmad HH. Round window otosclerosis: radiologic classification and clinical correlations. Otol Neurotol. 2011;32(3):384–92.
9. Marx M, Lagleyre S, Escude B, Demeslay J, Elhadi T, Deguine O, Fraysse B. Correlations between CT scan findings and hearing thresholds in otosclerosis. Acta Otolaryngol. 2011;131(4):351–7.
10. Goodhill V. The fixed malleus syndrome. Trans Am Acad Ophthalmol Otolaryngol. 1966;70:370–80.
11. Nakajima Nakajima HH, Ravicz ME, Rosowski Rosowski JJ, Peake WT, Merchant SN. Experimental and clinical studies of Experimental and clinical studies of malleus malleus fixation. Laryngoscope. 2005;115(1):147–54.
12. Martin C, Oletski A, Prades JM. Surgery of idiopathic malleus fixation. Otol Neurotol. 2009;30(2):165–9.
13. Hasso AN, Ledington JA. Traumatic injuries of the temporal bone. Otolaryngol Clin N Am. 1988;21:295–316.
14. Hough JVD, Stuart WD. Middle ear injury in skull trauma. Laryngoscope. 1968;78:899–937.
15. Swartz JD, Swartz NG, Korsvik H, et al. Computerized tomogmaphic evaluation of the middle ear and mastoid for posttraumatic hearing loss. Ann Otol Rhinol Laryngol. 1985;94:263–6.
16. Belluci RJ. Traumatic injury of the middle ear. Otolaryngol Clin North Am. 1983;16:633–50.
17. Watters KF, Rosowski JJ, Sauter T, Lee DJ. Superior semicircular canal dehiscence presenting as postpartum vertigo. Otol Neurotol. 2006;27:756–68. https://doi.org/10.1097/01.mao.0000227894.27291.9f.
18. Minor LB, Solomon D, Zinreich JS, Zee DS. Sound- and/or pressure-induced vertigo due to bone dehiscence of the superior semicircular canal. Arch Otolaryngol Head Neck Surg. 1998;124(3):249–58.
19. Arts HA, Adams ME, Telian SA, El-Kashlan H, Kileny PR. Reversible electrocochleographic abnormalities in superior canal dehiscence. Otol Neurotol. 2009;30:79–86.
20. Belden CJ, Weg N, Minor LB, et al. CT evaluation of bone dehiscence of the superior semicircular canal as a cause of sound- and/or pressure-induced vertigo. Radiology. 2003;226:337–43.
21. Dubrule F, Kohler R, Vincent C, Casselmann J. Two particular cases of superior semicircular canal dehiscence related to a procidence of the superior petrous sinus. J Neuroradiol. 2009;36:240–3.
22. Hirvonen TP, Weg N, Zinreich SJ, Minor LB. Highresolution CT findings suggest a developmental abnormality underlying superior canal dehiscence syndrome. Acta Otolaryngol. 2003;123:477–81.
23. Curtin HD. Superior semicircular canal dehiscence syndrome and multi-detector row CT. Radiology. 2003;226:312–4.
24. Branstetter BF 4th, Harrigal C, Escott EJ, et al. Superior semicircular canal dehiscence: oblique reformatted CT images for diagnosis. Radiology. 2006;238:938–42.
25. Silverstein H, Kartush JM, Parnes LS, Poe DS, Babu SC, Levenson MJ, et al. Round window reinforcement for superior semicircular canal dehiscence: a retrospective multi-center case series. Am J Otolaryngol. 2014;35:286–93.
26. Elliott SJ, Ni G, Verschuur CA. Modelling the effect of round window stiffness on residual hearing after cochlear implantation. Hear Res. 2016;341:155–67.
27. Bance M. When is a conductive hearing loss not a conductive hearing loss? Causes of a mismatch in air-bone threshold measurements or a "pseudoconductive" hearing loss. J Otolaryngol. 2004;33:135–8.

28. Mikulec AA, Poe DS. Operative management of a posterior semicircular canal dehiscence. Laryngoscope. 2006;116:375–8.
29. Brantberg K, Bagger-Sjoback D, Mathiesen T, Witt H, Pansell T. Posterior canal dehiscence syndrome caused by an apex cholesteatoma. Otol Neurotol. 2006;27:531–4.
30. Mondini C. Anatomica surdi nati sectio. De Bononiensi Scientarium et Artium Instituto atque Academia Commenarii. Banoniae. 1791;7:419.
31. Sato E, Nakashima T, Lilly D, et al. Tympanometric findings in patients with enlarged vestibular aqueducts. Laryngoscope. 2002;112:1642–6.
32. Nakashima T, Ueda H, Furuhashi A, Sato E, Asahi K, Naganawa S, Beppu R. Air bone gap and resonant frequency in large vestibular aqueduct syndrome. Am J Otol. 2000;21:671–4.
33. Zhou G, Gopen Q, Kenna M. Delineating the hearing loss in children with enlarged vestibular aqueduct. Laryngoscope. 2008;118:2062–6.
34. Merchant SN, Nakajima HH, Halpin C, Nadol JB Jr, Lee DJ, Innis WP, Curtin H, Rosowski JJ. Clinical investigation and mechanism of air-bone gaps in large vestibular aqueduct syndrome. Ann Otol Rhinol Laryngol. 2007;116(7):532–41.
35. Jackler R, De La Cruz A. The large vestibular aqueduct syndrome. Laryngoscope. 1989;99:1238–43.
36. Welling C, Slater P, Martyn M, et al. Sensorineural hearing loss after occlusion of the enlarged vestibular aqueduct. Am J Otol. 1999;20:338–43.
37. Cremers CW, Snik AF, Huygen PL, Joosten FB, Cremers FP. X-linked mixed deafness syndrome with congenital fixation of the stapedial footplate and perilymphatic gusher (DFN3). Adv Otorhinolaryngol. 2002;61:161–7.
38. Khetarpal U, Schuknecht HF. In search of pathologic correlates for hearing loss and vertigo in Paget's disease. A clinical and histopathologic study of 26 temporal bones. Ann Otol Rhinol Laryngol Suppl. 1990;145:1–16.
39. Monsell EM. The mechanism of hearing loss in Paget's disease of bone. Laryngoscope. 2004;114(4):598–606.
40. Juliano AF, Maya MM, Lo WW, Kovanlikaya I. Temporal bone tumors and cerebellopontine angle lesions. In: Som PM, Curtin HD, editors. Head and neck imaging. Philadelphia, PA: Mosby Elsevier; 2011. p. 1263–407.
41. May M. Tumors involving the facial nerve. In: May M, editor. The facial nerve. New York: Thieme; 1986. p. 455–67.
42. Mansour S, Nicolas K, Sbeity S. Triple ossicular fixation and semicircular canal malformations. J Otolaryngol. 2007;36(3):E31–4.
43. Bachor E, Just T, Wright CG, Pau HW, Karmody CS. Fixation of the stapes footplate in children: a clinical and temporal bone histopathologic study. Otol Neurotol. 2005;26(5):866–73.
44. Nandapalan V, Tos M. Isolated congenital stapes ankylosis: an embryologic survey and literature review. Laryngoscope. 2000;21:71–80.
45. Yuen HY, Ahuja AT, Wong KT, Yue V, van Hasselt AC. Computed tomography of common congenital lesions of the temporal bone. Clin Radiol. 2003;58(9):687–93.
46. Raveh E, Hu W, Papsin BC, Forte V. Congenital conductive hearing loss. J Laryngol Otol. 2002;116(2):92–6.
47. Hung KL, Tu TY, Tsai TL, Shiao AS. Congenital ossicular anomalies. J Chin Med Assoc. 2003;66(8):474–9.
48. Teunissen B, Cremers WR, Huygen PL, Pouwels TP. Isolated congenital stapes ankylosis: surgical results in 32 ears and a review of the literature. Laryngoscope. 1990;100(12):1331–6.
49. Dornhoffer JL, Helms J, Hoehmann DH. Stapedectomy for congenital fixation of the stapes. Am J Otol. 1995;16(3):382–6.
50. Albert S, Roger G, Rouillon I, Chauvin P, Denoyelle F, Derbez R, et al. Congenital stapes ankylosis: study of 28 cases and surgical results. Laryngoscope. 2006;116(7):1153–7.
51. Kurosaki Y, Tanaka YO, Itai Y. Malleus bar as a rare cause of congenital malleus fixation: CT demonstration. AJNR Am J Neuroradiol. 1998;19(7):1229–30.
52. Teunissen E, Cremers CW. Surgery for congenital anomalies of the middle ear with mobile stapes. Eur Arch Otorhinolaryngol. 1993;250(6):327–31.

53. House HP. Diagnostic aspects of congenital ossicular fixation. Trans Am Acad Ophthalmol Otolaryngol. 1956;60(6):787–90.
54. Staecker H, Merchant SN. Temporal bone pathology case of the month: congenital fixation of the incus. Am J Otol. 2000;21(1):137–8.
55. Hashimoto S, Yamamoto Y, Satoh H, Takahashi S. Surgical treatment of 52 cases of auditory ossicular malformations. Auris Nasus Larynx. 2002;29(1):15–8.
56. Selinsky CR, Kuhn JK. Congenital incus fixation to the fallopian canal. JAMA Otolaryngol Head Neck Surg. 2014;140(8):762–4.
57. Park HY, Han DH, Lee JB, Han NS, Choung YH, Park K. Congenital stapes anomalies with normal eardrum. Clin Exp Otorhinolaryngol. 2009;2(1):33–8.
58. Mansour S, Magnan J, Haidar H, Nicolas K, Louryan S. Middle ear cavity. In: Mansour S, Magnan J, Haidar H, Nicolas K, Louryan S, editors. Comprehensive and clinical anatomy of the middle ear. New York: Springer; 2013. p. 19–48.
59. Jahrsdoerfer RA. Congenital absence of the oval window. ORL J Otorhinolarygol Relat Spec. 1977;84:904–14.
60. Lambert PR. Congenital absence of the oval window. Laryngoscope. 1990;100:37–40.
61. Zeifer B, Sabini P, Sonne J. Congenital absence of the oval window: Radiologic diagnosis and associated anomalies. Am J Neuroradiology. 2000;21:322–7.
62. Briggs RJ, Luxford WM. Correction of conductive hearing loss in children. Otolaryngol Clin N Am. 1994;27:607–20.
63. Nance WE, Setleff R, McLeod A, Sweeney A, Cooper C, McConnell F. X-Linked mixed deafness with congenital fixation of the stapedial footplate and perilymphatic gusher. Birth Def. 1971;4:64–9.
64. Glasscock ME. The stapes gusher. Arch Otolaryngol. 1973;98:82–91.
65. Phelps PD, Reardon W, Pembrey M, Bellman S, Luxom L. X-Linked deafness, stapes gushers and a distinctive defect of the inner ear. Neuroradiology. 1991;33:326–30.
66. Snik AF, Hombergen GC, Mylanus EA, Cremers CW. Air-bone gap in patients with X-linked stapes gusher syndrome. Am J Otol. 1995;16:241–6.
67. Phleps PD, Reardon W, Pembrey M, et al. X-linked deafness, stapes gushers, and a distinctive defect of the inner ear. Neuroradiology. 1991;33:326–30.
68. Kumar G, Castello M, Bucman CA. X-linked stapes gusher; CT findings in one patient. Am J Neuroradiol. 2003;24:1130–2.
69. Talbot JM, Wilson DF. Computed tomographic diagnosis of X-linked congenital mixed deafness, fixation of the stapedial footplate, and perilymphatic gusher. Am J Otol. 1994;15(2):177–82.
70. Mansour S, Magnan J, Haidar H, Nicolas K, Louryan S. Facial nerve. In: Mansour S, Magnan J, Haidar H, Nicolas K, Louryan S, editors. Comprehensive and clinical anatomy of the middle ear. New York: Springer; 2013. p. 123–40.
71. Govaerts P, Casselman J, Daemers K, De Ceulaer G, Somers T, Offeciers F. Audiological findings in large vestibular aqueduct syndrome. Int J Pediatr Otorhinolaryngol. 1999;51:157–64.
72. Steinbach S, Brockmeier S, Kiefer B. The large vestibular aqueduct—case report and review of the literature. Acta Otolaryngol. 2006;126:788–95.
73. Au G, Gibson W. Cochlear implantation in children with large vestibular aqueduct syndrome. Am J Otol. 1999;20:183–6.
74. Lee K, Lee J, Isaacson B, et al. Cochlear implantation in children with enlarged vestibular aqueduct. Laryngoscope. 2010;120:1675–81.
75. Lagleyre S, Sorrentino T, Calmels MN, Shin YJ, Escude B, Deguine O, Fraysse B. Reliability of high-resolution CT scan in diagnosis of otosclerosis. Otol Neurotol. 2009;30(8):1152–9.

Methodology of CT-Imaging in ME Diseases

11

Contents

11.1 CT-Imaging

11.1.1 Multidetector Computed Tomography

High Resolution Computed Scanography (HRCT) is unanimously considered as the method of choice in imaging of middle ear pathologies. The acquisition of HRCT images is continuously evolving, especially on the new performing machines with multidetector techniques (MDCT). Nowadays, collimation values as small as 0.5–0.6 mm become routinely used and voxel sizes about 0.2 mm^3 permit the creation of a data volume that can be reconstructed along any required plane.

The otologist must be aware of a minimum knowledge about the adequate imaging techniques to be able to follow the contribution of imaging relative to the indication of a given pathology.

The standard acquisition plane and the most frequently used reconstruction planes, resumed in the table below, are the best planes to analyse the relevant anatomic structures of the temporal bone.

Routinely, CT is done without injection of iodine contrast; nevertheless, in special indications, as for glomus tumors, for example, injection can be indicated to determine the contrast uptake in the investigated lesion. CT of the temporal bone

S. Mansour et al., *Middle Ear Diseases*,
https://doi.org/10.1007/978-3-319-72962-6_11

includes the whole petrous bone of both sides, followed by a reconstruction of each ear with an adapted smaller field of view (FOV) of about 9–10 cm (initial FOV of about 22 cm).

The window width and level at 4000/800 permit the best discrimination of the different bony structures.

The main acquisition planes routinely done and the main reconstruction planes to do for the most frequent pathologies are described by the following and illustrated in Table 11.1.

1. The **Orbitomeatal plane** is the standard axial acquisition plane. The acquisition volume is covering the whole middle ear cleft from the base of the mastoid to the tegmen oriented along this orbitomeatal plane. This plane is successfully obtained, when the LSCC appears almost entirely on one slide.
2. **Reconstitution of the Orbitomeatal plane**: If the initial acquisition was deviating from the standard plane, it can be recovered by the reconstruction of multiple consecutive slides all over the cavity along a new reference line, that is inclined *on the sagittal plane* along the different parts of the LSCC.
3. The **Coronal plane** is routinely displayed for each ear, perpendicular to the axial plane, and showing well the tympanic membrane, the scutum, the second portion of the facial nerve, and the tegmen.
4. The plane of the **Ossicular V** is a coronal reconstruction based on a reference line that passes by the center of the footplate on the axial plane.
5. The **"Stapes Axial plane"** (**SAP** [1]) is obtained with the reference line drawn on the coronal image along the stapes axis (the stapes should be in place): essential for a good assessment of the whole stapes suprastructure, especially the footplate thickness.
6. The **Poeschl plane** is oriented along the axis of the SSCC to visualize it entirely on one slide and especially its bony cover [2, 3].
7. The **Stenvers plane** is oriented perpendicular to the Poeschl plane, perpendicular to the arc of the SSCC.
8. **The Sagittal oblique plane** along the axis of the incudomalleolar chain is the most adequate plane to judge any contact between the malleus head and the tegmen, also to demonstrate the AER in relation to the STR and the ET. It is not routinely done, however it is the plane of the surgeon's view when he is looking on the middle ear cavity during surgical intervention.

To favor continuous and successful radio-surgical correlations, the sagittal oblique reconstruction along the incudo-malleal axis should be "routinely" done and saved together with the whole data volume of the CT imaging that is delivered to the otosurgeon.

Table 11.1 The most relevant acquisition/reconstruction planes of the Temporal Bone CT

1. The Orbito-meatal Plane	**Key-image**
On the sagittal scout view: 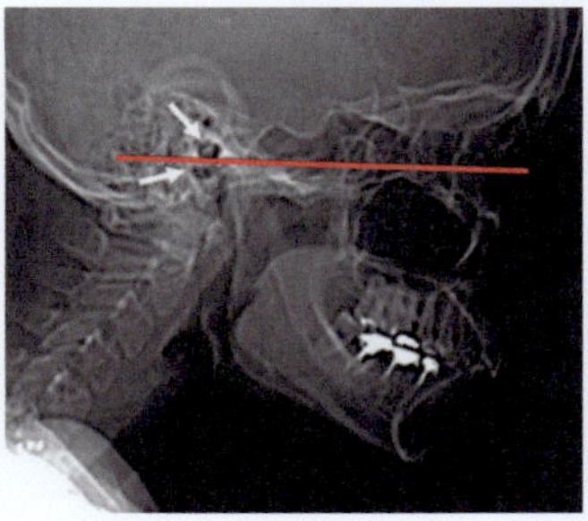	LSCC entirely seen (between the arrows) 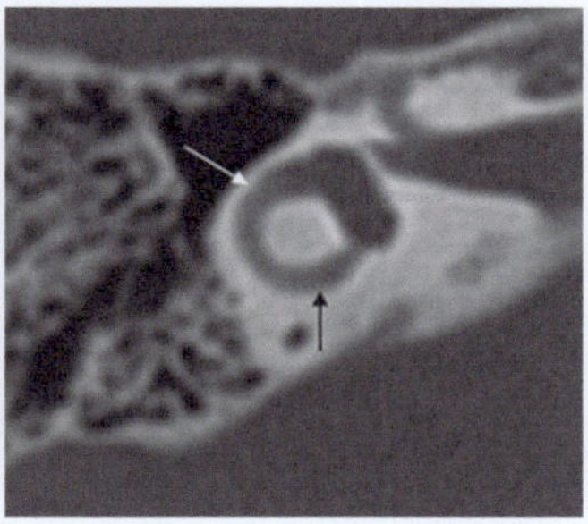
Ref. line between the EAC (arrows) and the center of orbit	**Standard Quality Criterium**
2. Recovering the Standard Orbito-meatal Plane	
In the sagittal plane: 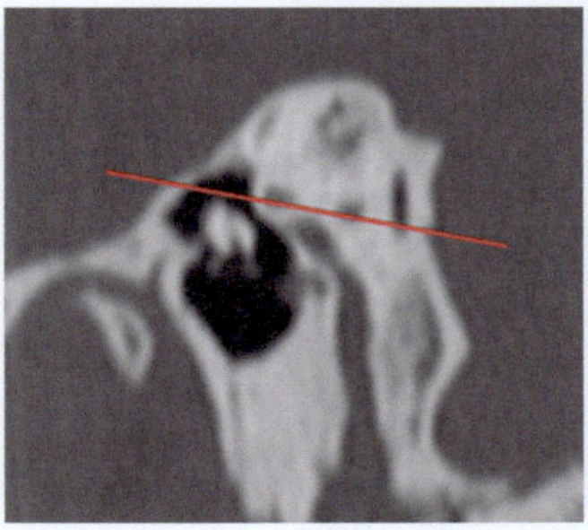	LSCC entirely seen (between the arrows) 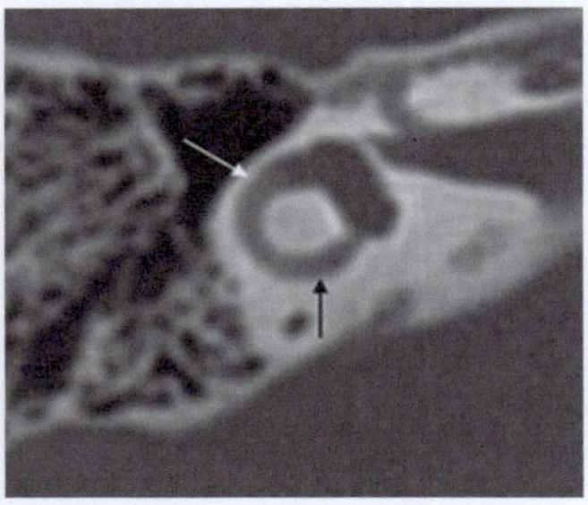
Ref. line along the arms of LSCC	**Standard Quality Criterium**
3. The Standard Coronal Plane	
On the standard axial images 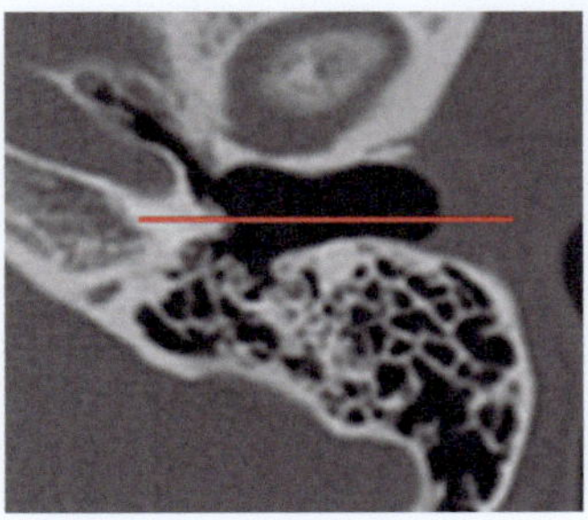	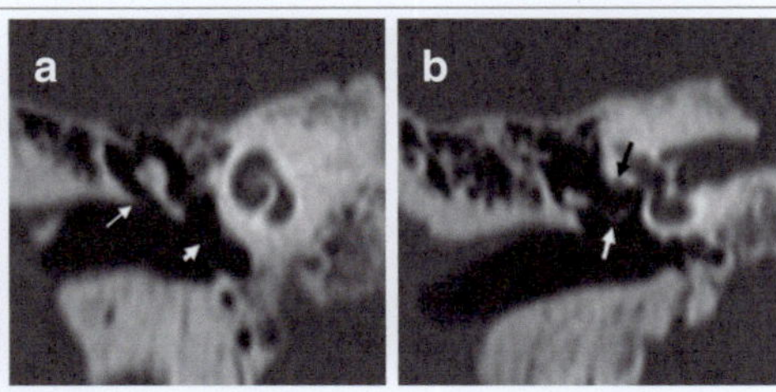 Good visibility of: a) scutum (long arrow), tympanic membrane (short arrow); b) ossicular chain (white arrow) and facial nerve (black arrow)
Ref. line strict coronal	**Search for:** Amputation of the scutum? TM retraction? Nerve VII Overhang?

(continued)

Table 11.1 (continued)

4. The Coronal Oblique Plane of the Ossicular V	
On the standard axial plane: 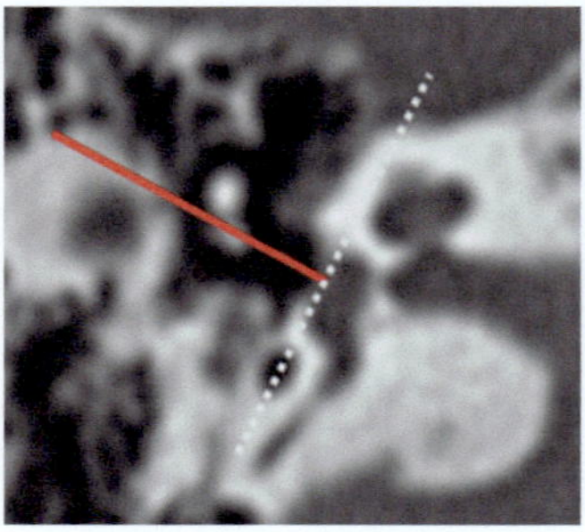 **Ref. line** perpendicular to the center of the footplate (dotted line) through the lenticular process of the incus	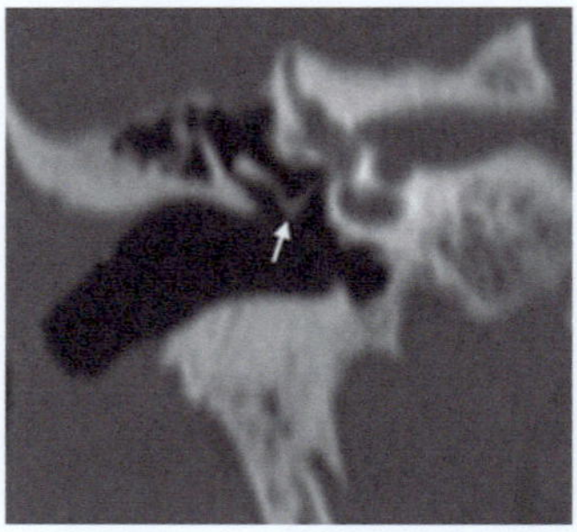 An intact ossicular V = incudostapedial continuity (arrow)
	Search for: Ossicular discontinuity?
5. The "Stapes axial plan" SAP	
on the coronal plane of the ossicular V (see plan 4 above): 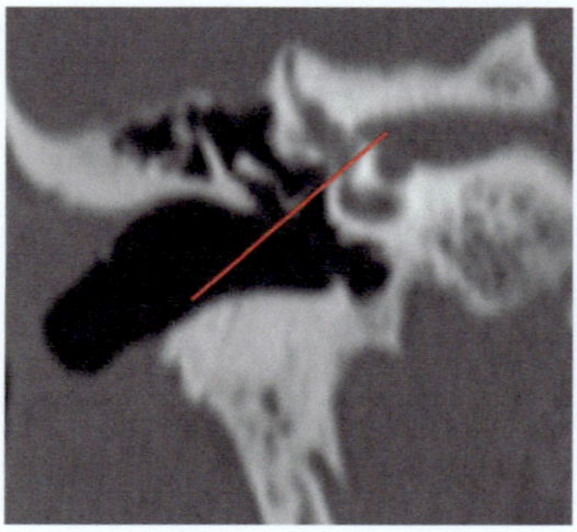 **Ref. line** passing by the lenticular V and the footplate, parallel to the axis of the stapes crura	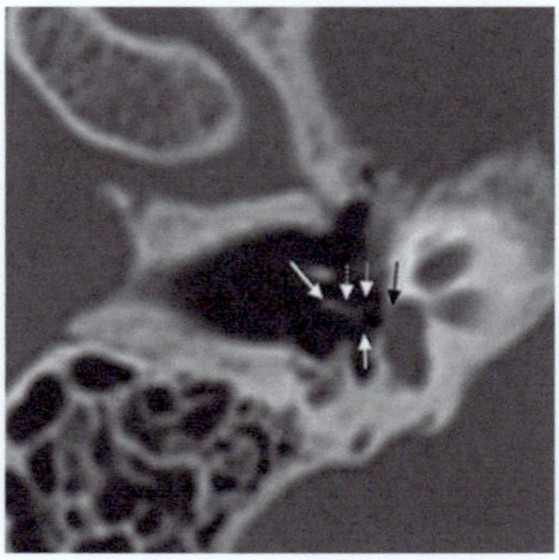 On the same image are seen: the lenticular process of the incus (long arrow), the head of the stapes (dashed arrow), the crura of the stapes (short white arrows) and the footplate (black arrow)
	Search for: Footplate thickness? OW size?

Table 11.1 (continued)

6. The Poeschl Plane	
On the standard axial plane 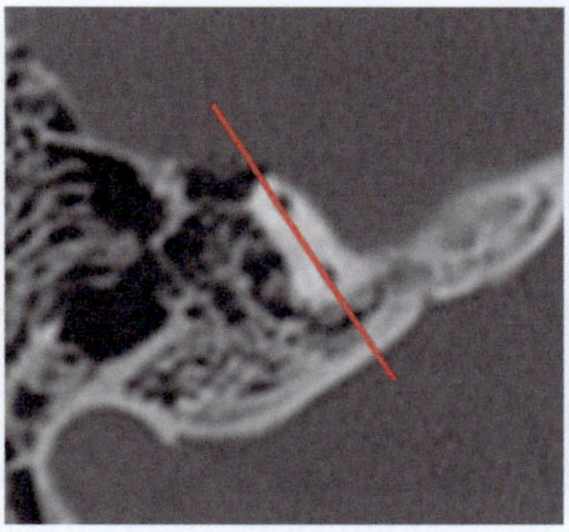 **Ref. line** parallel to the superior arch of the SSCC	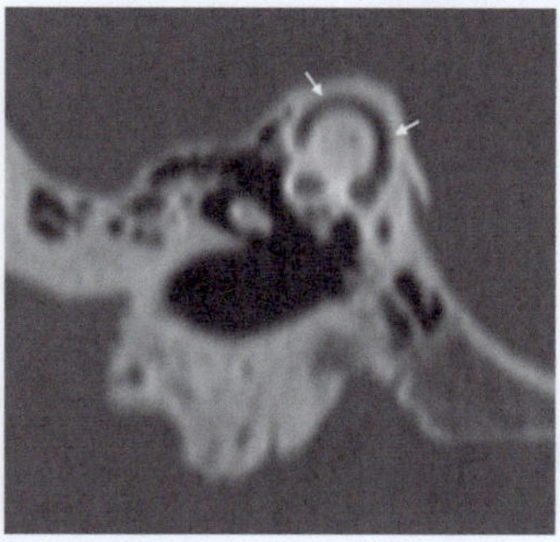 Visibility of the superior arch of the SSCC (between arrows) and its the bony cover
7. The Stenvers Plane	
On the standard axial plane 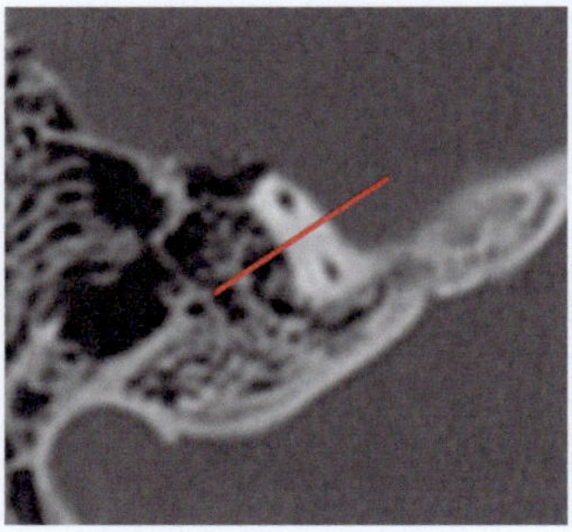	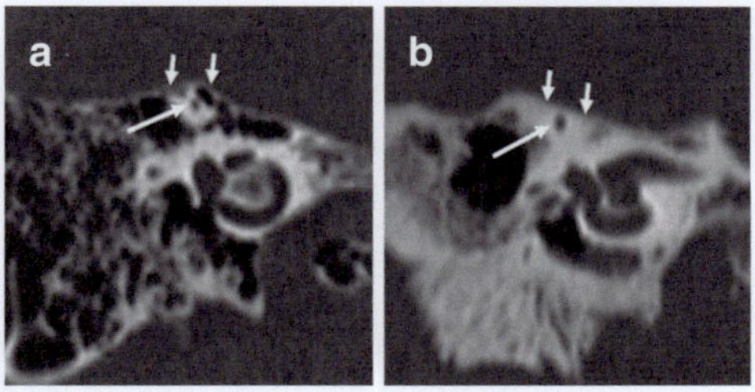 The bony cover above the superior arch of the SSCC (long arrows), in a) with a pneumatized tegmen (small arrows) , in b) with a sclerotic tegmen (small arrows)
Ref. line perpendicular to the superior arch of the SSCC	**(6) + (7) Search for :** Dehiscence of the SSCC?
8. The Sagittal Oblique Plane along the Incudomalleal Axis	
On the standard axial plane 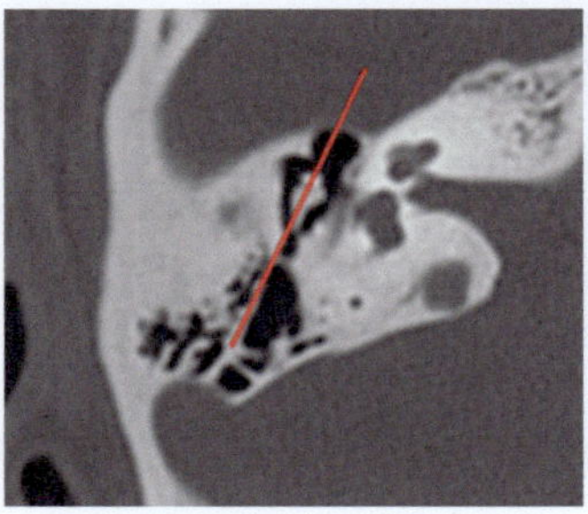	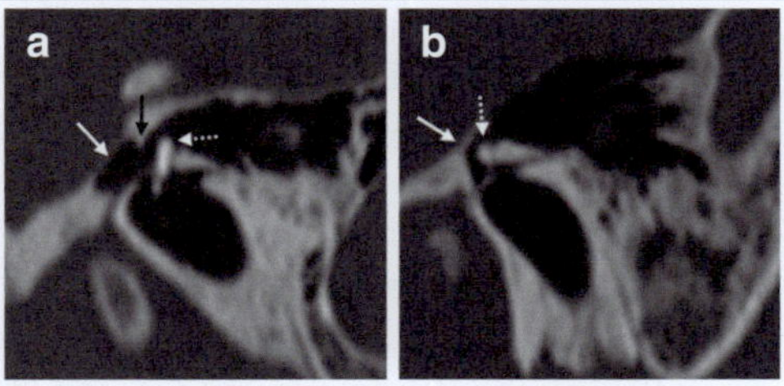 (a) Good visibility of the AER (white arrow), the cog (black arrow), malleus head (dashed arrow) (b) visibility of the distance between the malleus head (dashed arrow) and the anterior attic wall (white arrow)
Ref. line along the incudo malleal axis	**(8) Search for:** AER size and aeration

11.1.2 Systematic Reading

The reading of a CT of the temporal bone has to be methodic and systematic, even if it is oriented by the clinical context and the suspected pathology, in order not to miss any possible abnormal finding.

1. *First*: The quality of the acquisition must be confirmed, looking at the slice thickness and the acquisition plane to know if the given images can be considered as of standard quality
2. *Second*: The different anatomic structures have to be evaluated step by step, as the following:
   (a) ***The Mastoid***: pneumatization status (sclerotic, diploic, well pneumatized), aeration (well aerated/condensation images), bony septa (preserved or lytic), jugular bulb abnormalities, shape of the tegmen slope (on coronal images)
   (b) ***The EAC***: size (stenosis? atresia?), skin thickness, obliterations?, osseous borders (regular or lytic), relation to the sigmoid sinus, scutum (intact or amputated)?
   (c) ***The Tympanic Membrane***: Aspect (normal, lateralized, retracted, adhesive), thickness (thickened or thinned), perforation (size and site), calcifications
   (d) ***The Middle Ear Cavity***: aeration/condensations, osseous borders (intact, dehiscent, lytic)
   (e) ***The Ossicular Chain***: topography, continuity, discontinuity, ankylosis, stapes crura
      - in case of a proximity of the malleus head with the attic wall, the sagittal oblique plane has to be done to assess eventual fixity to the anterior attic wall (see plane 8, Table 11.1)
      - in case of doubt about discontinuity of the incudo-stapedial chain, reading of the standard axial plane should evaluate the incudostapedial jonction on several consecutive slides (Fig. 11.1)
   (f) ***The Oval Window*:**
      - Height (Fig. 11.2)
      - Footplate (thickness, size) evaluated according to the reconstruction of the Stapes Axial plane (plane 5 in Table 11.1)
      - Focus of the antefenestral region: if present, measurement of its density is to do. Extension to the endosteum of the cochlea is to look for.
   (g) ***The Round Window***: recess, inferior border, round window membrane, otosclerosis? tympanosclerosis? As the round window is almost vertically oriented, it appears consecutively on the axial slides from caudal to cranial (demonstrated in Fig. 11.3), passing successively by the inferior part of the RW (b), the RW membrane (c), and the superior limit of the round window at the level of the vestibular floor (d) [4].
   (h) ***The Facial Nerve***: three segments trajectory, size, dehiscence of the bony canal, overhang

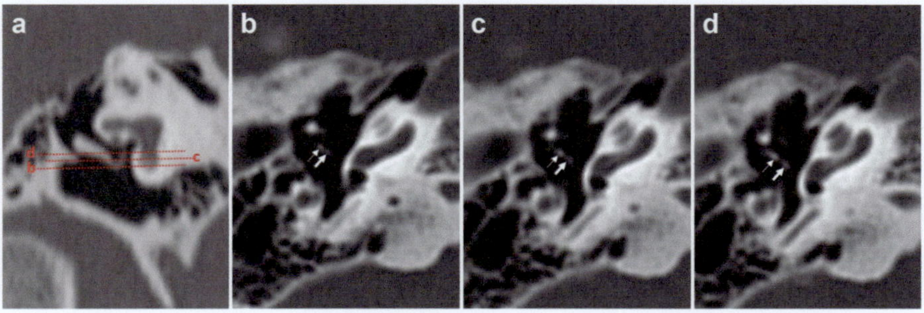

Fig. 11.1 Systematic assessment of the incudostapedial continuity on consecutive axial CT-images in caudo-cranial direction, as demonstrated in the first slide (**a**) with the corresponding reference lines on a coronal image. (**b**)-(**d**): Long process of the incus (thin arrow), head of the stapes (thick arrow): (**b**) at the deepest point of the incudostapedial junction, both extremities seem to be continuous, (**c**) the lenticular process and the head of the stapes can be individualized as two rounded ossicular structures, that are connected (**d**) the long process of the incus and the stapes head are separated structures

Fig. 11.2 According to Ukkola [4], the height of the oval niche is measured from a line (white line) that passes perpendicular to the footplate plane (black line) up to the inferior border of the facial nerve (double headed arrow). It is considered within normal limits when above 1.3 mm

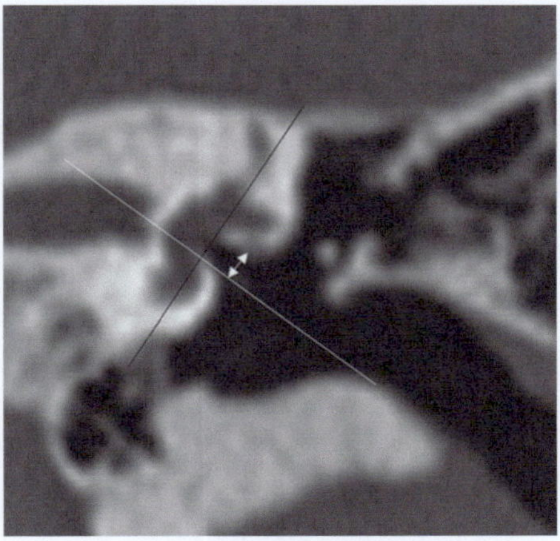

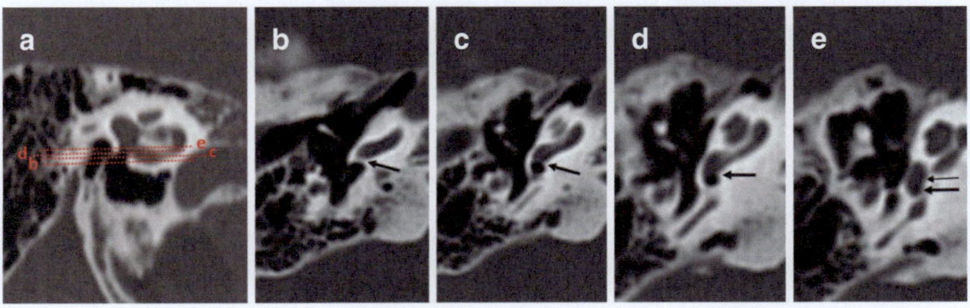

Fig. 11.3 Systematic assessment of the round window on consecutive axial CT-images in caudo-cranial direction [5], as demonstrated in the coronal oblique view with reference lines (**a**). (**b**) passing by the inferior edge of the round window (arrow), (**c**) and (**d**) passing consecutively by the round window membrane, which is normally a very thin structure (arrow). (**e**) top of the round window membrane (thick arrow), vestibule (thin arrow)

(i) ***The Inner Ear***: morphologic aspect of cochlea, vestibule and semicircular canals, variants of the morphology, dehiscence of the bony cover of the SCCs (Poeschl plane No 6, Stenvers Plane No 7 in Table 11.1) calcification? ossification?

(j) ***The IAC***: shape, osseous limits (regular or irregular), otosclerotic diverticulum?

This radiologic evaluation is confronted with the clinical informations to enlighten the differential diagnosis.

11.2 Cone Beam CT

Cone-beam CT (CBCT) is a relatively new imaging method already widely used in maxillofacial imaging. It offers major advantages because of its significantly lower irradiation doses than by MDCT (depending on the machines, the exposure is about 3–10 times less [6] and its very high spatial resolution due to isotropic voxel of a very small size (0.08–0.125 mm^3). Nevertheless, CBCT suffers from more noise and lesser density resolution due to the diminished energy of the radiation.

Promising results about the recognition of the anatomic details of the temporal bone structures have been mostly realized on temporal bone specimen [7–9], but these results are still not always reproducible in vivo, therefore the diagnostic imaging tasks of the ear by the CBCT remain under study. Until now, CBCT is still unable to replace the primary role of a diagnostic MDCT.

References

1. Garetier M, Rousset J, Gentric J-C, Koch G, Meriot P. Biometry of the normal stapes in high-resolution computed tomography: value of the stapes axial plane Poster No C-0351, ECR 2012, scientific paper.
2. Curtin HD. Superior semicircular canal dehiscence syndrome and multi-detector row CT. Radiology. 2003;226:312–4.
3. Branstetter BF 4th, Harrigal C, Escott EJ, et al. Superior semicircular canal dehiscence: oblique reformatted CT images for diagnosis. Radiology. 2006;238:938–42.
4. Ukkola-Pons E, Ayache D, Pons Y, Ratajczak M, Nioche C, Williams M. Oval window niche height: quantitative evaluation with CT before stapes surgery for otosclerosis. AJNR Am J Neuroradiol. 2013;34:1082–5.
5. Mansour S, Nicolas K, Ahmad HH. Round window otosclerosis: radiologic classification and clinical correlations. Otol Neurotol. 2011;32(3):384–92. https://doi.org/10.1097/MAO.0b013e3182096e80.
6. Loubele M, Bogaerts R, Van Dijck E, et al. Comparison between effective radiation dose of CBCT and MSCT scanners for dentomaxillofacial applications. Eur J Radiol. 2009;71:461–8.
7. Faccioli N, Barillari M, Guariglia S, et al. Radiation dose saving through the use of cone-beam CT in hearing-impaired patients. Radiol Med. 2009;114:1308–18.
8. Dahmani-Causse M, Marx M, Deguine O, Fraysse B, Lepage B, Escudé B. Morphologic examination of the temporal bone by cone beam computed tomography: comparison with multislice helical computed tomography. Eur Ann Otorhinolaryngol Head Neck Dis. 2011;128:230–5.
9. Révész P, Liktor B, Liktor B, Sziklai I, Gerlinger I, Karosi T. Comparative analysis of preoperative diagnostic values of HRCT and CBCT in patients with histologically diagnosed otosclerotic stapes footplates. Eur Arch Otorhinolaryngol. 2016;273(1):63–72.

Index

S. Mansour et al., *Middle Ear Diseases*,
https://doi.org/10.1007/978-3-319-72962-6

MIX
Papier aus verantwortungsvollen Quellen
Paper from responsible sources
FSC® C105338

If you have any concerns about our products,
you can contact us on
ProductSafety@springernature.com

In case Publisher is established outside the EU,
the EU authorized representative is:
Springer Nature Customer Service Center GmbH
Europaplatz 3, 69115 Heidelberg, Germany

Printed by Libri Plureos GmbH
in Hamburg, Germany